Breast Cancer: Diagnosis and Management

Breast Cancer: Diagnosis and Management

Edited by

J.M. Dixon

Consultant Surgeon and Senior Lecturer
Academic Office, Edinburgh Breast Unit
Western General Hospital
Edinburgh EH4 2XU, GB

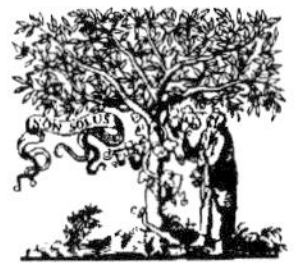

2000

Elsevier
Amsterdam - London - New York - Oxford - Paris - Shannon - Tokyo

ELSEVIER SCIENCE B.V.
Sara Burgerhartstraat 25
P.O. Box 211, 1000 AE Amsterdam, The Netherlands

First edition 2000

Library of Congress Cataloging in Publication Data
A catalog record from the Library of Congress has been applied for.

ISBN: 0-444-50011-1

♾ The paper used in this publication meets the requirements of ANSI/NISO Z39.48-1992 (Permanence of Paper).
Printed in The Netherlands.

Contributors

M. Aapro
Institut Multidisciplinaire d'Oncologie
Route du Muids 1
CH-1272 Genolier
Switzerland

M.J. Allen
Department of Medicine
Royal Marsden Hospital and Institute of Cancer Research
Fulham Road
London SW3 6JJ
UK

E.D.C. Anderson
Edinburgh Breast Unit
Western General Hospital
Edinburgh EH4 2XU
Scotland
UK

A.D. Baildam
Department of Surgery
South Manchester University Hospital
Nell Lane
West Didsbury
Manchester N20 8LR
UK

H. Bartelink
The Netherlands Cancer Institute/Antoni van Leeuwenhoek Huis
Plesmanlaan 121
1066 CX Amsterdam
The Netherlands

F. Bassi
European Institute of Oncology
Via Ripamonti 435
20141 Milan
Italy

P.I. Borgen
Breast Service
Department of Surgery
Memorial Sloan-Kettering Cancer Center
New York NY
USA

N.J. Bundred
University Department of Surgery
South Manchester University Hospital
Nell Lane
West Didsbury
Manchester M20 8LR
UK

D.A. Cameron
Department of Clinical Oncology
Western General Hospital
Edinburgh EH4 2XU
UK

K.C. Chan
Academic Department of Surgery
University Hospital of South Manchester
Nell Lane
Manchester M20 2LR
UK

U. Chetty
Edinburgh Breast Unit
Western General Hospital
Edinburgh EH4 2XU
UK

S. Ciatto
Centro per lo Studio e la Prevenzione Oncologica
Viale A. Volta 171
I-50131 Florence
Italy

R.E. Coleman
Yorkshire Cancer Research Department of Clinical Oncology
Weston Park Hospital
Whitham Road
Sheffield S10 2SJ
UK

J. Crown
St. Vincent's University Hospital
Elm Park
Dublin 4
Ireland

V.E. Currie
Memorial Sloan–Kettering Cancer Center
1275 York Avenue
New York NY 10021
USA

J.M. Dixon
Academic Office
Edinburgh Breast Unit
Western General Hospital
Edinburgh EH4 2XU
UK

V. Donati
Department of Plastic and Reconstructive Surgery
European Institute of Oncology
Via Ripamonti 435
20141 Milan
Italy

D.M. Eccles
Wessex Clinical Genetics Service
Princess Ann Hospital level G
Coxford Road
Southampton SO16 5YA
UK

I.O. Ellis
City Hospital NHS Trust
Hucknall Road
Nottingham NG5 1PB
UK

C.W. Elston
City Hospital NHS Trust
Hucknall Road
Nottingham NG5 1PB
UK

A. Evans
Breast Screening Training Centre
City Hospital NHS Trust
Hucknall Road
Nottingham NG5 1PB
UK

D.G. Evans
University Department of Medical Genetics and Regional Genetics Service
St Mary's Hospital
Hathersage Rd
Manchester M13 0JH
UK

M.H. Galea
Dept. of Surgery
Princess Margaret Hospital
Okus Road
Swindon
Wilts SN1 4JU
UK

V. Galimberti
Istituto Europeo di Oncologia
Via Ripamonti 435
Milan
Italy

C. Garusi
Department of Plastic and Reconstructive Surgery
European Institute of Oncology
Via Ripamonti 435
20141 Milan
Italy

G. Gasparini
Division of Medical Oncology
Azienda Complesso Ospedaliero
"San Filippo Neri"
Via Martinotti 20
00135 Rome
Italy

G. Gatti
European Institute of Oncology
Via Ripamonti 435
20141 Milan
Italy

W. Gatzemeier
European Institute of Oncology
Via Ripamonti 435
20141 Milan
Italy

R. Gennari
Division of Senology
European Institute of Oncology
Via Ripamonti 435
20141 Milan
Italy

F.J. Gilbert
Department of Radiology
Medical School
University of Aberdeen
Aberdeen AB25 2ZD
UK

M. Gion
Centre for the Study of Biological Markers of Malignancy
Regional General Hospital
Venice
Italy

R.A. Jensen
Vanderbilt University
Nashville TN
USA

J. Keen
St. Columba's Hospice
Challenger Lodge
Boswall Road
Edinburgh EH5 3RW
UK

C. Khoo
Wexham Park Hospital
Slough
Berkshire SLK2 4HL
UK

I. Kunkler
Department of Clinical Oncology
Western General Hospital NHS Trust
Crewe Road
Edinburgh EH4 2XU
UK

J.M. Kurtz
Radiation Oncology Division
University of Geneva
Geneva University Hospital
24 rue Micheli-du-Crest
1211 Geneva 14
Switzerland

A.H.S. Lee
City Hospital NHS Trust
Hucknall Road
Nottingham NG5 1PB
UK

R.C.F. Leonard
Department of Clinical Oncology
Western General Hospital
Crewe Road
Edinburgh EH4 2XU
UK

R.A. Linforth
University Department of Surgery
South Manchester University Hospital
Nell Lane
West Didsbury
Manchester M20 8LR
UK

J. Mackay
University of Cambridge
Department of Oncology
Box 193
Addenbrooke's Hospital
Cambridge CB2 2QQ
UK

P. Maguire
CRC Psychological Medicine Group
Christie Hospital NHS Trust
Stanley House
Wilmslow Road
Manchester M20 9BX
UK

J.L. Mansi
Division of Oncology
St. George's Hospital Medical School
Cranmer Terrace
London SW17 0RE
UK

A. Maraveyas
Division of Oncology
St. George's Hospital Medical School
Cranmer Terrace
London SW17 0RE
UK

A. Marando
Department of Plastic and Reconstructive Surgery
European Institute of Oncology
Via Ripamonti 435
20141 Milan
Italy

K. McPherson
Cancer and Public Health Unit
London School of Hygiene and Tropical Medicine
Keppel Street (Gower Street)
London WC1E 7HT
UK

M.J. Michell
SE London Breast Screening Programme
King's Healthcare NHS Trust
Denmark Hill
London SE5 9RS
UK

W.R. Miller
Edinburgh Breast Unit Research Group
Paderewski Building
Western General Hospital
Edinburgh EH4 2XU
UK

D.A.L. Morgan
Department of Clinical Oncology
City Hospital
Hucknall Road
Nottingham NG5 1PB
UK

F.E. Nussey
Department of Clinical Oncology
Western General Hospital
Crewe Road
Edinburgh EH4 2XU
UK

D.L. Page
Vanderbilt University
Nashville TN
USA

J.Y. Petit
Department of Plastic and Reconstructive Surgery
European Institute of Oncology
Via Ripamonti 435
20141 Milan
Italy

J.A. Petrek
Memorial Sloan–Kettering Cancer Center
1275 York Avenue
New York NY 10021
USA

B.R. Pieters
The Netherlands Cancer Institute/Antoni van Leeuwenhoek Huis
Plesmanlaan 121
1066 CX Amsterdam
The Netherlands

S.E. Pinder
City Hospital NHS Trust
Hucknall Road
Nottingham NG5 1PB
UK

R.M. Rainsbury
The Breast Unit
Royal Hampshire County Hospital
Winchester
Hampshire SO22 5DG
UK

M. Rietjens
Department of Plastic and Reconstructive Surgery
European Institute of Oncology (EIO)
Via Ripamonti 435
20141 Milan
Italy

A. Rodger
William Buckland Radiotherapy Centre
The Alfred Hospital
and Monash University
Melbourne
Australia

V. Sacchini
European Institute of Oncology
Via Ripamonti 435
I-20141 Milan
Italy

N.P.M. Sacks
Department ofAcademic Surgery
Royal Marsden Hospital
Fulham Rd
London SW3 6JJ
UK

D.M. Sibbering
Department of Surgery
Derby City General Hospital
Uttoxeter Road
Derby DE22 3NE
UK

M.J. Silverstein
USC/Norris Cancer Center
University of Southern California
1441 Eastlake Avenue, Room 7415
Los Angeles CA 900033
USA

J.F. Simpson
Vanderbilt University
Nashville TN
USA

I. Smith
Department of Surgery
Medical School
University of Aberdeen
Aberdeen AB25 2ZD
UK

I.E. Smith
Department of Medicine
Royal Marsden Hospital and Institute of Cancer Research
Fulham Road
London SW3 6JJ
UK

A.J. Spillane
Department of Academic Surgery
Royal Marsden Hospital
Fulham Rd
London SW3 6JJ
UK

M. Steel
Professor in Medical Science
School of Biology
University of St. Andrews
Bute Medical Building
St. Andrews
Fife KY16 9TS
Scotland
UK

A. Surbone
1045 31st Street N.W.
Washington DC 20007
USA

L.W. Turnbull
Centre for MR Investigations
Hull Royal Infirmary
Anlaby Road
Hull HU3 2JZ
UK

U. Veronesi
Division of Senology
European Institute of Oncology
Via Ripamonti 435
20141 Milan
Italy

O. Youssef
European Institute of Oncology (EIO)
Plastic and Reconstructive Surgery Department
Via Ripamonti 435
20.141 Milan
Italy

F. Zerwes
Istituto Europeo di Oncologia
Via Ripamonti 435
Milan
Italy

S. Zurrida
European Institute of Oncology
Via Ripamonti 435
20141 Milan
Italy

Contents

Introduction

Breast cancer continues to increase in frequency and approximately one million women world-wide are diagnosed with this disease each year. There have been major advances in our understanding and treatment of breast cancer and this has led to significant reductions in breast cancer mortality. Some of these advances have been slow to be translated into clinical practice. This book summarises our current knowledge of breast cancer and provides a succinct, didactic comprehensive approach outlining how women with suspected cancer should be investigated and once a diagnosis is established, they should be treated. It also explores new areas of diagnosis and management which are likely to be of increasing value in the future. The book is written by senior clinicians and scientists throughout Europe and the United States. It is aimed at all doctors involved in the investigation and management of patients with breast cancer. It should also be a valuable resource to breast care nurses, trainees and senior medical students.

M. DIXON

Breast Cancer: Diagnosis and Management
J.M. Dixon (Ed.)

CHAPTER 1

Magnetic resonance imaging: its role in the breast

L.W. Turnbull

1. Introduction

With the advent of Gadolinium based intravenous contrast agents, the development of purpose built surface coils for signal reception, the use of fast imaging techniques which allow temporal tracking of the contrast bolus and high-resolution fat suppressed 3D imaging which provides contiguous thin slice imaging of the entire breast, the Radiologist now has an additional powerful tool for breast examination. Technical limitations and personal preference have led to data acquisition at varying field strengths using a variety of techniques including gradient or spin echo sequences, acquired either 2 or 3 dimensionally, at time intervals varying from approximately 10 seconds to several minutes, with image processing carried out either by image subtraction or chemical-shift-selective, fat-suppression.

2 or 3D imaging possible depending on clinical problem and hence coverage of breast(s) required.

Despite large variations in technique magnetic resonance (MR) imaging has shown considerable promise in a number of areas of breast disease and although it has focussed on symptomatic, pre-operative or problem cases, research continues to expand the horizons of this investigation. This review will outline how the technique has developed recently and will define the requirement for breast MR and its optimal use in clinical management and treatment.

2. MR breast imaging

Following the introduction of the MR contrast agent dimeglumime gadopentetate (Gd-DTPA) the sensitivity of this technique for the detection of primary breast tumours has been widely studied [1–5]. Although most reports have consisted of pre-selected, symptomatic or problem cases, the sensitivity values have in general exceeded 90% with many now in excess of 95%. With increasing sophistication of breast MR and the detection of ever smaller lesions, the need for improved specificity has been paramount to prevent inappropriate biopsy or worse. Although previous reports have quoted widely ranging specificity values from 53 to 97%, current results now routinely exceed 80% [6–15]. However these studies are heavily biased towards symptomatic, pre-operative, post-menopausal women. As a consequence work continues to improve specificity so that dynamic contrast enhanced (DCE)-MRI may be applied with confidence to smaller lesions, particularly in pre-menopausal women in whom dense breast tissue frequently results in poor lesion visualisation by conventional X-ray mammography. To improve sensitivity and specificity, high-resolution thin slice (3D) imaging of the entire breast is optimal but is obtained at the expense of temporal resolution. Indeed in all protocols there is currently a trade off between temporal and spatial resolution, with the compromise dependent on the age of the patient, the clinical problem, the intended method of data analysis and the equipment employed. It is the task of the Radiologist to tailor the MR examination to the specific clinical question posed to optimise the information obtainable.

MR imaging of the breast has a sensitivity for cancer in recent studies in excess of 95% with a specificity of over 80%.

3. MRI methodology and reporting

Early studies attempted to distinguish between pathologies by measuring temporal signal intensity changes. A number of criticisms have been levied at these studies, in particular the case mix of breast pathology and technical problems related to statistical fluctuation and data sets [6–16]. In addition Weinreb et al. [17] commented on the similarity of enhancement, within 90 s after contrast injection, between benign lesions such as fibroadenomas, fibrocystic and inflammatory disease, recent excision sites, radial scars and sclerosing adenosis and pre-cancerous lesions including lobular carcinoma in situ and atypical ductal hyperplasia. This was confirmed by Kelcz [18] who showed that although the smallest increase in signal intensity by malignant lesions was 74%, 60% of all benign lesions exhibited a signal intensity increase of 75% or greater.

With the introduction of fast scanning techniques (FSPGR, 2D-FLASH, 2D-FFE) it is now possible to image pre-selected areas of the breast at a temporal resolution of as short as 2 s (10 and 42 s most commonly employed), allowing the signal intensity–time curve to be analysed in some detail. Methods for analysing such data continue to be refined with the objective of improving lesion classification and modelling pathophysiological processes. Such techniques vary considerably in complexity from the use of empirical techniques or mathematical descriptors, to fitting data to a pharmacokinetic model or more recently the use of neural networks.

DCE-MRI data can be analysed by empirical techniques, pharmacokinetic modelling, mathematical descriptors and neural networks.

Empirical techniques are the simplest, least labour intensive, and the most widely applied. These techniques used either alone or in combination examine contrast uptake relative to background, at pre-determined time points, which have been shown previously to provide best lesion discrimination [12,10,14,8,19]. However these are subject to some inaccuracy resulting from timing and speed of bolus injection and seldom allow for spurious data points secondary to artefacts. Pharmacokinetic modelling of DCE-MRI was originally performed on the central nervous system [20] and both 2 and 3 compartment models are broadly applicable to breast investigations [14–16,18,21–26]. However all make a number of assumptions concerning tracer mixing, constancy of tracer during the acquisition period, speed of flux of protons and all ignore potential contributions from a vascular component within the lesion itself and diffusion effects. Although these models provide an objective measure of various pathological parameters, namely permeability and contrast exchange rates between plasma and the extra-cellular and the extra-vascular space of a lesion, resulting in accuracy rates ranging from 53 to 95%, they do not exceed the diagnostic accuracy of an experienced Radiologist. However, they may provide valuable objective information for follow-up of chemotherapy or hormonal therapy. Mathematical descriptors primarily examine the heterogeneity of contrast uptake parameter values within a breast lesion with the aim of improving lesion classification. Results to date have been very encouraging. Issa et al. [23] reported a highly significant difference in the slope of a straight line fitted to the mean pixel intensity values obtained after segmentation of the distribution widths of values obtained from exchange rate parameter maps, between benign and malignant lesions. These results confirm the earlier work by Sinha et al. [24]. Recently supervised neural networks have been used to examine DCE-MRI data with a view to automating data analysis. Both back-propagation and probabilistic networks achieve a diagnostic accuracy of 90% compared to 78% for an experienced radiologist presented with signal intensity–time data only [25]. It is hoped that amalgamation of DCE-MRI with textural analysis information will further enhance lesion differentiation. Although these techniques are widely available their use is restricted to the research setting and less computer intensive reporting is generally favoured for routine work. Kuhl et al. [26], have recently reported on the classification accuracy of experienced radiologists subjectively assessing signal intensity–time curves. These curves were subdividing into those that demonstrated a straight or curved line (Type Ia and b); those with a sharp bend after the initial up slope with plateau thereafter (Type II); and those in which contrast washout was evident after an initial up slope (Type III). Using these criteria the diagnostic efficacy was 86%, with a sensitivity of 91% and a specificity of 83% respectively. This is similar to an earlier report by Knowles et al. [25] who quoted an accuracy rate of 76% for an experienced radiologist using signal intensity–time curves alone to differentiate benign from malignant lesions. The specificity value rose to 91% with the addition of morphological information from post-contrast fat-suppressed images.

> *Signal intensity–time curves provide good lesion classification accuracy.*

Fundamental to all methods of contrast uptake quantification is the method for determining the region of interest (ROI) for the lesion. No standardised method is currently in use although most workers utilise an ROI which encompasses the circumference of the lesion, as seen on DCE-MRI, whilst excluding areas of necrosis and surrounding fat [8,27,28]. While this is a common approach it is acknowledged that mean values from a large ROI may be inappropriate particularly for heterogeneous tumours. Many researchers now advocate selective sampling of the lesion based either on geometric, but perhaps more appropriately on enhancement properties. Gribbestad et al. [8] reported improved lesion differentiation using sub-region analysis but these were subjectively defined and the study numbers small. In contrast a larger study of 105 patients [29] analysed using selective pixel sampling revealed differences in the mean enhancement between benign and malignant lesions but the variability also increased resulting in similar classification accuracy compared to conventional whole lesion analysis. Liney et al. [30] have produced a computer algorithm which interrogates the entire lesion on a pixel-by-pixel basis to select a 9-pixel square area of greatest enhancement. Using this method the maximum percentage enhancement values for both benign and malignant lesions was greater than those obtained using a whole lesion ROI, potentially providing better lesion classification.

> *Fundamental to MRI assessment of lesions is quantification of contrast uptake in a region of interest over time.*

4. Extent of disease in the breast

One of the major roles of breast MR is the accurate staging of primary disease, involving determination of lesion extent including the presence of multi-focal/multi-centric disease and involvement of chest wall and contra-lateral breast. There is now substantial evidence of a good correlation between the findings at MR imaging and histology of resected specimens, with results exceeding those obtained by X-ray mammography or ultrasound [31,32].

> *MR breast imaging offers: excellent sensitivity for primary breast cancer; improved detection of multi-focal and multi-centric lesions; determination of chest wall invasion and contralateral disease.*

> *Breast MRI is accurate at determining disease extent within the breast.*

5. Invasive lobular carcinoma

This is also true of invasive lobular carcinoma which is consistently well staged by MR compared to X-ray mammography [33]. Similarly chest wall invasion can be diagnosed with confidence and reports from as early as 1986 quote alteration in patient management following MR, secondary to improved local staging and diagnosis of chest wall invasion [34–36]. However care must be exercised in the diagnosis of multi-focal disease as several reports have commented on inappropriate mastectomy in up to 28% of patients [37]. Of note these studies utilised 3D imaging of the breast at between 60 and 80 s following bolus GD-DTPA injection and the reduced temporal resolution may have contributed to the false-positive results.

> *Excellent correlation of tumour extent demonstrated by MR imaging and histopathology of resected specimens.*

6. MRI in younger women

The reported sensitivity and specificity values for X-ray mammography from the UK NHS breast screening programme for women aged 50 to 65 years has met expectations with values of 90 and 97% respectively. However initial results from the 40 to 49 year old cohort have been disappointing with a reduction in sensitivity and specificity [38]. In addition the interval cancer rate is greater than that for the routine breast-screening programme. The presence of relatively dense breast tissue is reported to be the prime cause of the above results and is a strong argument for the use of DCE-MRI. However the sensitivity of DCE-MRI in pre-menopausal women is as yet unknown and forms the basis of an on-going MRC funded study (MARIBS) [39] which is due to report early in the millennium. This study which compares DCE-MRI and conventional X-ray mammography, comprises an initial high-sensitivity examination followed by a high-specificity examination in equivocal cases, and will carry out a multi-parametric analysis of morphological features and quantitative parameters of contrast uptake. Reporting difficulties are anticipated due to menstrual cycle related changes which cause focal or diffuse enhancement with velocities beyond the malignant threshold [40,41] in many of the normal volunteers. These changes are most apparent in the 35–50 year age group, although of note contrast washout has not been reported during the course of these examinations and may allow discrimination. Similar reporting difficulties are anticipated with some forms of hormone replacement therapy.

> *MRI is being compared with mammography in young high-risk women as a method of screening.*

> *Menstrual cycle related changes may mimic focal or diffuse pathology on post-contrast MR images.*

7. Ductal carcinoma in situ

Ductal carcinoma in situ (DCIS) accounts for 15 to 20% of all detected malignancies and for 25 to 56% of all clinically occult cancers detected by X-ray mammography. Guidi et al. [42] previously demonstrated by immunoperoxidase staining for factor VIII related antigen, that tumour angiogenesis is present in patients with carcinoma in situ. Since then contrast-enhanced MR imaging has demonstrated focal areas or multiple foci of enhancement in a ductal distribution, or focal areas of enhancement with irregular borders. Gilles et al. carried out a comparative histopathological and MR study [43] using multiple T1-weighted spin-echo sequences acquired at 47 s intervals out to 4 min 42 s. He demonstrated neoangiogenesis in the stroma of all cases of noncomedo DCIS examined, but in only 22/24 cases of comedo DCIS, although of note one third of the total cases in this study demonstrated microinvasion. These results have been confirmed by Mendonca et al. [44] who acquired pre- and post-contrast high-resolution images ($512 \times 512 \times 32$ matrix; 16–18 cm field-of-view) at 90-s intervals following injection. Abnormal areas of enhancement, defined as those present on the first post-contrast sequence, were detected in 12/13 patients with either comedo or noncomedo DCIS. In neither study was there an association between subtype of DCIS and pattern of contrast enhancement. Similar results have also been reported by Greenstein Orel et al. [45].

MRI may have a role in detecting DCIS.

8. Impalpable cancers

Recent reports also suggest that MR imaging may be helpful in detecting clinically and mammographically occult breast tumours [46], but despite this potential usage no large-scale studies are available that would validate the application of this technique in asymptomatic patients. Twenty-two per cent of all breast cancer occurs in women under 50 years of age and many of these women have radiographically dense breasts. The false-negative rate of screening mammography in these patients is not known but as palpable cancer is only visible in 56% of women in this age group, cancer detection is likely to be limited. The MR screening trials of pre-menopausal genetically high-risk women that are currently on going in the UK and elsewhere may inform on this matter.

DCE-MRI data has also been applied to patients with equivocal cytology. In a study by Manton et al. [47] a three-compartment pharmacokinetic model was used to calculate the microvessel permeability surface area product and the extra-cellular, extra-vascular tissue volume fraction. Using the first of these parameters a diagnostic accuracy rate of 81% was achieved, whereas use of logistic regression analysis which included both of these variables and cytology grade provided a diagnostic accuracy rate of 91%. An unequivocal diagnosis was possible in 50% of cases potential halving the need for further biopsy.

MRI has a role in patients presenting with an occult primary breast lesion and in assessing patients with equivocal cytology.

9. Assessing effects of neoadjuvant chemotherapy

Neoadjuvant systemic chemotherapy followed by breast conservation surgery is gaining clinical acceptance for patients with locally advanced or large operable disease at presentation. Presurgical reduction in tumour volume can be achieved in as many as two thirds of patients allowing subsequent breast conserving treatment, as well as reducing the risk of tumour dissemination during surgery [48]. Evaluation of any residual tumour after initial chemotherapy by means of clinical examination, X-ray mammography or ultrasound is difficult because of chemotherapy-induced changes and can result in either over or under estimation in approximately 35% of cases [49]. In an early study by Gilles et al. [50] multiple T1-weighted spin-echo sequences were acquired before and at 42 s intervals after contrast infusion and any early enhancement was considered to represent tumour. In this study the extent of residual disease correlated with the histological findings in 16/18 patients. In the remaining patients intraductal extension and an in situ component were not identified. More sophisticated methods of monitoring treatment response are now in use. Pharmacokinetic modelling of TurboFLASH data acquired at a temporal resolution of 23 s, has shown a reduction in the redistribution constant k21 and more consistently a decrease in the amplitude of signal enhancement in patients with an associated histological response [51]. More recently using the RODEO sequence Abrahams et al. [52] evaluated 39 patients with stage II to IV disease prior to and following neoadjuvant chemotherapy. Treatment response was assessed by clinical examination, X-ray mammography, MR imaging and by serial sectioning of mastectomy specimens. Although mammography correlated with MR in only 52% of cases, and clinical assessment by medical and surgical oncologists agreed in only 52 and 55% of cases respectively, MR accurately predicted the pathological determination of residual tumour in 97% of patients. The pathophysiological features of tumour response have also been examined in short-term experiments in nude mice implanted with MCF7 human breast cancer [53]. These have shown increased leakage from permeable intratumoral capillaries indicating the induction of a specific angiogenic process associated with stress conditions that cause necrosis [53]. A marked rise in the extra-cellular volume fraction, indicating increased necrosis, and augmentation of the microvascular permeability as a result of stress-induced angiogenesis, has also been reported in response to tamoxifen [53]. Current results suggest that DCE-MRI will in the future be of major clinical importance for the noninvasive evaluation of neoadjuvant therapy.

MRI is the most accurate of the current imaging modalities at predicting response to primary chemotherapy.

10. Imaging the treated breast after breast conservation therapy

Following conservation therapy X-ray mammography is often confusing with the presence of asymmetrical soft tissue densities secondary to fluid collections, fat necrosis or fibrosis, stromal oedema, skin thickening or reticulation and the development of new calcifications. Fibrosis has been described in approximately 95% and new calcifications in between 14 and 28% of women after conservation therapy [54,55]. A number of workers [56–58] have separately reported on the high false-negative rate of conventional X-ray mammography, which ranges from 30 to 39% for recurrent tumour detection. This is thought to be due to the absence of malignant-type calcification within a densely glandular and distorted breast. However as salvage rate after tumour recurrence is significantly better after conservation therapy compared to mastectomy at 58% versus 21% at five years [59], improved methods of detection have been sought. A number of workers using techniques ranging from delayed post-contrast to high temporal resolution 3D T1-weighted imaging, analysed either by measurement of percentage enhancement versus time or pharmacokinetic modelling, have produced high levels of diagnostic accuracy ranging from 94 to 100% [60–64]. False positive results have included fat necrosis, severe post-radiotherapy change and proliferative dysplasia but false-negative results are infrequent. In this clinical setting morphological information is unhelpful [64] with 93% of benign lesions having a spiculated outline, a feature normally indicative of malignancy in primary pathology. Determination of contrast uptake is crucial to accurate diagnosis. Although sophisticated methods of data analysis generate excellent lesion discrimination, the simple calculation of an enhancement index (defined as the ratio I_{max}/I_{min}, where I_{max} is the maximum pixel signal intensity in the dynamic series and I_{min} is the average of the first three pixel signal intensities in the same series) will provide similarly diagnostic results. Despite

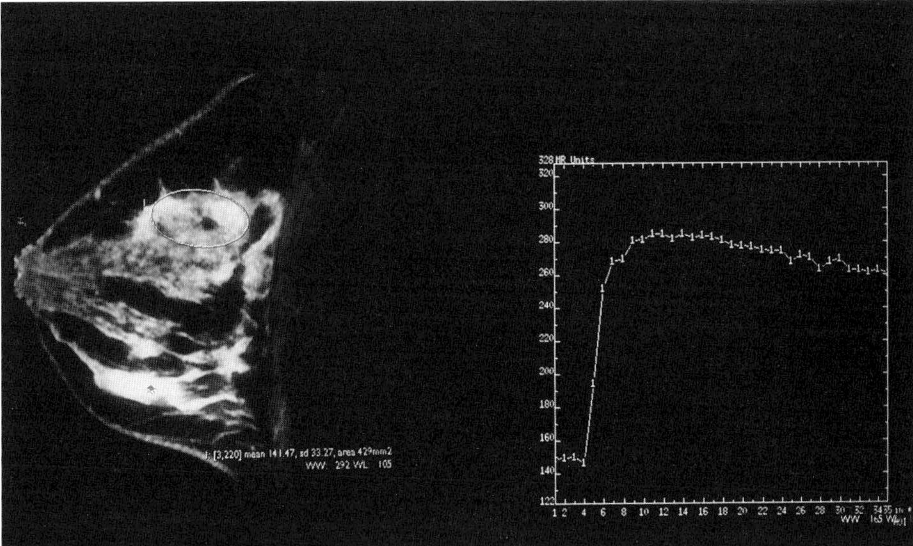

Fig. 1. High-resolution, post-contrast, fat-suppressed T1-weighted 3D FSPGR sagittal section from a pre-menopausal woman who presented with a palpable lump. X-ray mammography showed no abnormality, but diffuse, heterogeneous contrast uptake is seen on the post-contrast T1-weighted, fat-suppressed MR image in the upper half of the breast (RO1). The presence of rapid and intense (Type III signal intensity–time curve; insert) aided diagnosis.

these encouraging results there is a need to optimise breast coverage and spatial resolution whilst preserving the temporal resolution required for tissue differentiation. In 1998 Buckley et al. [65] examined the effect of image acquisition rate on the diagnostic efficacy. By serially removing data points from dynamic-enhanced FSPGR sequences obtained at a temporal resolution of 12 s, various acquisition rates were simulated. Significant differences in enhancement index between benign and malignant lesions were obtained between 24 and 264 s after contrast administration, indicating that the acquisition rate has a negligible effect on diagnostic efficacy. As a consequence it is possible to examine both breasts in their entirety during the same examination, enabling additional multifocal or second primary tumours to be detected. Using such an approach Murray et al. [66] employed subtracted 3D T1-weighted FLASH sequences acquired at 1, 2 and 3 min post-contrast injection and successfully distinguished all benign from malignant lesions. This is a highly specific and sensitive technique and as only a limited number of sequences are required, it is a highly cost effective method of examining the post-conservation breast. Ideally high-risk patients namely those with equivocal mammographic results, diagnosis at less than 35 years of age, an extensive intraductal component or comedo-type DCIS, as well as those in whom there is clinical concern benefit from DCE-MRI. However the timing of imaging in relation to conservation therapy would appear to be crucial. In 1993 Heywang et al. [67] examined the pattern and speed of enhancement at varying time intervals following radiotherapy in the only report on this subject in the current literature. She demonstrated that these results were only obtainable if MR imaging was delayed for at least 9 months after radiotherapy, by which time inflammatory changes which resulted in an overlap in the pattern and the speed of enhancement between benign and malignant lesions had resolved in the majority of patients. This time delay does not appear to be as important in patients who do not undergo radiotherapy. Soderstrom et al. [68] using a contrast enhanced 3D RODEO tech-

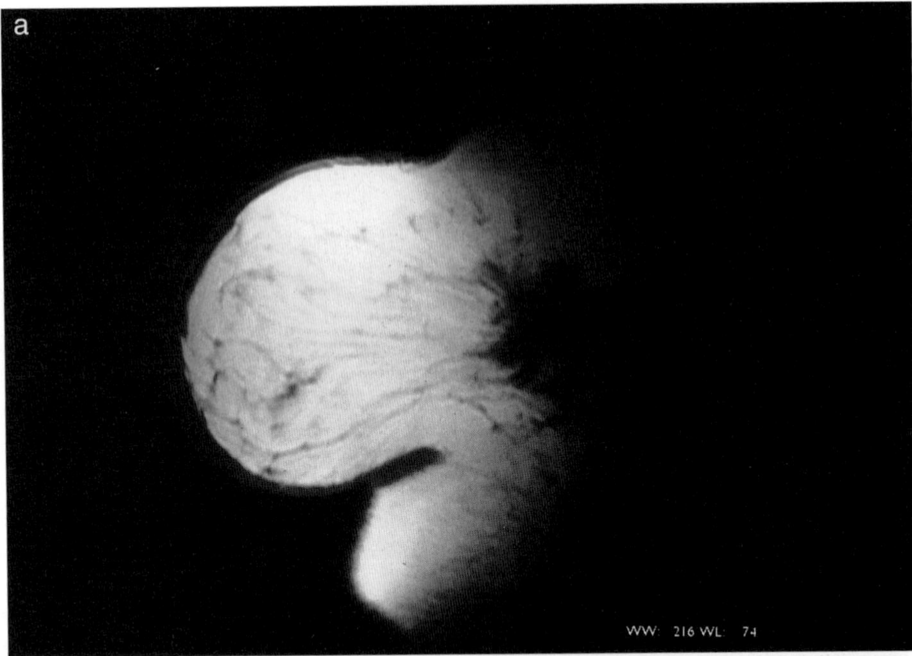

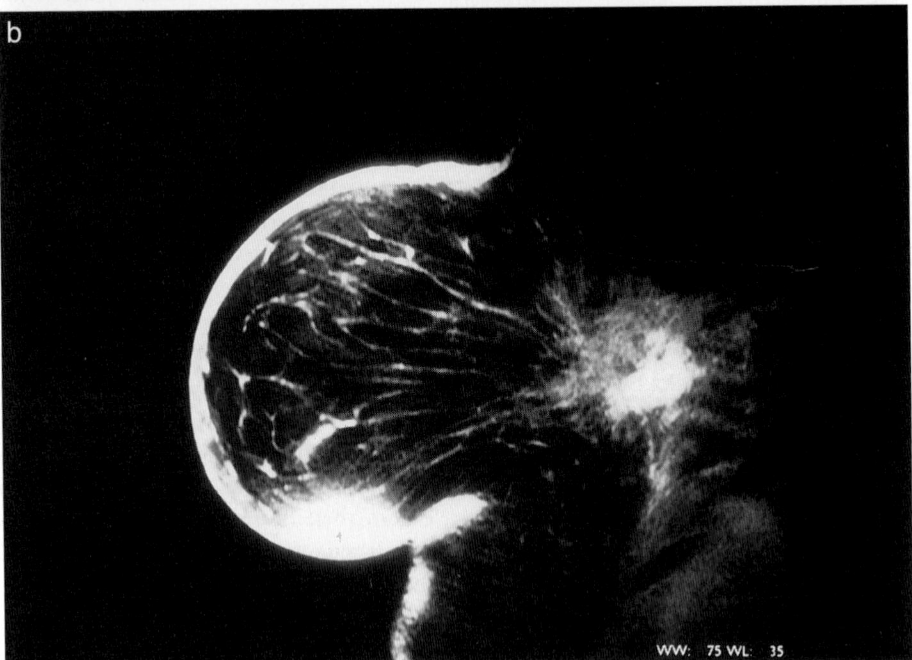

Fig. 2. Pre- (a) and post-contrast, fat-suppressed (b) T1-weighted images from a post-menopausal woman following conservation breast surgery. Whereas X-ray mammography was equivocal MR showed enhancement of a spiculated soft tissue mass secondary to recurrent tumour.

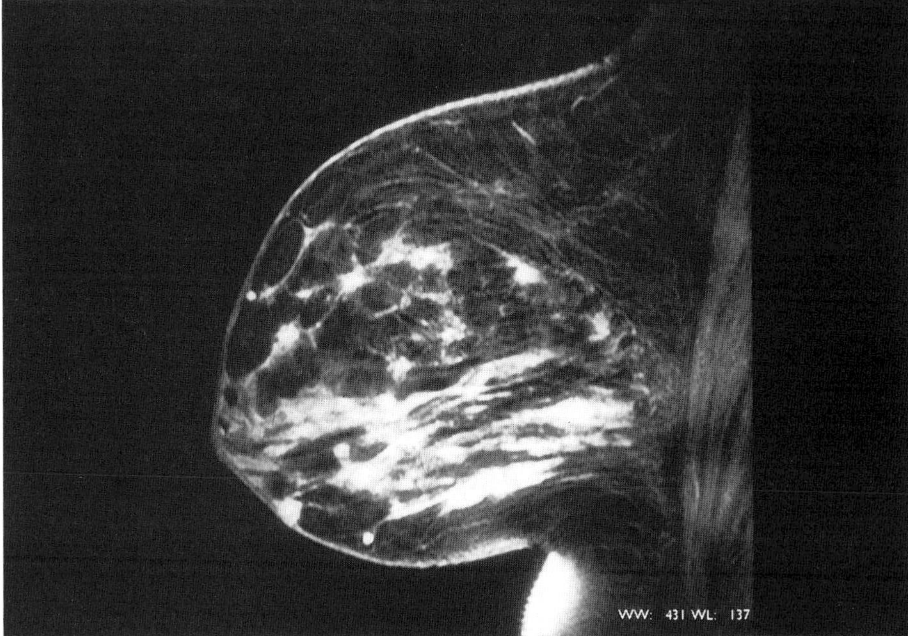

Fig. 3. Pre-menopausal women with X-ray mammographic evidence of DCIS. Post-contrast, fat-suppressed T1-weighted image shows the presence of abnormal contrast uptake and morphology.

nique examined 18 patients with either residual disease or positive excision margins, a mean of 10 months after wide local excision. Subsequent histopathological assessment of mastectomy specimens demonstrated accurate delineation of residual tumour in 84% of cases with mismatches due to microabscesses in 2 cases and failure to detect a retroareolar invasive lobular carcinoma in one case.

MRI is an accurate method of differentiating scar from local recurrence in the treated breast 9 months or more after treatment by radiotherapy.

Sensitivity and specificity of DCE-MRI for detection of recurrent tumour approaches 100% in patients imaged 9 months or more following radiotherapy.

11. Identifying silicone implant rupture

Concerns about the dangers of rupture of silicone-gel implants whether inserted for reconstructive or cosmetic purposes has prompted comparative studies of the efficacy of X-ray mammography, ultrasound and MR imaging for assessment of implant shell integrity. These have been undertaken using inversion recovery with short T1 sequences or chemical-shift-selective imaging which suppresses the signal from fat whilst maintaining the signal from silicone. Loss of implant integrity can be classified into silicone-gel bleed, characterised by an inverted teardrop sign on MR imaging; intracapsular rupture which gives rise to the linguine sign and extra-capsular rupture in which free silicone is seen in the soft tissues surrounding the implant. The sensitivity of MR for detection of silicone implant rupture has varied but most studies now report values around 95% with specificity values over 90% which exceed comparable results for ultrasound and X-ray mammography

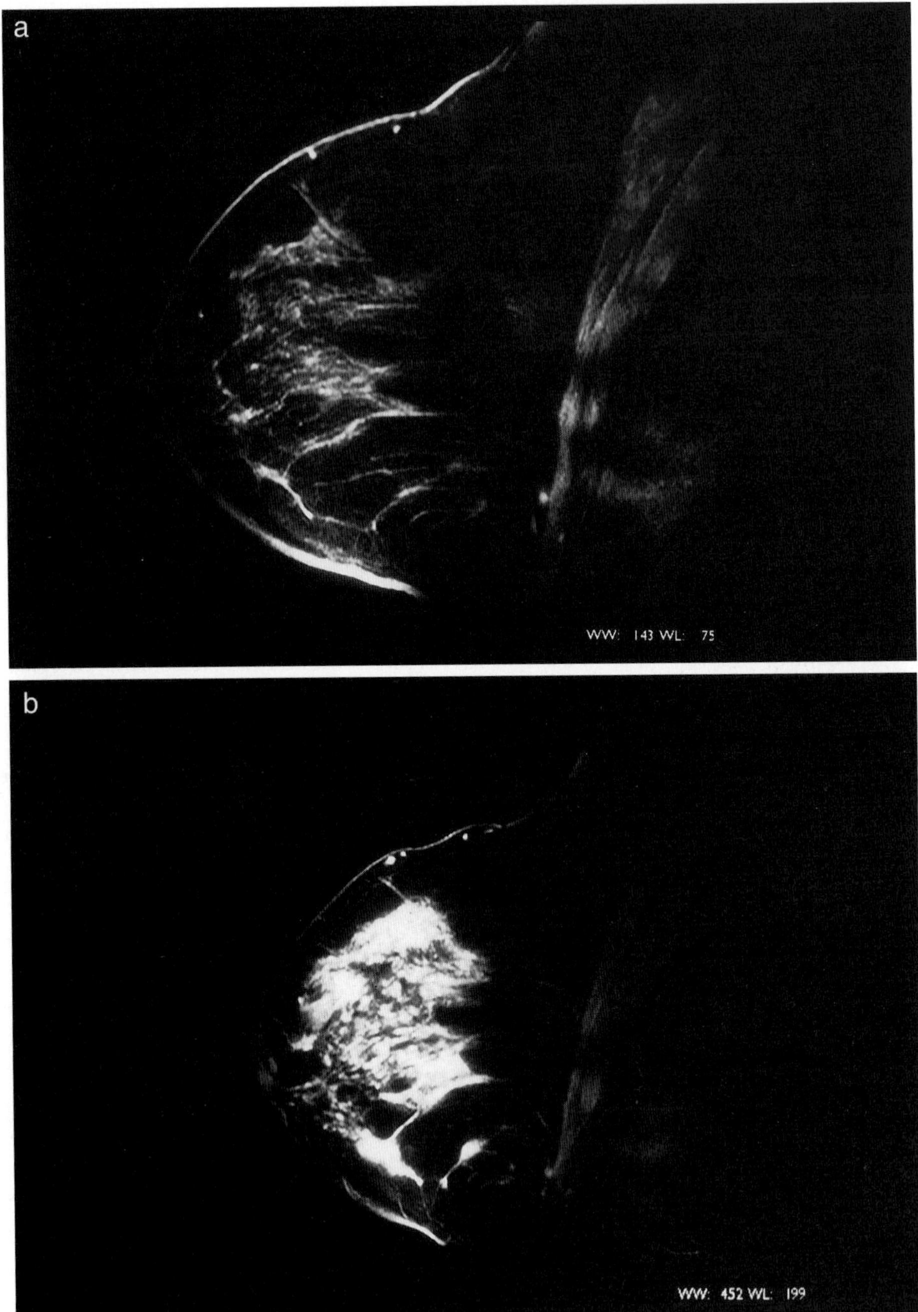

Fig. 4. Following commencement of continuous oestrogen replacement therapy, marked increase in the volume of breast parenchyma and extent of contrast enhancement is evident (a: pre-HRT; b: post-HRT).

[69–73]. In addition DCE-MRI is capable of detecting tumour recurrence in these patients with a high sensitivity, although the specificity values are reduced secondary to the presence of enhancing granulomas.

For suspected implant rupture MRI is the imaging modality of choice.

MR imaging of the breast now recommended for determination of implant shell integrity.

12. Localisation of lesions seen on MRI

With the increasing resolution of MR images and hence detection of ever smaller lesions, techniques are now evolving for localisation of lesions shown by MRI alone. These lesions present unique problems to the Radiologist as they may be detected only by transient contrast uptake and architectural distortion, a useful guide in X-ray mammography, may not be present. Unlike routine MR compression is required to allow accurate biopsy or localisation and the patient must be moved out of the system for needle insertion. Metal localisation needles give rise to susceptibility artefacts and hence check images cannot be obtained. A repeat contrast injection is required after needle insertion to confirm accurate positioning. With all these limitations it is not surprising that many techniques are in use, ranging from free-hand placement, use of surface markers, compression devices employing surface coils or alpha numeric plates within a fixed coil, to prototype stereotactic tables and the use of open magnets. As a consequence once the lesion has been detected careful retrospective review of X-ray mammograms with or without additional views and colour flow or contrast enhanced high-resolution ultrasound may offer a useful alternative, until reliable user and patient friendly devices become freely available.

Techniques are evolving to localise lesions seen only on MRI.

13. Conclusion

MR Imaging has already proved beneficial in planning appropriate surgical intervention in primary disease, accurate diagnosis of local tumour recurrence, monitoring treatment response and in determining implant shell integrity and with further refinement will develop an expanded role in other problematic areas such as investigation of microcalcification, treatment response and screening of pre-menopausal high-risk women in the near future.

References

1. Oellinger H, Heins S, Sander B (1993) Gd-DTPA enhanced MR breast imaging: the most sensitive method for multicentric carcinomas of the female breast. Eur Radiol, 3, 223–226.
2. Heywang SH, Wolf A, Pruss E, Hilbertz T, Eiermann W, Permanetter W (1989) MR imaging of the breast with Gd-DTPA: use and limitations. Radiology, 171, 95–103.
3. Kaiser WA (1992) MRM promises earlier breast cancer diagnosis. Diagn Imaging, 11, 44–50.
4. Doa TH, Rahmouni A, Campana F, Laurent M, Asselain B, Fourquet A (1993) Tumour recurrence versus fibrosis in the irradiated breast: differentiation with gadolinium-enhanced MR imaging. Radiology, 187, 751–755.
5. Fischer U, von Heyden D, Vosshenrich R (1993) Signal-verhalten maligner und benigner Läsionen in der dynamischen 2D-MRT der Mamma. Fortschr Geb Roentgenstr, 158, 287–292.
6. Gilles R, Guinebretiere JM, Shapeero LG (1993) Assessment of breast cancer recurrence with contrast-enhanced subtraction MR imaging: preliminary results in 26 patients. Radiology, 188, 473–478.
7. Boetes C, Barentsz JO, Mus RD, van der Sluis RF (1994) MR characterisation of suspicious breast lesions with the gadolinium enhanced Turbo FLASH subtraction technique. Radiology, 193, 777–781.
8. Gribbestad IS, Nilsen G, Fjosne HE (1994) Comparative signal intensity measurements in dynamic gadolinium-enhanced MR mammography. JMRI, 4, 477–480.
9. Kaiser WA, Zeitler E (1989) MR imaging of the

breast: fast imaging sequences with and without Gd-DTPA. Radiology, 170, 681–686.
10. Hulka CA, Smith BL, Sgroi DC (1995) Benign and malignant breast lesions: differentiation with echo-planar MR imaging. Radiology, 197, 33–38.
11. Stack JP, Redmond OM, Cobb MB (1990) Breast disease: tissue characterisation with Gd-DTPA enhancement profiles. Radiology, 174, 491–494.
12. Greenstein Orel S, Schnall MD, Powell CM (1995) Staging of suspected breast cancer: effect of MR imaging and MR-guided biopsy. Radiology, 196, 115–122.
13. Flickinger FW, Allison JD, Sherry RM, Wright JC (1993) Differentiation of benign from malignant breast masses by time–intensity evaluation of contrast-enhanced MRI. Magn Reson Imaging, 11, 617–620.
14. Buckley DL, Kerslake RW, Blackband SJ, Horsman A (1994) Quantitative analysis of multi-slice Gd-DTPA enhanced dynamic MR images using an automated simplex minimisation procedure. MRM, 32, 646–651.
15. Tofts PS, Berkowitz B, Schnall MD (1995) Quantitative analysis of dynamic Gd-DTPA enhancement in breast tumours using a permeability model. MRM, 33, 564–568.
16. Hoffmann U, Brix G, Knopp MV (1995) Pharmacokinetic mapping of the breast: a new method for dynamic MR mammography. MRM, 33, 506–514.
17. Weinreb JC, Newstead G (1995) MR imaging of the breast. Radiology, 196, 593–610.
18. Kelcz F, Santyr GE, Cron GO, Mongin SJ (1996) Application of a quantitative model to differentiate benign from malignant breast lesions detected by dynamic, gadolinium-enhanced MRI. JMRI, 6, 743–752.
19. Liney G, Turnbull LW (1999) Assessment of several quantitative measurements of dynamic contrast enhanced MRI in the differentiation of primary breast tumours. J Diagn Radiogr Imaging, 2, 81–87.
20. Tofts PS, Kermode AG (1991) Measurement of the blood–brain barrier permeability and leakage space using dynamic MR imaging, 1. Fundamental concepts. Magn Reson Med, 17, 357–367.
21. Hess T, Knopp MV, Brix G (1994) Pharmakokinetische Analyse der Gd-DTPA Anreicherung in der MRT beim Mammakarzinom. Fortschr Röntgenstr., 160, 518.
22. Hittmair K, Gomiscek G, Langenberger K (1994) Method for the quantitative assessment of contrast agent uptake in dynamic contrast-enhanced MRI. Magn Reson Med, 31, 567–571.
23. Issa B, Buckley DL, Mussurakis S, Horsman A (1997) Statistical analysis of contrast-enhanced breast images. 5th Scientific Meeting of ISMRM, Vancouver, p. 1049.
24. Sinha S, Lucas-Quesada FA, DeBuhl ND, Sayre J, Farria D, Gorczya DP, Bassett LW (1997) Multifeature analysis of Gd-enhanced MR images of breast lesions. JMRI, 7, 1016–1026.
25. Knowles AJ, Issa B, Burton S, Liney GP, Gibbs P, Turnbull LW (1998) Classification of benign and malignant disease by neural network analysis of dynamic imaging. Proceedings of Radiology, 1400, p. 83.
26. Kuhl CK, Mielcareck P, Klaschik S (1999) Dynamic breast MR imaging: are signal intensity time course data useful for differential diagnosis of enhancing lesions? Radiology, 211, 101–110.
27. Kaiser WA (1993) MR Mammography (MRM). Berlin, Springer, pp. 37–88.
28. Aronen HJ, Gazit IE, Louis DN (1994) Cerebral blood volume maps of gliomas: comparison of tumour grade and histologic findings. Radiology, 191, 41–51.
29. Mussurakis S, Gibbs P, Horsman A (1998) Primary breast abnormalities: selective pixel sampling on dynamic gadolinium-enhanced MR images. Radiology, 206, 465–473.
30. Liney G, Turnbull LW (1999) Dynamic contrast-enhanced MRI in the differentiation of breast tumours: the effect of region-of-interest. BJR, 72 (suppl), 37.
31. Davies PL, Staiger MJ, Harris KB, Ganott MA, Klementaviciene J, McCarthy KS, Tobon H (1996) Breast cancer measurements with magnetic resonance imaging, ultrasonography and mammography. Breast Cancer Res Treat, 37, 1–9.
32. Esserman L, Hylton N, Yassa L (1999) Utility of magnetic resonance imaging in the management of breast cancer: evidence for improved preoperative staging. J Clin Oncol, 17, 110–119.
33. Balen FG, Hall-Craggs MA, Mumtaz H, Wilkinson I, Scheidau A (1997) MRI of invasive lobular carcinoma of the breast. Proceedings of Radiology 1997, Birmingham, May, p. 51.
34. Deutch BM, Merchant TE, Scwartz LH, Powell CM, Liberman I, Dershaw DD (1993) Local staging of breast cancer by using MR imaging (abstr.) Radiology, 189 (P), 301.
35. Fischer U, Vosshenrich R, Kopka M, von Heyden D, Oestmann JW, Grabbe EH (1994) Preoperative MR mammography in patients with breast cancer: impact on therapy (abstr.) Radiology, 193 (P), 121.
36. Whitney WS, Herfkens RJ, Silverman J, Ikeda D, Brumbaugh J, Jeffreys S (1993) Gadolinium-enhanced spectral–spatial MR imaging for evaluation of breast carcinoma (abstr.) Radiology, 189 (P), 136.
37. Kramer S, Doinghaus K, Schulz-Wendtland R, Lang N, Bautz W (1997) The role of MR-mammography in the diagnosis of multicentricity in breast cancer. Proceedings of Radiology 1997, Birmingham, May, p. 51.
38. 3rd National Breast Cancer Trials Meeting, London, November 1998; Published by UK CCCR (Breast Cancer Subgroup).
39. Leach M (1997) National study of magnetic resonance imaging to screen women at genetic risk of breast cancer. Lancet, 350, 6.

40. Kuhl CK, Bieling HB, Gieseke K, Kreft BP, Sommer T, Lutterbey G, Schild HH (1997) Healthy premenopausal breast parenchyma in dynamic contrast-enhanced MR imaging of the breast: normal contrast medium enhancement and cyclic-phase dependency. Radiology, 203, 137–144.
41. Muller-Schimpfle M, Ohmenhäuser K, Stoll P, Dietz K, Claussenn CD (1997) Menstrual cycle and age: influence of parenchymal contrast medium enhancement in MR imaging of the breast. Radiology, 203, 145–149.
42. Guidi AJ, Fischer L, Harris JR, Schnitt SJ (1994) Microvessel density and distribution in ductal carcinoma in situ in the breast. J Natl Cancer Inst, 86, 614–619.
43. Gilles R, Zafrani B, Guinebretiere JM (1995) Ductal carcinoma in situ: MR imaging–histopathological correlation. Radiology, 196, 415–419.
44. Mendonca MH, Schnall MD, Orel S, Reynolds C (1996) High resolution MRI of ductal carcinoma in situ. 4th Scientific Meeting of the ISMRM, p. 347.
45. Greenstein Orel S, Mendonca MH, Reynolds C, Schnall MD, Solin LJ, Sullivan DC (1997) MR imaging of ductal carcinoma in situ. Radiology, 202, 413–420.
46. Tilanus Linthorst MMA, Obdeijn AIM, Bontenbal M, Oudkerk M (1997) MRI in patients with axillary metastases of occult breast carcinoma. Breast Cancer Res Treat, 44, 179–182.
47. Manton DJ, Coady AM, Knowles AJ, Turnbull LW (1999) Dynamic contrast-enhanced MRI following equivocal breast cytology: Using neural networks and logistic regression to maximise diagnostic efficacy. Proceedings of 7th Scientific Meeting of the ISMRM, Philadelphia, PA, 1999, p. 353.
48. Jacquillat C, Weil M, Auclerc G (1989) Neoadjuvant chemotherapy in the conservative management of breast cancer: a study of 252 patients. Recent Results Cancer Res, 115, 36.
49. Cocconi G, Di Blasio B, Alberti G (1984) Problems in evaluating response of primary breast cancer to systemic therapy. Breast Cancer Res Treat, 309–313.
50. Gilles R, Giunebretiere JM, Toussaint C (1994) Locally advanced breast cancer: contrast-enhanced subtraction MR imaging of response to preoperative chemotherapy. Radiology, 191, 633–638.
51. Knopp MV, Junkermann HJ, Hoffmann U, Sinn P, Himmelhan N, Zabel S, Juschka U, Hess T, Essig M, Brix G, van Kaick G (1996) Fast dynamic MR imaging for characterisation of breast lesions. Experiences of functional MR mammography. Proceedings of 4th Scientific Meeting of the ISMRM, New York, p. 353.
52. Abrahams DC, Jones RC, Jones SE (1996) Evaluation of neoadjuvant chemotherapeutic response of locally advanced breast cancer by magnetic resonance imaging. Cancer, 78, 91–100.
53. FurmanHaran E, Grobgeld D, Margalit R, Degani H (1998) Response of MCF7 human breast cancer to tamoxifen: evaluation by the three-time-point, contrast-enhanced magnetic resonance imaging method. Clin Cancer Res, 4, 2299–2304.
54. Libshitz HI, Montague ED, Paulus DD (1977) Calcifications in the therapeutically irradiated breast. AJR, 128, 1021.
55. Mendelson EB (1989) Imaging the post-surgical breast. Semin Ultrasound CT MR, 10, 154.
56. Stomper PC, Recht A, Berenberg AL, Jochelson MS, Harris JR (1987) Mammographic detection of recurrent cancer in the irradiated breast. AJR, 148, 39–43.
57. Hassell PR, Olivotto IA, Mueller HA, Kingston EW, Basco VE (1990) Early breast cancer: detection of recurrence after conservative surgery and radiation therapy. Radiology, 176, 731–735.
58. Dershaw DD, McCormick B, Cox L, Osborne MP (1990) Differentiation of benign and malignant local tumour recurrence after lumpectomy. AJR, 155, 35–38.
59. Harris JR, Recht A, Amalric R (1984) Time course and prognosis of local recurrence following primary radiation therapy for early breast cancer. J Clin Oncol, 2(1), 37–41.
60. Heywang SH, Hilbertz T, Beck R, Bauer WM, Eiermann W, Permanetter W (1990) Gd-DTPA enhanced MR imaging of the breast in patients with postoperative scarring and silicon implants. J Comput Assist Tomogr, 14, 348–356.
61. Lewis-Jones HG, Whitehouse GH, Leinster SJ (1991) The role of magnetic resonance imaging in the assessment of local recurrent breast carcinoma. Clin Radiol, 43, 197–204.
62. Hickman PF, Moore NR, Shepstone BJ (1994) The indeterminate breast mass: assessment with contrast-enhanced magnetic resonance imaging. Br J Radiol, 67, 14.
63. Kerślake RW, Fox JN, Carleton PJ (1994) Dynamic contrast-enhanced and fat suppressed magnetic resonance imaging in suspected recurrent carcinoma of the breast: preliminary experience. Br J Radiol, 67, 1158–1168.
64. Mussurakis S, Buckley DL, Bowsley SJ, Carleton PJ, Fox JN, Turnbull LW, Horsman A (1995) Dynamic contrast-enhanced MR imaging of the breast combined with pharmacokinetic analysis of Gd-DTPA uptake in the diagnosis of recurrence of early-stage breast carcinoma. Invest Radiol, 30, 650–662.
65. Buckley DL, Mussurakis S, Horsman A (1998) Effect of temporal resolution on the diagnostic efficacy of contrast-enhanced MRI in the conservatively treated breast. JCAT, 22, 47–51
66. Murray AD, Redpath TW, Needham G, Gilbert FJ, Brookes JA, Eremin O (1996) Dynamic magnetic res-

onance mammography of both breasts following local excision and radiotherapy for breast carcinoma. BJR, 69, 594–600.

67. Heywang-Koebrunner SH, Schlegel A, Beck R (1993) Contrast-enhanced MRI of the breast after limited surgery and radiation therapy. J Comput Assist Tomogr, 17, 891–900.
68. Soderstrom CE, Harms SE, Farrell RS, Pruneda JM, Flamig DP (1997) Detection with MR imaging of residual tumour in the breast soon after surgery. AJR, 168, 485–488.
69. Ahn CY, Shaw WW, Narayanan K (1993) Definitive diagnosis of breast implant rupture using magnetic resonance imaging. Plast Reconstr Surg, 94, 681–691.
70. Gorcyca DP, DeBruhl ND, Ahn CY (1994) Silicone breast implant ruptures in an animal model: comparison of mammography, MR imaging, US and CT. Radiology, 109, 227–232.
71. Rohrich RJ, Adams WP, Beran SJ (1998) An analysis of silicone-gel-filled breast implants: diagnosis and failure rates. Plast Reconstr Surg, 102, 2304–2308.
72. Goodman CM, Cohen V, Thornby U, Netscher D (1998) The life span of silicone gel breast implants and a comparison of mammography, ultrasound and magnetic resonance imaging in detecting rupture: a meta-analysis. Ann Plast Surg, 41, 577–585.
73. Chung KC, Greenfield MLVH, Walters M (1998) Decision-analysis methodology in the work-up of women with suspected silicone breast implant rupture. Plast Reconstr Surg, 102, 689–695.

Breast Cancer: Diagnosis and Management
J.M. Dixon (Ed.)

CHAPTER 2

Diagnosis: PET scanning and new techniques

Fiona J. Gilbert and Ian Smith

1. Positron emission tomography

Positron Emission Tomography (PET) is a 'functional' imaging technique that can be used to measure tumour metabolism, assess blood flow and quantitate oestrogen and progesterone receptor density [1]. While it can be used to detect breast cancer, it is not superior to conventional imaging methods of mammography, ultrasound and magnetic resonance imaging (MRI). It is the 'functional' attributes that have attracted researchers to this modality to try to gain further understanding of tumour kinetics in relation to growth, cell type and response to chemotherapy.

Elements, naturally occurring in the body such as oxygen, carbon, nitrogen and fluorine bombarded with protons or deuterons in a cyclotron, result in proton rich nuclei that decay by emitting positrons (positively charged electrons). The positrons travel a short distance (0.2–2.5 mm) [2] within the surrounding tissues before they collide with a local electron and undergo an annihilation reaction. Two gamma rays are emitted as a result of this, each of 511 keV at a 180° direction to each other. By placing the patient in the centre of a ring of gamma ray detectors it is possible to record the simultaneous emission of these gamma rays and with computer analysis produce a tomographic image of the source. The static PET images produced have poor anatomic detail and spatial resolution of 6–10 mm which is low compared with conventional imaging. However the dynamic image represents the rate of accumulation and the plateau concentration of the radioisotope allowing quantitative image analysis which reflects the underlying biological and physiological process. This has allowed PET to develop as a useful research tool in a variety of circumstances.

> *Positron Emission Tomography can measure tumour metabolism, blood flow and oestrogen receptor density in breast cancer.*

Many compounds can be labelled with positron emitting radionuclides without losing the chemical properties of the parent compound (Table 1) [3]. The most commonly used positron emitting tracer is the glucose analogue (^{18}F)fluoro-2-deoxy-D-glucose (^{18}F-FDG). This positron emitting compound is thought to accumulate in malignant cells for two main reasons. Firstly, malignant cells possess higher levels of the enzyme hexokinase [4–6] (an enzyme that catalyses a rate limiting step in the glycolytic pathway — the conversion of glucose to glucose-6-phosphate). If the positron emitting substance ^{18}F-FDG is provided as substrate for the hexokinase catalysed reaction, (^{18}F)fluoro-2-deoxy-D-glucose-6-phosphate

Table 1. Examples of radiopharmaceuticals used in PET

Parent compound	Radiopharmaceutical
Glucose	2-[^{18}F]fluoro-2-deoxy-D-glucose (^{18}F-FDG)
Water	^{15}O water ($H_2^{15}O$)
Oxygen	^{15}O oxygen ($^{15}O_2$)
Amino acids	^{11}C methionine
	^{11}C leucine
	^{13}N glutamate
	^{11}C tryptophan
	^{11}C valine
Ammonia	^{13}N ammonia ($^{13}NH_3$)
Oestrogen	16alpha-[^{18}F]fluoro-17beta-estradiol (FES)
Chemotherapeutic agents	^{18}F tamoxifen
	^{11}C carmustine
	^{18}F fluorouracil

is produced. This compound cannot be metabolised further. Therefore the rate limiting hexokinase catalysed reaction has effectively been isolated from the glycolytic pathway and thus the rate at which ^{18}F-FDG accumulates within the cell is proportional to the rate of cellular glycolysis [7,8]. Secondly, malignant cells have increased membrane Glut-1 and Glut-3 transporter proteins which allow malignant cells to accumulate glucose at higher rates than non-malignant cells [9].

^{18}F-FDG, a glucose analogue is the most commonly used radiotracer in breast cancer imaging. The rate at which ^{18}F-FDG accumulates within cells is proportional to the rate of glycolysis.

^{18}F-FDG was first used to differentiate benign from malignant breast lesions in 1992 [10] (Fig. 1). Since then a number of small series of patients have been published demonstrating 80–100% sensitivity for the detection of breast cancer and a wide range of specificity (Table 2) [3]. However the reason that PET will not replace conventional imaging in the diagnosis of breast cancer is that lesions less than 1.5 cm in size cannot reliably be detected [18]. Also false positives occur with metabolically active breast tissue such as benign breast change [14] and widespread carcinoma in situ which both cause increased activity which can mask a cancer [10]. The use of quantitative image analysis has improved the specificity of the technique allowing differentiation of tumour from metabolically active tissue [20]. A more interesting application of quantitative techniques has been the use of the differential absorption ratio (DAR) in comparing the uptake of ^{18}F-FDG in different tumours. This has allowed PET to be used as an independent prognostic indicator [19,23] with biologically more aggressive tumours with a high de novo tumour glycolytic rate correlating with a poor clinical outcome.

^{18}F-FDG PET has a high sensitivity for the detection of breast cancer but is unlikely to replace conventional imaging techniques.

PET has also been used with some success to monitor response to neo-adjuvant chemotherapy [19,23,24]. Conventional imaging i.e. mammography and ultrasound rely on morphological changes to take place within tumours following chemotherapy to demonstrate response to treatment. However PET is able to demonstrate changes in metabolism prior to any changes in morphology, and often within 10 days of treatment. In the study published by Wahl et al. [23] using PET to evaluate response to chemotherapy

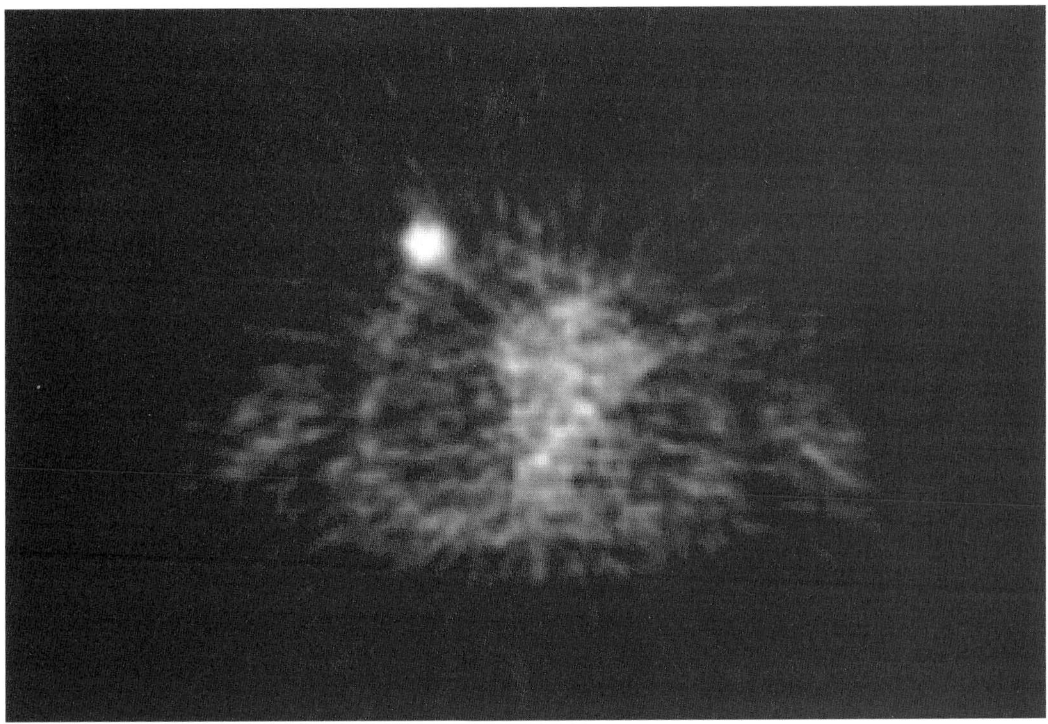

Fig. 1. ^{18}F-FGD PET image of breast cancer.

Table 2. PET studies to evaluate the primary breast lesion

Study	Number of breast lesions evaluated	Sensitivity	Specificity
Bolster et al. (1986) [11]	1	Not applicable	100%
Kubota et al. (1989) [12]	1	Not applicable	100%
Wahl et al. (1991) [13]	10	Not applicable	100%
Tse et al. (1992) [10]	14	80%	100%
Nieweg et al. (1993) [14]	20	91%	89%
Hoh et al. (1993) [15]	20	88%	33%
Adler et al. (1993) [16]	35	96%	100%
Bruce et al. (1995) [17]	15	93%	Not applicable
Dehdashti et al. (1995) [18]	32	88%	100%
Bassa et al. (1996) [19]	17	Not applicable	100%
Avril et al. (1996) [20]	72	83%	84%
Scheidhauer et al. (1996) [21]	30	91%	86%
Noh et al. (1998) [22]	31	100%	89%

in 11 patients, the 3 patients who did not respond to treatment were identified by PET at a much earlier time than conventional assessment. This was also confirmed in similar work from Bassa et al. [19]. Jansson et al. [24] showed that quantitative PET analysis documented response in 11 of 12 patients after the first course of chemotherapy. This has huge implications both for patient management and for the drug industry wishing to test novel chemotherapeutic agents.

PET imaging can detect response to chemotherapy earlier than conventional imaging and often after the first course of chemotherapy.

The experimental imaging of oestrogen receptor-positive (ER+) breast lesions has been accomplished using ^{18}F-radiolabelled oestrogen receptor ligands (^{18}FES). While allowing assessment of oestrogen receptor density it has allowed assessment of tumour response to tamoxifen therapy after as little as 7 days of treatment. However, only about 30% of tumours tested showed this oestrogen receptor positive imaging. Progesterone receptor (PR) ligands have not been as successful due to high hepatic uptake but second generation PR ligands are likely to be more effective and are ready for clinical evaluation [25]. These experimental techniques are unlikely to find a place in diagnostic imaging but could potentially be useful in identifying patients who might benefit from tamoxifen if there is any dubiety clinically.

Other agents have also been used to assess breast metabolism. L-(1-^{11}C)Tyrosine(^{11}C-TYR) measures the rate of protein synthesis and has been compared to ^{18}F-FDG. In a small series from Germany all 10 malignant lesions were identified with both ^{18}F-FDG and ^{11}C-TYR but visualisation was better with ^{18}F-FDG. However uptake in benign breast change was lower with ^{11}C-TYR suggesting this may be a more promising agent than ^{18}F-FDG [26]. Carbon-11-methionine (^{11}C-Met) has also been studied. In a series of 24 patients ^{18}F-FDG and ^{11}C-Met appeared equally effective in detecting residual and recurrent malignant tumours although ^{18}F-FDG uptakes were slightly higher. The problem with ^{11}C-labelled tracers is the very short half-life of the isotope, confining its use to the few centres with a cyclotron on site.

Although PET has many advantages as a research tool, it is unlikely to be used in diagnosis of breast cancer or its subsequent management. The technique is expensive and there are relatively few centres that are able to perform this technique. The radioisotopes all have a short half-life and with the exception of ^{18}F all need to be produced on site by a cyclotron adding considerably to the cost of the examination. PET will continue to be developed as a research tool that can be used to unravel information on tumour blood flow and metabolism and which could be used to test novel chemotherapeutic agents.

2. Scintimammography

The equipment required for this technique is available in most nuclear medicine departments and the radioisotopes are available commercially. This makes scintimammography possible in most hospitals offering it as a reasonable option for the diagnosis of breast cancer. It is a relatively inexpensive technique that has a high sensitivity in palpable lesions but unfortunately a low sensitivity in lesions less than 1 cm in size [27]. Despite the reasonably high specificity, the inability to reliably detect small lesions limits the value of the technique. Although it is often added to mammography and ultrasound it has similar sensitivity and specificity when compared to mammography and does not allow accurate diagnosis of lesions deemed indeterminate by other investigations. As it does not add significantly to other imaging investigations it has no role in the routine assessment of breast lesions.

Scintimammography is a widely available, inexpensive technique with high specificity but low sensitivity for lesions less than 1 cm in size. It has no role in the routine assessment of breast lesions.

Technetium-99m (^{99m}Tc) sestamibi (Fig. 2) was initially developed as a cardiac imaging agent to document myocardial blood flow. However following the observation that it is avidly taken by neoplastic breast tissue there have been a number of studies looking at the detection of breast cancer. ^{99m}Tc-sestamibi enters cancer cells by an active transport mechanism and stored in the mitochondria and the cytoplasm [28]. As there appears to be more mitochondria in metaboli-

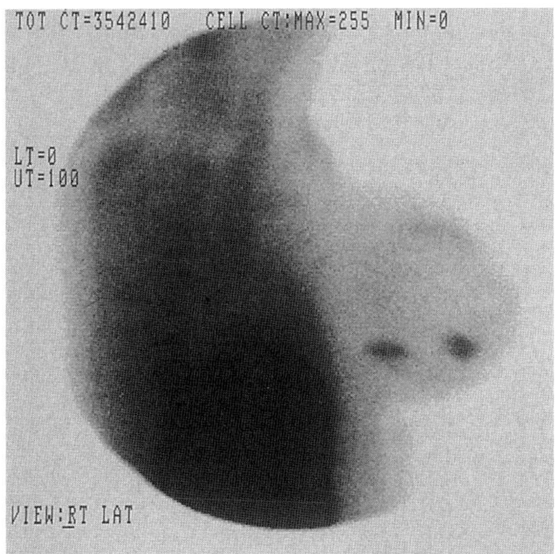

Fig. 2. ^{99m}Tc-sestamibi scintimammography showing multifocal breast cancer (courtesy of Dr John Buscombe, Royal Free Hospital, London).

cally active cancer cells than in surrounding normal tissue, ^{99m}Tc-sestamibi accumulates in cancer cells. However in one study there was a poor correlation with vessel counts and intracellular mitochondrial density but moderate correlation with desmoplastic activity and cellular proliferation [29] suggesting that mitochondrial density may not be important. The exact mechanisms by which ^{99m}Tc-sestamibi enters and exits neoplastic tissue is not yet fully understood.

> *The mechanism by which ^{99m}Tc-sestamibi enters and exits neoplastic cells is not fully understood.*

There has been a great deal of interest in the detection of the multidrug-resistant (MDR 1) phenotype in breast cancer. MDR 1 gene produces P-glycoprotein, a transmembrane protein which is believed to be responsible for the active removal of chemotherapy drugs from cancer cells. Technetium-99m sestamibi is a transport substrate of P-glycoprotein (Pgp) which appears to actively transport ^{99m}Tc-sestamibi out of tumour cells. High levels of Pgp result in rapid efflux of technetium-99m sestamibi and can be used in the in vivo identification of the MDR 1 phenotype [30–33]. This has been used to predict response to neo-adjuvant chemotherapy for locally advanced breast cancer. In a series of 39 patients with stage III disease 17 patients showed rapid efflux of ^{99m}Tc-sestamibi and 88% had a lack of tumour response to chemotherapy on subsequent histology. In contrast, only 36% with prolonged retention of sestamibi showed residual tumour. The rapid clearance of sestamibi may predict lack of response to chemotherapy [34].

> *Scintimammography may have an important role in assessing the resistance to chemotherapy.*

This assessment of efflux is potentially very useful in those patients being considered for chemotherapy either as primary treatment or in those patients who have relapsed.

Standard scintimammography has been used to monitor response to chemotherapy and when compared to X-ray mammography has similar accuracy [35]. It has also been used successfully to assess patients with suspected recurrent disease and found to be 85% accurate [36]. The assessment of recurrence can be very difficult using mammography, ultrasound and fine needle aspiration cytology and scintimammography can be used as an alternative to dynamic MRI in indeterminate lesions.

^{99m}Tc-Tetrofosmin (TF) (Fig. 3) is a lipophilic diphosphine compound routinely used for cardiac imaging. Extracardiac utilisation has occurred in patients with a variety of malignant neoplasms including breast cancer. The uptake mechanisms are similar to ^{99m}Tc-sestamibi and are also poorly understood. Tetrofosmin is also a substrate for P-glycoprotein, the multidrug resistance transporter and therefore similar uses for ^{99m}Tc-tetrofosmin and ^{99m}Tc-sestamibi are envisaged [37]. However, there are few controlled trials of the two agents so it is difficult to assess at present which might be more useful.

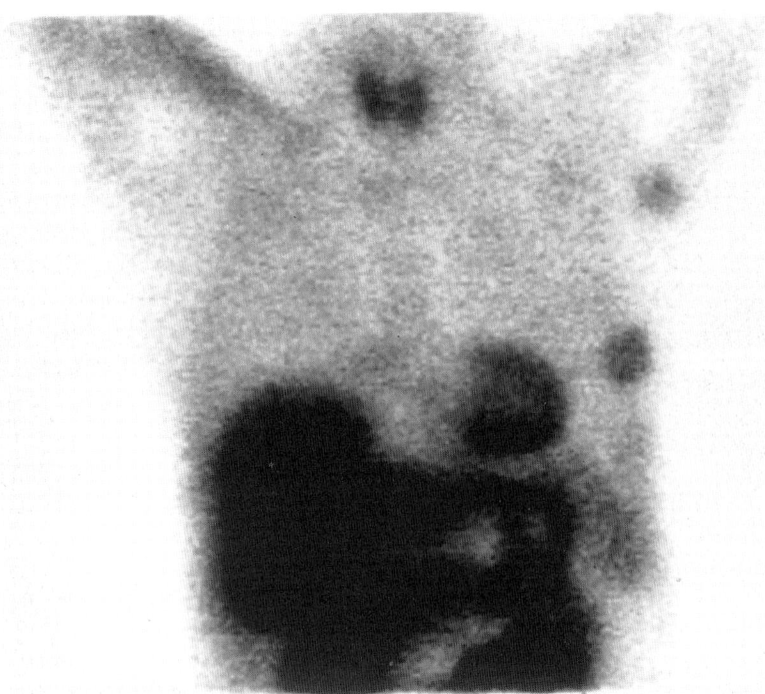

Fig. 3. ^{99m}Tc-Tetrofosmin scintimammography demonstrating breast cancer with positive axillary lymph nodes.

Several monoclonal antibodies are being investigated for identifying both primary breast cancer and axillary node metastases. Technetium-99m labelled SM3, an Imperial Cancer Research Fund murine monoclonal antibody and an anti-carcinoembryonic antigen antibody Fab fragment labelled directly onto technetium-99m have both been used with some success [38,39].

Various radiopharmaceuticals are used in scintimammography but ^{99m}Tc-sestamibi is the most widely used.

3. Electropotential measurements

Rapidly proliferating benign and neoplastic cells have electrically depolarised cell membranes compared to normal cells [40,41]. This effect is thought to extend from the cancerous area to the adjacent regions and is measurable at the skin surface above the lesion. A new modality based on the analysis of breast electropotentials by an array of specially designed sensors has been tested in an 8 centre trial in Europe. The results show a highly significant trend of progressive electrical changes depending on the proliferative characteristics of the biopsied tissue. This was not related to age or menopausal status. The depolarisation index gave a sensitivity of 90% and a specificity of 55% in women with palpable lesions. The test did not distinguish atypical or in situ disease from invasive cancer [42]. Further assessment is required of this new method of detection of breast cancer, particularly in relation to impalpable lesions.

4. Electrical impedance imaging

Electrical impedance imaging (Fig. 4) maps the local distribution of tissue impedance on the breast by applying a tiny electrical signal over a range of measured frequencies. The technology was developed in the 1980s and several studies have produced promising results [43]. In a series

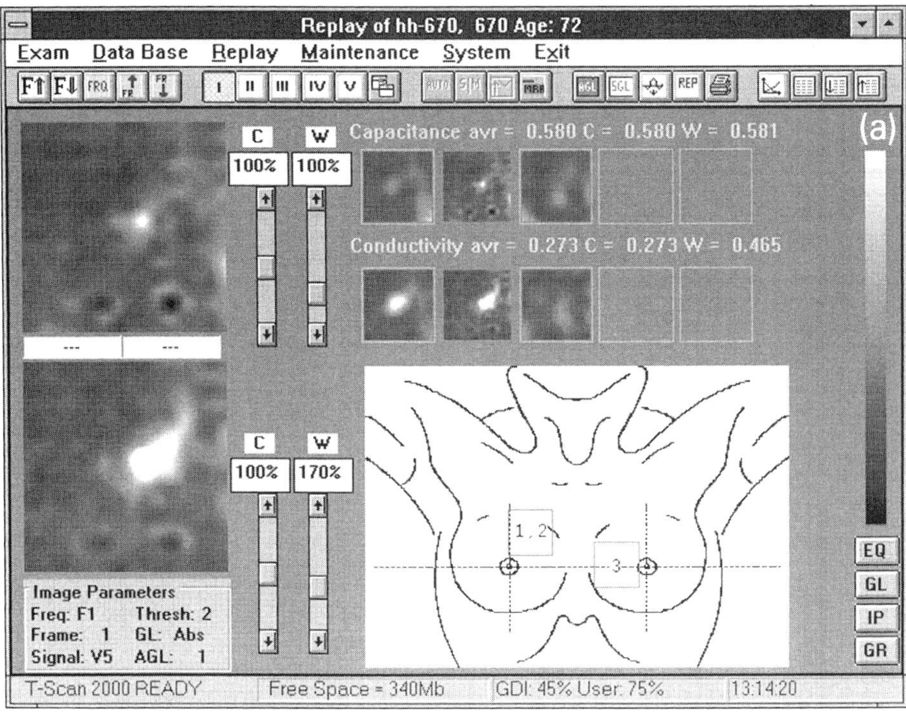

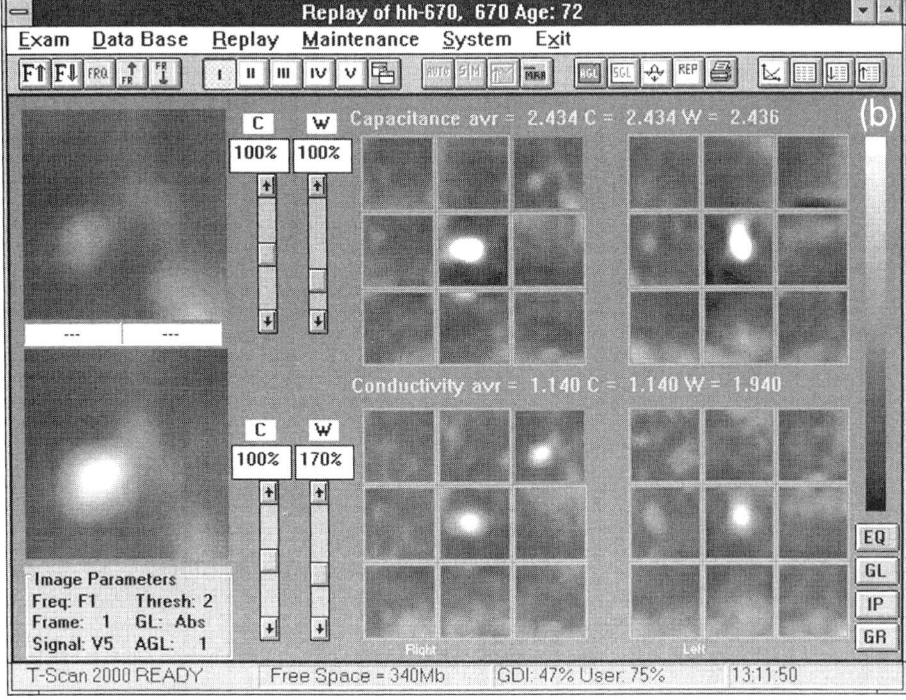

Fig. 4. T-scan electrical impedance whole breast (a) and targeted (b) examination showing an area of increased conductance and capacitance in the upper inner quadrant of the right breast due to carcinoma. Central area of brightness is due to the nipple. (Courtesy of Dr. Scott Fields, Hadassa University Hospital, Israel.)

of 470 patients from Israel the technique had a sensitivity of 74–85% and a specificity of 64–71% for the various groups of women examined. A greater sensitivity was seen in younger women with impalpable lesions and with invasive histology [44]. Like the previous technique, this novel approach warrants further investigation.

References

1. Wahl RL. Overview of the current status of PET in breast cancer imaging. Quart J Nucl Med 1998; 42: 1–7.
2. Cho ZH, Chan JK, Ericksson L et al. Positron ranges obtained from biomedically important positron-emitting radionuclides. J Nucl Med 1975; 16: 1174–1176.
3. Smith IC, Welch AE, Chilcott F, Heys SD, Sharp P, Eremin O. Gamma emission imaging in the management of breast disorders. Eur J Surg Oncol 1998; 24: 320–329.
4. Weber G. Enzymology of cancer cells (second of two parts). N Engl J Med 1977; 296: 541–551.
5. Tse N, Hoh C, Hawkins R et al. The application of positron emission tomographic imaging with fluorodeoxyglucose to the evaluation of breast disease. Ann Surg 1992; 216: 27–34.
6. Monakhov NK, Nelstadt EL, Shavioskli MM, Shvartsman AL, Neifakh SA. Physiochemical properties and isoenzyme composition of hexokinase from normal and malignant human tissues. J Natl Cancer Inst 1978; 61: 27–34.
7. Hawkins RA, Choi Y, Huang SC, Messa C, Hoh CK, Phelps ME. Quantitating tumour glucose metabolism with FDG and PET (editorial). J Nucl Med 1992; 33: 339–344.
8. Brock CS, Meikle SR, Price P. Does fluorine-18 fluorodeoxyglucose metabolic imaging of tumours benefit oncology? Eur J Nucl Med 1997; 24: 691–705.
9. Chung J, Lee YJ, Kim C, Choi SR, Kim M, Lee K et al. Mechanisms related to (^{18}F)fluorodeoxyglucose uptake of human colon cancers transplanted in nude mice. J Nucl Med 1999; 40: 339–346.
10. Tse N, Hoh C, Hawkins R et al. The application of positron emission tomographic imaging with fluorodeoxyglucose to the evaluation of breast disease. Ann Surg 1992; 216: 27–34.
11. Bolster JM, Vaalburg W, Paans AMJ et al. Carbon-11 labelled tyrosine to study tumour metabolism by positron emission tomography (PET). Eur J Nucl Med 1986; 12: 321–324.
12. Kubota K, Matsuzawa T, Amemiya A et al. Imaging of breast cancer with [F18]Fluorodeoxyglucose and positron emission tomography. J Comp Assist Tomogr 1989; 13: 1097–1098.
13. Wahl RL, Cody RL, Hutchins GD, Mudgett E. Primary and metastatic breast carcinoma: initial clinical evaluation with PET with radiolabeled glucose analogue 2-(18F)-fluoro-2-deoxy-D-glucose. Radiology 1991; 179: 765–770.
14. Nieweg OE, Kim EE, Wong WH et al. Positron emission tomography with fluorine-18-deoxyglucose in the detection and staging of breast cancer. Cancer 1993; 71: 3920–3925.
15. Hoh CK, Hawkins RA, Glaspy JA et al. Cancer detection with whole-body PET using 2-[18F]fluoro-2-deoxy-D-glucose. J Comp Assist Tomogr 1993; 17: 582–589.
16. Adler LP, Crowe JP, al-Kaisi NK, Sunshine JL. Evaluation of breast masses and axillary lymph nodes with [F-18] 2-deoxy-2-fluoro-D-glucose PET. Radiology 1993; 187: 743–750.
17. Bruce DM, Evans NT, Heys SD et al. Positron emission tomography: 2-deoxy-2-[18F]-fluoro-D-glucose uptake in locally advanced breast cancers. Eur J Surg Oncol 1995; 21: 280–283.
18. Dehdashti F, Mortimer JE, Siegel BA et al. Positron tomographic assessment of estrogen receptors in breast cancer: comparison with FDG-PET and in vitro receptor assays. J Nucl Med 1995; 36: 1766–1774.
19. Bassa P, Kim E, Inoue T et al. Evaluation of preoperative chemotherapy using PET with fluorine-18-fluorodeoxyglucose in breast cancer. J Nucl Med 1996; 37: 931–938.
20. Avril N, Dose J, Janicke F et al. Metabolic characterization of breast tumours with positron emission tomography using F-18 fluorodeoxyglucose. J Clin Oncol 1996; 14: 1848–1857.
21. Scheidhauer K, Scharl A, Pietrzyk U et al. Qualitative [18F]FDG positron emission tomography in primary breast cancer: clinical relevance and practicability. Eur J Nucl Med 1996; 23: 618–623.
22. Noh D, Yun I, Kim J et al. Diagnostic value of positron emission tomography for detecting breast cancer. World J Surg 1998; 22: 223–228.
23. Wahl RL, Zasadny K, Helvie M, Hutchins GD, Weber B, Cody R. Metabolic monitoring of breast cancer chemohormonotherapy using positron emission tomography: initial evaluation. J Clin Oncol 1993; 11: 2101–2111.
24. Jansson T, Westlin JE, Ahlstrom H, Lilja A, Langstrom B, Bergh J. Positron emission tomography studies in patients with locally advanced and/or metastatic breast cancer: a method for early therapy evaluation? J Clin Oncol 1995; 13: 1470–1477.
25. Jonson SD, Welch MJ. PET imaging of breast cancer with fluorine-18 radiolabeled estrogens and progestins. Quart J Nucl Med 1998; 42: 8–17.

26. Kole AC, Nieweg OE, Pruim J, Paans AM, Plukker JT, Hoekstra HJ, Schraffordt Koops H, Vaalburg W. Standardized uptake value and quantification of metabolism for breast cancer imaging with FDG and L-[1-11C]tyrosine PET. J Nucl Med 1997; 38: 692–696.
27. Prats E, Carril J, Herranz R, Merono E, Banzo J, Gtemegmmt YE. A Spanish multicenter scintigraphic study of the breast using Tc 99m MIBI. Report of results. Rev Espan Med Nucl 1998; 17: 338–350.
28. Buscombe J et al. Scintigraphic imaging of breast cancer: a review. Nucl Med Commun 1997; 18: 698–709.
29. Cutrone JA, Yospur LS, Khalkhali I, Tolmos J, Devito A, Diggles L, Vargas MP, Shitabata P, French S. Immunohistologic assessment of technetium-99m-MIBI uptake in benign and malignant breast lesions. J Nucl Med 1998; 39: 449–453.
30. Cordobes MD, Starzec A, Delmon-Moingeon L, Blanchot C, Kouyoumdjian JC, Prevost G, Caglar M, Moretti JL. Technetium-99m-sestamibi uptake by human benign and malignant breast tumor cells: correlation with mdr gene expression. J Nucl Med 1996; 37: 286–289.
31. Del Vecchio S, Ciarmiello A, Pace L, Potena MI, Carriero MV, Mainolfi C, Thomas R, D'Aiuto G, Tsuruo T, Salvatore M. Fractional retention of technetium-99m-sestamibi as an index of P-glycoprotein expression in untreated breast cancer patients. J Nucl Med 1997; 38: 1348–1351.
32. Vecchio SD, Ciarmiello A, Potena MI, Carriero MV, Mainolfi C, Botti G, Thomas R, Cerra M, D'Aiuto G, Tsuruo T, Salvatore M. In vivo detection of multidrug-resistant (MDR1) phenotype by technetium-99m sestamibi scan in untreated breast cancer patients [see comments]. Eur J Nucl Med 1997; 24: 150–159.
33. Kostakoglu L, Ruacan S, Ergun EL, Sayek I, Elahi N, Bekdik CF. Influence of the heterogeneity of P-glycoprotein expression on technetium-99m-MIBI uptake in breast cancer. J Nucl Med 1998; 39: 1021–1026.
34. Ciarmiello A, Del Vecchio S, Silvestro P, Potena MI, Carriero MV, Thomas R, Botti G, D'Aiuto G, Salvatore M. Tumor clearance of technetium 99m-sestamibi as a predictor of response to neoadjuvant chemotherapy for locally advanced breast cancer. J Clin Oncol 1998; 16: 1677–1683.
35. Maini CL, Tofani A, Sciuto R, Semprebene A, Cavaliere R, Mottolese M, Benevolo M, Ferranti F, Grandinetti ML, Vici P, Lopez M, Botti C. Technetium-99m-MIBI scintigraphy in the assessment of neoadjuvant chemotherapy in breast carcinoma. J Nucl Med 1997; 38: 1546–1551.
36. Cwikla JB, Buscombe JR, Parbhoo SP, Kelleher SM, Thakrar DS, Hinton J, Crow J, Deery A, Hilson AJ. Use of 99Tcm-MIBI in the assessment of patients with suspected recurrent breast cancer. Nucl Med Commun 1998; 19: 649–655.
37. Mainsi L, Rambaldi PF, Cuccrurullo V, Pecori B, Quarantelli M, Fallanca F, Del Vecchio E. Diagnostic and prognostic role of 99m-Tc-tetrafosmin in breast cancer. Quart J Nucl Med 1997; 41: 239–250.
38. Biassoni L, Granowska M, Carroll MJ, Mather SJ, Howell R, Ellison D, MacNeill FA, Wells CA, Carpenter R, Britton KE. 99mTc-labelled SM3 in the preoperative evaluation of axillary lymph nodes and primary breast cancer with change detection statistical processing as an aid to tumour detection. Br J Cancer 1998; 77: 131–138.
39. Goldenberg DM, Wegener W. Studies of breast cancer imaging with radiolabeled antibodies to carcinoembryonic antigen. Immunomedics Breast Cancer Study Group. Acta Med Austr 1997; 24: 55–59.
40. Binggeli R, Weinstein RC. Membrane potentials and sodium channels: hypotheses for growth regulation and cancer formation based on changes in sodium channels and gap junctions. J Theor Biol 1986; 123: 377–401.
41. Marino AA, Iliev IG, Schwalke MA, Gonzalez E, Marler KC, Flanagan CA. Association between cell membrane potential and breast cancer. Tumour Biol 1994; 15: 82–89.
42. Cuzick J, Holland R, Barth V, Davies R, Faupel M, Fentiman I, Frischbier HJ, LaMarque JL, Merson M, Sacchini V, Vanel D, Veronesi U. Electropotential measurements as a new diagnostic modality for breast cancer. Lancet 1998; 352: 359–363.
43. Piperno G et al. Breast cancer screening by impedance measurements. Frontiers Med Biol Engng 1990; 2(2): 111–117.
44. Moskovitz O (Laver). Electrical impedance imaging of the breast. Eur Radiol 1997; 7: S82.

Breast Cancer: Diagnosis and Management
J.M. Dixon (Ed.)

CHAPTER 3

Diagnostic techniques: FNAC and core biopsy of palpable lesions

Stefano Ciatto

1. Introduction

Fine needle aspiration cytology (FNAC) and core biopsy (CB) are currently used in the differential diagnosis of breast cancer. Nevertheless their exact role and place in the diagnostic process is often misunderstood. Both techniques are often over- or underused and/or their reliability is overestimated. In this chapter the utility of both techniques is summarised and a flow chart for their use in the current practice is provided.

2. Fine needle aspiration cytology

FNAC is performed with a variety of thin needles (19 to 23 G) with no substantial differences in results. Needles with a transparent barrel are recommended to identify blood contamination early so needling can be stopped. A free hand technique using a needle connected to an aspiration source (syringe, automatic aspirator) is preferred to using a syringe holder as it allows a better feel of tissue consistency and permits accurate sampling. Ten to 20 passes of the needle are usually sufficient to obtain an adequate sample, moving the needle in different directions. More details on the technique can be found elsewhere [1].

2.1. FNAC: who should do the sampling?

Discussion concerning who should do the sampling; whether it should be a clinician or a pathologist has concluded that whoever does the FNAC sampling the operator must be fully trained and carrying out the technique regularly. Anybody carrying out breast examination regularly can be trained and should be able to perform FNAC sampling. Training is simple (a few days) but there is a long learning curve and regular audit of results must show satisfactory levels of sensitivity and specificity.

FNAC requires a trained operator and continued experience.

2.2. FNAC: reporting categories

A variety of reporting categories have been used for FNAC, and this has caused problems when comparing different centres and made meta-analyses of diagnostic accuracy almost impossible. The most commonly used reporting system is that proposed by the EC [2] with 5 categories (C1 = inadequate, C2 = negative, C3–5 = abnormalities of increasing predictivity). This classification is used in the present report. Another problem which may arise in comparing different series is

Table 1. Positive predictive value (PPV) of FNAC [3]

Cytologic report	Benign	Cancer	PPV
Atypia (C3)	146	142	0.493
Suspicious (C4)	19	372	0.951
Positive (C5)	2	500	0.996
Total	167	1014	0.858

that the predictive value of 'abnormal' categories is not always known. The positive predictive value (PPV) for each category of abnormality must be known in each centre to allow proper clinical use of these categories. For example (see Table 1) reports with a PPV > 99% might well prompt immediate treatment, without waiting for histologic confirmation, whereas reports with a PPV of 50–60% should prompt biopsy with treatment requiring histologic confirmation.

FNAC should be reported according to fixed categories of known predictive value.

2.3. FNAC: inadequate or acellular samples

Inadequate samples (acellular FNAs) are expected at FNAC and their occurrence depends on a number of variables. Cancers are more cellular and acellular rates for cancers should be approximately half those of benign lesions. As the proportion of cancers in FNAC series varies, comparisons of inadequacy rates must be performed for benign or malignant lesions separately [4]. Acellular rates drop with multiple sampling, and repeat sampling is used routinely in some centres or is performed based on naked eye or microscopic evaluation of fresh unstained smears. Applying negative pressure reduces the acellular rate, especially for benign lesions. A controlled study comparing aspiration with no aspiration [5] showed no difference in cancer cases but reduced the number of inadequate samples to half in benign lesions (13.6 vs. 24.4%) when aspiration was used. Inadequacy rates are also strongly correlated with operator experience. When several operators are performing FNAs, checking their inadequacy rate should be part of a regular audit: performance below standards (commonly an acellular rate of 10% or more for cancer cases and 20% or more for benign cases) should prompt retraining. Inadequate samples or acellular FNAs should not influence diagnostic judgement and it should not be assumed to be a negative report. If a lesion is clinically or mammographically suspicious and the FNA is acellular, it should be repeated or a biopsy performed.

- *Acellular rates of aspirators should be audited at regular intervals.*
- *Acellular FNAs should not be assumed to show no evidence of cancer. Where other assessments suggest a lesion is suspicious of cancer then FNA should be reported or a biopsy performed.*

2.4. FNAC: sensitivity

When inadequate samples are excluded sensitivity in reported series ranges from 87 to 98% [6]. False negatives may be due to missing the lesion (normal tissue adjacent to cancer is sampled): this may occur when free hand sampling is used for a small cancer particularly those that appear larger at palpation than they are on imaging. In such cases image guided aspiration is recommended to ensure exact positioning of the needle. False negatives can result from a reading error by the cytopathologist or can occur in a well differentiated cancer which shows limited cellular atypia. When an adequate sample is obtained, quality control of reports of these samples (i.e. smears should be reported again by a second cytologist) should be undertaken at regular intervals.

2.5. FNAC: specificity

FNAC is one of the most specific tests presently available for breast cancer diagnosis. False posi-

Table 2. Flow chart of the diagnostic process for palpable masses

Step 1: Palpation	
– plain benign (e.g. lipoma) >	STOP
– dubious >	go to step 2
– plain malignant	go to biopsy (through step 2)
Step 2: Imaging (mammography or ultrasonography depending on age)	
– plain benign (e.g. cyst, lipoma) >	STOP
– dubious >	go to step 3
– plain malignant	go to biopsy (through step 3)
Step 3: Cytology (free-hand or US-guided)	
– inadequate	repeat or ignore and base decision on step 1 and 2
– negative	follow-up of dubious cases at both step 1 and 2
– abnormal	go to biopsy whatever result at step 1 and 2

tives should be less than 5% [4] and false positives are generally associated with reporting categories of low predictive value e.g. C3. Reports of borderline abnormalities in cytological smears are often confirmed at review, but are rarely associated with 'atypical' lesions, such as atypical ductal or lobular hyperplasia. An excess of false positive reports should prompt a quality review in the laboratory, with a panel review and discussion of smears and verification of the PPV of each reporting category. As false positives are rare and the PPV of any abnormality (C3–5) is usually over 0.6 [3], cytologic abnormality of any grade should prompt a biopsy for histologic confirmation.

> *FNAC is highly specific: any FNAC abnormality should prompt a biopsy. A malignant report (C5) may prompt immediate treatment.*

2.6. Role of FNAC in current practice

The role of and the indication for FNAC depends on the aim with which FNAC is used. If FNAC is performed to confirm malignancy and to allow immediate treatment (by-passing a two-step approach or a frozen biopsy) then it can be limited to the few cases (3–5% in an average clinical setting) with a strong suspicion of cancer at palpation/imaging.

In contrast, if FNAC is used in an effort to increase sensitivity by reducing false benign reports at palpation/imaging, then it should be used in all cases considered benign/borderline on palpation/imaging. Such a policy will result in an increase in costs and unnecessary FNACs will be performed. The proportion of subjects undergoing FNAC will increase and there may be an increase in the total cancer detection rate of approximately 5% [4]. The use of FNAC as part of the diagnostic flow chart is outlined in Table 2. FNAC is indicated in all cases with questionable (not certainly benign) findings and in cases with a strong suspicion of malignancy on palpation/imaging. In the former group FNAC will select cases for biopsy (C3–C4) and will select cases for immediate treatment (C5). As false negative FNACs are expected in up to 10% of cancer cases [4], a negative (C2) FNAC report should not stop a biopsy which is indicated because of a strong suspicion of malignancy on palpation/imaging.

> *FNAC of lesions of uncertain interpretation may reduce unnecessary biopsies or false benign reports at palpation/imaging.*

2.7. Quality control of FNAC performance

FNAC performance should be monitored according to a series of parameters suggested by the EC [2] (Table 3). When FNAC performance does

Table 3. EC parameters for FNAC quality assurance [2]

Absolute sensitivity (C5)	> 60%
Complete sensitivity (C3 + C4 + C5)	> 80%
Specificity (including non-biopsied)	> 60%
Positive predictive value (C5)	> 98%
False negative rate	< 5%
False positive rate	< 1%
Inadequate rate (overall)	< 25%
Inadequate rate (samples from cancers)	< 10%
Suspicious rate (C3 + C4)	< 20%

not reach the standards, action must be taken to improve quality. For example, an excess of inadequate samples may be due either to sampling technique or to smear reading. Checking parameters at each stage (sample taker or reader) may help to find the cause, and individuals scoring below specific standards should be retrained.

3. Core biopsy (CB)

CB biopsy removes a core of breast tissue using a percutaneous approach in an outpatient setting, following infiltration with local anaesthesia. Different techniques have been developed, but those obtaining a larger amount of tissue, such as the suction mammotome technique or more recently the ABBI system, are generally restricted to non-palpable lesions. For palpable lesions the classic method adopts a 14–20 G needle fitted in an automated biopsy gun. The needle is directed using a free-hand approach or under image guidance; the latter method is advisable for smaller/deeply located lesions which appear larger at palpation compared to their actual size on imaging. One or more cores may be taken but for most lesions, if the needle is properly positioned, one core may be sufficient. As for FNAC, CB requires training.

3.1. CB: inadequate sampling

CB has a low rate of inadequate samples [7], and this is one of its major advantages over FNAC.

3.2. CB: sensitivity

In palpable lesions, precise needling and full utilisation of 'long throw' (2.2 cm excursion) needles, means sensitivity is extremely high, over 95% [7]. False negatives are rare but may be more frequent when a single core is taken and may arise in 'difficult' cancer cases such as lobular carcinoma with single cancer cells diffusely infiltrating normal tissue.

3.3. CB: specificity

As usual for histopathology, specificity is very high. False positives are extremely rare, providing that pathologists are aware of the limits of the technique. For example, in the presence of a radial scar, normal tubules distorted by the scar process may mimic tubular carcinoma but as the core offers only a partial view of the lesion pathologists should be careful in reporting these lesions on core biopsies. The same is true for in situ and invasive lesions: a report of an in situ lesion on core biopsy requires confirmation by surgical excision, as scattered foci of infiltration are missed in approximately half of cases by CB.

3.4. Role of CB

CB is being used successfully all over the world and is being increasingly used in current practice. Unfortunately, CB has been often used as an alternative to bad quality FNAC, but this is not its role. FNAC is a diagnostic test, which is simple and cheap, it can be reported immediately and should be available at all breast clinics. It is an important part of the current diagnostic process and combined with palpation and imaging (the so called 'triple diagnosis') represents the standard diagnostic approach to breast abnormalities. In current practice 5 to 10% of women referred for symptoms undergo FNAC. In contrast, CB is a relatively complex diagnostic test, which is more costly (it costs 5 to 10 time more than FNAC), requires local anaesthesia and is not available at all breast clinics (it requires a trained operator, and many lesions are best sampled under US guidance).

- *Core biopsy should never be used as an alternative to poor quality FNAC.*
- *Core biopsy is more accurate but more complex and more costly when compared to FNAC.*

CB is performed whenever a histologic diagnosis is needed and to reduce the need for open biopsy. For example: a) CB has no diagnostic role in the presence of a strong suspicion of malignancy at palpation and imaging as with a positive (C5) report FNAC has a PPV of over 99%; b) CB may be necessary when the diagnosis after a triple approach is still uncertain, e.g. a lesion consistent with fibroadenoma at palpation/imaging and an indeterminate (C3) report at FNAC (PPV less than 50%); c) the use of preoperative (neoadjuvant) chemotherapy requires a CB to obtain tissue for tumour characterisation and a histologic diagnosis; d) CB is preferred as an alternative to frozen section biopsy (routinely used in most southern european countries) as it is simpler, cheaper, possibly more accurate and allows a full discussion of diagnosis and treatment options prior to surgery.

- *Core biopsy is used following triple diagnosis to avoid unnecessary open biopsy.*
- *Core biopsy is a cheaper, simpler and better alternative to frozen section biopsy.*
- *Core biopsy has an important role in histologic assessment of patients prior to treatment by primary medical therapy.*

3.5. Quality control of CB performance

In cases undergoing surgery, quality control is based on correlations between the CB and the final histologic diagnosis on the surgical specimen. For cases assumed to be benign on CB, follow-up is advisable to confirm that the lesion is stable over time. CB accuracy must be high to be useful with a specificity > 99% and a sensitivity > 95% suggested as suitable levels for quality control standards.

References

1. Catania S, Ciatto S. Breast cytology: instruments and technique. In: Catania S, Ciatto S, eds. Breast Cytology in Clinical Practice. London: Martin Dunitz 1992; pp. 11–60.
2. European Guidelines for Quality Assurance in Mammographic screening. de Wolf CJM, Perry NM, eds. Brussels/Luxembourg: European Commission – Europe Against Cancer Programme 1996.
3. Ciatto S, Cecchini S, Grazzini G et al. Positive predictive value of fine needle aspiration cytology of breast lesions. Acta Cytol 1989; 33: 894–898.
4. Ciatto S, Cariaggi P, Bulgaresi P et al. Fine needle aspiration cytology of the breast: review of 9533 consecutive cases. Breast 1993; 2: 87–90.
5. Ciatto S, Catania S, Bravetti P et al. Fine needle cytology of the breast: a controlled study of aspiration versus non-aspiration. Diagn Cytopathol 1991; 7: 125–127.
6. Ciatto S, Catania S. Fine needle aspiration cytology of solid masses. In: Catania S, Ciatto S, eds. Breast Cytology in Clinical Practice. London: Martin Dunitz 1992; pp. 75-79.
7. Parker SH, Burbank F, Jackman RJ et al. Percutaneous large-core breast biopsy: a multi institutional study. Radiology 1994; 193: 359–364.

Breast Cancer: Diagnosis and Management
J.M. Dixon (Ed.)

CHAPTER 4

FNAC and core biopsy of impalpable lesions

Michael J. Michell

1. Introduction

Non operative diagnosis of impalpable mammographically detected lesions using image guided needle biopsy allows pre-operative planning of definitive treatment and effective pre-operative counselling for women with malignant lesions. Many women with benign lesions may be spared diagnostic surgical excision. The minimum standard for the UK National Breast Screening Programme is for more than 70% women with impalpable or palpable cancers to have a positive pre-operative diagnosis either by fine needle aspiration cytology (FNAC) or by needle core biopsy (CB) [1].

2. Multidisciplinary assessment

All cases should undergo a thorough work up including both imaging and clinical examination prior to image guided needle biopsy. The imaging characteristics of a suspicious lesion should be demonstrated using further mammography, including spot compression views for small spiculate lesions or areas of parenchymal distortion and fine focus magnification views to allow detailed analysis of areas of microcalcification.

Ultrasound should also be used to assess the characteristics of soft tissue masses. From the imaging characteristics, both the differential diagnosis and the probability of malignancy can be determined. This information is essential when considering the results of image guided needle biopsy and deciding on management — the multidisciplinary team must be confident that the needle biopsy findings are consistent with the differential diagnosis suggested by the imaging features.

All suspicious breast lesions should undergo full imaging work up to characterise the lesion and determine the probability of malignancy before needle biopsy.

3. Image guidance

Needle biopsy of impalpable breast lesions is carried out using either ultrasound or X-ray stereotactic guidance. Most soft tissue masses in the breast are visible using modern high frequency apparatus with a frequency range up to 10–13 MHz. Ultrasound is therefore the image guidance method of choice for such lesions and allows real-time demonstration of the needle traversing the lesion [2]. X-ray stereotaxis is used for microcalcifications, areas of parenchymal distortion or small soft tissue masses which cannot be adequately visualised by ultrasound. Stereotactic localisation can be carried out with the patient in either the upright [3–6] or prone positions (Fig. 1). Upright 'add on' stereotactic units are

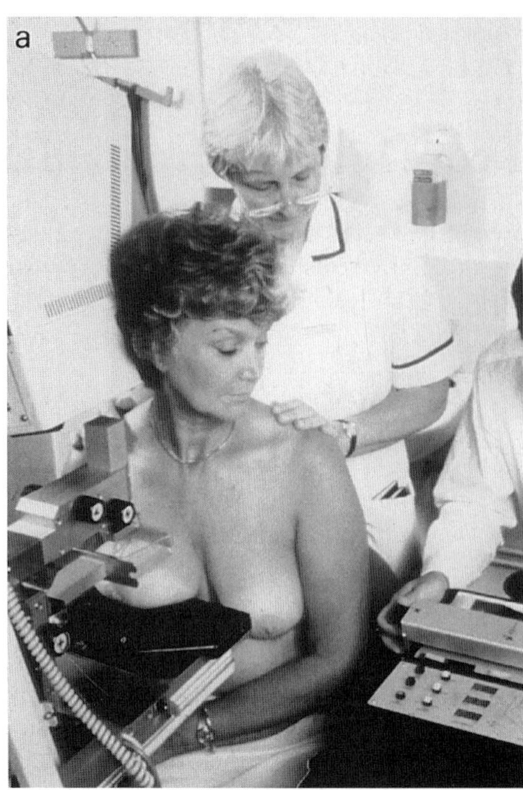

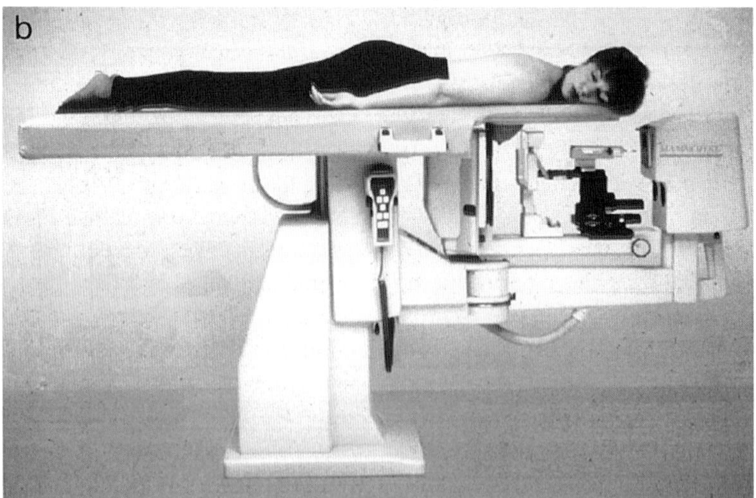

Fig. 1. (a) Upright stereotactic apparatus. (b) Prone stereotactic table.

more widely available and less expensive than dedicated prone stereotactic units. The main advantages of dedicated prone stereotactic apparatus are that the breast is in a more stable position with less likelihood of movement [7] and the patient is unable to see the procedure.

A vaso-vagal episode is extremely unusual in the prone position. Digital imaging is used with prone biopsy systems and is now becoming available for use with upright systems. The advantages of digital imaging for breast biopsy work are rapid (< 5 seconds) acquisition of stereotactic images for targeting, and manipulation of the digital images including magnification, image reversal and contrast adjustment for improved visualisation of target abnormalities.

- *Ultrasound is the image guidance method of choice for soft tissue masses.*
- *Stereotaxis is used for microcalcification, architectural distortion and small masses which cannot be adequately visualised using ultrasound.*

4. Sampling

The breast may be sampled either to produce material for cytological analysis — Fine Needle Aspiration Cytology (FNAC), or histological analysis, Core Biopsy (CB). FNAC is performed using a 21–23G needle. For CB, an automated core biopsy gun is used most commonly with a 14G needle — 14G needles have been shown to produce better samples than 18G or 16G needles but a 16G needle may be required for penetration through breast tissue where resistance is encountered due to benign breast change and fibrosis. More recently, several devices have become available which allow image guided sampling of larger volumes of breast tissue [8] — they include vacuum assisted core biopsy [9–11] (mammotome), the ABBI (Advanced Breast Biopsy Instrumentation) [12,13] and Site Select PBB (Percutaneous Breast Biopsy) [14] systems.

5. Ultrasound guided needle biopsy

The patient is positioned to provide optimal access to the area to be biopsied. This may involve for example raising and supporting the left side for biopsy of lesions situated in the lateral aspect of the left breast. In many patients, particularly for lesions in the lateral or upper parts of the breast, visualisation of the lesion and subsequent needle biopsy is easier if the ipsilateral arm is raised and rested above the head. If space allows, an assistant works from the opposite side of the couch to the radiologist.

5.1. Ultrasound guided FNAC [15]

The lesion is demonstrated and the surrounding breast tissue is immobilised by applying pressure with the palm of the hand holding the probe. Using the other hand, the skin adjacent to the probe where the needle puncture is to be made is cleaned. For FNAC, infiltration of the skin with local anaesthetic may be used. The FNAC needle, attached by a short connecting tube to a 10 cc syringe held by the assistant, is introduced into the breast and its relationship to the position of the target lesion is demonstrated on the ultrasound image. The needle is introduced along the long axis of the ultrasound probe and will be easily visualised along its length if it is kept as parallel to the surface of the ultrasound probe as possible (Fig. 2). The needle should also be kept parallel to the chest wall to minimise any risk of damage to chest wall structures. The needle tip is guided into the lesion and an image is taken to record that the needle is correctly positioned. The needle is then moved back and forth within the lesion with simultaneous rotation and with negative pressure being applied by the assistant. Aspiration is continued until material is seen within the hub of the needle; the aspirate is then delivered onto slides and dry and wet preparations made in accordance with instructions from the cytopathologist. If local circumstances allow, it is helpful to have the cellularity of the specimens checked by a cytology technician or pathologist immediately following the procedure. Two or three separate aspirates are obtained in order to increase the chance of obtaining a diagnostic cellular sample.

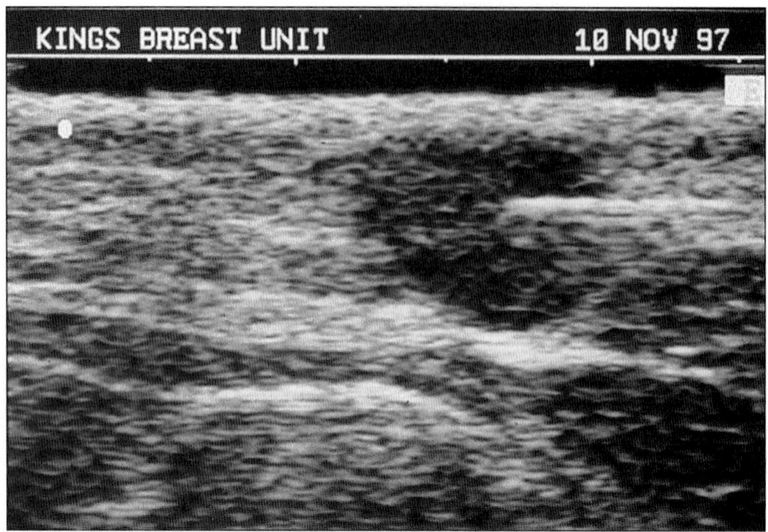

Fig. 2. Ultrasound guided FNAC — the needle is parallel to both the chest wall and the ultrasound probe.

5.2. Ultrasound guided CB [16]

The lesion is demonstrated and the surrounding breast tissue immobilised in the same way as for FNAC. After cleaning the skin, local anaesthetic (4.5 ml 1% lignocaine with 0.5 ml 10% sodium bicarbonate) is infiltrated both superficially and deeply in the breast down to the lesion. A 2–3 mm skin incision is made to allow insertion of the core biopsy needle along the direction of the long axis of the ultrasound probe; the point of needle entry should be 1–1.5 cm away from the edge of the ultrasound probe to allow the needle to be positioned at the required depth in relation to the lesion while ensuring that the biopsy needle remains parallel to both the ultrasound probe and the chest wall. The biopsy needle is advanced until the tip is a few mm proximal to the edge of the lesion (Fig. 3). Correct positioning can be checked by moving the ultrasound probe slightly above and below the level of the needle to check that the needle is not likely to pass over the edge of the lesion. The core biopsy gun is then fired and the needle is visualised passing through the lesion. A check image with the needle through the lesion is recorded. The needle is withdrawn and the specimen is delivered into formal saline.

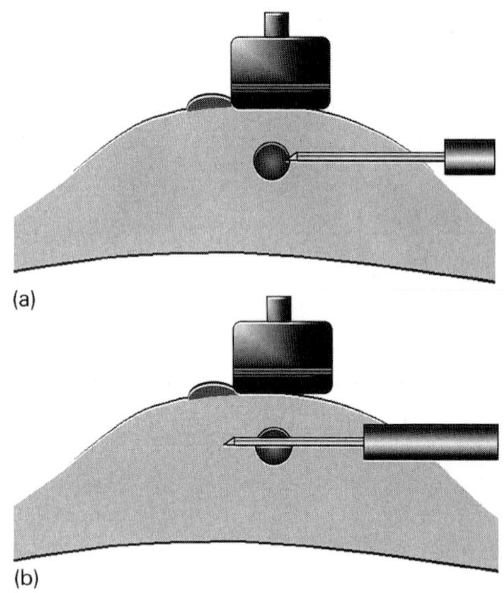

Fig. 3. Ultrasound guided core biopsy. (a, b) The needle tip is positioned just proximal to the lesion. (c, d) The needle has traversed the lesion.

One to two passes are sufficient in most cases to obtain diagnostic material from soft tissue masses. At the end of the procedure, firm pressure is applied by the assistant over the site of the biopsy to ensure haemostasis.

> *For ultrasound guided needle biopsy, the biopsy needle should be kept parallel to the chest wall and in line with the long axis of the ultrasound probe, to ensure optimal visualisation of the biopsy needle in relation to the target lesion and to avoid any risk of damage or injury to chest wall structures.*

6. Stereotactic guided needle biopsy

6.1. Stereotactic FNAC [17–19]

For needle biopsy using an add on stereotactic device with a conventional upright mammography machine, the patient is seated. A superior approach with the breast positioned for the cranio caudal view is suitable for most lesions but latero-medial, medio-lateral or oblique approaches may be needed for lesions that are inferiorly positioned or are situated laterally in the axillary tail region. After demonstrating the lesion on a scout film, paired stereotactic views are obtained with the X-ray tube angled 15 degrees either side of the central straight tube position. The position of the lesion on the stereotactic views is used to determine the position of the needle guide in the X and Y axes so that when a needle of known length is introduced through the guide into the breast, the needle tip will be correctly positioned within the lesion. The skin is cleaned and superficial infiltration with local anaesthetic may be carried out. The sampling needle (21G or 23G) is inserted through the needle guide and into the breast so that the needle hub is against the guide. Check stereotactic films are taken to ensure correct positioning of the needle in relation to the target lesion — if the position is not correct, the needle is repositioned and further check films are obtained (Fig. 4). When the needle position is correct, aspiration is carried out by simultaneously rotating and passing the needle repeatedly in and out of the lesion, Different areas of the lesion are sampled by moving the needle guide 2–3 mm in the X and Y axes — up to 5 aspirates are usually obtained. The aspirate is delivered onto slides in the same way as described for US FNAC.

6.2. Stereotactic core biopsy

Stereotactic guided CB may be carried out with upright stereotactic apparatus [20]. Targeting of the lesion is carried out in the same way as for FNAC. A small skin nick is made to allow insertion of the core biopsy needle. Having checked the position of the needle tip, the needle is withdrawn approximately 5 mm so that the needle tip is just proximal to the lesion before firing — the biopsy port will then traverse the lesion on firing, ensuring accurate tissue sampling. It is important to ensure that there is sufficient tissue deep to the needle tip following firing so that the needle tip does not hit the surface of the cassette holder. Most published series of stereotactic guided CB involve use of a dedicated prone table [21–23]. Using this equipment, the patient lies in the prone oblique position and the breast passes through a round aperture in the table. For lesions which are very posteriorly positioned or which lie in the region of the axillary tail, access can be improved by passing the ipsilateral arm and shoulder girdle through the aperture. The direction of the X-ray beam is horizontal and stereotactic views are obtained by rotating the tube 15 degrees either side of the central position. The digital X-ray images obtained are displayed on a computer screen within approximately 5 seconds of exposure. Target areas for biopsy are selected on the computer screen and the position and angulation of the biopsy needle/gun holder are adjusted automatically. A 14G needle is used and after insertion under local anaesthetic, check films are taken to ensure correct positioning. Check films can also be taken after firing the biopsy gun to ensure that the lesion has been traversed by the needle (Fig. 5). Five or more core samples are usually obtained. When sampling areas of microcalcification, specimen radiography of the core samples is carried out to ensure that tissue containing microcalcification has been obtained.

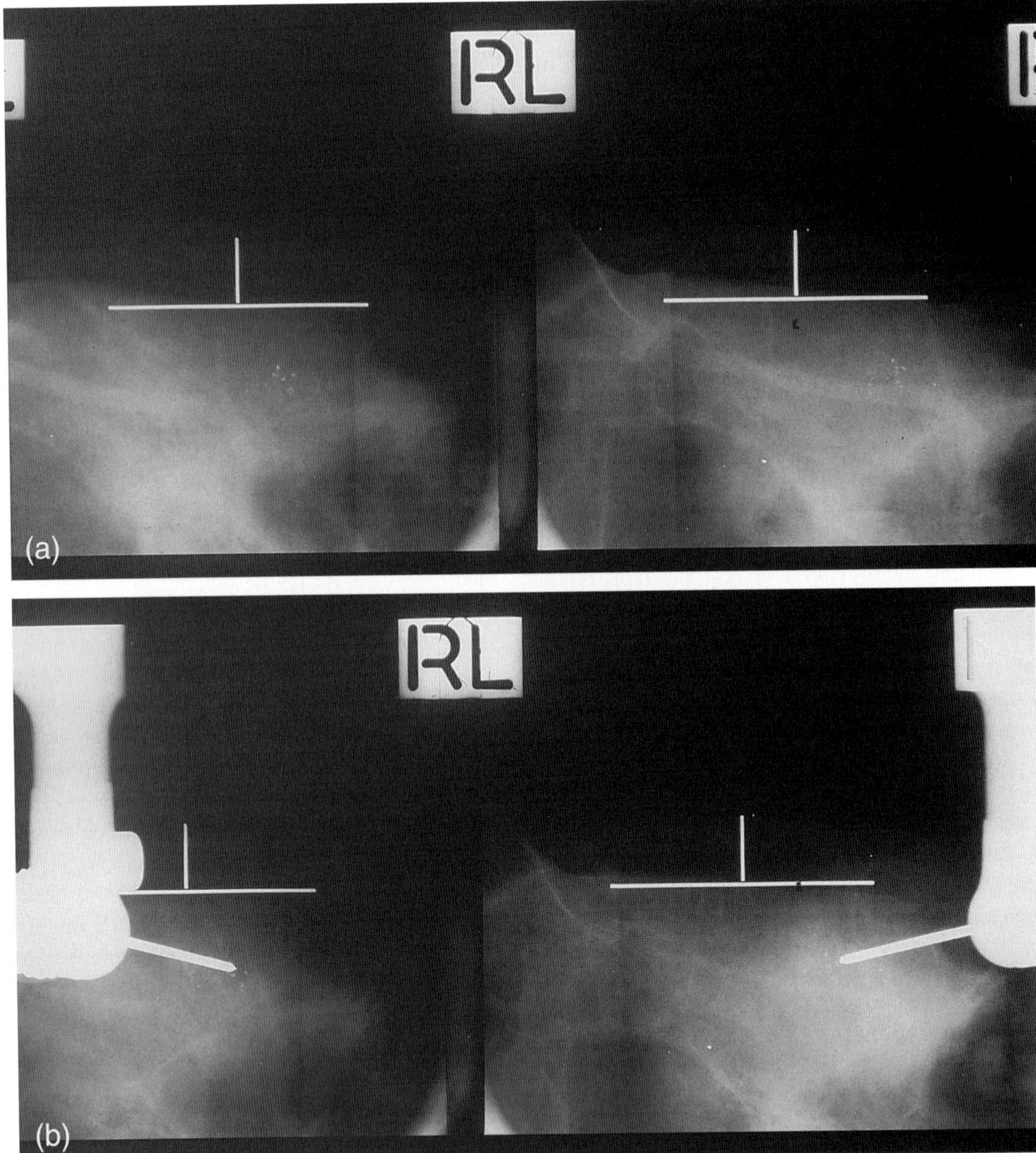

Fig. 4. Upright stereotactic FNAC. (a) A cluster of microcalcification is seen in the stereotactic images. (b) The check films show the needle positioned correctly within the cluster of microcalcification.

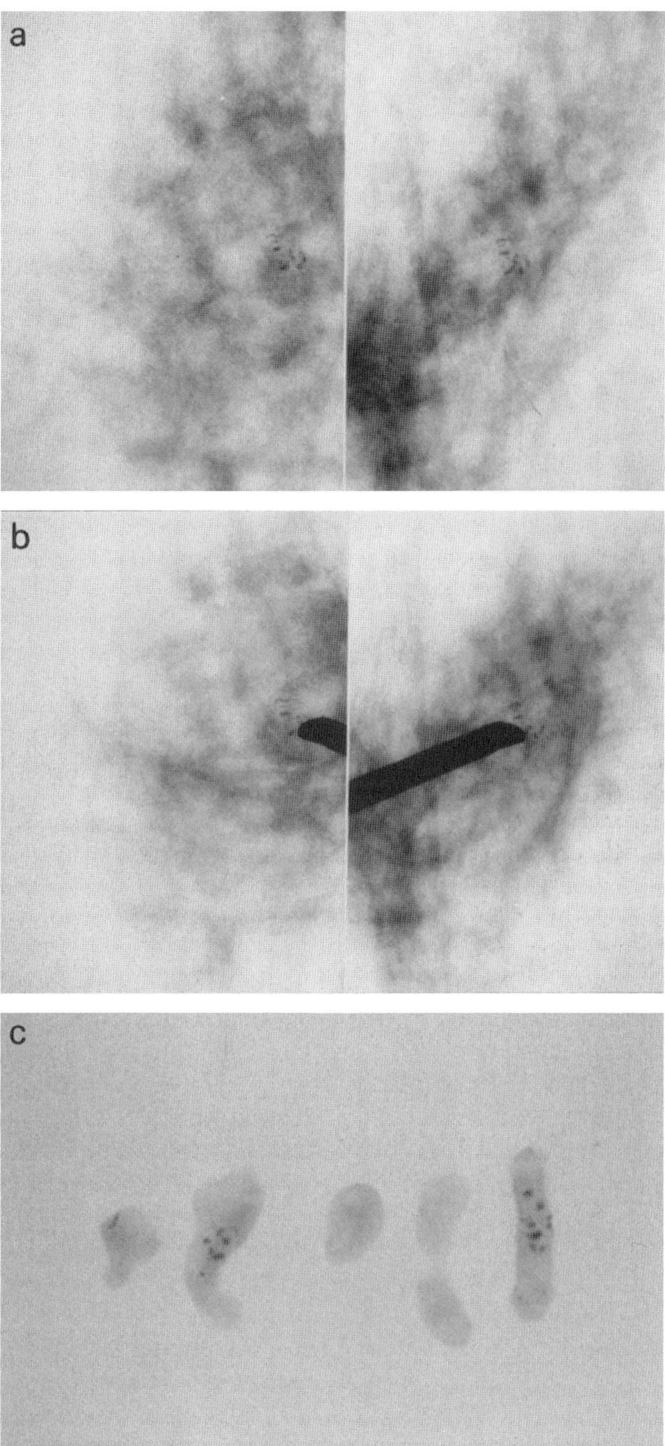

Fig. 5. Prone stereotactic 14G core biopsy. (a) A small cluster of microcalcification is shown on the digital stereotactic images. (b) The needle tip is shown proximal to the microcalcification. (c) The specimen X-ray confirms the presence of calcification in the core specimens.

7. Large volume sampling techniques

7.1. Vacuum assisted core biopsy (mammotome) [24,25]

The mammotome vacuum assisted core biopsy system may be used with an 11G or 14G needle probe. Most published results of the mammotome system describe its use with prone stereotactic apparatus, although it can be used for sampling lesions under ultrasound guidance. The probe incorporates a vacuum channel which applies negative pressure to the biopsy port and thereby sucks the adjacent breast tissue into the port for sampling. The biopsy probe is introduced into the breast and positioned using imaging guidance — deep local anaesthetic containing adrenaline is used. The vacuum is used to suck breast tissue into the biopsy port; a rotating cutting cylinder then passes down within the probe and separates the biopsy material from the surrounding tissue — the biopsy specimen is then delivered by withdrawing the cutting cylinder while applying negative pressure and delivering the specimen, while the main probe remains within the breast. Multiple specimens are obtained by rotating the biopsy probe within the breast so that the biopsy port is applied to different areas of breast tissue. Any haematoma which collects in the biopsy cavity is rapidly evacuated by the vacuum. In case the whole mammographic abnormality has been removed, a small metal marker clip is introduced through the biopsy probe and deployed at the biopsy site.

7.2. The ABBI and PBB biopsy devices [26]

Both involve insertion, using prone stereotactic imaging guidance, of a large bore cutting cylinder which cuts a core of tissue containing the mammographic abnormality. The diameter of the ABBI sampling device is up to 20 mm, the diameter of the PBB device 15 mm. The PBB device differs from the ABBI system in having a cutting blade at the leading edge of the biopsy probe allowing it to be placed against the proximal edge of the lesion before sampling.

The relative merits and the use of such large volume breast biopsy techniques in clinical practice are subject to ongoing debate and research [27,28].

8. Choice of sampling technique

The choice of sampling method should be determined by both the accuracy of the technique as measured by sensitivity and specificity, the information required for malignant lesions, cost and patient comfort. The accuracy of image guided FNAC has been shown to vary widely between different centres. The accuracy of cytology depends on an adequate cellular sample being obtained from the target lesion and interpretation by a suitably trained breast cytopathologist. FNAC has been successfully used by some centres but its effectiveness has been limited by inadequate sample rates of 10–30%, and equivocal sample rates of 20–30% where a definitive benign or malignant diagnosis cannot be made. Poor cytology specimens are more likely to be obtained from certain poorly cellular lesions such as sclerosing fibroadenomas and microcalcification due to fibrocystic change. A further limitation of cytology is its inability to distinguish between invasive from non invasive cancer and to determine the grade and type of the invasive tumours. The availability of automated core biopsy guns and the publication of results from several centres showing very high sensitivity and specificity has resulted in the more widespread use of image guided CB [29,30]. A recent review [31] of 31 published series of image guided breast biopsy shows that a higher sensitivity and specificity are obtained using CB compared to FNAC. No difference in patient discomfort between FNAC and CB has been demonstrated [32]. The interpretation of the biopsy material does not require a specially trained cytologist and information regarding the invasive nature and grade of a tumour can be obtained in most malignant soft tissue lesions. For malignant microcalcification, if an invasive tumour is present, 14G CB will detect the invasive element in approximately 40% of cores.

Sensitivity for certain lesions is dependent on the number of samples taken — for spiculate masses, one or two needle passes are required; for low suspicion, punctate non-branching microcalcification or for stellate areas of parenchymal distortion six or more passes are required to achieve satisfactory levels of sensitivity [33,34].

The advantages of core biopsy compared to FNAC for non palpable lesions are:

- *Higher sensitivity and specificity.*
- *Lower inadequate and equivocal sample rates.*
- *Diagnosis of invasive tumour, tumour type and grade.*

Use of the larger volume sampling techniques may be effective in further reducing the equivocal sample rate and increasing the sensitivity for the detection of invasive tumour. Breast units carrying out image guided needle biopsy of non palpable lesions should audit their results so that they can determine the accuracy of the biopsy techniques used and thus develop local protocols for appropriate patient management.

9. Patient management

Following image guided needle biopsy, further patient management is decided at a multidisciplinary meeting where the imaging findings are discussed together with the results of needle biopsy by both radiologist, cytopathologist and surgeon. In order to reach a definite diagnosis on which a management decision can be based, there must be compatibility between the biopsy findings and the differential diagnosis suggested by the imaging work up. It is very useful, therefore, for a breast unit to have a clear management protocol for non palpable suspicious mammographic abnormalities.

For lesions with a greater than 90% probability of malignancy such as spiculate mass or highly suspicious microcalcification, a malignant needle biopsy enables definitive therapeutic surgery to be planned. If a benign or equivocal needle biopsy result is obtained in such lesions, either repeat needle biopsy or diagnostic surgery following needle localisation should be planned.

For stellate areas of parenchymal distortion with no central mass, where there is a 50% chance of malignancy, therapeutic surgery can be planned if a malignant CB is obtained; diagnostic excision should be offered with a benign or equivocal CB result because of the lack of data on the negative predictive value of benign CB for such lesions. For low suspicion lesions such as low density circumscribed soft tissue masses and localised punctate microcalcification, the pathologist and radiologist must be confident that an adequate sample has been obtained by needle biopsy and that a definitive benign diagnosis is demonstrated which is compatible with the mammographic appearances in order to offer reassurance with no diagnostic surgery. For microcalcification, this clearly means that calcium must be demonstrated within the core biopsy specimens. Cases where an inadequate or equivocal needle biopsy result is obtained should be offered either repeat needle biopsy or diagnostic surgery. When the core biopsy shows features of atypical ductal hyperplasia, diagnostic surgical excision should be offered because surgical histology will demonstrate the presence of either in-situ or invasive cancer in 30–40% of cases [35,36].

Following image guidance breast needle biopsy, management is decided at a multi-disciplinary meeting where the imaging findings are considered together with the results of FNAC or Core Biopsy — the needle biopsy result must be compatible with the differential diagnosis suggested by the imaging work up.

References

1. NHS Breast Screening Radiologists Quality Assurance Committee. Quality Assurance Guidelines for Radiologists. Sheffield: NHSBSP Publications. 1997, No 15, pp 13.
2. Parker SH, Stavros AT. Interventional breast ultrasound. In Parker SH, Jobe WE, eds. Percutaneous Breast Biopsy. New York, Raven Press, 1993, pp. 129.
3. Dowlatshi K, Gent MJ, Schmidt R, Jokich PM, Biobbo M, Sprenger E. Non palpable breast tumours: diagnosis with stereotaxis localisation and fine needle aspiration. Radiology 1989; 170: 427–433.
4. Helvie MA, Baker D, Adler DD et al. Radiographically guided fine needle aspiration of non palpable breast lesions. Radiology 1990; 174: 657–661.
5. Dent DM, Kirkpatrick AE, McGoogan E, Chetty U, Anderson TJ. Stereotaxic localisation and aspiration cytology of impalpable breast lesions. Clin Radiol 1989; 40: 380–382.
6. Ciatto S, Roselli de Turco M, Bravetti P. Non palpable breast lesions: stereotactic fine needle aspiration cytology. Radiology 1989; 173: 57–59.
7. Parker SH, Lovin JD, Jobe WE et al. Stereotactic breast biopsy with a biopsy gun. Radiology 1990; 176: 741–747.
8. Michell MJ. Image guided breast biopsy – technical advances. Br J Radiol 1998; 71: 908–909.
9. Berg WA, Krebs TL, Compassi C, Magder LS, Sun CC. Evaluation of 14 and 11 gauge directional, vacuum assisted biopsy probes and 14 gauge biopsy guns in a breast parenchymal model. Radiology 1997; 205(1): 203–208.
10. Meyer JE, Smith DN, Dipiro PJ et al. Stereotactic breast biopsy of clustered microcalcifications with a directional, vacuum assisted device. Radiology 1997; 204(2): 575–576.
11. Leiberman L, Smolkin JH, Derhaw DD, Morris EA, Abramson AF, Rosen PP. Calcification retrieval at stereotactic, 11 gauge directional vacuum assisted breast biopsy. Radiology 1998; 208(1): 251–260.
12. D'Angelo PC, Galliano DE, Rosemurgy AS. Stereotactic excisional breast biopsies utilized the advanced breast biopsy instrumentation system. Am J Surg 1997; 174(3): 297–302.
13. Ferzli GS, Hurwitz JB. Initial experience with breast biopsy utilising the advanced breast biopsy instrumentation (ABBI) system. Surg Endoscopy 1997; 11(4): 393–396.
14. Denton ERE, Michell MJ, Nash RM, Bingham M. Use of the site select percutaneous breast biopsy device. The Breast 2000; 9: 107–109.
15. Sneige N, Fornage BD, Saleh G. Ultrasound guided fine needle aspiration of non palpable breast lesions: cytologic and histological findings. Am J Clin Pathol 1994; 102(1): 98–101.
16. Parker SH, Jobe WE, Dennis MA et al. US guided automated large core breast biopsy. Radiology 1993; 187(2): 507–511.
17. Azavedo E, Svane G, Aver G. Stereotactic fine needle biopsy in 2594 mammographically detected non palpable lesions. Lancet 1989; 1(8646): 1033–1036.
18. Bibbo M, Scheiber M, Cajulis R, Keeber CM, Wied GL, Dowlatchi K. Stereotaxic fine needle aspiration cytology of clinically occult malignant and pre-malignant breast lesions. Acta Cytol 1988; 32(2): 193–201.
19. Fajardo LL, Davis JR, Wiens JL, Trego DC. Mammographically guided stereotactic fine needle aspiration cytology of non palpable breast lesions: prospective comparison with surgical biopsy results. Am J Roentgenol 1990; 155(5): 977–981.
20. Caines JS, McPhee MD, Konok GP, Wright BA. Stereotaxic needle core biopsy of breast lesions using a regular mammographic table with an adaptable stereotaxic device. Am J Roentgenol 1994; 163(2): 317–321.
21. Parker SH, Lovin JD, Jobe WE, Burke BJ, Hopper KD, Yakes WF. Non palpable breast lesions: stereotactic automated large core biopsies. Radiology 1991; 180(2): 403–407.
22. Elvecrog EL, Lechner MC, Nelson MT. Non palpable breast lesions: correlation of stereotaxic large core needle biopsy and surgical biopsy results. Radiology 1993; 188(2): 453–455.
23. Gisvold JJ, Goellner JR, Grant CS et al. Breast biopsy: a comparative study of stereotaxically guided core and excisional techniques. Am J Roentgenol 1994; 162(4): 815–820.
24. Burbank F, Parker SH, Fogarty TJ. Stereotactic breast biopsy: improved tissue harvesting with the mammotome. Am J Surg 1996; 62(9): 738–744.
25. Burbank F. Stereotactic breast biopsy of atypical ductal hyperplasia and ductal carcinoma in-situ lesions: improved accuracy with directional, vacuum assisted biopsy. Radiology 1997; 202(3): 843–847.
26. Liberman L. Advanced Breast Biopsy Instrumentation (ABBI): analysis of published experience (commentary). A J R 1999; 172: 1413–1416.
27. Parker SH. The advanced breast biopsy instrumentation: Another Trojan horse? Am J Roentgenol 1998; 171(1): 51–53.
28. Ferzli GS. Letter. J Am Coll Surgeons 1997; 185: 604–605.
29. Britton PD, Flower CD, Feeman AH et al. Changing to core biopsy in an NHS breast screening unit. Clin Radiol 1997; 52(10): 764–767.
30. Litherland JC, Evans AJ, Wilson AR et al. The impact of core biopsy on the pre operative diagnosis rate of screen detected breast concerns. Clin Radiol 1996; 51(8): 562–565.
31. Britton PD. Fine needle aspiration or core biopsy. The Breast 1999; 8: 1–4.

32. Denton ERE, Ryan S, Beaconfield T, Michell MJ. Image Guided Breast Biopsy: analysis of pain and discomfort related to technique. The Breast 1999; 8: 257–260.
33. Rich PM, Michell MJ, Humpherys S, Howes GP, Nunnerley HB. Stereotactic 14G Core biopsy of non palpable breast cancer: what is the relationship between the number of core samples taken and the sensitivity for detection of malignancy. Clin Radiol 1999; 54: in press.
34. Liberman L, Dershaw DD, Rosen PP, Abramson AF, Deutch BM, Hann LE. Stereotaxic 14 Gauge breast biopsy: how many specimens are needed? Radiology 1994; 192(3): 793–795.
35. Liberman L, Cohen MA, Dershaw DD, Abramson AF, Hann LE, Rosen PP. Atypical ductal hyperplasia diagnosed at stereotaxic core biopsy of breast lesions: an indication for surgical biopsy. AJR 1995; 164(5): 1111–1113.
36. Moore MM, Margett C, Hanks JB et al. Association of breast cancer with the finding of atypical ductal hyperplasia at core breast biopsy. Ann Surg 1997; 225(6): 726–733.

Breast Cancer: Diagnosis and Management
J.M. Dixon (Ed.)

CHAPTER 5

Open biopsy: indications and complications

M.H. Galea

1. Diagnosis: Open biopsy: indications and complications

All women presenting with a palpable breast abnormality and those with screen detected abnormalities will be subject to 'triple assessment'; this is a multi modality approach to diagnosis consisting of clinical assessment, diagnostic imaging and diagnostic FNAC (fine needle aspiration cytology)/core biopsy [1]. Imaging and cyto/histopathology can be semi-qualitatively scored (Table 1). Scoring focuses the assessor and is of help to the clinical team in ensuring consistent protocol driven patient management pathways.

If the abnormality appears benign on all assessment modalities (R2/C2/B2) either a conservative approach or excision may be decided upon depending on local protocols or patient preference. If the abnormality appears malignant (R5/C5/B5) a definitive cancer operation can be discussed with the woman. If a definitive diagnosis cannot be made by the combination of clinical examination, imaging and FNAC/core biopsy because of inconsistency between results then an open biopsy is necessary. In practice the number of women needing an open biopsy should be small as the increasing use of core biopsy for both palpable and particularly impalpable abnormalities with its greater specificity over FNAC has helped clinicians become more confident in 'non-operative' diagnosis [2,3].

> *Failure of triple assessment to provide an accurate 'non-operative' diagnosis is the indication for proceeding to an open biopsy.*

2. Indications for an open biopsy of a palpable abnormality

(1) C3/C4/C5 obtained from a abnormality that clinically and on imaging is benign (R2). There is a recognised false positive rate for malignant cytology (C5) of about 2 : 1000 to 1 : 3000. Specific clinical entities that can make interpretation difficult are occasional fibroadenomas, pregnancy and after radiotherapy. In this situation core biopsy is recommended; if the pathology confirms malignancy (B5) wide local excision/mastectomy and axillary node surgery can be discussed. If the pathology is benign or equivocal (B2/B3/B4) an open excision biopsy is recommended (and usually by this stage requested by the woman) to confirm a benign diagnosis. If the abnormality is over 4 cm an incisional biopsy may be preferred if it is thought likely that the lesion will prove to be

Table 1. Scoring of diagnostic imaging and diagnostic cytology/core biopsy

Score	Degree of suspicion	Mammographic/ultrasound appearance
Diagnostic imaging (R1–5)		
1	Normal appearance	No abnormality seen
2	Consistent with a benign abnormality	Scar, well circumscribed mass with halo or large calcification, multiple well rounded masses, lesion containing fat, benign and bilateral calcification, duct ectasia, haematoma
3	Equivocal (but probably benign)	Distortion, positional shadow, clusters of round calcifications, solitary defined mass of intermediate density, unilocular simple cyst, cyst with solid elements or irregular wall, solid mass with lobulated margin
4	Suspicious of malignancy	Ill defined or irregular dense mass, spiculated lesion with central mass, cluster of fine, punctate or granular calcifications, distortion with no central mass
5	Consistent with malignancy	Spiculate lesion with central mass +/− microcalcifications, comedo microcalcifications, irregular hypoechoic mass interrupting breast architecture with or without distortion, distal shadowing, vertical orientation, lymphadenopathy
Diagnostic cytology (C1–5)		
1	No epithelial cells present	
2	Benign epithelial cells present	
3	Equivocal (but probably benign; a predominantly benign background with one or two atypical cells seen)	
4	Suspicious of malignancy (predominantly a picture of cells with loss of cohesion, varied sizes and nuclear pleomorphism)	
5	Malignant	
Diagnostic core biopsy (B1–5)		
1	Normal breast tissue	
2	Benign lesion	
3	Hyperplastic/borderline lesion present	
4	Severe atypia/Carcinoma in situ	
5	Malignancy	

benign and that removing it would cause an unsightly cosmetic result.

(2) C2 from an abnormality that clinically or on imaging is equivocal or suspicious (R3/R4/R5). Core biopsy may confirm the abnormality to be malignant and allow definitive cancer surgery. If, however, the pathology is benign (B2) or borderline (B3/B4) open excision biopsy is necessary.

(3) Repeat C1 cytology in a patient unwilling to allow a core biopsy if there is any suspicion clinically or on imaging (R3/R4/R5).

(4) Clinical anxiety despite benign imaging (R2) and cytology (C2)/pathology (B2).

(5) Frank blood staining of cyst aspirate or repeated filling of same cyst. Ultrasound may not suggest anything other than a simple cyst but excision biopsy is advised to exclude a rare intracystic malignancy.

(6) There will always be some women who despite benign triple assessment will chose to have their 'lump' excised. The number varies with individual series but is in the order of approximately 15–20%; if these women are

reviewed at 3 months this figure increases.

(7) There are a small number of women who will fail triple assessment because they will not allow needle aspiration or core biopsy for personal reasons or fears and will choose preferentially to have an open biopsy and excision of the abnormality.

The excision of a benign feeling lump assessed as benign on imaging and cytology/core biopsy because of patient choice or local protocol is *not* considered a diagnostic open biopsy; it is for the purposes of discussion in this chapter on diagnosis considered a therapeutic procedure.

3. Indications for an open biopsy of an impalpable abnormality

Most of these women will come through breast cancer screening programmes or have incidental abnormalities picked up on mammography for other reasons. In order to minimise the benign/malignant biopsy ratio and to ensure screening morbidity is kept to a minimum the open biopsy rate needs to be kept low. This has been increasingly helped by the widening use of ultrasound and stereoguided core biopsy in preference to cytology allowing better and more frequent 'non-operative' diagnosis [4].

(1) Suspicious microcalcification (R3/R4/R5) not adequately accounted for on core biopsy. Either no microcalcification or too few of the calcifications are seen in the biopsy sections or the pathology maybe borderline. If the pathology is 'atypical hyperplasia' open excision is always necessary as frequently the definitive pathology of the biopsy in up to half of patients will show in situ or invasive disease.

(2) Suspicious parenchymal change (R3/R4/R5) not adequately accounted for on core biopsy. The core may demonstrate an area of fat necrosis or radial scar but open excision is usually advised to exclude malignancy.

(3) Suspicious mass (R3/R4/R5) not adequately accounted for on cytology or core biopsy. A C2/C3 cytology/B2 benign core cut would still require an open excision biopsy.

(4) Extensive suspicious microcalcification (R3/R4/R5) that may necessitate a mastectomy as treatment. Open biopsy of more than one quadrant will define the extent of any underlying problem and help plan future management.

(5) Some women when called back for screening assessment will become extremely anxious and request excision either prior to allowing any further 'invasive' assessment or afterwards.

The influence of ultrasound or stereoguided core biopsy on the diagnosis of impalpable screen detected abnormalities is illustrated in Fig. 1.

4. Techniques for open biopsy

Open biopsy of a breast abnormality may be performed either as an incisional biopsy or more commonly an excisional biopsy.

4.1. Incisional biopsy

This is uncommonly performed now because a definitive diagnosis and immunohistochemistry can usually be obtained with a core biopsy. If it is considered appropriate an incision is made directly over the abnormality along the lines of resting skin tension and the biopsy taken as a wedge with a knife. After haemostasis the wound is closed as for an excision biopsy. For a superficial abnormality this can be done under local anaesthetic.

4.2. Excisional biopsy

The intention is to remove the lump/lumpy area/localised abnormality in its entirety but with a minimal margin.

4.2.1. Palpable abnormalities

If the abnormality is superficial and less than 2 cm excision is easily performed under local

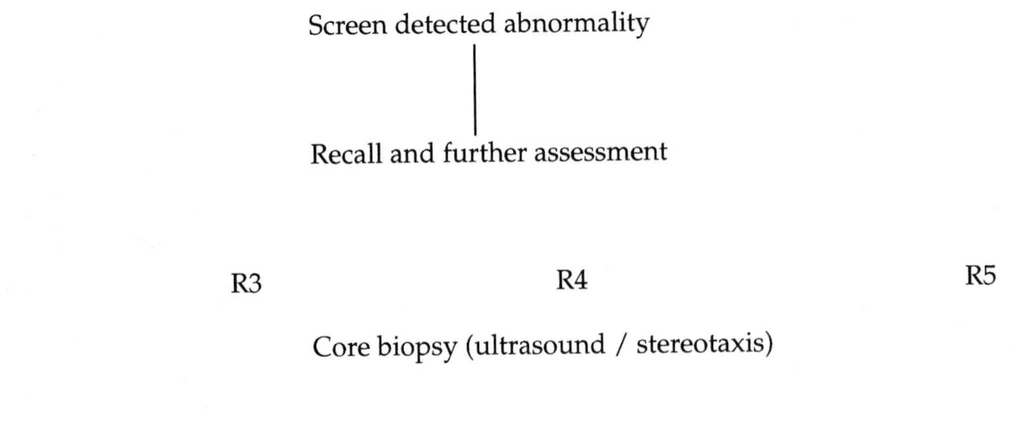

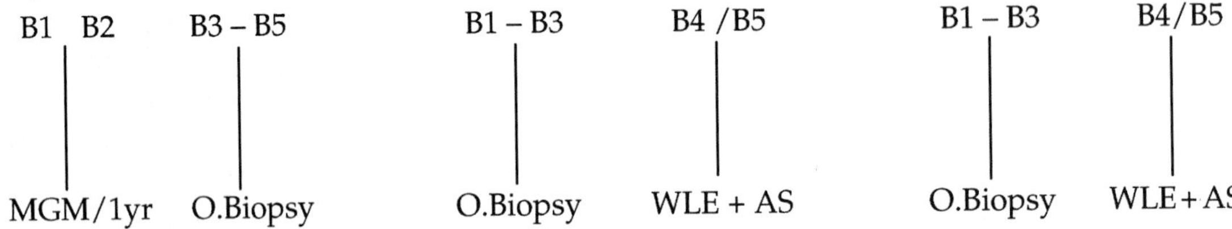

Fig. 1. Core biopsy in the assessment and diagnosis of screen detected impalpable abnormalities. MGM = mammogram; WLE = wide local excision; AS = axillary surgery.

anaesthetic. It is advisable to carefully and clearly mark out the abnormality with the woman in the position she will be asked to adopt on the operating table before the local anaesthetic is infiltrated as the volume can make the lump more difficult to feel.

Otherwise a general anaesthetic is used. For abnormalities close to the areola a circumareolar incision leaves an excellent cosmetic result. Elsewhere site the scar along the lines of resting skin tension. Sometimes a lump easily felt pre-operatively can appear less obvious once an incision is made through the skin. It is advised that the operator fixes the lump to be excised firmly between thumb and index finger and an incision is made through all the covering tissues down onto the lump. It can then be grasped safely and excised in total using either knife or scissors or a combination of the two. Do not pull too hard and distort the area as this can lead to over excision. If there is any suspicion the lump may be malignant, orientate the specimen clearly and ensure that the pathologist has details of the orientation.

Secure haemostasis with diathermy or ties if necessary. Drains are rarely if ever required after biopsy. Close the breast defect providing this causes no significant distortion. If it does do not, close the skin wound in two layers with an absorbable suture; take the tension on the dermal tissue and close skin with an absorbable continuous subcuticular suture.

5. Impalpable abnormalities

Prior to surgery the abnormality has to be localised using either ultrasound or mammographic stereotaxis. If visible on ultrasound this is the preferred method. The timing of localisation prior to surgery depends on local logistics and the method of localisation. Methods of localisation include injection of blue dye, injection of radio-isotope labelled colloid, wire localisation or ultrasound

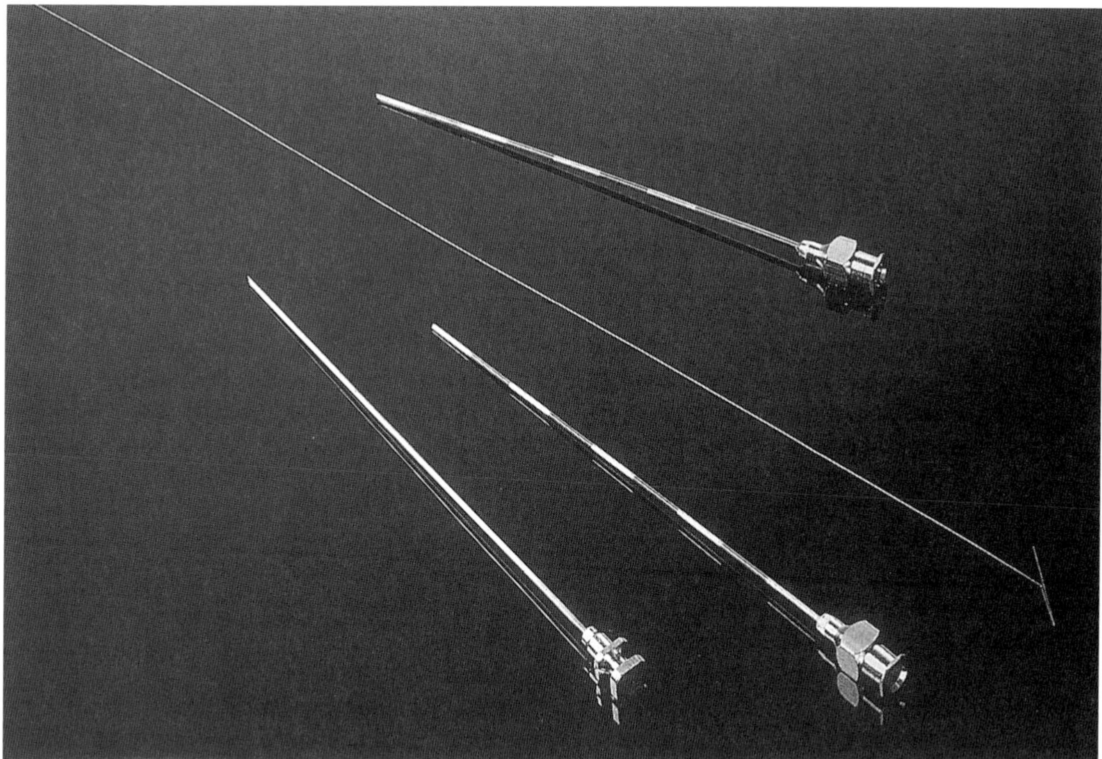

Fig. 2. The Nottingham Wire localisation apparatus.

guided inked marking of the skin overlying a superficial abnormality. The commonest method used is wire localisation. There are a number of wires manufactured each with advantages and disadvantages. A commonly used system is the Nottingham Wire (Fig. 2). This is a fine wire which maximises patient comfort while in situ; when the patient/breast is anaesthetised the wire is strengthened with a sleeve which makes it easily palpable within the breast. Although it has a T shape at its end to prevent migration it is easily removed from the specimen and does not interfere with assessment by the pathologist.

Following placement of the wire true lateral and craniocaudal films are performed to confirm positioning. These must come to the operating theatre with the patient.

Excision can be performed under general or local anaesthetic depending on patient preference, anaesthetic risk, position of the abnormality in the breast and the relative breast size. Local anaesthetic is preferred from a health economist viewpoint; it is more commonly the technique of choice in the USA/Scandinavia than in the UK.

The skin incision should be made directly over the site of the abnormality and not to follow the wire down from its insertion. Site the scar along the lines of skin tension; lesions adjacent to and up to 4 cm away from the areola margin can be removed through a peri-areolar incision. Once through the skin elevate it off the breast by dissection in the subcutaneous plane. Hold back the skin edges over the abnormality with a small self-retaining retractor. Using a blade make two incisions parallel to the long axis of the wire. Deepen as necessary to ensure the abnormality is contained within the cylinder of breast tissue excised. This is made easier if the abnormality becomes 'palpable' during the operation. With a grasping forceps the cylinder of tissue which

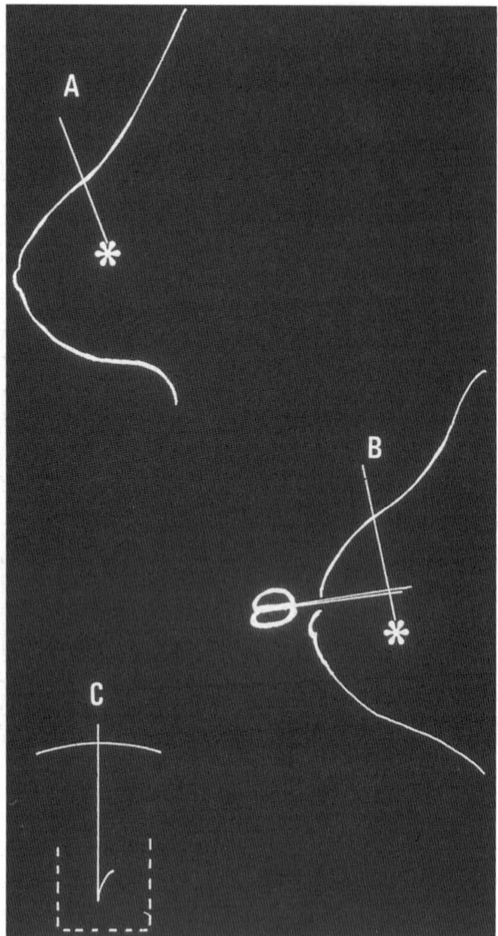

Fig. 3. Excision biopsy of an impalpable abnormality illustrating that the skin incision should be sited directly over the abnormality minimising the distance travelled through the breast and that the surgical intention is to remove a cylinder of tissue containing the abnormality.

contains the wire is excised by dividing distally (sometimes the wire overshoots the marked abnormality by many centimetres making distal dissection less straight forward (Fig. 3). Lifting the distal end out of the wound allows the surgeon to work towards the proximal end of the wire. Once the specimen is ready to come out the wire can be divided with wire cutters. Carefully orientate the specimen, mark in three axes and X-ray. The best pictures are obtained with paddle compression (Fig. 4). Marking varies according to individual preferences; radio-opaque clips are preferred. Information about orientation and marking should be accurately conveyed to the pathologist. Specimen orientation is important in directing further cavity dissection either at the time of surgery or at a later date if the margins prove to be close or involved. If during the procedure the abnormality is palpable and the surgeon is confident the lesion has been removed then the cavity is closed while waiting for the specimen X-ray. If it is not palpable, carry out haemostasis while the specimen X-ray is awaited. The X-ray may be shown to a radiologist or returned promptly to the theatre for the surgeon to see and compare with the pre-operative films. If the abnormality is contained within the specimen closure can be completed. If a cylinder is excised as described, closure of the cavity by apposing the two longitudinal axes walls is straightforward. Closure is otherwise as for a palpable breast lump.

The above describes a diagnostic open biopsy; intentionally the amount of resected breast should be small but if the abnormality is small and there is a high index of radiological/cytopathological suspicion, a wider excision (aiming for a 1 cm margin of clearance) is performed.

> *The intention of an open biopsy is to remove the abnormality in its entirety.*

6. Microdochectomy

A microdochectomy operation is performed for the indications given below and excises a portion of a diseased duct for both pathological assessment and to stop the discharge. It can be considered a form of open biopsy. If the patient has an associated breast lump its assessment and diagnosis always takes precedent over a nipple discharge.

The indications for a microdochectomy are:

(1) Blood stained nipple discharge from a single duct.

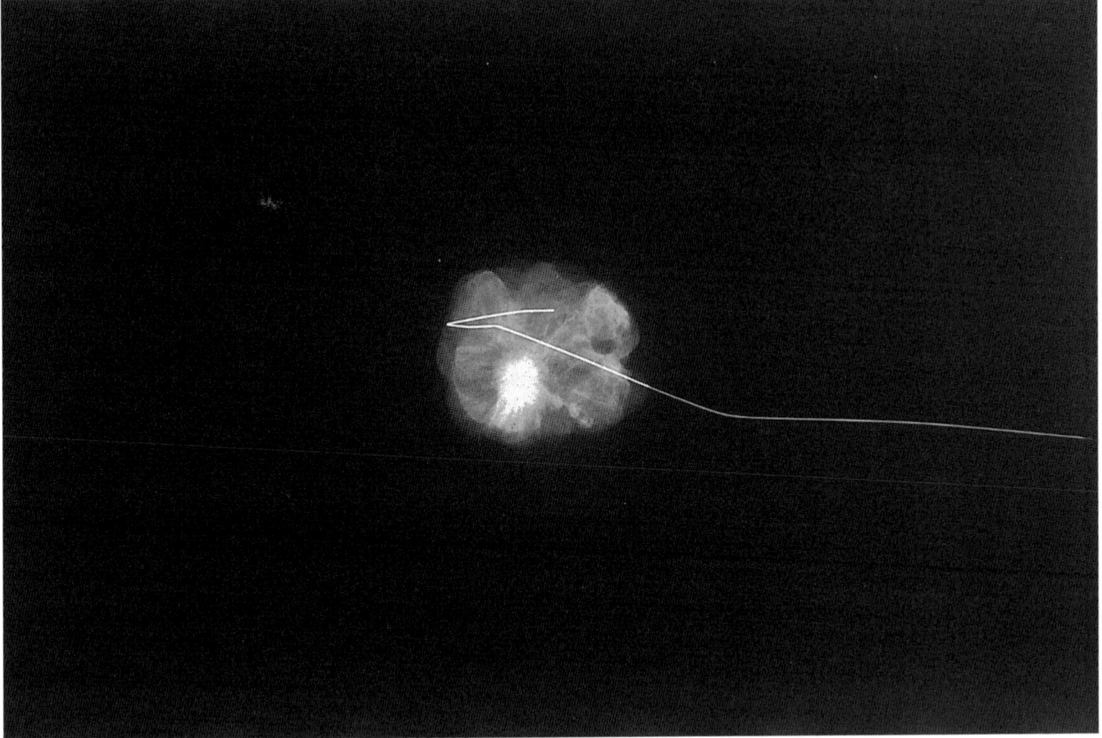

Fig. 4. Specimen X-ray of resected localisation biopsy with Nottingham Wire and localised abnormality in situ.

(2) Persistent or troublesome nipple discharge from a single duct.

(3) Periductal mastitis associated with a troublesome ectatic duct and/or a mammary fistula.

The operation is most easily carried out under general anaesthetic as infiltration with local can distort the subareolar duct system. If there is the suggestion of associated infection peri-operative antibiotics are advised. The antibiotics used should have anaerobic cover.

After skin preparation the breast is gently squeezed to express the discharge. A probe is placed into the discharging duct. With the probe in the duct a circumareolar incision is made centred over the abnormal duct. If it is a central duct, site the incision inferiorly to maximise cosmetic outcome. Deepen the dissection down to the probe and dissect up/down parallel to and along the long axis of the probe. Proximally excise the duct up to the back of the nipple and distally aim to excise about 2–3 cm of duct unless there is an obvious abnormality deeper in the breast tissue. Obtain haemostasis and close the wound in layers.

7. Complications

7.1. Specific

7.1.1. Unable to find the abnormality

Previously palpable: This is rare if the surgeon has examined the patient pre-operatively with the patient lying in the same position as on the operating table and accurately marks the skin overlying the abnormality. If the skin has been accurately marked any abnormality is usually easily located once the skin has been incised.

If truly impalpable once through the skin it is unlikely that the abnormality will turn out to be significant. The lump may have been a cyst inadvertently burst during injection of local anaesthetic. If there is truly nothing to feel excise a small area from under the skin incision and close.

Previously impalpable: Review the localisation films and carefully palpate the excision cavity. If the abnormality was a mass lesion or parenchymal distortion it may be palpable; if so excise, orientate the specimen and repeat the specimen X-ray to ensure excision of the required abnormality. If the abnormality has not been excised and the mammographic abnormality is impalpable a 'best guess' as to the likely position of the abnormality is made from the two localisation films and further tissue excised. If at this point the abnormality is still not in the resected specimens, secure haemostasis and abandon the procedure. The odds of missing an invasive carcinoma are small. Explain the difficulties to the patient and arrange for a repeat mammogram 6–12 weeks. If the abnormality is still present and still considered worthy of assessment repeat the localisation procedure.

7.1.2. Wire dislodged in the breast

This is uncommon and occurs in fatty breasts. If the abnormality remains transfixed identifying the area to be excised is not difficult. If however the wire has been dislodged towards the skin and is sitting above/proximal to the abnormality one can 'best guess' where the abnormality is by examining the localisation films. If excision of the abnormality is not successful proceed as above.

7.1.3. Wire kinked

For localisation techniques that use a fine wire this can be a problem as it may not be possible to pass the strengthening sleeve over the wire. Without this additional rigidity it is impossible to feel the wire and an excision is taken from where the abnormality is thought to be as assessed from the localisation films. Alternatively try following the wire down from the skin puncture. Kinking can be avoided by gently pulling the wire away from the breast; this effectively straightens the wire and allows the strengthening sleeve to slide easily over it and up to the end.

7.1.4. Poor localisation

Reasons why the abnormality in the breast may be poorly localised include:

- Difficult areas such as deep on the chest wall or high up in the axillary tail;
- Difficult breasts such a very small breasts;
- The mammographic abnormality is less defined on the stereotactic films than on the original films;
- Poor radiological technique;
- Wire migration;
- Patient is unable to tolerate the procedure through to completion.

Poorly localised abnormalities are more difficult to excise. If lateral and cranio-caudal views following localisation are available 'best-guessing' the position of the abnormality is the best approach. If the abnormality proves difficult to find abandon the procedure and repeat the mammogram at 6–12 weeks to reassess.

7.2. General

7.2.1. Bruising and haematoma

Through small incisions haemostasis can sometimes be difficult to secure. It is easy to burn skin edges with diathermy cautery and care must be taken. Some degree of bruising is common after open biopsy and the patient should be appropriately informed prior to hospital discharge. If at the time of surgery haemostasis is difficult a small suction drain can be used for 2–4 hr combined with padding and a pressure dressing. Because of the mobility of the breast on the chest wall obtaining a useful pressure dressing is difficult; it should not be delegated to the scrub nurse.

The painful accumulation of a sizeable volume of blood evident as an obvious haematoma occurs in about 2% of patients. Depending on the post operative stay in hospital it may not become apparent until the patient has returned home.

Some patients will return immediately; if tense and painful, evacuation and washout is advised as this will ensure the breast will settle much more quickly. Others will return for results at 1–2 weeks post operatively with a haematoma and very bruised breast; this group are best managed conservatively advising that it will be some weeks before the breast softens and the bruising fades.

If there are any signs of superadded infection antibiotics are necessary.

7.2.2. Wound infection

Post operative wound infection rates are approximately 4%. There are no indications that these rates are influenced by wound drainage or type of anaesthesia. There is no need for peri-operative antibiotics for open biopsy of either palpable or impalpable abnormalities unless the patient is having a microdochectomy for periductal mastitis or mammary fistula.

> *The morbidity of an open biopsy is both physical and psychological; it is important to keep the open biopsy rate as low as possible by striving hard to achieve an accurate 'non-operative' diagnosis using triple assessment.*

References

1. Galea M, Blamey R. Diagnosis by team work; an approach to conservatism. In: Stewart H, Anderson T, Forrest A, eds. Breast Disease New Approaches. British Medical Bulletin. Churchill Livingstone 1991; pp. 295–304 (chapter).
2. Andreu FJ, Sentis M, Castaner E et al. The impact of stereotactic large-core needle biopsy in the treatment of patients with nonpalpable breast lesions: a study of diagnostic accuracy in 510 consecutive cases. Eur Radiol 1998; 8(8): 1468–1474.
3. Furhman G, Cederbom G, Bolton J et al. Image guided core-needle breast biopsy is an accurate technique to evaluate patients with non palpable breast abnormalities. Ann Surg 1998; 227(6): 932–939.
4. Litherland J, Evans A, Wilson A et al. The impact of core-biopsy on pre-operative diagnosis rate of screen detected breast cancers. Clin Radiol 1996; 51(8): 526-5.

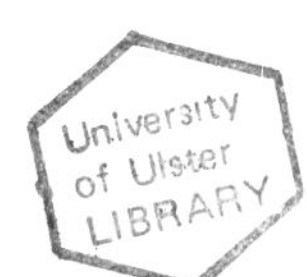

Breast Cancer: Diagnosis and Management
J.M. Dixon (Ed.)

CHAPTER 6

Pathology of breast cancer: in situ and invasive disease. Histological classification, tumour grade and other histological factors

S.E. Pinder, A.H.S. Lee, C.W. Elston and I.O. Ellis

1. Ductal carcinoma in situ (DCIS)

In populations where mammographic breast screening is performed DCIS accounts for approximately 15 to 20% of breast carcinomas [1]. As a result of the apparent increase in DCIS incidence from 5% of symptomatic practice, a great deal of interest has arisen in techniques for predicting the biological behaviour and in systems for classification of the disease process. Although the clinical significance of DCIS has been questioned [2] it is generally accepted to be a precursor of invasive cancer [3]. It is however acknowledged that not all DCIS progresses inevitably towards invasive malignancy.

- *DCIS is the main precursor of invasive breast cancer and has increased in frequency of detection due to use of mammographic screening.*

A spectrum of atypical intraductal epithelial proliferative diseases is recognised histopathologically from atypical ductal hyperplasia (ADH) to ductal carcinoma in situ (DCIS) and it is clear that there is difficulty in achieving good reproducibility of diagnosis in the diagnosis of ADH versus low grade DCIS [4,5]. These problems can often be resolved through adherence to strict criteria along with training and guidance but disagreements in the definitions of these early lesions may still occur [5]. The majority of cases are readily classifiable if pathologists adhere to the view [6] that ADH is a lesion of cellular changes typical of DCIS in less than two separate duct spaces [7]. Thus ADH is a small microfocal lesion. It has been argued that the overall size of the lesion is more important than the number of duct spaces involved [8]. Two mm in size has previously been used as a cut-off point for differentiating between ADH and DCIS; a lesion less than 2 mm in overall size indicating ADH. The Armed Forces Institute of Pathology criteria for DCIS have now been updated [9] and the 2 mm size criterion is now invoked only when assessing non-necrotic atypical intraductal proliferations i.e. those with features of low grade DCIS. High grade intraductal proliferations qualify as DCIS, regardless of size.

- *The distinction of benign and malignant in situ epithelial proliferations is currently set between ADH and low grade DCIS and is based on arbitrary criteria of size and number of duct spaces involved.*

1.1. Classification of DCIS

As noted above the apparently increased incidence in DCIS seen since the advent of mammographic screening has led to increased interest in histopathological features of DCIS which may predict behaviour. In the past DCIS was classified largely on architecture alone into comedo, solid, cribriform and micropapillary patterns. Subsequently some groups have proposed categorisation based on combined architectural or cytological features, others have recommended cytonuclear features alone should be used and yet others that necrosis should be assessed, alone or in combination with cytonuclear grade. In 1996 a European Union Working Group on Breast Screening Pathology recommended classification into high, intermediate and low grade DCIS [10].

- *Classification systems of DCIS based on cytonuclear grading, supported by assessment of other features such as cellular architecture and necrosis, can predict outcome.*

Tumour cells in high nuclear grade DCIS have pleomorphic, irregularly spaced, usually large nuclei (Fig. 1a). Nuclear contours are irregular with coarse chromatin and prominent nucleoli. Mitoses are often frequent. The growth pattern in high grade DCIS may be varied; a solid pattern is the most common with sheets of cell filling the duct with central comedo type necrosis which frequently contains amorphous calcification. This may be confined to the nipple ducts and may present with Paget's disease of the nipple. High nuclear grade DCIS may also form micropapillary and cribriform structures. There is rarely any organisation or polarisation of cells around cribriform structures or covering micropapillae.

Low grade DCIS is composed of monomorphic, evenly-spaced cells (Fig. 1b). The nuclei are usually small, roughly spherical and centrally-placed with inconspicuous nucleoli. Mitoses are few. There is rarely individual cell necrosis. The lesion most commonly has a cribriform or micropapillary architecture; both are frequently present within the same tumour although the cribriform pattern is usually more common. There is frequently polarisation of tumour cells covering the micropapillae or lining the intercellular lumina. Low grade DCIS is less frequently of solid pattern. In some cases it may not be possible to distinguish between low grade solid DCIS and LCIS and in this situation the lesions should be classified as a combined lesion.

A lesion is classified as being of intermediate grade type when the nuclei are mildly to moderately pleomorphic and there is less variation in cell size and shape than seen in high nuclear grade disease and the neoplastic cells lack the monotony and polarisation of the low grade type. The growth pattern may be solid, cribriform, or micropapillary.

A small proportion of cases of DCIS may show features of more than one nuclear grade but this is relatively rare, particularly when compared to the commonly seen variation in architectural pattern. Thus one of the advantages of classification by nuclear grade is that DCIS is usually of pure cytological type. If heterogeneity in cytological grade is present the case is classified according to the highest nuclear grade present.

2. Microinvasive carcinoma

Microinvasive carcinoma is rare. The process is one in which the dominant lesion is DCIS but with one or more foci of infiltration of the non-specialised interlobular stroma, *none of which measures more than 1 mm in diameter* [11]. 'Cancerisation of lobules', as seen when carcinoma extends into lobular structures with expansion of the acini (but remains within the basement membrane of the ductal system), should not be over-diagnosed as invasion. Nevertheless cases of pure high or intermediate nuclear grade DCIS and those with comedo type necrosis should be sampled extensively to exclude foci of invasion. Stains for smooth muscle actin may also assist in the diagnosis, with an absence of immunoreactive myoepithelial cells in areas of invasion.

When these strict criteria for microinvasive carcinoma of the breast are adhered to, the incidence of metastatic disease in axillary lymph

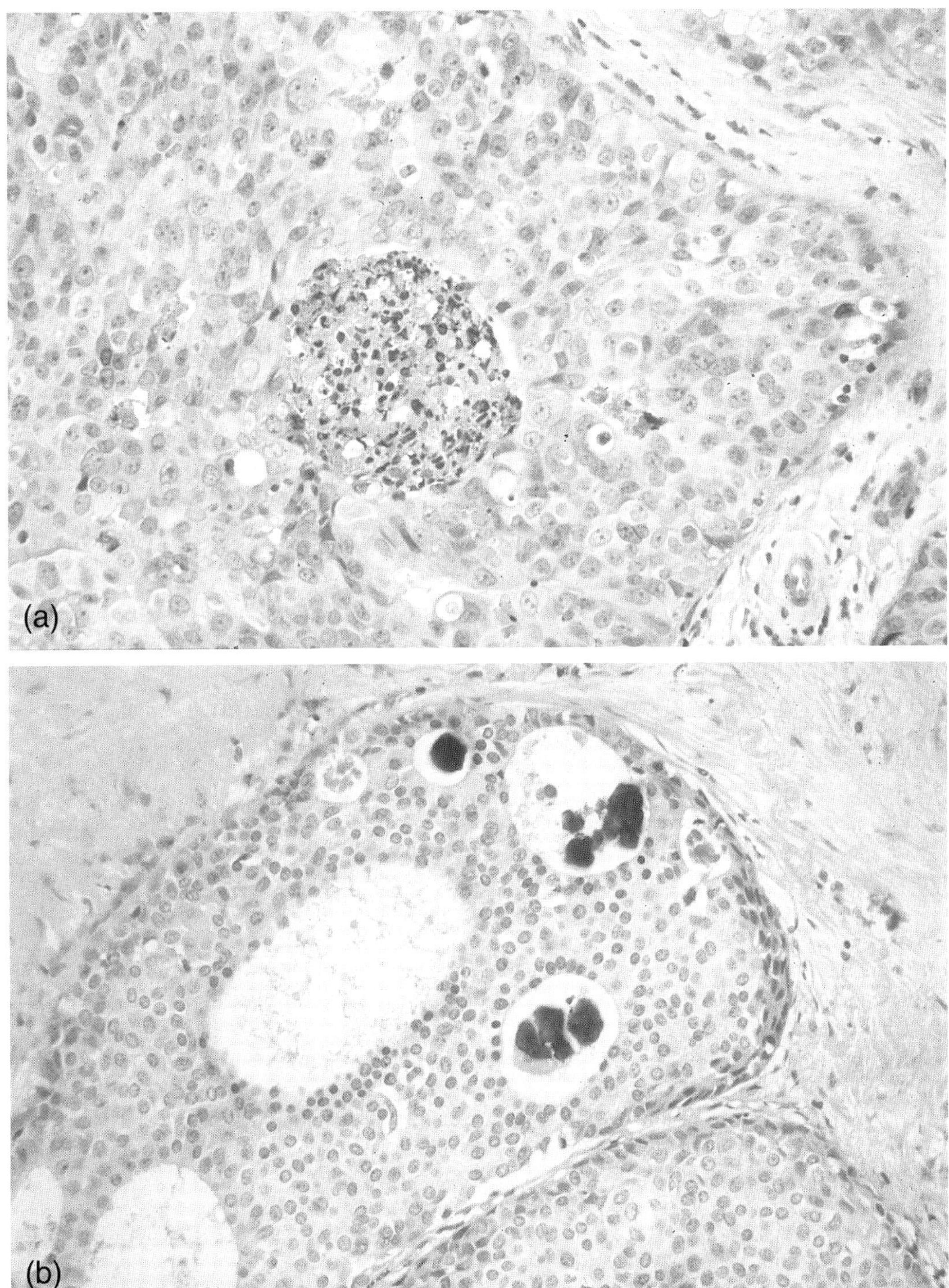

Fig. 1. Photomicraphs of high grade (a) and low grade (b) DCIS showing the difference in cytonuclear characteristics.

nodes is very low and the condition is thus managed clinically as a form of DCIS. It should be noted that (rarely) in pure DCIS metastatic foci may be found due to missed occult foci of invasion for example in extensive disease.

- *The definition of microinvasive carcinoma is very restrictive and this condition is consequently exceptionally rare.*

3. Invasive breast carcinoma

Historically, the main role of the histopathologist lay in the establishment of a diagnosis of breast cancer from surgical biopsy or frozen section. Apart from the examination of loco-regional lymph nodes for the presence or absence of metastases it was unusual for any other prognostic information to be supplied, or indeed requested. However in the last few decades the treatment of breast cancer has undergone dramatic changes and a much wider range of both local and systemic therapeutic options is now available. The advent of mammographic breast screening has resulted in an increase in tumours which are more likely to have a favourable outcome. Unfortunately some patients with breast cancers still present relatively late in the course of the disease. It has become increasingly important to assess prognosis for each patient and to devise an appropriate therapeutic plan.

- *The prognosis of an individual patient with breast cancer can be predicted by histological assessment of the tumour and regional lymph nodes.*

Many of the histological features which provide valuable prognostic information can be obtained by thorough careful examination of histological sections [12]. The following factors are all relatively simple to assess and have been shown to provide clinically relevant prognostic information, with the proviso that attention is paid to diagnostic guidelines and protocols.

Table 1. Pathological staging of breast cancer

Stage 1:	All lymph nodes sampled tumour free.
Stage 2:	Tumour seen in a low axillary node only or in an internal mammary node only or in 3 or less nodes in axillary sample
Stage 3	Tumour seen in apical node or low axillary plus internal mammary nodes or 4 or more nodes in axillary sample

4. Lymph node stage

Involvement of loco-regional lymph nodes in invasive breast cancer is clearly an important prognostic factor. It is, however, apparent that the clinical assessment of the presence of disease in axillary lymph node is not sufficiently accurate for therapeutic use [13] and the evaluation of lymph node stage must be based on careful and thorough histological examination of excised nodes.

- *Lymph node stage should be determined by histological examination of resected lymph node and not by clinical examination.*

Patients who have histologically confirmed metastatic deposits in loco-regional lymph nodes have a significantly poorer prognosis than those without nodal disease [12,14–19]; 10 year survival is reduced from 75% for node negative patients to 25–30% for those with nodal disease. Outcome of patients with invasive breast carcinoma is also related to the number and the level of lymph nodes involved. Patients can be divided into 3 groups for therapeutic purposes based on the number of nodes involved; those with none, those with 1–3 positive nodes and those with 4 or more containing metastatic deposits (Table 1). The greater the number of nodes involved the poorer the patient survival [20,21] (Fig. 2). Similarly, nodal disease in the higher levels of the axilla, specifically the apex, carries a worse prognosis [19,22].

The extent of axillary surgery in patients with breast cancer however is controversial. Highly

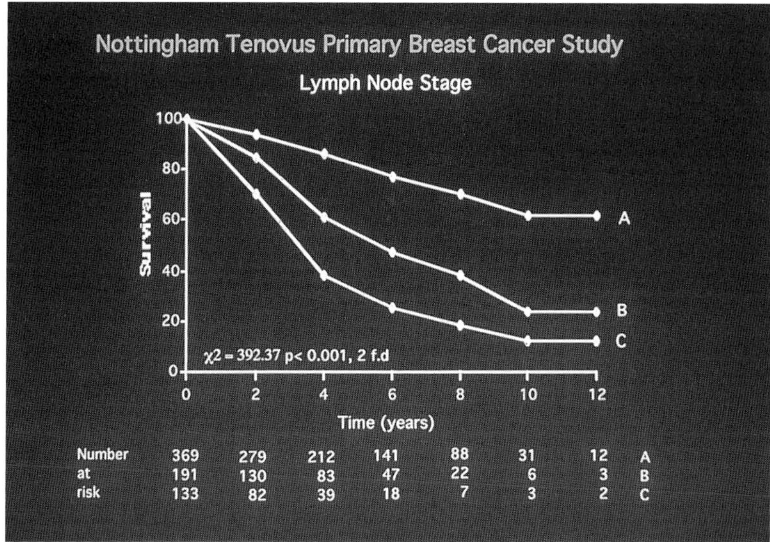

Fig. 2. Survival of patients in the Nottingham Tenovus series according to lymph node stage.

significant prognostic information can be obtained by a lymph node sampling method with examination of a node from the low axilla, apex of axilla and second intercostal space [18,23–25]. There has, however, been considerable debate regarding the extent of axillary lymph node dissection with arguments in favour of both axillary sampling [26,27] and axillary clearance [28,29] in the recent past. A greater number of nodes can be obtained at clearance compared with sampling, but the price for the additional prognostic information is the greater post operative morbidity, including reduced shoulder mobility, neuropathy and chronic lymphoedema [30].

In the last few years sentinel node biopsy has been widely advocated and there are now sufficient studies for the concept to have be validated in invasive breast cancer [31–34]. The basis of the concept is that the lymphatic system draining a tumour will dictate in which lymph node the first deposit of metastatic disease will develop. Whether the sentinel lymph node is involved or not will therefore reflect the status of the axilla of patients with invasive breast cancer. If the sentinel lymph node contains metastatic disease, then further surgery or radiotherapy can be considered. If it is uninvolved, the remaining lymph nodes in that group should be free of tumour. Early series have shown that if only one node contains metastatic carcinoma it is almost always the sentinel node and that this node is frequently the sole site of metastasis. One weakness of some of these studies, however, is that the sentinel node has been examined more intensively than the other lymph nodes and thus metastases in non-sentinel nodes may have been missed [35–37]. A proportion of cases with false negative sentinel lymph nodes (i.e. sentinel lymph node negative with metastases elsewhere in the axilla) will also be found and to date this varies from 1 to 11% [33,35–38].

- *Sentinel lymph node biopsy may allow targeted rigorous histological assessment and will increase the detection of early micrometastatic disease which is currently of uncertain clinical significance.*

The histopathological method for examination of the sentinel node is of vital importance. The data on prognostic value of axillary nodal status is based largely on series in which one slice from each axillary node has been examined using routinely stained tissue sections and clinical therapy decisions have been based on this information. Other techniques can increase the sensitivity of detection of metastatic disease, in essence by examining more of any individual lymph node. Thus each lymph node can be separately or completely embedded and multiple sections ('serial sectioning') of all the tissue embedded can also increase the chance of identifying metastases [39–41]. The use of immunohistochemistry also increases detection [40,42,43] by increasing the area of the node examined and also be making the metastases easier to see. Not surprisingly immunohistochemistry and serial sections increase the detection of metastases in sentinel lymph node biopsies [44,45]. Use of the reverse transcriptase polymerase chain reaction (RT–PCR) has also been proposed.

The role of these more sensitive histopathological methods for detecting deposits is controversial. There is some evidence that the size of the deposit in lymph nodes is of prognostic significance [40,43,46–49]. There is conflicting data on whether the position, in the marginal sinus or parenchyma, of the metastasis is important [39,41,50,51]. There is however neither an agreed definition for these small deposits nor a universal methodology for their detection, making comparison of published results impossible. Definitions of 'occult' or 'micro'-metastases used have included: metastases less than 2 mm, metastases found on review that were initially missed, deposits shown only in deeper histological sections and metastases identified only with immunohistochemistry for cytokeratins. Many of the larger studies have shown a worse prognosis for patients with 'micro'-metastases compared with node negative patients in univariate analysis [39,40,42,43,52] although the effect is more clear for disease-free survival than overall survival. Further large series with clear description of the technique of detection and definitions of the size and site of any small metastatic deposits in the lymph nodes are required before the true prognostic import of 'micro'-metastases can be determined.

Some authors have advocated intra-operative frozen sections or imprint cytology of axillary lymph nodes. Conventional frozen sections have in our opinion an unacceptably high false negative rate of 10 to 30% [37,53–55] in routine practice in most hands. More intensive intra-operative assessment with serial sections and immunohistochemistry has been described, but this is extremely time-consuming, very labour intensive and thus costly. Some studies have found acceptably low false negative rates of 2 to 3% with intra-operative imprint cytology [34,53] but many have been able to achieve this level of accuracy [55].

Pragmatically our current practice is to cut all axillary lymph nodes into slices about 3 mm thick perpendicular to the long axis (to maximise the assessment of the marginal sinuses) and to examine each node in a single cassette. Very large obviously involved nodes have one section taken. The majority of nodes are completely embedded in one cassette although some larger nodes may have only alternate slices embedded.

5. Tumour size

As, at least in part, a time-dependent factor, tumour size has been shown convincingly to influence prognosis [14,17,21,56,57], patients with small tumours have a better long-term survival than those with large lesions. The projected relapse-free survival rates 20 years after initial treatment in the study from the Memorial–Sloan Kettering Cancer Centre [58] are shown in Table 2

Table 2. Relapse-free survival rates 20 years after initial treatment

Tumour size	Survival
< 10 mm	88%
11–13 mm	73%
14–16 mm	65%
17–22 mm	59%

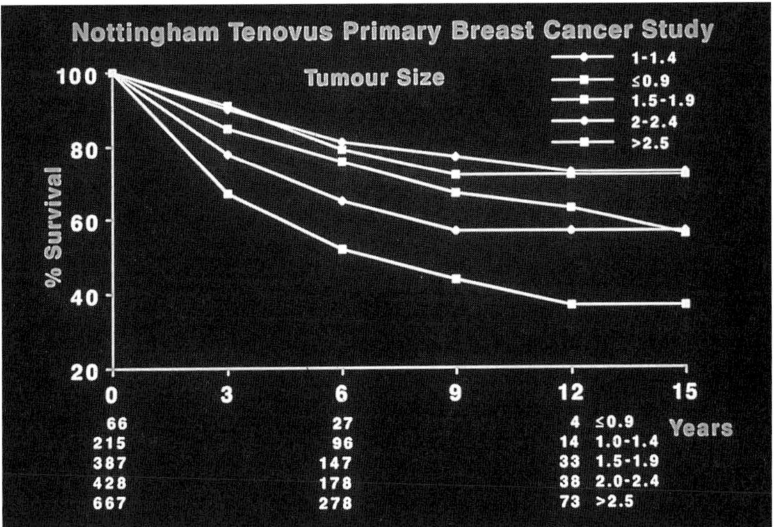

Fig. 3. Survival of patients in the Nottingham Tenovus series according to tumour size.

and the survival of patients in the Nottingham series in Fig. 3.

- *Increasing tumour size is associated with a poorer prognosis and forms the basic rationale for breast cancer screening.*

The size of tumours should be assessed for prognostic purposes on pathological specimens; clinical measurement is notoriously inaccurate. If an estimate of clinical tumour size is required for therapeutic planning it should be performed by ultrasonography. Size of the surgically excised tumour is measured in the laboratory in three planes to the nearest millimetre using a ruler, initially in the fresh state. The measurements are confirmed after fixation and the greatest dimension is taken as the tumour size. Tumour extent should be checked a third time on the histological sections using the stage micrometre of the microscope. This is particularly important for DCIS or tumours with a large in situ component and for small lesions, such as those measuring less than 1 cm in size. Even when the measurement of tumours is carried out by local rather than central review pathologists correlations with prognosis are seen [17,21,57] emphasising the inherent strength of tumour size as a prognostic factor. However as size decreases so the risk of errors in measurement increases, and inconsistencies between histopathologists' measurements from tissue sections have been reported [5,59].

Tumour size has become an important quality assurance measure for breast screening programmes [60–62], used in part to judge the ability of radiologists to detect impalpable carcinomas on mammography. In the NHS BSP a target of 15 small tumours per 10,000 women screened in the prevalent round is expected [62]. It is, therefore, vital that pathologists measure tumour diameter as accurately as possible to provide accurate data for audit. Our own indicate that the cut of point of 10 mm is not necessarily the best discriminator for good prognosis and the more significant size in life table analysis is 15 mm.

6. Differentiation

Historically the classification of carcinoma of the breast was restricted to division into in situ and invasive carcinoma. It is now clear that it is valuable to further divided invasive carcinomas histologically according to their differentiation; this may be achieved in two ways, by assessing histological grade and histological type.

- *Histological grading and typing are methods of tumour classification based on morphology and differentiation.*

7. Histological grade

Greenhough [63] undertook the first recognised study of histological grading of breast cancer over 70 years ago. Eight morphological features were examined in a somewhat subjective way, but he nevertheless showed a strong correlation with so-called 'cure'. Scarff and colleagues re-examined the method in 1928 and found that only 3 factors, tubule formation, nuclear pleomorphism and hyperchromatism were of importance [64]. This technique has subsequently formed the basis of most grading systems for invasive breast carcinoma, whether they use multiple histological features [21,65–69] or only nuclear appearances [70–72]. Despite the diversity of methods employed, very many studies have demonstrated the significant association between grade and survival.

- *Histological grading is a simple semiquantitative method, based on histological assessment of tubular differentiation, nuclear pleomorphism and mitotic frequency, which can provide powerful prognostic information.*

The acceptance of histological grade into routine practice has been slow in large part due to lack of clinical demand. However there was also a perception that grading was of poor reproducibility and consistency [73]. A substantial number of studies have now reported acceptable levels of observer variability [74–77] but it is clear that grading must be carried out by trained histopathologists and in particular they should work to an agreed protocol on well-fixed material. One of the fundamental problems with systems used in previous studies is the lack of strictly defined written criteria; Bloom and Richardson [67] made an invaluable contribution to grading breast cancers with the addition of numerical scoring (although clear criteria for cut off points were not described). Subsequent modifications to the above method have been made to introduce greater objectivity [69].

The same 3 characteristics of the tumour are evaluated in present routine practice as were described in Patey and Scarff's original work; these are tubule formation, nuclear pleomorphism and mitotic count. A numerical scoring system on a scale of 1–3 is now used to ensure that each factor is assessed individually. The proportion of lumina/acinar formation in the tumour is assessed for the tubule score. Reference to the size, regularity of nuclear size and shape of normal epithelial cells in adjacent breast tissue is used for the pleomorphism score. However the most important modifications to earlier descriptions of grading methodology concern the evaluation of mitotic figures and these amendments are both qualitative and quantitative. Care is taken to count only clearly defined mitotic figures; hyperchromatic and pyknotic nuclei are ignored since they are more likely to represent apoptotic than dividing cells. Quantitatively a more accurate assessment is now undertaken than identification of "about 2 or 3 mitoses per high power field" (HPF) [67]. In particular it is now recognised that the area of a single HPF may vary by as much as six-fold from one microscope to another [78] and mitotic counts are standardised to a fixed field area. Using this system any microscope can be calibrated to obtain reproducible and comparable data.

The sum of the scores for each component (each 1 to 3) is used to assign the overall histological grade. A grade 1 tumour has scores for tubules, pleomorphism and mitoses adding to 3, 4 or 5, a grade 2 to 6 or 7 and a tumour is classified as 3 if the sum of the scores is 8 or 9 (Table 3; Fig. 4). To date in the Nottingham–Tenovus Pri-

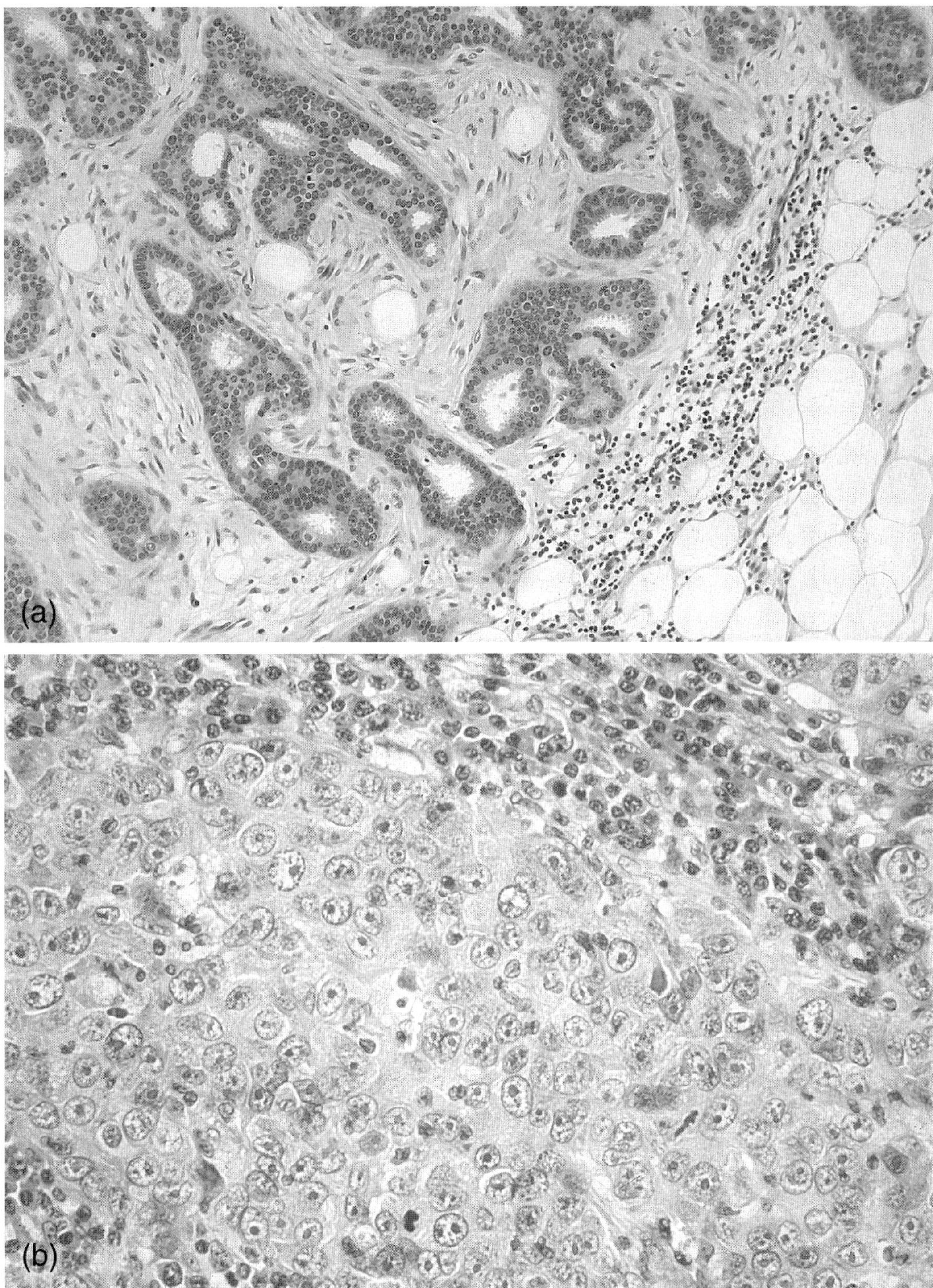

Fig. 4. Photomicrographs of a grade 1 tumour (a), note prominent tubule formation, small regular nuclear size and lack of mitoses, and a grade 3 tumour (b), note the absence of tubule formation, large pleomorphic nuclei and numerous mitotic figures.

Table 3. Outline methodology for histological grading (Nottingham method)

Feature	Score
Tubule formation	
Majority of tumour (> 75%)	1
Moderate degree (10–75%)	2
Little or none (< 10%)	3
Nuclear pleomorphism	
Small, regular uniform cells	1
Moderate increase in size and variability	2
Marked variation	3
Mitotic counts	
Dependent on microscope field area	1–3

Table 4. Survival of patients in the Nottingham Tenovus series according to histological grade

	Number of patients (%)	10 year survival (%)
Grade 1	620 (20)	86.5
Grade 2	1084 (35)	60.5
Grade 3	1402 (45)	48.8
Total	3106	

mary Breast Cancer Series the overall survival figures and distribution of histological grade are shown in Table 4 and Fig. 5. It should be noted that the majority of the patients in this series (which began accrual in the 1970's) have been symptomatically detected. Histological grade has been convincingly proven to be associated with prognosis based on life table analysis with long term follow-up in Nottingham; survival worsens with increasing (higher) grade [69]. This method for histological grading described above has been adopted for use in the pathological data set of the United Kingdom screening programme and in the USA and Europe.

8. Histological type

The histological appearances of invasive mammary carcinoma vary widely [16,79,80] and a large number of histological types have been described. It is evident that this information on type provides prognostic information [80,81]. The diagnostic criteria for different entities have been described in detail in several publications [79–82]. It should be noted that there is, however, a considerable subjective element to histological typing and there is not yet any universal agreement between histopathologists for all tumour types. In the UK National Health Service Breast Screening Programme pathology quality assurance scheme the consistency of diagnosis of histological type has been disappointingly low [5]; indicating adherence to protocols could be improved. This poor reproducibility may explain in part the varying proportions of types seen in published series. Nevertheless the favourable prognosis of certain histological types of invasive carcinoma of the breast is well established. Tubular carcinoma [83–85], mucinous carcinoma [86,87], invasive cribriform carcinoma [88], medullary carcinoma [89,90], infiltrating lobular carcinoma [91] and tubulo-lobular carcinoma [92] (Fig. 6) have all been reported to have a better prognosis than carcinomas of ductal/no special type (NST). There are, however, relatively few long-term comprehensive follow-up studies examining survival of patients with different histological types of invasive breast carcinoma.

A relative excess of tubular, mucinous, medullary and infiltrating lobular carcinomas has been reported in patients surviving at least 25 years after mastectomy compared with those having survived less than 10 years [93]. These findings were subsequently confirmed, and papillary and invasive cribriform carcinomas were added to those found amongst long term survivors [94]. It is also well recognised that a relative excess of these 'special type' tumours is seen in cancers detected in the prevalent round of mammographic breast screening [95,96].

- *Special histological types of breast cancer have an excellent long term prognosis.*

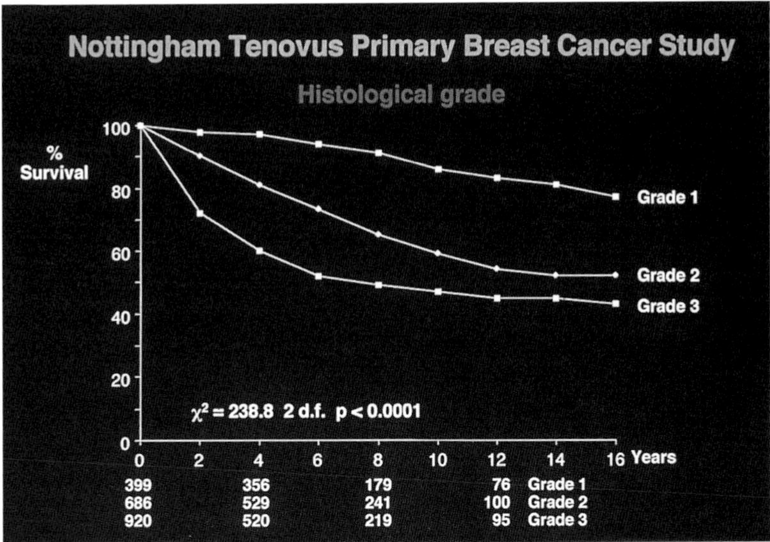

Fig. 5. Survival of patients in the Nottingham Tenovus series according to histological grade.

Further evidence from Nottingham has confirmed that histological type can provide prognostic information [81]. The prognosis of the special types, pure tubular, invasive cribriform and mucinous was again shown to be excellent. Additional categories of tubular mixed carcinoma and mixed ductal NST with special type were also found to be worth recording; these type categories confer a better prognosis than a classification of NST carcinoma. In most series these mixed categories not been recognised separately from NST lesions but they account for more than 15% of cases in symptomatic series and valuable information is lost if they are overlooked.

As noted above, early studies indicated that medullary carcinomas had a good (or even excellent) prognosis and this has become accepted dogma [89,90,97,98], despite a failure of other series to confirm finding [89,99–101]. However, some of the latter studies have demonstrated a survival advantage of medullary carcinoma over those of NST grade 3 morphology [81,100,101].

Infiltrating lobular carcinoma has a slightly better prognosis than ductal NST carcinoma does overall [81,91], although the 10 year survival of 54% implies no more than a moderate outcome. Dixon and colleagues [102], however, found significant differences in survival between morphological sub-types of lobular carcinoma and this has been subsequently confirmed [81]. Thus alveolar lobular carcinoma has a good prognosis (60–80% 10 year survival) and the classical type of invasive lobular carcinoma a moderate prognosis (50–60% 10 year survival) but mixed lobular and solid lobular variants have a poor prognosis (< 50% at 10 years) [103]. Conversely tubulo-lobular carcinoma has an excellent prognosis (> 80% 10 year survival) in our experience [103].

Thus it is clear that patients with invasive carcinoma of the breast can be stratified into broad prognostic groups according to their histological type [103]. The excellent (> 80% 10 year survival) prognosis group comprises tubular, invasive cribriform, mucinous and tubulo-lobular carcinomas. The good (60–80% 10 year survival) group is composed of tubular mixed, mixed ductal NST with special type and alveolar lobular carcinomas. The average group (50–60% 10 year survival) includes classical lobular, invasive papillary, medullary and atypical medullary carcinoma and the poor prognosis group (< 50% 10 year

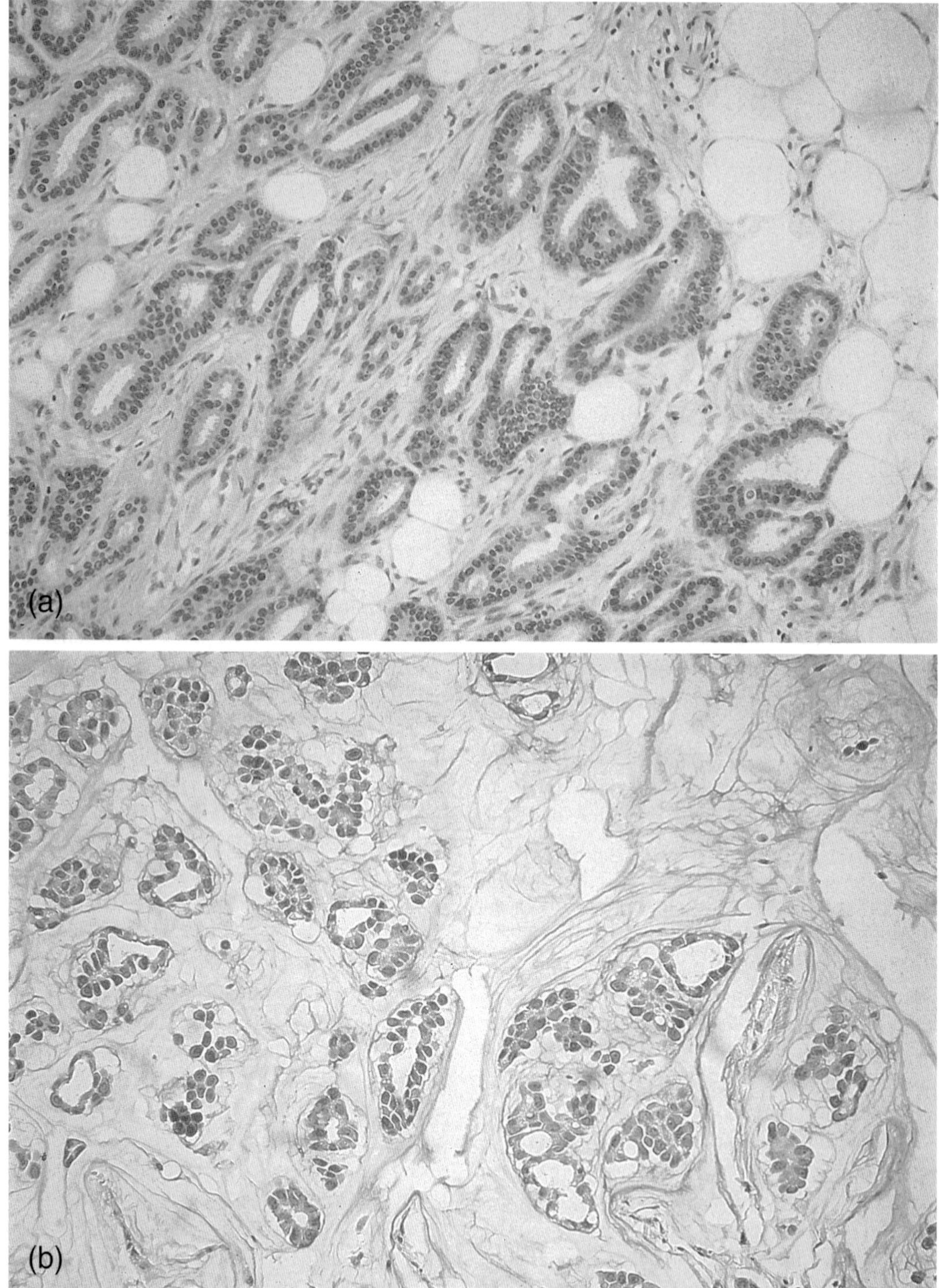

Fig. 6. Photomicrographs of some special types of breast cancer: tubular (a), mucinous (b), medullary (c) and lobular (d). Note their differing morphological structure.

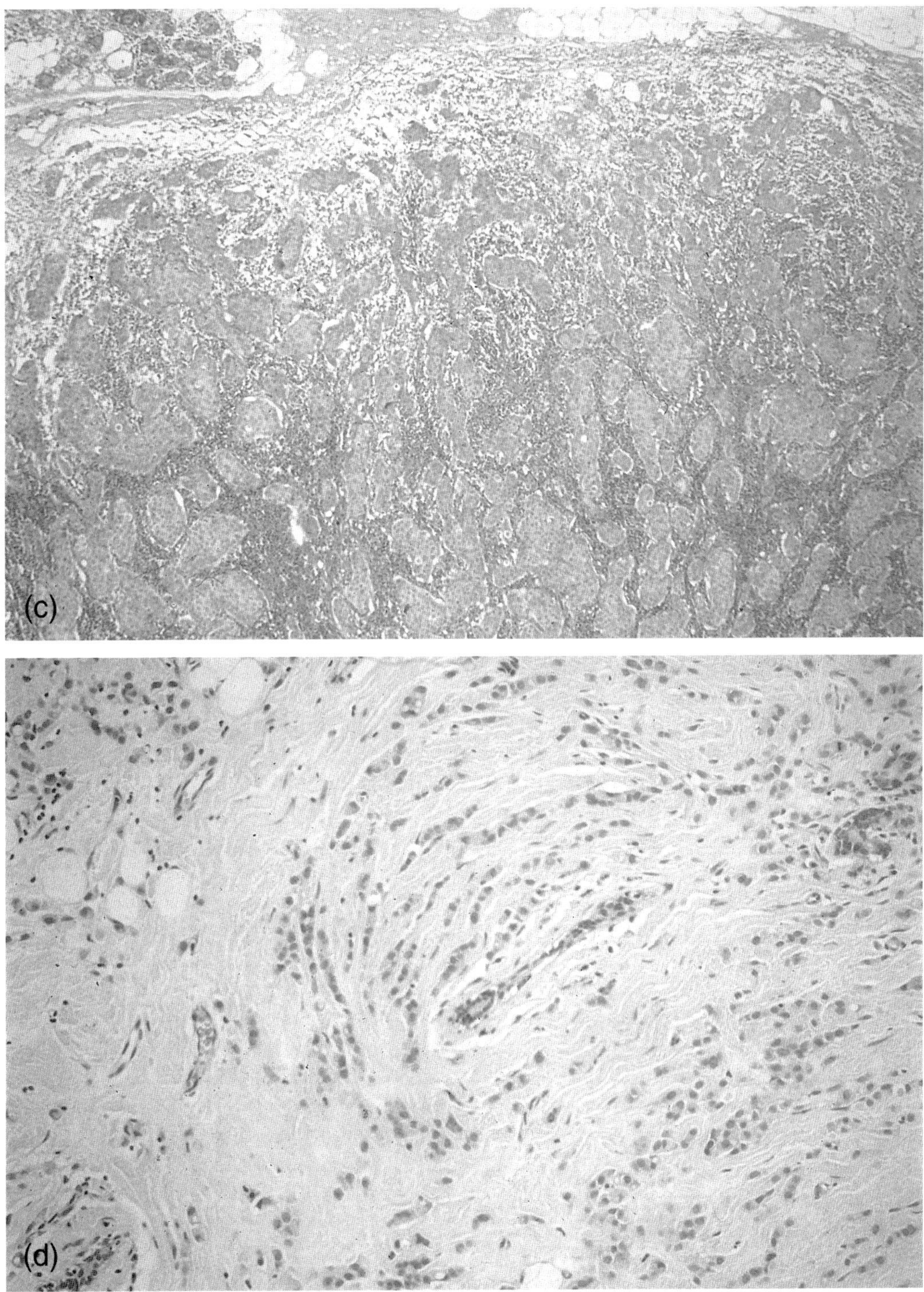

Fig. 6 (continued).

survival) is composed of ductal NST, mixed ductal and lobular, lobular mixed and solid lobular carcinomas.

9. Other histological features

9.1. Extranodal spread

The prognostic significance of extranodal spread of carcinoma into adipose tissue surrounding axillary lymph nodes is uncertain. It has been suggested that this feature carries a poor prognosis [104] particularly in patients with up to 3 nodes involved but not those with 4 or more involved nodes [105]. Other groups have found no additional effect to lymph node disease of extranodal tumour [106] with no intrinsic prognostic significance [107].

9.2. Vascular invasion

Tumour emboli may be identified within thin-walled vascular channels adjacent to an invasive carcinoma. In the breast it is impossible to determine reliably whether such spaces are lymphatic spaces, capillaries or venules and we used the broad term 'vascular invasion'. Muscular blood vessels are very rarely involved. Some studies have found no significant correlation between lympho-vascular invasion and prognosis [93,108] whilst others have shown that the presence of vascular invasion predicts for both recurrence [26,109,110] and survival [111–114]. Such discrepancies may be, in part, explained by the wide variation in the frequency of vascular invasion (20–54%). This itself may be partly explained by the difficulty in distinguishing vessels from artefactual soft tissue spaces, particularly in sub-optimally fixed specimens. Care must be taken to avoid misinterpretation of both DCIS and shrinkage artefact as vascular invasion [114,115]. However if strict criteria are applied the reproducibility of the evaluation of vascular invasion has been shown to be satisfactory [21,114]. Even in series where the authors have questioned their own reproducibility they have reported complete agreement in over 85% of cases [116].

Vascular invasion is strongly related with loco-regional lymph node disease [114,115,117]. Indeed some groups have claimed that it can provide prognostic information as powerful as lymph node stage [110]. There is certainly a correlation between the presence of vascular invasion and early recurrence in lymph node negative patients [109,110,118]. Vascular invasion is also related to long-term survival, and in our hands this effect is independent of lymph node stage in multivariate analysis [114]. The most important clinical application of vascular invasion, however, is its power as a predictor of local recurrence following conservation therapy [26,109,114,118] and as a marker of flap recurrence after mastectomy [119].

9.3. Extent of DCIS

The extent of DCIS associated with the invasive tumour is extremely variable and indeed the assessment of its degree is highly subjective. A prominent DCIS component within an invasive carcinoma has been said to be a feature indicating a better prognosis with a decreased frequency of nodal metastases [120,121]. It seems likely however that the DCIS component is of greater importance in the management of patients undergoing breast conserving surgery. The principal risk factor for relapse of disease after such surgery is large residual tumour burden, the main source of which is an extensive in situ component (EIC) [122]. Schnitt et al. have defined EIC as the presence of DCIS in an invasive carcinoma which occupies 25% or more of the overall tumour mass and which extends beyond the confines of that main mass [123]. They have found that invasive breast carcinomas with EIC have a considerably higher local recurrence rate than those without extensive DCIS. Significantly a significant proportion of such cases relapse as invasive disease. Extensive DCIS appears to be a much less important factor for local recurrence than completeness of excision.

9.4. Tumour necrosis

Tumour necrosis is a relatively common feature in invasive breast cancers which may be accompanied as it resolves by fibrosis. The prognostic value of tumour necrosis has been described in only a few studies and its presence noted to be associated with decreased survival and early treatment failure [21,124,125]. Necrosis is said to be almost entirely confined to NST carcinomas and is seen most frequently in those of high histological grade [80,126]. Unfortunately, a precise definition is not included in most of the studies in which it is reported and terms such as 'extensive' have been utilised, which makes confirmation of the results in new series impossible.

9.5. Stromal fibrosis and elastosis

Stromal fibrosis is frequently seen, in varying amounts, in invasive mammary carcinoma [125, 127]. The prognostic significance is uncertain. It has been associated variously with a poorer survival [125,128], a favourable prognosis [129] and to have no effect on outcome [93]. The data on stromal fibrosis in breast cancer is confounded by the related effects of tumour type; fibrosis is very frequently seen, for example, in low grade tubular carcinomas but may also be identified in those of high grade and no special type.

There are also conflicting data on the prognostic significance of stromal elastosis which is a feature of many breast lesions, both benign and malignant. It may be diffusely seen throughout a tumour or in a peri-ductal distribution [130]. Some authors have suggested that its presence is correlated with a good prognosis [131,132] but this has not been confirmed in other studies [133,134]. Elastosis is again often associated with tumour types having an excellent or good prognosis (such as tubular, invasive cribriform and tubular mixed) [81] indicating that it is not an independent prognostic factor.

10. Nottingham prognostic index

Many of the histological features described above been examined in a large number of publications as possible prognostic factors, indeed this area of research has grown exponentially in the last 10 years or so. It is now well recognised that prognostic factors can be used to select the most appropriate treatment for an individual breast cancer patient. In particular, patients with an excellent prognosis can avoid unnecessary adjuvant treatment and women with a very poor prognosis can receive more aggressive therapies [135]. Clinical series and therapeutic trials can be compared reliably if the distribution of patients by likely outcome can be predicted. Prognostic factors also have an important role in the identification of patients who may respond or be resistant to specific therapies.

- *Combining prognostic factor data in the form of a prognostic index gives excellent stratification of patients into prognostic groups.*

Although lymph node stage is the most commonly promulgated prognostic factor in mammary cancer, it is a relatively poor discriminator; neither a group of patients with near to 100% survival nor one with near to 100% mortality can be identified. Similarly, despite histological grade being the complex morphological outcome of losses and gains of a multitude of markers, neither stage nor grade alone is sufficiently discriminatory on which to base definitive therapy. A combination of features is more valuable than any one factor alone. In multivariate analysis in our Unit the 3 features which are of greatest prognostic import are histological grade, lymph node stage and tumour size. These have been combined into the Nottingham prognostic index (NPI) [18], with appropriate weighting from the statistical analysis. This is calculated as:

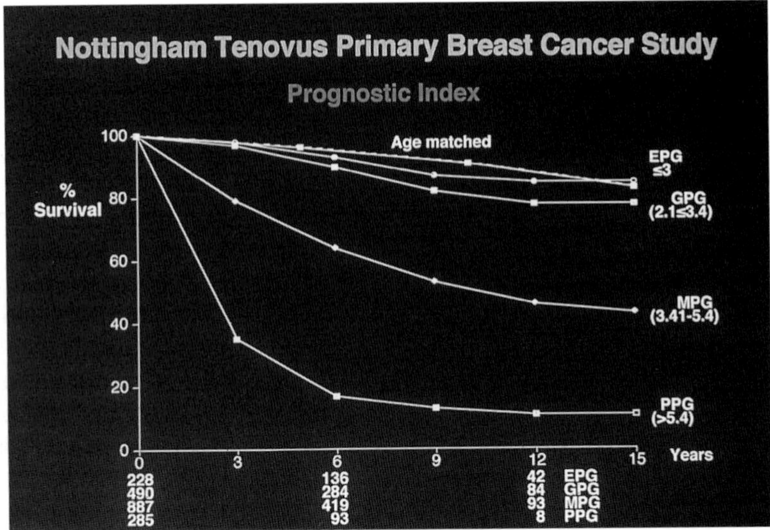

Fig. 7. Survival of patients in the Nottingham Tenovus series according to Nottingham Prognostic Index score.

- *NPI = size × 0.2 (in cm) + lymph node stage (1–3) + histological grade (1–3).*

The NPI has been subsequently confirmed prospectively [12] in studies from Nottingham and elsewhere [136] as providing robust information on patients with operable primary breast carcinoma. (Fig. 7). Cut off points of 3.4 and 5.4 are used to categorise the patients into 3 groups and to manage their disease. Women with a NPI of 3.4 or less have a good survival and receive no adjuvant systemic treatment. Those patients with a score greater than this have systemic treatment and receive hormone therapy if their tumour is oestrogen receptor positive.

Thus prognostic indices for invasive carcinoma can be devised which make use of a great deal of valuable histological prognostic data. These can be directly used to aid in clinical management and patient counselling and are more robust than utilising any one prognostic factor alone. At present the features recognised as providing robust prognostic information in invasive breast cancer (histological grade, lymph node stage and tumour size) are assessed and reported routinely by the histopathologist.

References

1. Pinder SE, Ellis IO. Atypical ductal hyperplasia, ductal carcinoma in situ and in situ atypical apocrine proliferations of the breast. Curr Diagn Pathol 1996; 3: 235–242.
2. Fisher ER, Sass R, Fisher B, Wicherham L, Paik SM. Pathologic findings from the National Surgical Adjuvant Breast Project (protocol 6). I. Intraductal carcinoma (DCIS). Cancer 1986; 57: 197–208.
3. Frykberg ER, Bland KI. Overview of the biology and management of ductal carcinoma in situ of the breast. Cancer 1994; 74: 350–361.
4. Rosai J. Borderline epithelial lesions of the breast. Am J Surg Pathol 1991; 15: 209–221.
5. Sloane JP, Ellman R, Anderson TJ et al. Consistency of histopathological reporting of breast lesions detected by screening: findings of the U.K. National External Quality Assessment (EQA) Scheme. U. K. National Co-ordinating Group for Breast Screening Pathology. Eur J Cancer 1994; 30: 1414–1419.
6. Schnitt SJ, Connolly JL, Tavassoli FA et al. Interobserver reproducibility in the diagnosis of ductal proliferative breast lesions using standardized criteria. Am J Surg Pathol 1992; 16: 1133–1143.
7. Page DL, Rogers LW. Carcinoma in situ (CIS). In: Page D, Anderson, TJ, Ed. Diagnostic Histopathology Of The Breast. New York: Churchill Livingstone, 1987: pp. 157-192.
8. Tavassoli FA, Norris HJ. A comparison of the results of long-term follow-up for atypical intraductal

hyperplasia and intraductal hyperplasia of the breast. Cancer 1990; 65: 518–529.
9. Tavassoli FA. Atypical hyperplasia: a morphologic risk factor for subsequent development of invasive breast carcinoma. Cancer Invest 1992; 10: 433–441.
10. European Community. European Guidelines for Quality Assurance in Mammographic Screening. (Second Ed.) Luxembourg: Office for Official Publications of the European Communities, 1996.
11. National Co-ordinating Committee for Breast Screening Pathology. Pathology Reporting in Breast Cancer Screening, Second Edition. NHS Breast Screening Program, 1995.
12. Galea MH, Blamey RW, Elston CW, Ellis IO. The Nottingham Prognostic Index in primary breast cancer. Breast Cancer Res Treat 1992; 22: 207–219.
13. Barr LC, Baum M. Time to abandon TNM staging of breast cancer? Lancet 1992; 339: 915–917.
14. Cutler WJ, Black MM, Mort T, Hartveit S, Freeman C. Further observations on prognostic factors in cancer of the female breast. Cancer 1969; 24: 653–667.
15. Ferguson DJ, Meier P, Karrison T et al. Staging of breast cancer and survival rates: an assessment based on 50 years of experience with radical mastectomy. JAMA 1982; 248: 1337–1341.
16. Fisher ER, Gregorio RM, Fisher B. The pathology of invasive breast cancer. A syllabus derived from findings of the national surgical adjuvant breast cancer project (protocol no 4). Cancer 1975; 36: 1–85.
17. Elston CW, Gresham GA, Rao GS et al. The Cancer Research Campaign (Kings/Cambridge) Trial for Early Breast Cancer - pathological aspects. Br J Cancer 1982; 45: 655–669.
18. Haybittle JL, Blamey RW, Elston CW et al. A prognostic index in primary breast cancer. Br J Cancer 1982; 45: 361–366.
19. Veronesi U, Galimberti V, Zurrida S et al. Prognostic significance of number and level of axillary node metastases in breast cancer. The Breast 1993; 2: 224–228.
20. Nemoto T, Vana J, Bedwani RN. Management and survival of female breast cancer: results of a national survey by the American College of Surgeons. Cancer 1980; 45: 2917–2924.
21. Fisher ER, Sass R, Fisher B et al. Pathologic findings from the National Surgical Adjuvant Project for breast cancers. X. Discriminants for Tenth year treatment failure. Cancer 1984; 53: 712–723.
22. Handley RF. Observations and thoughts on carcinoma of the breast. Proc R Soc Med 1972; 65: 437–444.
23. Blamey RW, Davies CJ, Elston CW et al. Prognostic factors in breast cancer: the formation of a prognostic index. Clin Oncol 1979; 5: 1–10.
24. Todd JH, Dowle C, Williams MR et al. Confirmation of a prognostic index in primary breast cancer. Br J Cancer 1987; 56: 489–492.
25. DuToit RS, Locker AP, Ellis IO, Elston CW, Blamey RW. Evaluation of the prognostic value of triple node biopsy in early breast cancer. Br J Surg 1990; 77: 163–167.
26. Locker AP, Ellis IO, Morgan DAL, Elston CW, Mitchell A, Blamey RW. Factors influencing local recurrence after excision and radiotherapy for primary breast cancer. Br J Surg 1989; 76: 890–894.
27. Steele RJG, Forrest APM, Gibson T. The efficacy of lower axillary sampling in obtaining lymph node status in breast cancer: a controlled randomized trial. Br J Surg 1985; 72: 368–369.
28. O'Dwyer PJ. Editorial. Axillary dissection in primary breast cancer; the benefits of node clearance warrant reappraisal. BMJ 1992; 302: 360–361.
29. Cabanes PA, Salmon RJ, Vilcoq JR. Value of axillary dissection in addition to lumpectomy and radiotherapy in early breast cancer. Lancet 1992; 339: 1245–1248.
30. Ivens D, Hoe AL, Podd TJ, Hamilton CR, Taylor I, Royle GT. Assessment of morbidity from complete axillary dissection. Br J Cancer 1992; 66: 136–138.
31. Albertini JJ, Lyman GH, Cox C, Yeatman T, Balducci L, Ku NN, Shivers S, Berman C, Wells K, Rapaport D, Shons A, Horton J, Greenberg H, Nicosia S, Clark R, Cantor A, Reintgen DS. Lymphatic mapping and sentinel node biopsy in the patient with breast cancer. JAMA 1996; 276: 1818–1822.
32. Giuliano AE, Kirgan DM, Guenther JM, Morton DL. Lymphatic mapping and sentinel lymphadenectomy for breast cancer. Ann Surg 1994; 220: 391–401.
33. Nwariaku FE, Euhus DM, Beitsch PD, Clifford E, Erdman W, Mathews D, Albores-Saavedra J, Leitch MA, Peters GN. Sentinel lymph node biopsy, an alternative to elective axillary dissection for breast cancer. Am J Surg 1998; 176: 529–531.
34. Rubio IT, Korourian S, Cowan C, Krag DN, Colvert M, Klimberg VS. Sentinel lymph node biopsy for staging breast cancer. Am J Surg 1998; 176: 532–535.
35. Borgstein PJ, Pijpers R, Comans EF, van Diest PJ, Boom RP, Meijer S. Sentinel lymph node biopsy in breast cancer: Guidelines and pitfalls of lymphoscintigraphy and gamma probe detection. J Am Coll Surg 1998; 186: 275–283.
36. Giuliano A, Jones R, Brennan M, Statman R. Sentinel lymphadenectomy in breast cancer. J Clin Oncol 1997; 15: 2345–2350.
37. Veronesi U, Paganelli G, Viale G, Galimberti V, Luini A, Zurrida S, Robertson C, Sacchini V, Veronesi P, Orvieto E, De Cicco C, Intra M, Tosi G, Scarpa D. Sentinel lymph node biopsy and axillary dissection in breast cancer: Results in a large series. J Natl Cancer Inst 1999; 91: 368–373.
38. Krag D, Weaver D, Ashikaga T, Moffat F, Klimberg VS, Shriver C, Feldman S, Kusminsky R, Gadd M,

Kuhn J, Harlow S, Beitsch P. The sentinel node in breast cancer. A multicenter validation study. New Engl J Med 1998; 339: 941–946.

39. International (Ludwig) breast cancer study group. Prognostic importance of occult axillary lymph node micrometastases from breast cancers. Lancet 1991;335:1565-1568.

40. Nasser IA, Lee AKC, Bosari S, Saganich R, Heatley G, Silverman ML. Occult axillary lymph node metastases in 'node-negative' breast carcinoma. Hum Pathol 1993; 24: 950–957.

41. Wilkinson EJ, Hause LL, Hoffman RG, Kuzma JF, Rothwell DJ, Donegan WL, Clowry LJ, Almagro UA, Choi H, Rimm AA. Occult axillary lymph node metastases in invasive breast carcinoma: characteristics of the primary tumor and significance of the metastases. Pathol Ann 1982; 17: 67–91.

42. Hainsworth PJ, Tjandra JJ, Stillwell RG, Machet D, Henderson MA, Rennie GC, McKenzie IFC, Bennett RC. Detection and significance of occult metastases in node-negative breast cancer. Br J Surg 1993; 80: 459–463.

43. McGuckin MA, Cummings MC, Walsh MD, Hohn BG, Bennett IC, Wright RG. Occult axillary node metastases in breast cancer: their detection and prognostic significance. Br J Cancer 1996; 73: 88–95.

44. Cserni G. Metastases in axillary sentinel lymph nodes in breast cancer as detected by intensive histopathological work-up. J Clin Pathol 1999; 52: 922–924.

45. Veronesi U, Galimberti V, Zurrida S, Merson M, Greco M, Luini A. Prognostic significance of number and level of axillary node metastases in breast cancer. Breast 1993; 2: 224–228.

46. Clayton F, Hopkins CL. Pathologic correlates of prognosis in lymph node positive breast carcinomas. Cancer 1993; 71: 1780–1790.

47. Fisher ER, Palekar A, Rockette H, Redmond C, Fisher B. Pathologic findings from the national surgical adjuvant breast project (protocol no. 4). V. Significance of axillary nodal micro- and macrometastases. Cancer 1978; 42: 2032–2038.

48. Huvos AG, Hutter RVP, Berg JW. Significance of axillary macrometastases and micrometastases in mammary cancer. Ann Surg 1971; 173: 44–46.

49. Rosen PP, Saigo PE, Braun DW, Weathers E, Fracchia AA, Kinne DW. Axillary micro- and macrometastases in breast cancer. Ann Surg 1981; 194: 585–591.

50. Friedman S, Bertin F, Mouriesse H, Benchabat A, Genin J, Sarrazin D, Contesso G. Importance of tumor cells in axillary sinus margins ('clandestine' metastases) discovered by serial sectioning in operable breast carcinoma. Acta Oncol 1988; 27: 483–487.

51. Hartveit F, Lilleng PK. Breast cancer: two micrometastatic variants in the axilla that differ in prognosis. Histopathology 1996; 28: 241–246.

52. de Mascarel I, Bonichon F, Coindre JM, Trojani M. Prognostic significance of breast cancer axillary lymph node micrometastases assessed by two special techniques: reevaluation with longer follow-up. Br J Cancer 1992; 66: 523–527.

53. Fisher CJ, Boyle S, Burke M, Price AB. Intraoperative assessment of nodal status in the selection of patients with breast cancer for axillary clearance. Br J Surg 1993; 80: 457–458.

54. Galimberti V, Zurrida S, Zucali P, Luini A. Can sentinel node biopsy avoid axillary dissection in clinically node-negative breast cancer patients? Breast 1998; 7: 8–10.

55. van Diest PJ, Torrenga H, Borgstein PJ, Pijpers R, Bleichrodt RP, Rahusen FD, Meijer S. Reliability of intraoperative frozen section and imprint cytological investigation of sentinel lymph nodes in breast cancer. Histopathology 1988; 35: 14–18.

56. Carter DL, Allen C, Henson DE. Relation of tumour size, lymph node status, and survival in 24,270 breast cancer cases. Cancer 1989; 63: 181–187.

57. Neville AM, Bettelheim R, Gelber RD et al. Predicting treatment responsiveness and prognosis in node-negative breast cancer. J Clin Oncol 1992; 10: 696–705.

58. Rosen PP, Groshen S. Factors influencing survival and prognosis in early breast carcinoma (TINOMO-TININO). Assessment of 644 patients with median follow up of 19 years. Surg Clin N Am 1990; 70: 937–962.

59. Beahrs OH, Shapiro S, Smart C et al. Summary report of the Working Group to review the National Cancer Institute - American Cancer Society Breast Cancer Demonstration Detection projects. J Nat Cancer Inst 1979; 62: 641–709.

60. Hartman WH. Minimal breast cancer: an update. Cancer 1984; 53: 681–684.

61. Tabar L, Duffy SW, Krusemo VB. Detection method tumour size and node metastases in breast cancers diagnosed during a trial of breast cancer screening. Eur J Cancer Clin Oncol 1987; 23: 959–962.

62. Royal College of Radiologists. QA Guidelines for Radiologists. NHSBSP Publications. 1990.

63. Greenhough RB. Varying degrees of malignancy in cancer of the breast. J Cancer Res 1925; 9: 452–463.

64. Patey DH, Scarff RW. The position of histology in the prognosis of carcinoma of the breast. Lancet 1928; i: 801–804.

65. Bloom HJG. Prognosis in carcinoma of the breast. Br J Cancer 1950; 4: 259–288.

66. Bloom HJG. Further studies on prognosis of breast carcinoma. Br J Cancer 1950; 4: 347–367.

67. Bloom HJG, Richardson WW. Histological grading

and prognosis in breast cancer. Br J Cancer 1957; 11: 359–377.

68. Contesso G, Nouriesse H, Friedman S et al. The importance of histologic grade in long-term prognosis of breast cancer: a study of 1010 patients, uniformly treated at the Institut Gustave-Roussy. J Clin Oncol 1987; 5: 1378–1386.
69. Elston CW, Ellis IO. Pathological prognostic factors in breast cancer. I. The value of histological grade in breast cancer: experience from a large study with long term follow up. Histopathology 1991; 19: 403–410.
70. Hartveit F. Prognostic typing in breast cancer. BMJ 1971; 4: 253–257.
71. Black MM, Barclay THC, Hankey BF. Prognosis in breast cancer utilising histologic characteristics of the primary tumour. Cancer 1975; 36: 2048–2055.
72. Le Doussal V, Tubiana-Hulin M, Friedman S, Hacene K, Spyratos F, Brunet M. Prognostic value of histologic grade nuclear components of Scarff Bloom Richardson (SBR). An improved score modification based on a multivariate analysis of 1262 invasive ductal breast carcinomas. Cancer 1989; 64: 1914–1921.
73. Gilchrist KW, Kalish L, Gould VE et al. Interobserver reproducibility of histopathological features in stage II breast cancer. An ECPG study. Br Cancer Res Treat 1985; 5: 3–10.
74. Fisher ER, Redmond C, Fisher B. Histological grading of breast cancer. Pathol Annu 1980; 15: 239–251.
75. Hopton DS, Thorogood J, Clayden AD, MacKinnon D. Observer variation in histological grading of breast cancer. Eur J Surg Oncol 1989; 15: 21–23.
76. Robbins P, Pinder S, de Klerk N et al. Histological grading of breast carcinomas: A study of interobserver agreement. Hum Pathol 1995; 26: 873–879.
77. Frierson HFJ, Wolber RA, Berean KW et al. Interobserver reproducibility of the Nottingham modification of the bloom and Richardson histologic grading scheme for infiltrating ductal carcinoma. Am J Clin Pathol 1995; 103: 195–198.
78. Ellis P, Whitehead R. Mitosis counting - a need for reappraisal. Hum Pathol 1981; 12: 3–4.
79. Ellis IO, Elston CW. Diagnostic Histopathology of the Breast. In: Diagnostic Histopathology of Tumours. London, Edinburgh: Churchill Livingstone, 1995.
80. Page DL, Anderson TW. Diagnostic Histopathology of the Breast. Edinburgh: Churchill Livingstone, 1987.
81. Ellis IO, Galea M, Broughton N et al. Pathological prognostic factors in breast cancer. II. Histological type. Relationship with survival in a large study with long-term follow-up. Histopathology 1992; 20: 479–489.
82. Royal College of Pathologists Working Group. Pathology Reporting in Breast Cancer Screening. J Clin Pathol 1991;44:710-725.
83. McDivitt RW, Boyce W, Gersell D. Tubular carcinoma of the breast. Am J Surg Pathol 1982; 6: 401–411.
84. Cooper HS, Patchefsky AS, Krall RA. Tubular carcinoma of the breast. Cancer 1978; 42: 2334–2342.
85. Carstens PHB, Greenberg RA, Francis D, Lyon H. Tubular carcinoma of the breast. A long term follow up. Histopathology 1985; 9: 271–280.
86. Lee BJ, Hauser H, Pack GT. Gelatinous carcinoma of the breast. Surg Gynecol Obstet 1934; 59: 841–850.
87. Clayton F. Pure mucinous carcinomas of the breast: morphologic features and prognostic correlates. Hum Pathol 1986; 17: 34–39.
88. Page DL, Dixon JM, Anderson TJ et al. Invasive cribriform carcinoma of the breast. Histopathology 1983; 7: 525–536.
89. Bloom HJG, Richardson WW, Fields JR. Host resistance and survival in carcinoma of the breast: A study of 104 cases of medullary carcinoma in a series of 1411 cases of breast cancer followed for 20 years. BMJ 1970; 3: 181–188.
90. Ridolfi RL, Rosen PP, Port A et al. Medullary carcinoma of the breast - a clinicopathological study with a ten year follow up. Cancer 1977; 40: 1365–1385.
91. Haagensen CD, Lane, Lattis R, Bodian C. Lobular neoplasia (so called lobular carcinoma in situ) of the breast. Cancer 1978;42:737-769.
92. Fisher ER, Gregorio RM, Redmond C, Fisher B. Tubulolobular invasive breast cancer: A variant of lobular invasive cancer. Hum Pathol 1977; 8: 679–683.
93. Dawson P, Ferguson DJ, Karrison T. The pathologic findings of breast cancer in patients surviving 25 years after radical mastectomy. Cancer 1982; 50: 2131–2138.
94. Dixon JM, Page DL, Anderson TJ et al. Long term survivors after breast cancer. Br J Surg 1985; 72: 445-448.
95. Anderson TJ, Lamb J, Donnan P et al. Comparative pathology of breast cancer in a randomised trial of screening. Br J Cancer 1991; 64: 108–113.
96. Ellis IO, Galea MH, Locker A et al. Early experience in breast cancer screening: emphasis on development of protocols for triple assessment. The Breast 1993; 2: 148–153.
97. Moore OS, Foote FWJ. The relatively favourable prognosis of medullary carcinoma of the breast. Cancer 1949; 2: 635–642.
98. Richardson WW. Medullary carcinoma of the breast. A distinctive tumour type with a relatively good prognosis following radical mastectomy. Br J Cancer 1956; 10: 415–423.

99. Cutler SJ, Black MM, Fried GH et al. Prognostic factors in cancer of the female breast. Cancer 1966; 19: 75–82.
100. Pedersen L, Holck S, Schiodt T. Medullary carcinoma of the breast. Cancer Treat Rev 1988; 5: 53–63.
101. Fisher ER, Kenny JP, Sass R et al. Medullary cancer of the breast revisited. Breast Cancer Res Treat 1990; 16: 215–229.
102. Dixon JM, Anderson TJ, Page DL, Lee D, Duffy SW. Infiltrating lobular carcinoma of the breast. Histopathology 1982; 6: 149–161.
103. Pereira H, Pinder SE, Sibbering DM et al. Pathological prognostic factors in breast cancer IV. Should you be a typer or grader? A comparative study of two prognostic variables in operable breast cancer. Histopathology 1995; 27: 219–226.
104. Cascinelli N, Greco M, Bufalino R et al. Prognosis of breast cancer with axillary node metastases after surgical treatment only. Eur J Cancer Clin Oncol 1987; 23: 795–799.
105. Mambo NC, Gallager HS. Carcinoma of the breast. Prognostic significance of extranodal extension of axillary nodes. Cancer 1977; 39: 2280–2285.
106. Fisher ER, Gregorio RM, Redmond C et al. Pathologic findings from the National Surgical Adjuvant Breast Project. III. The significance of extranodal extension of axillary metastases. Am J Clin Pathol 1976; 65: 439–449.
107. Hartveit F. The routine histological investigation of axillary lymph nodes for metastatic breast cancer. J Pathol 1984; 143: 187–191.
108. Sears HF, Janus C, Levy W, Hopson R, Creech R, Grotzinger P. Breast cancer without axillary metastases. Are there subpopulations. Cancer 1982; 50: 1820–1827.
109. Roses DF, Bell DA, Fotte TJ, Taylor R, Ratech H, Dubin N. Pathologic predictors of recurrence in stage I (TINOMO) breast cancer. Am J Clin Pathol 1982; 78: 817–820.
110. Bettelheim R, Penman HG, Thornton-Jones H, Neville AM. Prognostic significance of peritumoral vascular invasion in breast cancer. Br J Cancer 1984; 50: 771–777.
111. Nime FA, Rosen PP, Thaler HT, Ashikari R, Urban JA. Prognostic significance of tumour emboli in intramammary lymphatics in patients with mammary carcinoma. Am J Surg Pathol 1977; 1: 25–30.
112. Nealon TF, Nkongho A, Grossi CE et al. Treatment of early cancer of the breast (T1NOMO and T2NOMO) on the basis of histological characteristics. Surgery 1981; 89: 279–289.
113. Dawson PJ, Karrison T, Ferguson DJ. Histological features associated with long-term survival in breast cancer. Hum Pathol 1986; 17: 1015–1021.
114. Pinder S, Ellis IO, O'Rourke S, Blamey RW, Elston CW. Pathological prognostic factors in breast cancer. III. Vascular invasion: relationship with recurrence and survival in a large series with long term follow up. Histopathology 1993; 24: 41–48.
115. Orbo A, Stalsberg H, Kunde D. Topographic criteria in the diagnosis of tumor emboli in intramammary lymphatics. Cancer 1990; 66: 972–977.
116. Gilchrist KW, Gould VE, Hirschl S et al. Interobserver variation in the identification of breast carcinoma in intramammary lymphatics. Hum Pathol 1982; 13: 170–172.
117. Davis BW, Gelber R, Goldhirsh A et al. Prognostic significance of peritumoral vessel invasion in clinical trials of adjuvant therapy for breast cancer with axillary node metastases. Hum Pathol 1985; 16: 1212–1218.
118. Rosen PP, Saigo PE, Brown DW, Weathers E, DePalo A. Predictors of recurrence in stage I (TINOMO) breast carcinoma. Ann Surg 1981; 193: 15–25.
119. O'Rourke S, Galea MH, Euhuf D et al. An audit of local recurrence after simple mastectomy. Br J Surg 1994; 81: 386–389.
120. Matsukuma A, Enjoji M, Toyoshima S. Ductal carcinoma of the breast. An analysis of the proportion of intraductal and invasive components. Pathol Res Pract 1991; 87: 62–67.
121. Silverberg SG, Chitale AR. Assessment of the significance of proportion of intraductal and infiltrating tumor growth in ductal carcinoma of the breast. Cancer 1973; 32: 830–837.
122. Van Dongen JA, Fentiman IS, Harris JR et al. In situ breast cancer: the EORTC consensus meeting. Lancet 1989; ii: 25–27.
123. Schnitt SJ, Connelly JL, Harris JR et al. Pathologic predictors of early local recurrence in stage I and stage II breast cancer treated by primary radiation therapy. Cancer 1984; 53: 1049–1057.
124. Carter D, Elkins RC, Pipkin RD, Abbey H, Shepard RH. Relationship of necrosis and tumour border to lymph node metastases and 10 year survival in carcinoma of the breast. Am J Surg Pathol 1978; 2: 39–46.
125. Parham DM, Robertson AJ, Brown RA. Morphometric analysis of breast carcinoma: association with survival. J Clin Pathol 1988; 45: 517–520.
126. Fisher ER, Palikar AS, Gregario RM, Redmond C, Fisher B. Pathologic findings from the National Surgical Adjuvant project for breast cancers (protocol no.4) IV Significance of tumor necrosis. Hum Pathol 1978; 9: 523–530.
127. Underwood JC. A morphometric analysis of human breast carcinoma. Br J Cancer 1972; 26: 234–237.
128. Black R, Prescott R, Bers K et al. Tumour cellularity, oestrogen receptors and prognosis in breast cancer. Clin Oncol 1983; 9: 311–318.

129. Sistrunk WE, MacCarty. Life expectancy following radical amputation for carcinoma of the breast — a clinical and pathological study of 218 cases. Ann Surg 1922;75:61-69.

130. Parfrey NA, Doyle CT. Elastosis in benign and malignant breast disease. Hum Pathol 1985; 16: 674–676.

131. Shivas AA, Douglas JG. The prognostic significance of elastosis in breast carcinoma. J R Coll Surg 1972; 17: 315–320.

132. Masters JR, Millis RR, King RJB, Rubens RD. Elastosis and response to endocrine therapy in human breast cancer. Br J Cancer 1979; 39: 536–539.

133. Robertson AJ, Brown RA, Cree IA, MacGillivray JB, Slidders W, Beck JS. Prognostic value of measurement of elastosis in breast carcinoma. J Clin Pathol 1981; 34: 738–743.

134. Rasmussen BB, Pederson BV, Thorpe SM, Rose C. Elastosis in relation to prognosis in primary breast carcinoma. Cancer Res 1985; 45: 1428–1430.

135. Clark GM. Do we really need prognostic factors for breast cancer? Breast Cancer Res Treat 1994; 30: 117–126.

136. Brown JM, Benson EA, Jones M. Confirmation of a long-term prognostic index in breast cancer. The Breast 1993; 2: 144–147.

Breast Cancer: Diagnosis and Management
J.M. Dixon (Ed.)

CHAPTER 7

Screening: historical perspective

Stefano Ciatto

1. Introduction

Screening for breast cancer has a long history: the first controlled trial was performed in the 1960's [1] and following this many other studies were carried out, based on either a randomised or case-control design, and have provided evidence of the efficacy of screening in reducing breast cancer mortality. Based on that evidence service screening has been implemented in several regions/countries and data from these provide further evidence of the characteristics and effects of screening as a current preventive policy in population settings.

A large amount of data are now available, which allow precise definition of how and when screening should be performed. Many questions remain to be answered and require further investigation. This chapter will discuss the aspects of screening on which most experts agree as there is sufficient supporting evidence. Remaining questions and perspectives for the future will be the object of another chapter.

2. Efficacy

Several case-control and randomised studies have reported a significant reduction in breast cancer mortality in the screening arm compared to controls [2]. Today, there is no question as to the efficacy of mammographic screening, and the only scientific debate surrounds its cost–effectiveness and efficacy in different age groups.

> *Mammographic screening reduces breast cancer mortality.*

3. Cost–effectiveness

Screening costs are relatively high and the priority of mammographic screening with respect to other health care issues has been questioned [3]. Criticism has mainly surrounded the limited impact of screening in reducing overall mortality but this is to be expected as a wide variety of diseases contributes to overall mortality. Any impact on a single cause will result in a limited reduction in overall mortality. In population based European screening programmes the cost of screening a woman is between 40 and 60 US$. Estimates of the cost per year of life saved by screening varies in the literature based on different assumptions and on different scenarios. When real data from organised population based programmes are used, the costs are acceptable when compared to the cost of other public health care interventions [4].

> *The cost per year of life saved by screening is similar to that of other health care interventions.*

4. Age categories to be screened

While the benefit of screening in women aged 50 year or more is established, there remains controversy as to whether women between 40 and 49 years of age should be screened. Results in this age group have been variable in controlled trials. This is at least partially due to the lack of statistical power of single studies, none of which was specifically designed to demonstrate efficacy in the 40–49 years age subgroup. Meta-analyses, pooling data from different studies, have been used to avoid the lack of statistical power but problems have arisen. The inclusion/exclusion in meta-analyses of the Canadian NHSS study led to a long and still unresolved debate on whether this study should be included or excluded [5,6]. No concerns have arisen about including the HIP study [1] which was based on 'old fashioned', very poor quality mammography which any radiologist would now reject.

A recent overview was performed in 1996 [7]. The overall reduction in mortality from breast cancer included data from all randomised trials was 15% and did not reach statistical significance (95% C.I. 0.71–1.01). The efficacy of screening on breast cancer mortality in women aged 40–49 years is thus smaller than in older women. Many explanations have been given for such a finding. A shorter sojourn time due to a faster growth rate has been postulated for younger women [8,9] although such a finding is not confirmed by differences in survival when breast cancer patients aged 40–49 years are compared to an older age group [10]. The finding that interval cancers are not more aggressive than screen detected cancers [11] suggests that the failure of screening to detect cancers is mostly due to a lack of sensitivity rather than to faster cancer growth. A lower sensitivity of mammograpy due to a higher frequency of radiologically dense breasts in younger women has been recognised for some time in symptomatic women [12] and seems a more reasonable explanation for problems screening younger women, where smaller cancers may be easily masked by dense breast tissue.

A complication with the interpretation of screening efficacy in younger women is that data are generally calculated for women age 40–49 'at entry' in the trial, and not 'at diagnosis'. In fact some women entering the study before the age of 50 years will have their cancer detected at screening beyond the age of 50. As the open question is "shall we screen before the age of 50 years?", censoring cases detected over the age of 50 years would seem appropriate. This does however introduce another bias, as these are some cancers which in the absence of screening would have been detected over the age of 50 years, but are detected before age 50 [13].

Whatever the explanation, the evidence on the efficacy of screening women aged 40–49 years is insufficient to support population based screening in this age group and for this reason screening in Europe is generally restricted to women between the ages of 50 to 69 [14]. In view of a moderate reduction in mortality in recent overviews, in younger women mammography on an individual basis can be difficult to refuse if requested by women aged 40–49 years, providing that information is given about the possible problems with mammography which includes false reassurance and potential delayed self-referral if symptoms are present.

New prospective studies of screening women aged 40–49 years are ongoing and will provide further evidence on screening efficacy and will influence recommendations for population based screening in this age group. Major difficulties in such studies include ensuring sufficient numbers of women are enrolled and reducing the contamination in the control arm (it is difficult to avoid provision of mammography if requested in women aged 40–49 years in some countries). The study will need to run for 10 years before complete data are available.

Mortality reduction by screening varies according to age: 25–30% for women over 50 years, and approximately 15% for women aged 40–49 years.

5. Rescreening interval

The optimal interval between screens is not yet established. A significant reduction in breast cancer mortality has been achieved with different screening intervals, which vary from one to three years. A rescreening interval of one year will maximise sensitivity but will increase costs (often to an unacceptable level with respect to existing resources) and reduce the specificity of the screening programme. Whether an increase of sensitivity will translate into increased efficacy or will simply change the ratio of screen detected to interval cancers is still unclear. A rescreening interval of 2–3 years is currently recommended [2,14] for women aged over 50 years as this balances costs and sensitivity. The 3-year rescreening interval in the national screening program in the UK was adopted as the available resource did not allow a shorter interval; an excess of interval cancers in the third year has been observed [15,16].

A rescreening interval of one year has been suggested for prospective studies of women between 40 and 49 years of age to maximise sensitivity and efficacy.

> *The choice of screening interval is a compromise between costs and sensitivity. EC guidelines recommend an interval of 2–3 years for women over 50 years of age.*

6. Number of mammographic views

A single oblique view was adopted in the Swedish two countries trial which reported a significant reduction in mortality [17]. The reduction in costs using a single view instead of two views is limited, and is approximately 20%. At the same time reduced sensitivity (increased masking effect of breast density) and increased recall rate (asymmetries due to superimposed densities which might be clarified by an additional view) have been reported [18,19]. Currently, two views are recommended at the first screen [14], whereas a single oblique view is adopted most frequently at repeat screens, when a previous mammogram is available for comparison, and is reasonable in subjects with fibrous–fatty breasts in whom the risk of a masking effect by parenchymal densities is lower.

> *Two view (oblique + cranio-caudal) mammography is the standard for the first screening examination.*

7. Single or double reading

Double reading is recommended to maximise sensitivity. Increased sensitivity in the range of 5% has been demonstrated [20], together with a small but acceptable increase in recall rates. Double reading is valuable in training and useful when using readers of limited experience if an expert reader is also involved. With expert readers the cost/benefit ratio are limited as the costs of double reading and the increased recall rate is counterbalanced by only a small increase in sensitivity, if any, which is limited to cases missed due to fatigue or loss of attention. The impact of double reading should be constantly monitored in a screening programme, as its value may change over time.

> *Double reading offers an opportunity for training of inexperienced readers and is recommended as it produces an increase in sensitivity.*

8. Monitoring screening programmes

The efficacy of mammographic screening has been demonstrated in prospective studies where dedicated (mostly full-time) expert operators have worked in centres with a high quality performance. This maximises screening efficacy.

As service screening is implemented on a regional or national basis, screening is de-cen-

Table 1. Parameters of screening performance recommended by the EC guidelines [14]

Performance parameter	Acceptable	Desirable
a. Initial screening		
– participation rate	60%	> 75%
– recall rate	< 7%	< 5%
– cancer detection rate × 100 women screened	3 × IR [a]	> 3× IR [a]
– invasive cancers < 10 mm × 100 invasive ca. detected		25%
– benign open biopsy rate × 1000 women screened	< 5	< 4
– benign/malignant biopsy ratio	< 2 to 1	< 1 to 1
b. Subsequent screening		
– participation rate	60%	> 75%
– recall rate	< 5%	< 3%
– cancer detection rate × 100 women screened	1.5 × IR [a]	
– invasive cancers < 10 mm × 100 invasive ca. detected		25%
– benign open biopsy rate × 1000 women screened	< 3.5	< 2
– benign/malignant biopsy ratio	< 1 to 1	< 0.5 to 1

[a] IR = expected incidence rate in the absence of screening.

tralised to peripheral units, using existing mammographic facilities. The latter may not be adequate for screening purposes, and reaching satisfactory performance standards (especially high mammographic quality and adequate training of operators) may require considerable extra resources. Screening performance may not equal that of dedicated screening centres, and doubts have arisen about cost/effectiveness of population screening. Great attention must be paid to the quality assurance of any screening programme, to identify problems and ensure proper action is taken to solve them.

Direct assessment of screening efficacy is not possible, as any reduction in mortality takes years to be seen and evaluation through a case-control design requires a large population observed for a long period. Surrogate early indicators of screening efficacy have been suggested [11], which can now be used to monitor a newly implemented programme from its inception. To ensure the quality of screening performance such indicators should be regularly monitored. Guidelines for quality assurance of mammographic screening have been issued by the European Community [14] and provide indicators for quality control of incidence and detection, cytopathology, pathology, and mammography. Standards for indications of screening performance are summarised in Table 1.

References

1. Shapiro S, Venet W, Strax P, Venet L. Periodic screening for breast cancer; the Health Insurance Plan Project and its sequelae 1963–86. Baltimore: Johns Hopkins University Press, 1988.
2. Wald N, Chamberlain J, Hackshaw A. Report of the European Society for Mastology: Breast Cancer Screening Evaluation Committee. Breast 1993; 2: 209–216.
3. Baum M. The breast screening controversy. Eur J Cancer 1996; 32: 9–11.
4. De Koning HJ, Coebergh JWW, van Dongen JA. Current controversies in Cancer: Is mass screening for breast cancer cost-effective? Eur J Cancer 1996; 32: 1835–1844.
5. Mettlin CJ, Smart CR. The Canadian National Breast Screening Study: an appraisal and implications for early detection policy. Cancer 1993; 72: 1461–1465.
6. Baines CJ. The Canadian National Breast Screening Study: a perspective on criticism. Ann Intern Med 1994; 120: 326–334.
7. Report of the Organizing Committee and Collaborators of the Falun Meeting. Int J Cancer 1996;68:693-699.
8. Chen HH, Duffy SW, Tabar L. A Markov chain method to estimate the tumor progression rate from preclinical to clinical phase, sensitivity and positive predictive value for mammography in breast cancer screening. Statistician 1996; 45: 307–317.

9. Tabar L, Fagerberg G, Chen HH et al. Efficacy of breast cancer screening by age: new results from the Swedish two-county trial. Cancer 1995; 75: 2507–2517.
10. Ciatto S, Cecchini S, Iossa A, Grazzini G. T category and operable breast cancer prognosis. Tumori 1989; 75: 18–22.
11. Paci E, Ciatto S, Buiatti E et al. Early indicators of efficacy of breast cancer screening programmes. Results of the Florence District programme. Int J Cancer 1990; 46: 198–202.
12. Ciatto S. Breast cancer diagnosis. In: Veronesi U (ed.), Clinical Oncology, Breast Cancer, Baillière Tindall, London, 1988, pp. 155-174.
13. De Koning HJ, Boer R, Warmerdam PG et al. Quantitative interpretation of age-specific mortality reductions from the Swedish breast cancer screening trials. J Natl Cancer Inst 1995; 87: 1217–1223.
14. European Guidelines for Quality Assurance in Mammography Screening. De Wolf CJM, Perry N, eds. Brussels/Luxembourg: European Commission 1996.
15. Woodman CBJ, Threfall AG, Boggis CRM, Prior P. Is the three year breast screening interval too long? Occurrence of interval cancers in NHS Breast Screening Programme's North Western region. Br Med J 1995; 310: 224–228.
16. Day N, McCann J, Camilleri-Ferrante C. Monitoring interval cancers in breast screening programmes: The East Anglian experience. J Med Screen 1995; 2: 180–185.
17. Tabàr L, Fagerberg G, Duffy SW, Day N. The swedish two county trial of mammographic screening for breast cancer. Recent results and calculation of benefit. J Epidemiol Commun Health 1989; 43: 107–112.
18. Bryan S, Brown J, Warren R. Mammography screening: An incremental cost effectiveness analysis of two views versus one view procedures in London. J Epidemiol Commun Health 1995; 49: 70–78.
19. Anttinen I, Pamilo M, Rolha M et al. Baseline screening mammography with one versus two views. Eur J Radiol 1989; 9: 241–243.
20. Ciatto S, Rosselli Del Turco M, Morrone D et al. Independent double reading of screening mammograms. J Med Screen 1995; 2: 99–101.

Breast Cancer: Diagnosis and Management
J.M. Dixon (Ed.)

CHAPTER 8

Screening: current view

Andrew Evans

1. Introduction

The Swedish controlled trials have shown that mammographic screening can produce a 28% to 31% reduction in population mortality from breast cancer in women aged 50–69 [1]. Recent attention has concentrated on refining the screening and assessment processes, establishing, measuring and maintaining the quality of national programmes and defining the utility of screening women under 50 and over 69 years of age.

Screening by mammography reduces mortality by 28–31% in women aged 50–69 years.

2. Number of views

Two view mammography without physical examination is the screening modality of choice at both prevalent and incident screens. The use of two views especially when using a high film density is associated with increased small invasive cancer detection compared to single view mammography (> 50% increase in invasive cancers < 10 mm in size) [2,3]. Invasive lobular cancers are particularly likely to be visible on one view only [4]. The use of two views results in lower recall rates and increased specificity [5,6]. The cost saving associated with fewer assessments largely offsets the extra costs of using two views when compared with a single view [5].

Two view mammography should be performed at every screening episode.

3. Mammography reading

Double reading of mammograms results in a 5% increase in cancer detection [7]. If double reading is performed without consensus this should intuitively result in a decrease in the specificity of screening and increase costs, while double reading with consensus should increase both sensitivity and specificity. In practice radiologist double read differently depending on whether consensus is used or not and this results in similar recall rates using either method [8]. Double reading by radiologists is expensive when considering the relatively modest increase in cancer detection. Alternative strategies include the use of trained radiographers as second readers or the use of computer aided diagnosis (CAD). It has been demonstrated that with suitable training radiographers can read films with the same specificity and sensitivity as radiologists [9]. Full field digital mammography is now at an advanced stage of development and is likely to be in widespread use by 2005. This will facilitate the routine use of CAD. At present, CAD has been shown to be successful at identifying and classifying microcalcification [10]. CAD of other mammographic abnormalities is proving more difficult. A recent study comparing single reading of a test set with single reading with CAD prompting showed no significant benefit when films were read by experienced screening radiologists [11].

Double reading with arbitration is the ideal method of mammographic screening.

4. Frequency of screening

The majority of screening programmes advocate a screening frequency of 2 years for women over the age of 50. The ideal screening frequency is governed by the lead time of screening (the average time by which a diagnosis of cancer is advanced by screening) which can be calculated from screening cancer detection and interval cancer rates. The lead time of screening for women over 50 is just over 3 years [12]. Interval cancer rates have been shown to rise steeply in the third year after screening reaching over 80% of the naturally occurring incidence [13]. Interval cancer rates have been shown to be commoner in younger women [14]. These facts support the need for a 2-year screening interval, particularly in women aged 50–60 years. Provisional findings from the UKCCCR frequency trial (SE Pinder, personal communication) show that annual screening finds smaller tumours compared with a 3 yearly interval but that annual screening did not influence nodal involvement. This result has caused the cost effectiveness of 2 yearly screening to be questioned. There are however problems with the design and results of the frequency trial: one centre did not stage the axilla and annual screening was with single view mammography only, which decreases the sensitivity for small invasive cancer detection.

2 years is the ideal screening interval for women over 50 but may not be as cost effective as 3 yearly screening.

5. Hormone replacement therapy and mammographic screening

It has been known for some time that Hormone Replacement Therapy (HRT) increase the mammographic background density in about a third of women [15]. It is also widely known that cysts and fibroadenomas continue to develop and grow in post menopausal women taking HRT and that focal/asymmetric increases in mammographic density frequently occur [16]. Only in recent years has attention been given to quantifying the effect HRT may have on the sensitivity and specificity of mammographic screening. A recent study has suggested that at incident round screening women are more likely to recalled and that recall is less specific in women on HRT, particularly if HRT was commenced since the previous screen [17]. A study from Scotland has also demonstrated an adverse effect of HRT on the sensitivity of mammographic screening. Women taking HRT at the time of screening were more than twice as likely to present with an interval cancer within 1 year of screening [18]. Recent conflicting results of the effect of HRT on mammography [19,20] are likely to be due to different HRT preparations and routes of administration having different effects on the breast. It has been shown that continuous combined HRT use has a much higher relative risk of causing new mammographic density than cyclically combined or oestradiol only HRT [21]. The recent study showing no HRT effect on mammographic sensitivity or specificity contained many women using topical HRT preparations only and very few women on continuous combined HRT preparations [19].

HRT reduces the sensitivity of and specificity of screening mammography.

6. Screening women under the age of 50

Recent results from the Malmo and Gothenburg randomised controlled trials have shown statistically significant breast cancer mortality reductions of 36% and 45% in women randomised when under 50 years of age [22,23]. Meta-analysis of all randomised controlled trials, even when the Canadian Trial is included confirm a statistically significant benefit of 16%. Both the Gothenburg and Malmo studies used a short screening interval and 2 views in the majority of patients. Both trials also used modern mammographic technique and had a large number of screening rounds. Unfortunately both studies did not screen the control group at 50 so at least part of the mortality benefit may have been due to screening of the study group when they were over 50 even though they were randomised under 50 years of age. The UK randomised age trial which is currently in progress screens women aged 40–42 and no screening of the study group will occur after the age of 48 until both the control and study group are screened when aged 50–53. When the results of this study are known the data will be clean and not contaminated by over 50s screening in one arm of the study. The UK age trial consists of annual mammographic screening of the study group but unfortunately only single view mammography is being used.

The Malmo and Gothenburg studies confirmed earlier findings that the lead time of screening in women under 50 is short (2.26 years). The incidence of cancer in women in their 40s is half that seen in women in their 50s yet recall rates are similar in both age groups indicating a decrease in the specificity of recall when screening younger women are compared to women over 50 years of age.

This means that although screening younger women almost certainly reduces breast cancer mortality, to achieve this reduction, it is necessary to screen younger women twice as often (every 18 months) to find only half the number of cancers. This indicates that screening women under 50 will be much less cost effective than screening women over the age of 50. This needs to be balanced against the greater life years gained per breast cancer death prevented, and the benefit to society of preventing breast cancer deaths in women who are still likely to have dependant children. It does however seem unlikely that national breast screening programmes will obtain government funding for screening of women under 50 years of age.

> *Screening women under 50 reduces breast cancer mortality but may not be cost effective.*

7. Screening women over 70 years of age

No randomised controlled trials of mammographic screening have shown a mortality benefit in women over 70 years of age. However, none of the randomised trails were specifically designed to look at the effect of screening in this age group, and few women in this age group were included in Swedish trials. A recent non-randomised trial of women aged 68–83 suggested a 40% mortality reduction but the findings were not statistically significant [24]. A pilot project in the UK has shown that women aged 65–69 have a high uptake rate and that cancer detection rates are high [25]. It should therefore be concluded that screening women over 70 has not been shown to be of benefit rather than screening women over 70 is of no benefit.

> *There is no conclusive evidence that screening women over 70 is effective.*

8. The assessment process

Modern screen reading assessment aims to make a non-operative diagnosis in all women with a significant screen detected abnormality. Women without a significant abnormality or a benign abnormality can then be promptly returned to routine screening, while women with proven malignancy can make informed choices concerning treatment options. Screening assessment should be carried out by a multi-disciplinary team consisting of a radiologist, clinician, radiographer, breast care nurse and pathologist [26]. Management decisions should be taken at a multidisciplinary meeting.

Recent technological advances have improved screening assessment dramatically. This has resulted in less benign surgical biopsies, improved preoperative diagnosis of malignancy and reduced short term recall rate. The most significant changes have been the introduction of automated gun core biopsy [27] and vacuum assisted biopsy devices [28], prone and upright digital stereotactic equipment and improved breast ultrasound equipment. 14g image guided core biopsy of screen detected abnormalities should enable a preoperative diagnosis of invasive cancers in over 95% of cases. Diagnosing DCIS non-operatively is more difficult [29]. Although the use of digital stereotactic equipment now means that specimen X-ray confirmation of correct sampling can be obtained in $> 85\%$ of cases using prone or upright equipment, it is common for cores from DCIS lesions to be reported as atypical ductal hyperplasia (ADH) or suspicious of malignancy. This is because insufficient abnormal ductal tissue has been obtained to enable the pathologist to make a definitive diagnosis. The use of a vacuum assisted mammotomy device has been shown to increase calcification yield, decrease ADH core results from DCIS and decrease the need for repeat biopsy [28,30]. Vacuum assisted mammotomy is well tolerated but is significantly more expensive than core biopsy. Although the mammographic lesion is often removed at mammotomy requiring the placement of a metallic localisation clip, residual malignancy is usually present pathologically. Mammotomy should therefore be viewed as a diagnostic, not a therapeutic tool.

High frequency ultrasound (13 Mhz) enables the detection of nearly all screen detected mass lesions. Although the use of grey scale features and power doppler has improved benign/malignant differentiation [31,32], all discrete solid lesions recalled for assessment should undergo image guided core biopsy. High frequency ultrasound and power doppler examination now enables the visualisation of an abnormality at the site of most screen detected calcification clusters. Ultrasound can sometimes be used to biopsy such lesions.

Breast MRI is occasionally useful in defining the extent of screen detected cancer [33], especially if other methods are unhelpful or contradictory.

High quality ultrasound and image guided biopsy enables sensitive and specific screening assessment.

9. Quality assurance

The only way to maintain a uniformly high quality breast screening service is through a central system of quality assurance (QA). Such a QA system should set minimum and expected standards [34], monitor performance and encourage excellence. Failure to meet standards should lead to prompt action such as retraining or changes in policy followed by re-evaluation. Monitoring performance is of no value if poor performance is tolerated and goes uncorrected. Monitoring performance and maintaining expertise is easier in large units which work to agreed protocols.

QA should incorporate all facets of the screening process including equipment, radiography, radiology, pathology, surgery, breast care nursing and administration.

In the UK screening units undergo regular visits by a multidisciplinary team which evaluate all aspects of the units performance [35]. Some of QA standards of the UK NHS Breast Screening Programme are listed in table 2.

References

1. Nystrom L, Rutqvist L, Wall S et al. Breast cancer screening with mammography; overview of Swedish randomised trials. Lancet 1993; 341: 973–978.
2. Blanks RG, Moss SM, Wallis MG. Use of two view mammography compared with one view in the detection of small invasive cancers: Further results from the

National Health Service breast screening programme. J Med Screen 1997; 4: 98–101.
3. Young KC, Wallis MG, Ramsdale. Mammographic film density and detection of small breast cancers. Clin Radiol 1994;49:461-465.
4. Cornford EJ, Wilson ARM, Athanassiou E. Mammographic features of invasive lobular and invasive ductal carcinoma of the breast: a comparative analysis. Br J Radiol 1995; 68: 450–453.
5. Wald N, Murphy P, Major P, Parkes C, Townsend J, Frost C. UKCCCR multicentre randomised controlled trial of one and two view mammography in breast cancer screening. BMJ 1995; 311: 1189–1193.
6. Moss S, Michell M, Patnick J, Johns L, Blanks R, Chamberlain J. Results from the NHS breast screening programme 1990-1993. J Med Screen 1995; 2: 186–190.
7. Ciatto S, Turco MD, Morrone D et al. Independent double reading of screening mammograms. J Med Screen 1995; 2: 99–101.
8. A comparison of cancer detection rates achieved by breast cancer screening programmes by number of readers, for one and two view mammography: results from the National Health Service breast screening programme. J Med Screen 1998;5:195-201.
9. Pauli R, Hammond S, Cooke J, Ansell J. Radiographers as film readers in screening mammography: an assessment of competence under test and screening conditions. Br J Radiol 1996; 69: 10–14.
10. Jiang Y, Nishikawa RM, Wolverton DE et al. Malignant and benign clustered microcalcifications: Automated feature analysis and classification. Radiology 1996; 198: 671–678.
11. Thurfjell E, Thurfjell MG, Egge E, Bjurstam N. Sensitivity and specificity of computer assisted breast cancer detection in mammographic screening. Acta Radiol 1998; 39: 384–388.
12. Tabar L, Fagerberg G, Chen H, Duffy S, Gad A. Screening for breast cancer in women aged under 50: mode of detection, incidence, fatality, and histology. J Med Screen 1995; 2: 94–98.
13. Woodman CBJ, Threlfall AG, Boggis CRM, Prior P. Is the three year breast screening interval too long? Occurrence of interval cancers in NHS breast screening programmes north western region. BMJ 1995; 310: 224–226.
14. Threlfall AG, Woodman CBJ, Prior P. Breast screening programme: should the interval between tests depend on age. Lancet 1997; 349: 472.
15. Crlak D, Wong CH. Mammographic changes in post menopausal women undergoing hormone replacement therapy. Am J Roentgenol 1993; 161: 1177–1183.
16. Doyle GJ, McLean L. Unilateral increase in mammographic density with hormone replacement therapy. Clin Radiol 1994; 49: 50–51.
17. Litherland JC, Evans AJ, Wilson ARM. The effect of hormone replacement therapy on recall rate in the National Health Breast Screening Programme. Clin Radiol 1997; 52: 276–279.
18. Litherland JC, Stallard S, Hole D, Cordiner C. The effect of hormone replacement therapy on the sensitivity of screening mammograms. Clin Radiol 1999; 54: 285–288.
19. Thurfjell EL, Holmberg LH, Persson. Screening mammography: sensitivity and specificity in relation to hormone replacement therapy. Radiology 1997;203:339-341.
20. Rosenberg RD, Hunt WC, Williamson MR et al. Effects of age, breast density, ethnicity, and estrogen replacement therapy on screening mammographic sensitivity and cancer stage at diagnosis: review of 183,134 screening mammograms in Albuquerque, New Mexico. Radiology 1998; 209: 511–518.
21. Persson I, Thurfjell E, Holmberg L. Effect of estrogen and estrogen-progestin replacement regimens on mammographic breast parenchymal density. J Clin Oncol 1997; 15: 3201–3207.
22. Bjurstam N, Bjorneld L, Duffy SW et al. The Gothenburg Breast Screening Trial. First results on mortality, incidence and mode of detection for women ages 39-49 years at randomization. Cancer 1997; 80: 2091–2099.
23. Reduced breast cancer mortality in women under age 50: Updated results from the Malmo mammographic screening program. JNCI Monograph 1997;22:63-68.
24. Van Jijck JA, Verbeek AL, Beex LV et al. Breast cancer mortality in a non-randomised trial on mammographic screening in women over age 65. Internat J Cancer 1997; 70: 164–168.
25. Rubin G, Garvican L, Moss S. Routine screening of women aged 65-60 for breast cancer screening: results of first year of pilot study. BML 1998; 317: 388–389.
26. Ellis I, Galea M, Locker A et al. Early experience in breast cancer screening: emphasis on development of protocols for triple assessment. The Breast 1993; 2: 148–153.
27. Parker SH, Burbank F, Jackman RJ et al. Percutaneous large-core breast biopsy: a multi-institutional study. Radiology 1994; 193: 359–364.
28. Burbank F. Stereotactic breast biopsy of atypical ductal hyperplasia and ductal carcinoma in situ lesions: improved accuracy with directional, vacuum-assisted biopsy. Radiology 1997; 202: 843–847.
29. Liberman L, LaTrenta LR, Van Zee KJ et al. Stereoactic core biopsy of calcifications highly suggestive of malignancy. Radiology 1997; 203: 673–677.
30. Philpotts LE, Shaheen NNA, Lange RC, Lee CH. Comparison of rebiopsy rates after stereotactic core needle biopsy of the breast with 11-gauge vacuum suction probe versus 14-gauge needle and automatic gun. AJR 1999; 172: 683–687.

31. Cilotti A, Bagnolesi P, Moretti M et al. Comparison of the diagnostic performance of high-frequency ultrasound as a first or second-line diagnostic tool in non-palpable lesions of the breast. Eur Radiol 1997; 7: 1240–1244.
32. Raza S, Baum JK. Solid breast lesions: evaluation with power Doppler. Radiology 1997; 203: 164–168.
33. Boetes C, Mus RD, Holland R et al. Breast tumours: comparative accuracy of MR imaging relative to mammography and ultrasound for demonstrating extent. Radiology 1995; 197: 743–747.
34. NHSBSP Quality assurance guidelines for radiologists. May 1997.
35. NHSBSP Guidelines on quality assurance visits. October 1998.

Breast Cancer: Diagnosis and Management
J.M. Dixon (Ed.)

CHAPTER 9

Genetics of breast cancer

Michael Steel

1. Introduction

1.1. Familial breast cancer in perspective

Many of to-day's surgeons were taught at medical school that there is no hereditary element in common cancers; that the genetic contribution to oncology is confined to rare familial syndromes like retinoblastoma, neurofibromatosis and familial adenomatous polyposis. Even now, it is not unusual to meet families affected by multiple cases of breast cancer, who have had to overcome scepticism and outright resistance from their doctors, before obtaining access to specialist cancer genetics services.

In reality, evidence that family history can be a significant risk factor for breast cancer (and for colorectal, prostate, ovarian and most other common cancers) has been available for decades; in some cases, for over a century. It is rather difficult to see why this has so often been overlooked because obvious 'breast cancer families' are not excessively rare and the clustering of cases among close relatives has certainly been recognised by the family members themselves. Nevertheless, multi-case families of the kind described by Broca in 1866 (Fig. 1) [1] account for only a modest proportion of the genetic contribution to breast cancer and discrepancies between the findings of epidemiological and classical genetic studies in this field have perhaps served to muddy the waters.

2. Population data

Since the 1980's, many population-based surveys have been undertaken to assess the incidence of breast cancer among women whose mothers, sisters and/or more distant relatives have had the disease, comparing it with the rate among control women (without affected relatives) from the same population group [2–6]. In virtually all cases, the findings agree that as the number of affected relatives increases, so does breast cancer risk. With few exceptions, they also show that the earlier the onset of disease in a blood relative, the greater the risk to other family members. Table 1 documents the generally accepted ranges for lifetime risk amplification, given specified family histories. Though much of the data derives from the USA or Northern Europe, where the incidence of breast cancer is high, the proportional effect of a positive family history appears to be the same in Mediterranean countries and in the Far East where, overall, breast cancer is much less common [7]. The strength of the familial associations in all populations studied suggests that genetic factors are of major importance in some 5–10% of breast cancers, particularly in cases with early onset.

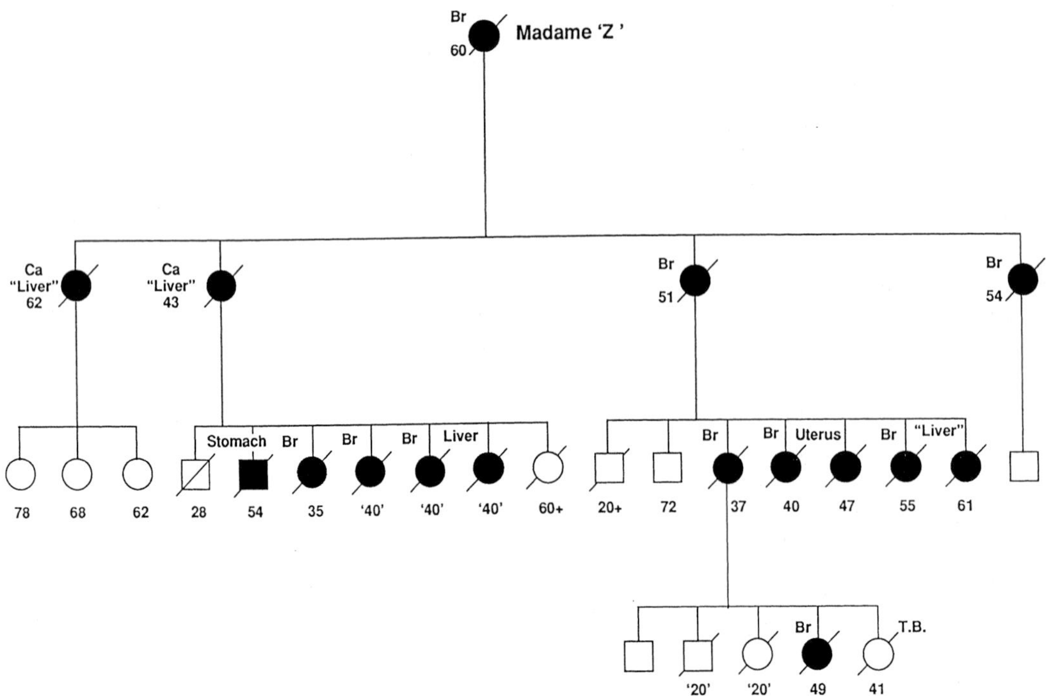

Fig. 1. A breast cancer family recorded by the French physician Paul Broca in 1866. This was probably his own wife's family. Filled symbols indicate cases of cancer. Round symbol = female, square = male. Diagonal slash = deceased. 'Br' = breast. Figures under each symbol indicate that individual's age at death or at the time of Broca's study. Note that, in addition to the concentration of affected family members, breast cancer clearly tended to occur at an early age.

Table 1. Lifetime risks of breast cancer according to family history

Relatives with breast cancer	Increase in risk
Mother or sister diagnosed under 35	2.5×
Mother or sister diagnosed over 35	1.5–2.0×
2 first degree relatives, average age at diagnosis <55	2.5–3.0×
2 first degree relatives, average age at diagnosis >55	1.5–2.0×
3 first or second degree relatives diagnosed < 60	2.5–4.0×
4 first or second degree relatives diagnosed at any age	4.0–5.0×
Male first degree relative affected at any age	2.5× (female), 6× (male)

These estimates of risk apply to a woman under 35. An older woman will have lived through some of the risk period so her chances of carrying a 'breast cancer gene' will have diminished.

A first degree relative is mother, sister or daughter; second degree is grandmother, aunt or niece. It is implied that, where there are several affected relatives, they are on the same side of the family. A relative with bilateral breast cancer counts as two cases for calculating genetic risk.

The presence of one or more cases of ovarian cancer among relatives, in addition to breast cancers, greatly increases risk estimates. Cases of prostate, bowel, pancreatic, thyroid, endometrial and laryngeal cancers on the same side of the family, particularly if they are of early onset, may also indicate a higher risk of familial breast cancer.

Strictly speaking, we should make allowance for absolute family size. Two affected sisters may be less significant in a sibship of twelve than in a sibship of three. However, since the figures listed above are intended only as approximations, they take no account of unaffected relatives. Several computer programmes have been devised that make more sophisticated risk estimates from complete family trees.

- *Less than 5% of breast cancers occur within 'obvious' families with multiple early-onset tumours but genetic factors make* **some** *contribution to many more cases.*

3. Segregation analysis

The population-based approach documents and quantifies the familial clustering of breast cancer but does not formally identify the explanation as genetic rather than environmental and certainly does not specify any underlying genetic mechanism (single gene or polygenic, dominant or recessive). These issues can only be addressed by the process known as 'segregation analysis', which estimates the probability that an observed distribution of disease could have arisen through any given mechanism. In practice, segregation analysis has usually been applied to collections of unusually large multi-case breast cancer families because this increases the statistical power of the exercise. It does, however, introduce an element of selection, which means that the findings may not apply, unmodified, to breast cancer in general.

According to the great majority of segregation studies [8], the most plausible basis for familial clustering of breast cancer is a single gene effect, transmitted as a Mendelian autosomal dominant but with limited penetrance. In practical terms, this means that the cancer risk is inherited from only one parent — either mother or father — but that development of cancer is not inevitable among those who inherit (and transmit) the 'cancer gene' (Fig. 2).

- *The genetic contribution to breast cancer is mainly via single genes, inherited as autosomal dominants but with limited penetrance. Not all carriers will develop cancer.*

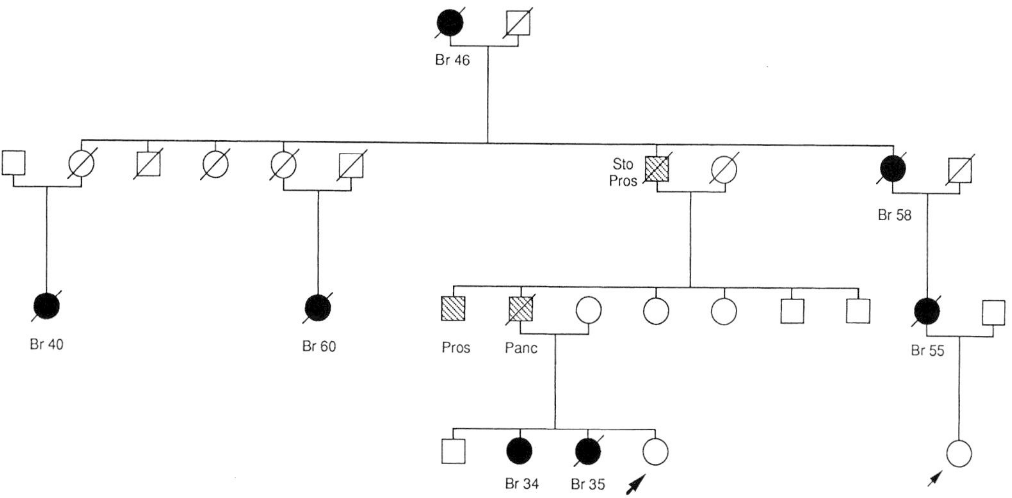

Fig. 2. A more typical breast cancer family. Two members of this family (arrowed) independently sought advice about possible genetic risks. One knew that her two sisters had developed the disease in their thirties. The other knew that her mother and maternal grandmother had been affected. On extending the family tree they were found to have a common great grandmother (who had died from breast cancer) and there were two further cases of breast cancer in their parents' generation. Note that genetic predisposition to breast cancer appears to have been transmitted by two successive males, both of whom developed epithelial cancers (not breast), as did a third male in the same branch of the family. The breast cancer patients who died at age 40 and 60 years seem to have inherited the risk through their mothers, who were unaffected. These mothers may illustrate non-penetrance of the trait. Alternatively, one or both of the daughters may have developed sporadic breast cancer, unconnected with any genetic risk.

Table 2. Familial breast cancer syndromes

Gene implicated (location)	Syndrome and its features
p53 (Chromosome 17p)	Li-Fraumeni syndrome. Early onset breast cancer in females plus (both sexes) sarcomas, brain tumours, adrenal carcinomas, usually in childhood.
PTEN (Chromosome 10q)	Cowden's syndrome. Skin hamartomas, breast cancer, bowel polyps (may be juvenile), thyroid adenomas/carcinomas, meningiomas.
BRCA1 (Chromosome 17q)	Early onset breast cancer, substantial risk of ovarian cancer. Real (but smaller) risk of bowel and prostate cancers.
BRCA2 (Chromosome 13q)	Early onset breast cancer, including risk in males. Risk of ovarian cancer but lower than for BRCA1. Excess of endometrial, bowel, bladder, renal, laryngeal, pancreatic cancers. Probably also increased risk of lymphomas and melanomas.

4. Gene hunting

That outcome would be consistent with just one gene accounting for all multi-case breast cancer families. However the same result would have been obtained if a different gene were implicated in each family. There could, therefore, be many 'breast cancer genes', each liable to mutation at many different sites and all displaying autosomal dominant transmission. Clearly, the challenge was to map and identify these genes.

There are essentially two routes to locate an unknown gene. The first is the 'candidate gene' approach. From a knowledge of the biology of the associated disease or perhaps by extrapolation from an animal model, an inspired guess is made and one or more genes are selected for intensive analysis, in the hope of finding mutations that coincide with the disorder. In familial breast cancer, the p53 gene was targeted in this way and was indeed found to underlie a very small number of cases, usually within the Li-Fraumeni cancer family syndrome (Table 2) [9,10].

The second, and more commonly followed, route is genetic linkage mapping. This makes use of highly variable human DNA sequences whose chromosomal locations are known with great precision. These markers are used to trace the transmission of chromosomal segments through the generations of a family. Because there is crossing-over and interchange of material between paired chromosomes at meiosis, in the formation of germ cells (sperm and egg), only DNA sequences that lie physically very close together on the same chromosome will stay together through the generations. The object of linkage mapping is to ask, "within a family affected by a single-gene disorder, what DNA markers are consistently inherited along with the disease?" The answer should provide a chromosomal map location for the causal gene. It then becomes a manageable task to search for genes within that chromosomal region and ultimately to find one that shows mutations in affected individuals.

Advances in molecular biology techniques in recent years have increased the power of genetic linkage analysis but in the late 1980's and early 1990's there were formidable obstacles to its use in mapping breast cancer genes. Since breast cancer is common, it is very likely that any large multi-case family will include one or more affected individuals with sporadic (i.e. non-genetic) disease. Furthermore, given that penetrance of the trait is less than 100%, some mutation carriers will be unaffected. Hence the match between disease and gene will be far from perfect. Even worse, in order to generate convincing evidence of linkage, it is usually necessary to combine data from several affected families. Should there be more than one gene causing similar patterns of familial breast cancer, then combining data from different families may obscure, rather than confirm, a map location. All of these problems (among others) were, in fact, encountered and the successful identification of even a few breast cancer genes must be regarded as something of a triumph. The effort required pooling of resources (particularly DNA samples from very large families with many cases of early onset breast cancer) from many centres throughout the world [11]. That consortium activity is continuing with the intention of finding further relevant genes.

- *Some important breast cancer genes remain to be discovered and international collaborative studies of affected families are ongoing.*

4.1. Known breast cancer genes

BRCA1, the first human breast cancer locus identified through linkage analysis, was mapped to the long arm of chromosome 17 in 1990 [12]. By 1994 the gene itself had been characterised so that mutations in some affected families could be demonstrated [13]. It is a very large gene, distributed in 24 exons over 100 kilobases of DNA, encoding a protein of 1,863 amino acids which appears to have multiple functions. The protein is normally found in the nucleus and forms complexes with other proteins involved in DNA repair after radiation-induced damage [14].

More than two hundred distinct BRCA1 mutations have been identified in breast cancer families. They include very large deletions, splice site changes (eliminating an exon from the transcript), frame-shifts caused by small insertions or deletions, and single base substitutions (usually introducing a stop codon and thereby truncating the protein product) [15].

BRCA2 was mapped and isolated by following up the clue that breast cancer families with an affected male generally do not show linkage to the BRCA1 locus [16]. Male breast cancer is rare (about 1% of the female incidence) but is significantly over-represented among multi-case families (where the other cases are predominantly female). From a collection of such families, linkage to a site on chromosome 13 was established and BRCA2 was identified in little over a year [17]. It is an even larger gene than BRCA1, with 27 coding exons and a protein product of over 3000 amino acids. Like BRCA1 it probably performs a number of functions, is normally confined to the nucleus and appears to be involved in repair of damaged DNA [18]. Although important in the discovery of BRCA2, male cases are not seen in most breast cancer families attributable to this gene, while a few have subsequently been identified in BRCA1 mutation families. Over one hundred separate mutations have been found in BRCA2 and, as in the case of BRCA1, most cause truncation of the product.

In contrast to some other large genes such as APC, new mutations in BRCA1 and BRCA2 are exceptionally rare and many have evidently been passed down, unaltered, through successive generations over several centuries [19]. Equally curious is the fact that neither BRCA1 nor BRCA2 commonly undergoes somatic mutation in breast or other tumours. Despite their roles in familial breast cancer and some similarity in putative function, there is very little sequence homology between BRCA1 and BRCA2 and the two proteins evidently do not interact directly [18].

PTEN (also known as MMAC) is the gene implicated in Cowden's syndrome and in a number of other rare genetic disorders characterised by a remarkable range of signs and symptoms [20]. The gene, located on chromosome 10q, has nine exons. Mutations can occur at any position and, as yet, no clear correlation has been established between the site or nature of the mutation and the clinical consequences [21].

- *Four human 'breast cancer' genes are known, affecting different families:*
  BRCA1 on chromosome 17;
  BRCA2 on chromosome 13;
  p53 on chromosome 17;
  PTEN on chromosome 10.
- *Individually, mutations in any of these genes are rare in most populations.*
- *Molecular screening for mutations in any of these genes is currently difficult.*

5. Contribution of known genes to familial breast cancer

Throughout the USA and most of Europe, germline mutations in BRCA1 and BRCA2 are each believed to occur in just over one per thousand of the population [22,23]. Mutations in p53 and PTEN are probably much less common. Collectively, therefore, these genes could not account for 5–10% of all breast cancers. This leaves a disconcerting gap between the estimates of the genetic component in breast cancer derived from epidemiological studies and the aggregate frequency of known breast cancer genes.

The gap becomes even wider when it is appreciated that a very substantial percentage of women carrying BRCA1 or BRCA2 mutations never develop cancer — i.e. penetrance of the trait is much less than 100%. Irrefutable evidence has followed the discovery of certain recurrent 'founder' mutations in genetically homogeneous groups, notably Ashkenazi Jews, among whom specific mutations, denoted by BRCA1 185delAG (deletions of two base pairs adenine and guanine at position 185 in the base pair sequence) and BRCA2 6174delT, are each carried by more than 1% of the population [24]. Similarly, in Icelanders, BRCA2 999del5 outnumbers all other BRCA1 and BRCA2 mutations [25]. In such settings it is possible to screen the general population, rather than selected families. It emerges that many inherited BRCA1 or BRCA2 mutations are found in the absence of any striking family history of cancer [26]. This has now been confirmed in a survey of apparently sporadic breast cancer patients in the UK [23]. It therefore appears that, in those unusual families where breast cancer incidence is extremely high, there may be additional factors that compound the risks associated with BRCA1 or BRCA2 mutations.

- *In some population groups (e.g. Ashkenazi Jews, Icelanders) particular mutations in BRCA1 or BRCA2 may be relatively common. Special molecular screening procedures may be appropriate for them.*

In both BRCA1 and BRCA2 mutation-carriers there is an increased risk of epithelial ovarian cancer (usually of serous type) but this seems to apply to some families more than others, perhaps depending on the site and nature of the mutation. Information on this point is not yet sufficiently firm to use the molecular findings as a guide to management (for example in reaching a decision about prophylactic oophorectomy). As indicated in Table 2, several other types of cancer show increased incidence in BRCA1 — and especially BRCA2 — families.

- *In many 'breast cancer' families there is also an increased risk of other tumours, notably ovarian cancer.*

6. Unknown breast cancer genes

There are almost certainly more genes, yet to be identified, that account for some very obvious family clusters of breast cancer. Because BRCA1 and BRCA2 mutations are associated with certain characteristic clinical and pathological patterns in multi-case families (Tables 2 and 3), the search for 'BRCA3' is concentrating on families where these features are absent — i.e. on families with relatively late-onset breast cancer of low pathological grade and oestrogen-receptor positive, with neither affected males nor cases of ovarian cancer.

Even if that search is successful, it is clear that the gap between the incidence of genetically-determined breast cancer, (as derived from epidemiological surveys) and the frequency of BRCA1, BRCA2 and 'BRCA3', in most populations, cannot be bridged. Much of the genetic contribution to breast cancer must come from rather common genes — perhaps combinations of very common genes — that confer relatively modest increases in cancer risk [23]. Indeed it can be argued that genes conferring a two- or three-fold increase in lifetime risk may be implicated in the majority of breast cancers. Since they will

Table 3. Features of BRCA1- and BRCA2-associated breast cancers [32]

Age of onset:	About 50% under age 50 (compared with only ~ 20% of sporadic cases). But can present at any age.
Risk of second primary (breast):	4–6% per year.
Oestrogen receptor status:	Majority negative, regardless of age at diagnosis.
Pathological type:	Almost always invasive ductal (no special type).
Pathological grade:	Tend to be high (usually 3), with high mitotic index. BRCA1 tumours show absence of tubule formation and other features that may lead to classification as 'medullary' or 'atypical medullary' (particularly for BRCA1 tumours)

While the above features apply to BRCA1 and BRCA2 tumours as a group, there are always exceptions and pathological appearances, oestrogen receptor status etc. cannot be taken as strong evidence for or against involvement of one of these genes in any individual case.

not generate obvious multi-case families, segregation analysis and genetic linkage are not likely to prove efficient techniques for locating genes of this type.

7. Implications for breast cancer genetics

Except for those communities where founder mutations are genuinely common, family history will, for the immediate future, be the mainstay of genetic risk assessment. In clinical practice, cancer genetics services (counselling and surveillance) are generally becoming available to women whose lifetime risk of breast cancer is (statistically) increased two and a half times above that of the general population. Among these will be a subset — perhaps a quarter — with really strong family histories and in these families the chances of identifying a mutation in BRCA1 or BRCA2 will be around 50%. As the family history becomes less striking, so the chances of finding a mutation in a known gene decline. Until molecular and/or other screening techniques become much more efficient, it is inevitable that the majority of women eligible to attend breast cancer family clinics are not at increased risk. For example, in the UK and many other countries, at least two thirds of patients who develop breast cancer under the age of thirty-five carry no mutation in a known breast cancer gene. Their first degree relatives cannot be distinguished from the minority whose affected mother or sister is the only indication of a BRCA1 or BRCA2 mutation in that family.

Conversely, if most BRCA1 or BRCA2 mutations confer a 50–60% lifetime risk of breast cancer (in line with recent estimates) then a substantial proportion of carriers will have no affected mother or sister and, on the basis of family history alone, are unlikely to be recognised as requiring special surveillance. This problem of unrecognised genetic risk is exacerbated by the trend towards smaller families.

8. Gene–environment interactions

Where penetrance of a genetic trait is less than 100%, questions arise about factors that may modify the gene effect. Many environmental or 'lifestyle' influences are known to be relevant to sporadic breast cancer and there is much current interest in assessment of their role in familial cases. As yet, there are few hard data. Until proved otherwise, it is assumed that prolonged use of hormonal contraception or of hormone replacement therapy will increase still further a pre-existing genetic risk, though there is evidence that 'the pill' reduces the risk of ovarian cancer among BRCA1 mutation-carriers [27]. Trials of Tamoxifen as a preventive agent in women at risk of breast cancer have given conflicting results to date. An American study showed a clear protective effect [28] but UK and Italian trials do not yet show any benefit [29,30]. The picture may become clearer with longer follow-up. Only general advice about diet — encouraging the eating of fresh fruit and vegetables — can be given, and that mainly because of the broad health benefits rather than proven efficacy in familial breast cancer.

- *Environmental factors probably modify inherited breast cancer risk. Dietary and hormonal influences may be important but hard evidence is awaited.*

The possible role of 'modifying genes' must also be considered. There are well-recognised genetic variations, for example, in biochemical pathways that regulate the production or action of hormones and in enzymes that detoxify environmental carcinogens [31]. Genes involved in these functions might be among the factors compounding the risks associated with BRCA1 and BRCA2 mutations or could even be low-penetrance breast cancer genes in their own right.

- *Other genes may interact with BRCA1 or BRCA2 to modify cancer risk. If these modifiers can be identified it may be possible to give more accurate risk estimates to individual carriers of BRCA1 or BRCA2 mutations.*

9. Conclusions

The hope that finding breast cancer genes would resolve all the problems of familial breast cancer has not been fulfilled. The known genes are large and contain a bewildering array of mutations. Not all carriers of known mutations develop cancer and not all inherited cancer risk is accounted for by known mutations. Identification of those at increased genetic risk is a very inexact process, with much room for improvement in both sensitivity and specificity. Nevertheless much more progress has been made in the past ten years than in all the preceding centuries and optimism about significant advances over the next ten years is not out of place.

References

1. Broca P. Traite des Tumeurs. Paris: P. Asselin, 1866.
2. Lynch HT, Guirgis HA. Genetics and breast cancer. New York: Van Norstrand Reinhold, 1981.
3. Schneider NR, Williams WR, Chaganti RSK. Genetic epidemiology of familial aggregation of cancer. Adv Cancer Res 1986; 47: 1–36.
4. Bain C, Speizer FE, Rosner B et al. Family history of breast cancer as a risk indicator for the disease. Am J Epidemiol 1980; 11: 301–308.
5. Iselius L, Slack J, Littler M, Morton NE. Genetic epidemiology of breast cancer in Britain. Ann Hum Genet 1991; 55: 151–159.
6. Colditz GA, Willett WC, Hunter DJ et al. Family history, age and risk of breast cancer. JAMA 1993; 270: 338–343.
7. Steel CM. Cancer of the breast and female reproductive tract. In Rimoin DL, Connor JM, Pyeritz RE, Eds. Emery and Rimoin's Principles and Practice of Medical Genetics, 3rd Edition. New York: Churchill Livingstone, 1996, pp. 1503-1523.
8. Steel CM, Thompson AM, Clayton J. Genetic aspects of breast cancer. Br Med Bull 1991; 47: 504–518.
9. Malkin D, Li FP, Strong LC et al. Germ-line p53 mutations in a familial syndrome of breast cancer, sarcomas and other neoplasms. Science 1990; 250: 1233–1238.
10. Srivastava S, Zou Z, Pirollo K et al. Germ-line transmission of a mutated p53 gene in a cancer-prone family with Li-Fraumeni syndrome. Nature 1990; 348: 747–749.
11. Easton D, Bishop DT, Ford D et al. Genetic linkage analysis in familial breast and ovarian cancer: results from 214 families. Am J Hum Genet 1993; 52: 678–681.
12. Hall JM, Lee MK, Newman B et al. Linkage of early onset familial breast cancer to chromosome 17q21. Science 1990; 250: 1684–1689.
13. Miki Y, Swensen J, Shattuck-Eidens DJ et al. A strong candidate for the breast and ovarian cancer susceptibility gene BRCA1. Science 1994; 266: 66–71.
14. Paterson JWE. BRCA1: a review of structure and putative functions. Dis Markers 1998; 13: 261–274.
15. Couch FJ, Weber BL. Mutations and polymorphisms in the familial early onset breast cancer (BRCA1) gene. Breast cancer information core. Hum Mutat 1996; 8: 8–18.
16. Stratton MR, Ford D, Neuhausen S et al. Familial male breast cancer is not linked to the BRCA1 locus on chromosome 17q. Nat Genet 1994; 7: 103–107.
17. Wooster R, Bignell J, Lancaster J et al. Identification of the breast cancer susceptibility gene BRCA2. Nature 1995; 378: 789–792.
18. Gayther SA, Ponder BAJ. Clues to the function of

the tumour susceptibility gene BRCA2. Dis Markers 1998; 14: 1–8.
19. Szabo C, King M-C. Population genetics of BRCA1 and BRCA2. Am J Hum Genet 1997; 60: 1013–1020.
20. Starink TM. The Cowden syndrome: a clinical and genetic study in 21 patients. Clin Genet 1986; 29: 222–233.
21. Liaw D, Marsh DJ, Li J et al. Germline mutations of the PTEN gene in Cowden disease, an inherited breast and thyroid cancer syndrome. Nat Genet 1997; 16: 64–67.
22. Ford D, Easton DF, Peto J. Estimates of the gene frequency of BRCA1 and its contribution to breast and ovarian cancer incidence. Am J Hum Genet 1995; 57: 1457–1462.
23. Peto J, Collins N, Barfoot R et al. Prevalence of BRCA1 and BRCA2 gene mutations in patients with early-onset breast cancer. J Natl Cancer Inst 1999; 91: 943–949.
24. Roa BB, Boyd AA, Volcik K, Richards CS. Ashkenazi Jewish population frequencies for common mutations in BRCA1 and BRCA2. Nat Genet 1996; 14: 185–187.
25. Thorlacius S, Olafsdottir G, Trygvadottir L et al. A single BRCA2 mutation in male and female breast cancer families in Iceland with varied cancer phenotypes. Nat Genet 1996; 13: 117–119.
26. Struewing JP, Hartge P, Wacholder S et al. The risk of cancer associated with specific mutations of BRCA1 and BRCA2 among Ashkenazi Jews. N Engl J Med 1997; 336: 1401–1408.
27. Narod SA, Risch H, Moslehi R et al. Oral contraceptive use reduces the risk of hereditary ovarian cancer. N Engl J Med 1998; 339: 424–428.
28. Fisher B. National Surgical Adjuvant Breast and Bowel Project breast cancer prevention trial: a reflective commentary. J Clin Oncol 1998; 17: 1632–1638.
29. Powles TJ. Re Tamoxifen for prevention of breast cancer: report of the National Surgical Adjuvant Breast and Bowel Project P-1 study. J Natl Cancer Inst 1999; 91: 730.
30. Bruzzi P. Tamoxifen for the prevention of breast cancer: important questions remain unanswered and existing trials should continue. BMJ 1998; 316: 1181–1182.
31. Friend S. Breast cancer susceptibility testing: realities in the post-genomic era. Nat Genet 1996; 13: 16–17.
32. Lakhani SR, Jacquemeier J, Sloane JP et al. Multifactorial analysis of differences between sporadic breast cancers and cancers involving BRCA1 and BRCA2 mutations. J Natl Cancer Inst 1998; 90: 1138–1145.

Breast Cancer: Diagnosis and Management
J.M. Dixon (Ed.)

CHAPTER 10

High risk women: the role of histology

David L. Page, Jean F. Simpson and Roy A. Jensen

1. Introduction

Concepts and terminology of lesions implicating cancer risk found within otherwise benign breast biopsies remain controversial for some clinicians. However, there is a broad consensus [1–3], and this presentation will focus on widely accepted terms and their clinical utility. The validity of these terms derives from linkage of histologic criteria to epidemiologic outcome studies that demonstrate breast cancer risk implications. Several epidemiologic studies using the same or similar criteria have found quite similar results [4–8], verifying this approach.

2. Histological risk lesions

There are three elements of importance in this linkage of histopathologic criteria to epidemiologically verified clinical outcomes:

(1) Diagnoses of specifically defined atypical hyperplasia (AH, lobular [ALH] or ductal [ADH] types) avoid over-diagnosis of carcinoma in situ of lobular or ductal types, thereby avoiding unnecessary surgery or radiotherapy and reducing anxiety linked to the term 'carcinoma'.

(2) It is recognized that the great majority of women who undergo biopsy do not have any or only a slight increase in risk of later breast cancer [9]. Prior to these studies of histologic risk factors, it was widely believed that any woman undergoing a surgical breast biopsy had an increased risk of later breast cancer [10].

(3) Perhaps of least importance, each of the specifically defined patterns of AH is associated with about a 4 times increased risk of cancer in the ensuing 10–15 years after biopsy. There is increasing understanding of some differences between ALH and ADH, although each recognizes a similar risk when diagnosed between the ages of 35 to 55 years [11].

The absolute risk of developing cancer in women with atypical hyperplasia after age 40 to 45 is approximately 10% in the first 15 years. The risk of cancer is at any site in either breast.

Considering that all women, particularly in high risk geographic areas such as North America and most of Europe are at a significant risk of developing breast cancer, increased risk indicators in these regions must be understood to be relative, comparing a woman or group of women to similar women. Many have accepted that a risk double that of comparable women is a useful boundary for guiding clinical concern and management. Indeed, even a doubling of risk has little personal impact when viewed in short time segments such as the next year: for example, most women in

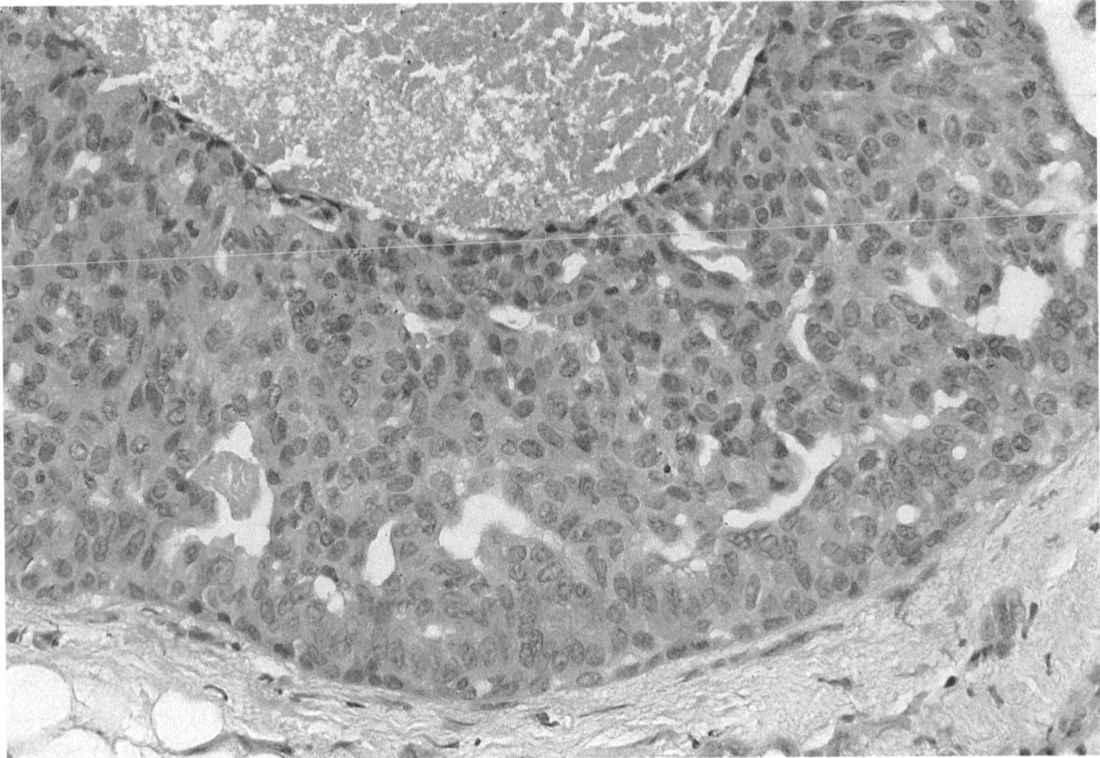

Fig. 1. Hyperplasia of usual type (florid) without atypia. Note well developed slit-like lumina between the cells and variability of the individual cells. The central material may be the result of cellular necrosis but may also be the result of cell secretions. In any case, this detritus does not change the diagnosis from ordinary florid hyperplasia without atypia.

high risk geographic areas have approximately a 1 in 1,000 risk of developing invasive breast cancer in the next twelve months after their 40th birthday [9]. If the risk continues to accrue in the ten years between the 40th and 50th birthdays, the overall, actual risk for that period of 120 months is about 1.5% [9,12]. The translation of relative risks (the concept to be discussed below and usually presented) to these absolute risks is expressed by Dupont and Plummer [13] and is part of the 'Gail Model' [14] that has been used to choose patients for breast cancer prevention trials.

The magnitude of risk, the period of time it is operative, and the locality of the risk are extremely important concepts. All of the lesions discussed here indicate a general increase in risk with subsequent cancers appearing anywhere in either breast (Table 1). Also, we believe that the term "high risk" should not be used unless the risk approaches at least 4–5 times that of the general population. Looking at Table 1 with the various levels of relative risk, it is clear that the highest (small DCIS and LCIS) risk lesion recognizes a magnitude of relative risk of about 10 times. The absolute risk for the moderately increased risk lesions (ALH and ADH) is approximately 10% in specific settings, e.g. for women recognized at time of biopsy to have these lesions in their mid-forties followed over the next ten to fifteen years. This absolute risk of about 10% for the development of invasive breast cancer compares to women without these lesions who have a 2–2 1/2 percent absolute risk over the same period of time. Other papers review these numbers in greater detail which essentially is an exercise of transferring relative risk determined in epidemi-

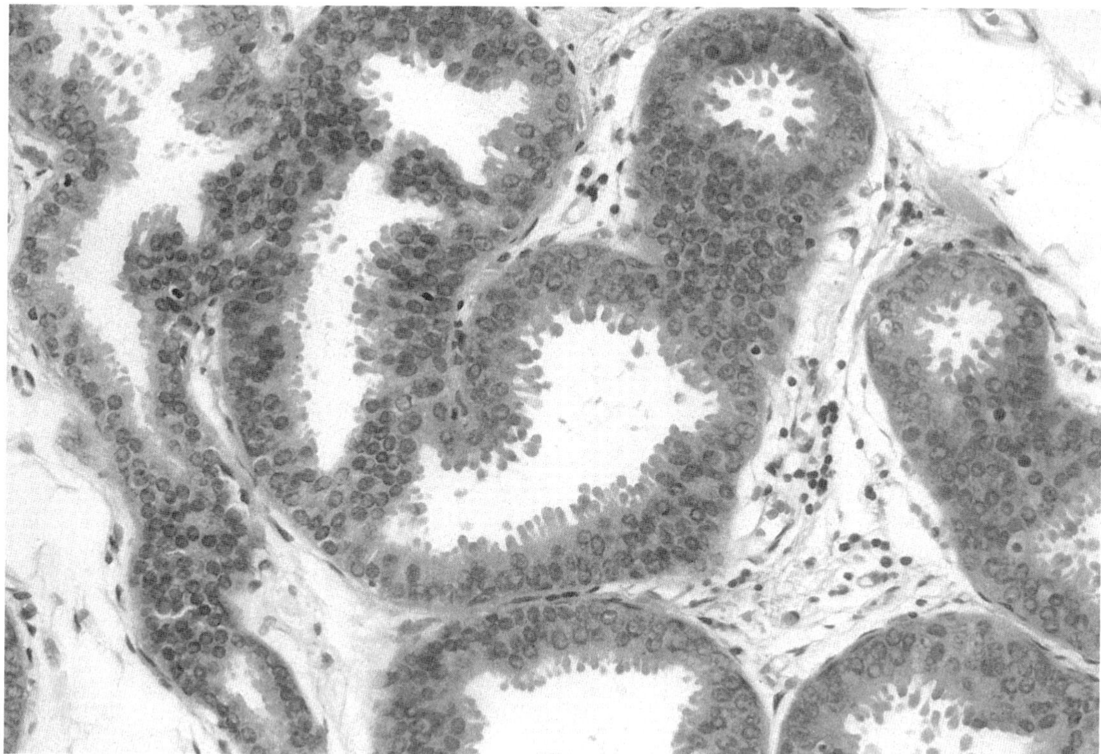

Fig. 2. Columnar alteration of cells in a lobular unit. These cells have attained cytologic characteristics of concern (nuclear enlargement, hyperchromasia and pattern similarity). However, when confined to enlarged lobular units without characteristic patterns of atypical hyperplasia, these changes have little significance with regard to cancer risk.

ologic follow-up studies to absolute risk figures for counselling individual women. It is mandatory to recognize that these risks have only been verified in the age group of women between 35 and 55–60. Women who are either younger or older probably have a different risk. Younger women do not have any verified risk because so few have been biopsied and found to have ADH or ALH lesions. There is a continuing confirmation of slight differences between ADH and ALH, in particular a decreasing risk for ALH after age 55 [7].

Atypical ductal and lobular hyperplasias are associated with a 4–5 times elevated relative risk of developing breast cancer compared to an age matched population without this condition.

Risk can be expressed in different ways. If women in their 40s have a cancer risk of 2% over the next 15 years then a relative risk of 1.5 or a 50% of elevation of risk produces a 3% absolute risk over this 15 year time period.

Beginning in the mid 1980s it became widely accepted that the majority of women undergoing benign breast biopsy have no increased risk of subsequent breast cancer, and that a minority of these women may be identified at some risk of later breast cancer on the basis of histologic patterns of disease, [7,15,16] (Table 1). Any study that has looked at hyperplastic or proliferative lesions within the breast has identified an increased risk for women who have such lesions. However, with the exception of the uncommon specifically

Table 1. Relative risk for invasive breast carcinoma based on pathologic examination of benign breast tissue

No increased risk
Women with the following lesions are at no greater risk for invasive breast carcinoma than women who have not had a breast biopsy:
- Adenosis (other than sclerosing adenosis)
- Duct ectasia
- Fibroadenoma without complex features [a]
- Fibrosis
- Mild hyperplasia without atypia [b]
- Ordinary cysts (gross or microscopic)
- Simple apocrine change or papillary apocrine change

Slight increased risk (1.5–2.0 times)
Women with the following lesions have a slightly increased risk for invasive breast carcinoma compared with women who have not had a breast biopsy:
- Fibroadenoma with complex features [a]
- Moderate or florid hyperplasia without atypia
- Sclerosing adenosis [c]
- Solitary papilloma without coexistent atypical hyperplasia [d]
- Radial scars/complex sclerosing lesions, multiple [e]

Moderately increased risk (4.0–5.0 times)
Women with the following lesions have a moderately increased risk for invasive breast carcinoma compared with women who have not had a breast biopsy:
- Atypical ductal hyperplasia [b,f]
- Atypical lobular hyperplasia

Markedly increased risk (8.0–10.0 times)
Women with the following lesions have a high risk for invasive breast carcinoma compared with women who have not had a breast biopsy:
- Ductal carcinoma in situ [g]
- Lobular carcinoma in situ

[a] Fibroadenomas are associated with relative risks of the range of 1.7, but patients without proliferative epithelial changes around the fibroadenoma or a positive family history do not appear to have increased risk [18] with the exception of one study which showed a relative risk of cancer for complex fibroadenomas approaching three times. Complex fibroadenomas contain cysts larger than 3 mm, sclerosing adenosis, epithelial calcifications and/or papillary apocrine changes.
[b] Mild epithelial hyperplasia without atypia of usual pattern is identified when the epithelial proliferation is 3–4 cell layers thick (as opposed to the usual 2) and does not bridge or distend the lumen. More extensive changes are called moderate and florid where distension and filling of the lumens is seen [24]. Irregularity of nuclear size pattern and placement characterize these lesions. Atypical ductal hyperplasia has some but not all of the features of ductal carcinoma in situ and includes the features noted in the text [25,32].
[c] Well developed examples of sclerosing adenosis are associated with a relative risk at the level of about 1.7 with or without associated hyperplasia and are likely to be higher when combined with specifically defined lesions of atypical ductal or atypical lobular hyperplasia [38].
[d] Although not specifically and precisely defined, it seems that papilloma by itself is associated with a similar risk to that of the moderate and florid hyperplasia. Atypia within a papilloma may indicate a greater risk for local development of later invasive carcinomas [17].
[e] A recent study [3] indicates that radial scar lesions when multiple are associated with an elevated risk of breast cancer and this is further elevated when other increased risk lesions are also present.
[f] Most of the studies which have follow-up beyond 7–8 years have found risk for atypical hyperplasia in the range of 4–5 times. This risk is operative over a period of 10–15 years with women and after that time, it probably approaches the risk of women of their own age who have not had a history of atypia. Marshall et al. reported a higher risk in premenopausal women with atypical lobular hyperplasia which reduced remarkably after menopause or age 55 [7].

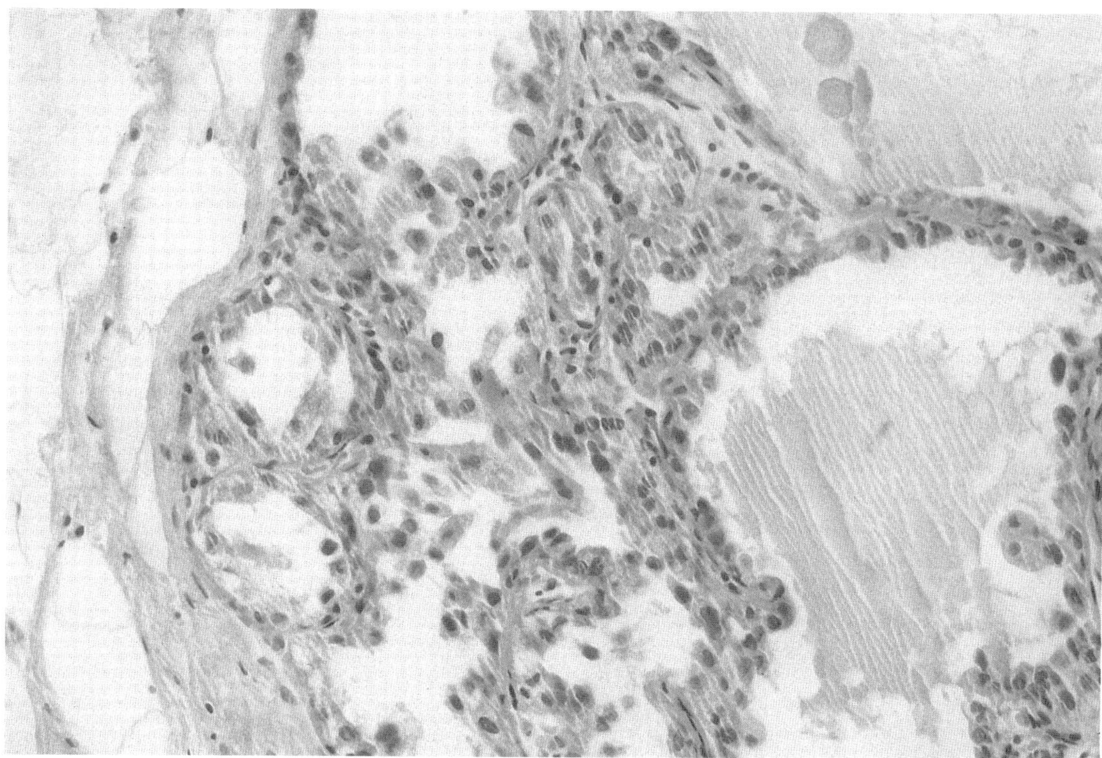

Fig. 3. Hypersecretory change with nuclear atypia. There is foamy cytoplasm and secretion of milk-like material into slightly distended lumins with "budding out" of nuclei with enlargement. These changes may be associated with atypical ductal hyperplasia and ductal carcinoma in situ elsewhere, but if confined to lobular units have little clinical significance except that the secreted material may form benign calcifications seen on mammography.

defined atypical hyperplasias, none of these obtain clinical significance, i.e. is greater than a doubling of risk compared to similar women in the same population. Careful definition of atypical hyperplastic lesions has identified high risk groups of women [7,11,15–17]. Fibroadenomas have also been approached in the same way noted above by trying to stratify the 1.4–1.7 times increased risk found for all fibroadenomas. A single large study indicates elements occurring within the fibroadenomas identify women at a slight increased risk for breast cancer (Figs. 1–3), leaving approximately 70% of women with fibroadenomas without an increased risk [18] (Table 2).

The majority of women undergoing biopsy for benign breast conditions have no significantly increased risk of breast cancer.

In situ "lobular" lesions present special problem with terminology. This is because recently performed studies in fairly large groups of pa-

[g] This category refers specifically to small, less than 5–7 mm and usually by definition, greater than 2–3 mm in overall size. In one study, 28 women with these low grade lesions who received no treatment after biopsy had a relative risk of 9.1 times over a period of 25 years compared to age matched women in the general population. Allowing for the fact that some of these lesions might have been removed by biopsy, it is the local occurrence of invasive carcinoma in almost 50% of these women in a premammographic era [29] together with the data from Betsill et al. [33] that gives us the best natural history of these lesions.

Table 2. Features associated with fibroadenoma that elevate breast cancer risk

(1) Complex histology: any combination of apocrine change, cysts, sclerosing adenosis and/or calcification (epithelial-related).
(2) Usual patterns of hyperplasia, moderate and florid in surrounding parenchyma (similar to women without fibroadenoma).
(3) History of breast cancer in first degree relative (slightly higher than the history of cancer in a relative alone).
This leaves somewhat over 70% of women with fibroadenoma with no demonstrable increase of cancer risk.

Note, most of the risk is probably expressed 10–15 years following diagnosis [18].

tients from the NSABP, Columbia University and Nashville [19,20] have shown that lesser changes within lobular units indicate a lesser risk than fully developed lesions which may are considered as lobular carcinoma in situ [19,21–23]. In this way, the term "carcinoma" can be avoided in the majority of these cases and these lesions. Thusly, they must be understood to mean increased risk only. Some accept lobular neoplasia as a clinically useful term encompassing all of these changes. While it is understandable as a broad category, it still includes the concept of the higher risk lesions. The term 'atypical lobular hyperplasia' is preferred as it cannot be understood to mean other than a risk indicator, and provides the clinician with more specific information on the magnitude of the risk.

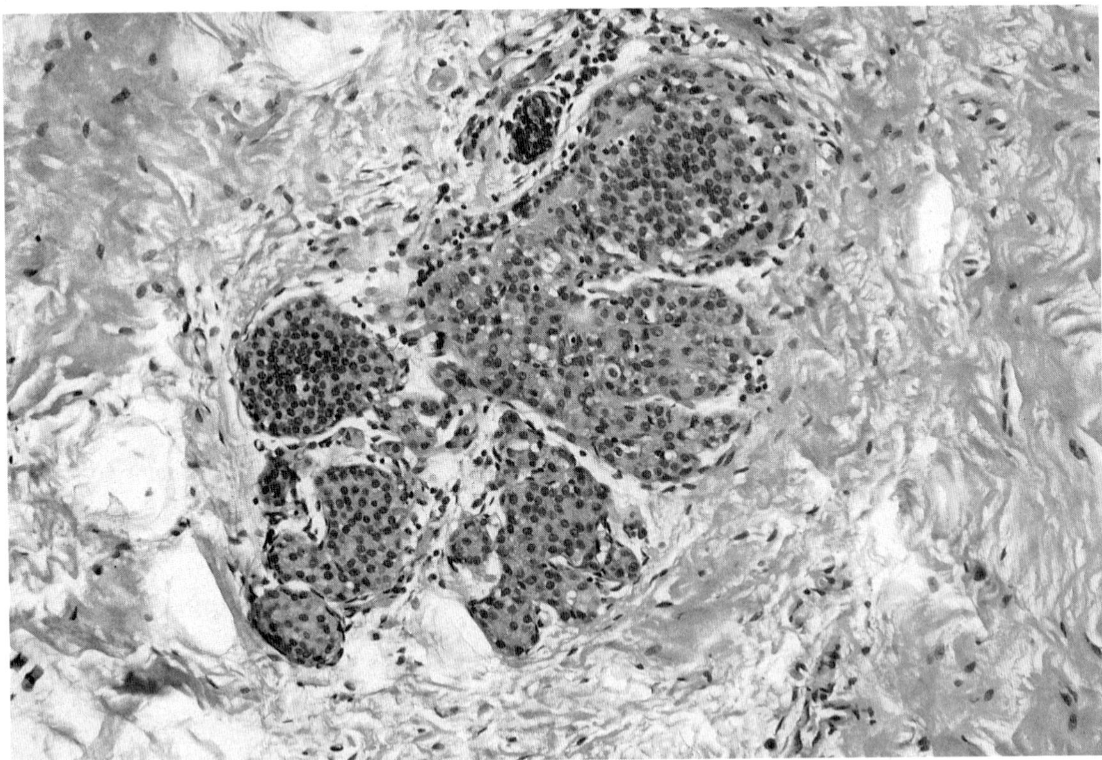

Fig. 4. Atypical lobular hyperplasia with defining, characteristic rounded cells of lobular neoplasia. This is a slightly unusual example of this entity with dilatation of several spaces in a lobular unit. Inclusion of other spindled cell types and a lack of extensive distension means that this lesion does not fulfil the criteria of LCIS.

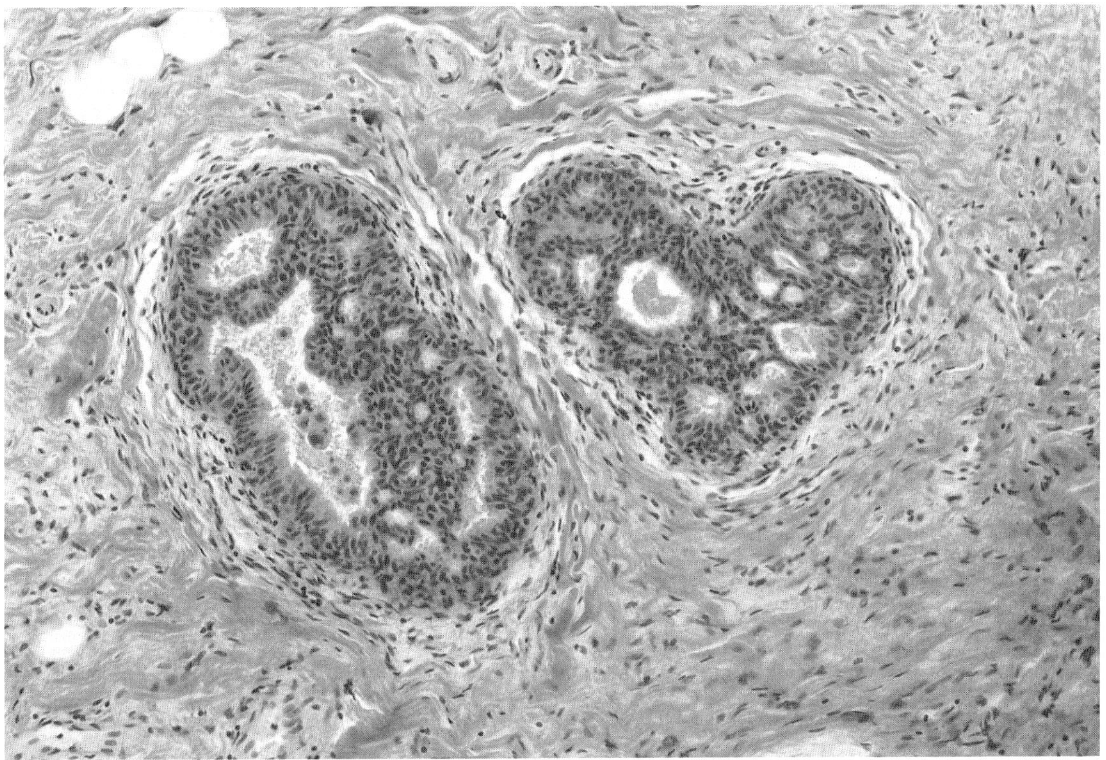

Fig. 5. Atypical ductal hyperplasia. Note that although two epithelial spaces are involved, there are some normally polarized cells just above the region of the basement membrane facing the lumen. The uniformity of the central cell population and the formation of rigid spaces in a circumscribed and relatively confined area complete the diagnosis of this change.

Histologic Lesions on Biopsy Associated with slight cancer risk elevation — Magnitude of risk probably not clinically meaningful, but reliably about 50–80% elevated for 10–15 years (relative risk compared to similar women is 1.5–1.8 times). These include well-developed patterns of moderate and florid usual type epithelial hyperplasia; sclerosing adenosis; subsets of fibroadenoma; papilloma(s); and possibly multiple, large and recurrent cysts.

3. Histologic criteria

3.1. Atypical ductal hyperplasia (ADH) and atypical lobular hyperplasia (ALH)

From the first studies in the 1980s the histologic definition of ADH has included an extent criterion based on the minimum criteria for DCIS [6,15]. In order to foster interobserver agreement, this was stated as necessitating involvement of two spaces with a completely uniform population of cells, i.e. no cells remaining similar to normally polarized luminal cells [24,25]. When the histologic pattern and cytologic features were more extensive, then small, non-comedo examples of DCIS would be easily diagnosed [26–28]. These criteria produced importantly different outcomes in women

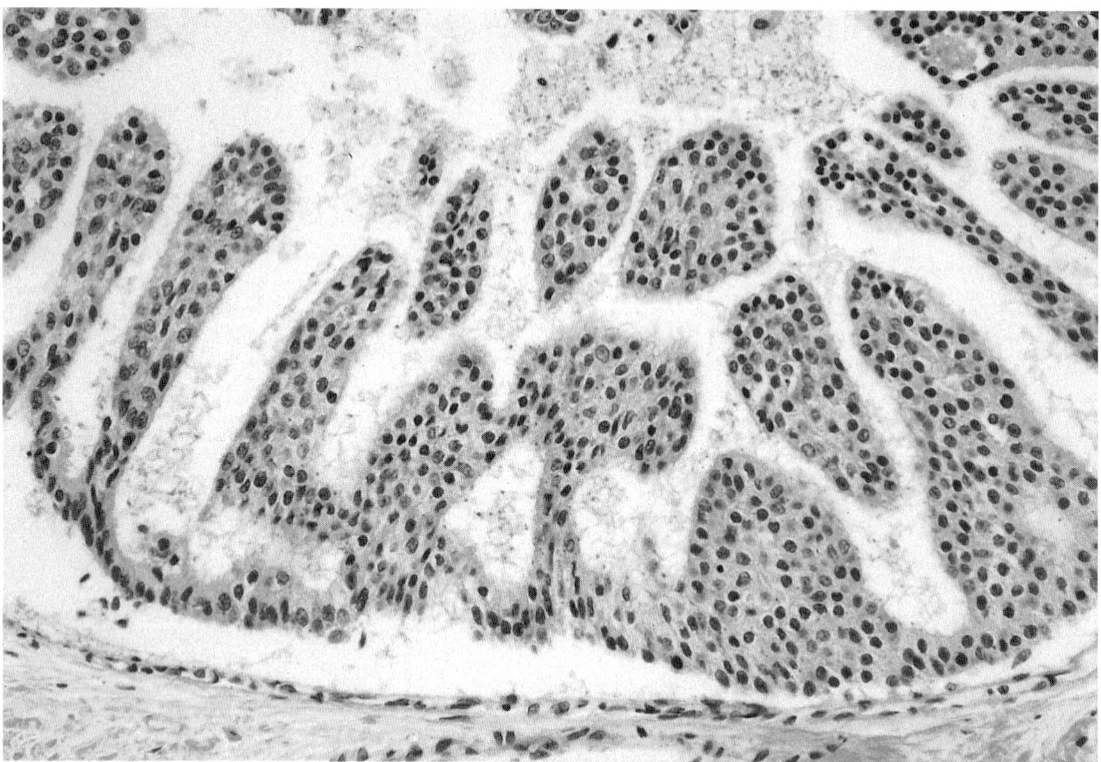

Fig. 6. Well-developed and low grade micropapillary ductal carcinoma in situ. This pattern is seldom well-confined. It is usually associated with extensive disease although it can be relatively circumscribed in a few adjacent lobular units. The pattern is presented here to contrast it with many other micropapillary forms that do not have this significance.

having biopsy alone with frequent evolution to invasive cancer in women with inadequately removed DCIS [29], and only an increased risk of breast cancer anywhere in the breasts for ADH. Most ADH lesions are confined to a single lobular unit, although the unit may extend over 3–4 mm in largest size. It became recognized that overall size was a helpful criterion for ADH [15]. For both ADH [24] and ALH [19,30] the criteria are more complex than most histopathologic exercises because the extent of the characteristic cells, as well as the overall extent of involved area are considered (Figs. 4 and 5). Also, lesser and non-formally atypical lesions are not defined on the same spectrum and are considered usual pattern 'ductal' hyperplasias (moderate and florid) which have their own characteristic features. When the varied cytology and diverse cell placement of usual hyperplasia is present, then ADH should not be diagnosed [31,32].

Making the distinction between limited lesions that indicate a minor to moderate degree of general increased cancer risk, atypical ductal hyperplasia, and ductal carcinoma in situ has also produced an important clinical benefit which is seldom discussed. That is, lesions defined as minimal ductal carcinoma in situ (Fig. 6) by the Memorial Study of 1978 [33] and the Nashville Study of 1982 [34] were obviously being consistently underdiagnosed in widely varied settings in the 1950s and 1960s. During the 1970s it was our impression that ductal carcinoma in situ was being over-diagnosed, with any case that had some of the features of ductal carcinoma in situ and included a few cells present within rigid arches within an otherwise completely normal space being considered DCIS. In some settings these lesions continue to be called ductal carcinoma in situ but if they are carefully reported as having a limited and very small size, the limited rate of subsequent cancer development can be recognized. For some larger DCIS lesions local excision with clear margins without subsequent radiotherapy may be appropriate treatment [35–37].

3.2. Other histologic changes

Table 1 indicates various histologic diagnoses and their association with risk along with explanatory rates. Note well that these risks operate over a finite time period of 10 to 20 years after their identification. After that the risk for cancer becomes closer to that of women of similar age without a history of a breast biopsy.

Also, the common finding of breast density, fibrosis and cysts, most often seen in perimenopausal women should not be regarded as a disease. This is because there is no regularly identified and clinically useful association with pain or breast cancer risk. However, it still remains possible that excessive and large cyst development may be associated with some increased breast cancer risk, and this association awaits careful clinical studies of women with palpable breast cysts.

4. Atypical lesions without specific definition

There are many lobulocentric lesions with increased nuclei which garner attention because of atypical and enlarged nuclei. Such lesions usually have apocrine or lactational/secretory features and have no known clinical significance with regard to recognizing increased risk (Figs. 2 and 3).

There are a range of benign conditions which have a 50–80% elevated relative risk compared to similar women and this risk last for 10–15 years. Well developed patterns of moderate and florid usual type epithelial hyperplasia, sclerosing adenosis, subsets of fibroadenomas, papillomas and cysts.

References

1. Fitzgibbons PL, Henson DE, Hutter RV (1998) Benign breast changes and the risk for subsequent breast cancer: an update of the 1985 consensus statement. Cancer Committee of the College of American Pathologists. Arch Pathol Lab Med, 122, 1053–5.
2. Page DL, Dupont WD (1998) Benign breast diseases and premalignant breast disease. Arch Pathol Lab Med, 122, 1048–1050.
3. Jacobs TW, Byrne C, Colditz G, Connolly JL, Schnitt SJ (1999) Radial scars in benign breast-biopsy specimens and the risk of breast cancer. N Engl J Med, 340, 430–6.
4. Dupont WD, Page DL (1985) Risk factors for breast cancer in women with proliferative breast disease. N Engl J Med, 312, 146–151.
5. Dupont WD, Parl FF, Hartmann WH et al. (1993) Breast cancer risk associated with proliferative breast disease and atypical hyperplasia. Cancer, 71, 1258–1265.
6. Page DL, Dupont WD, Rogers LW, Rados MS (1985) Atypical hyperplastic lesions of the female breast. A long follow-up study. Cancer, 55, 2698–2708.
7. Marshall LM, Hunter DJ, Connolly JL et al. (1997) Risk of breast cancer associated with atypical hyperplasia of lobular and ductal types. Cancer Epidemiol Biomarkers Prev, 6, 297–301.
8. London SJ, Connolly JL, Schnitt SJ, Colditz GA (1992) A prospective study of benign breast disease and risk of breast cancer. Jama, 267, 941–944.
9. Fitzgibbons PL, Henson DE, Hutter RVP, Canc Comm Coll Am P. (1998) Benign breast changes and the risk for subsequent breast cancer — An update of the 1985 consensus statement. Arch Pathol Lab Med, 122, 1053–1055.
10. Kelsey JL, Gammon MD (1990) Epidemiology of breast cancer. Epidemiol Rev, 12, 228–240.
11. Page DL, Jensen RA, Simpson JF (1998) Premalignant and malignant disease of the breast: the roles of the pathologist. Mod Pathol, 11, 120–8.
12. Ries LAG, Kosary CL, Hankey BF, Miller BA, Edwards BK (1998) SEER Cancer Statistics Review: 1973–1975. Bethesda, MD: National Cancer Institute.
13. Dupont WD, Plummer WD (1996) Understanding the relationship between relative and absolute risk. Cancer, 77, 2193–2199.
14. Gail MH, Brinton LA, Byar DP et al. (1989) Projecting individualized probabilities of developing breast cancer for white females who are being examined annually. JNCI, 81, 1879–1886.
15. Tavassoli FA, Norris HJ (1990) A comparison of the results of long-term follow-up for atypical intraductal hyperplasia and intraductal hyperplasia of the breast. Cancer, 65, 518–529.

16. London SJ, Connolly JL, Schnitt SJ, Colditz GA (1992) A prospective study of benign breast disease and the risk of breast cancer. Jama, 267, 941–4.
17. Page DL, Salhany KE, Jensen RA, Dupont WD (1996) Subsequent breast carcinoma risk after biopsy with atypia in a breast papilloma. Cancer, 78, 258–66.
18. Dupont WD, Page DL, Parl FF et al. (1994) Long-term risk of breast cancer in women with fibroadenoma. N Engl J Med, 331, 10–15.
19. Page DL, Kidd TE, Dupont WD, Simpson JF, Rogers LW (1991) Lobular neoplasia of the breast: Higher risk for subsequent invasive cancer predicted by more extensive disease. Hum Pathol, 22, 1232–1239.
20. Bodian CA, Perzin KH, Lattes R (1996) Lobular Neoplasia: long term risk of breast cancer in relation to other factors. Cancer, 78, 1024–1034.
21. Fisher ER, Costantino J, Fisher B et al. (1996) Pathologic findings from the National Surgical Adjuvant Breast Project (NSABP) Protocol B-17. Five-year observations concerning lobular carcinoma in situ. Cancer, 78, 1403–16.
22. Page DL, Dupont WD (1990) Anatomic Markers of Human Premalignancy and Risk of Breast Cancer. Cancer, 66, 1326–1335.
23. Rosen PP, Braun DWJ, Lyngholm B, Urban JA, Kinne DW (1981) Lobular carcinoma in situ of the breast: preliminary results of treatment by ipsilateral mastectomy and contralateral breast biopsy. Cancer, 47, 813–819.
24. Jensen RA, Page DL (1998) Epithelial Hyperplasia. In: Elston CW, Ellis IO, eds. The Breast. Edinburgh: Churchill Livingstone, 65–90.
25. Page DL, Rogers LW (1992) Combined histologic and cytologic criteria for the diagnosis of mammary atypical ductal hyperplasia. Hum Pathol, 23, 1095–1097.
26. Page DL, Dupont WD (1991) Histologic indicators of breast cancer risk. Bull Am Coll Surg, 76, 16–23.
27. Scott MA, Lagios MD, Axelsson K, Rogers LW, Anderson TJ (1997) Page DL. Ductal carcinoma in situ of the breast: Reproducibility of histological subtype analysis. Hum Pathol, 28, 967–973.
28. Lagios MD, Silverstein MJ (1997) Ductal carcinoma in situ. The success of breast conservation therapy: a shared experience of two single institutional nonrandomized prospective studies. Surg Oncol Clin N Am, 6, 385–92.
29. Page DL, Dupont WD, Rogers LW, Jensen RA, Schuyler PA (1995) Continued local recurrence of carcinoma 15–25 years after a diagnosis of low grade ductal carcinoma in situ of the breast treated only by biopsy. Cancer, 76, 1197–1200.
30. Simpson JF, Page DL (1998) Lobular Neoplasia. In: Elston CW, Ellis IO, eds. The Breast. Churchill Livingstone, Edinburgh, 91–106.
31. Page DL, Anderson TJ, Rogers LW (1988) Epithelial hyperplasia. Churchill Livingstone, Edinburgh, 1, 120–156.
32. Schnitt SJ, Connolly JL, Tavassoli FA et al. (1992) Interobserver reproducibility in the diagnosis of ductal proliferative breast lesions using standardized criteria. Am J Surg Pathol, 16, 1133–1143.
33. Betsill WL Jr., Rosen PP, Lieberman PH, Robbins GF (1978) Intraductal carcinoma. Long-term follow-up after treatment by biopsy alone. Jama, 239, 1863–1867.
34. Page DL, Dupont WD, Rogers LW, Landenberger M (1982) Intraductal carcinoma of the breast: Follow-up after biopsy only. Cancer. Cancer, 49, 751–758.
35. Silverstein MJ, Lagios MD, Groshen S et al. (1999) The influence of margin width on local control of ductal carcinoma in situ of the breast. N Engl J Med, 340, 1455–1461.
36. Page DL, Simpson JF (1999) Ductal carcinoma in situ — The focus for prevention, screening, and breast conservation in breast cancer. N Engl J Med, 340, 1499–1500.
37. Lagios MD, Margolin FR, Westdahl PR, Rose MR (1989) Mammographically detected duct carcinoma in situ. Cancer, 63, 618–624.
38. Jensen RA, Page DL, Dupont WD, Rogers LW (1989) Invasive breast cancer risk in women with sclerosing adenosis. Cancer, 64, 1977–83.

Breast Cancer: Diagnosis and Management
J.M. Dixon (Ed.)

CHAPTER 11

Genetic testing in breast cancer patients: options for gene carriers and high risk women

James Mackay

1. Introduction

Recent identification of two high penetrance breast cancer genes, BRCA1 [1] and BRCA2 [2], has raised unrealistic public and professional expectations of the clinical utility of testing for cancer genes. There are important messages to give to breast cancer patients and their families who are seeking advice on genetic testing. There are a variety of management options available today for unaffected women at high risk.

2. Mutation search and genetic testing

Both BRCA1 and BRCA2 are long genes. The former is 5592 base pairs and the latter 10,254 base pairs in the coding region. Mutations are distributed throughout the entire length of both genes [1–6]. In order to offer genetic testing the relevant mutation needs to be identified in each family. This involves taking a blood sample from an affected family member with either breast or ovarian cancer and then searching for a mutation. Once the mutation has been found in the affected family member, then direct genetic testing can be offered to other unaffected family members to determine if they have inherited the mutated (or faulty) copy, or have inherited the unmutated (good) copy of the gene [7].

Genetic testing is a two-stage process:

(1) identification of the faulty gene in an affected family member and then

(2) offering a direct genetic test to unaffected members.

There are several different techniques in use in clinical genetics laboratories to identify mutations, with varying sensitivity and specificity. Many of the techniques used have a high false negative rate of up to 20% [8]. One technique — direct sequencing of the whole gene — has a low false negative rate but picks up a significant number of genetic alterations of unknown significance. These mutations may not increase cancer susceptibility risk and they do not therefore help clarify the risk to unaffected individuals in the family. There is concern that identifying these genetic variants of unknown significance may raise anxiety in patients and their families [9].

In a number of populations including Ashkenazi Jews [10–13] and the Icelandic population [14,15], there are a small number of mutations which are found more frequently than in other populations, so-called 'founder mutations'. Mutation searching within these populations is therefore easier [16]. Most cancer genetic centres, however, continue to follow the management strategy outlined above.

There has been a lack of consensus among

providers of cancer genetic services in defining the criteria on which to offer to search for BRCA1 or BRCA2 mutations. One of the main determinants of success will be cost effectiveness of mutation searching, determined by the balance between the cost of screening each gene and the mutation pick-up rate within each gene. At the moment, with current mutation searching techniques used in most clinical genetics laboratories, mutation pick-up rate remains low even in families with a strong family history of breast and ovarian cancer. Ongoing research should clarify the chance of identifying a mutation based on the strength of the family history, and more accurate searching techniques are being developed which will improve the cost effectiveness of testing.

Most clinical laboratories have a low pick-up rate for BRCA1 and 2 mutations at the moment. Many unaffected individuals in high risk families are not currently offered genetic testing.

3. The implications of identifying a mutation in a breast cancer patient

Although the number of known mutation carriers throughout the world remains relatively low, it is gradually increasing as mutation searching in both research and clinical laboratories becomes available in more and more countries. Managing patients who have been shown to carry a mutation is difficult because there is a dearth of treatment outcome data in known gene carriers. There is an urgent need to put in place large multinational collaborative studies to address the important treatment questions. The recent EORTC hereditary breast cancer task force [17] has been set up to act as a catalyst to these studies.

The risk of developing a new primary breast cancer in the contralateral breast in any woman with breast cancer is around 0.8%/year [18]. The absolute risk in an individual of developing a second primary breast cancer therefore depends on the age of diagnosis, and the survival of that individual. The lifetime risk of developing a second primary breast cancer in gene carriers is over 50% [19–21], at least double that of non-gene carriers.

Offering a prophylactic contralateral mastectomy to a known gene carrier presenting with primary breast cancer, or to an individual presenting with primary breast cancer from a family known to carry a mutation but who has not yet herself been tested, seems a reasonable course of action. Many women from high risk families make that decision as soon as their breast cancer is diagnosed.

This option may be less attractive to women who have finished their definitive primary breast cancer treatment, often many years ago, and are then identified as gene carriers. The available options become more complicated in women where primary local treatment was wide local excision and radiotherapy. Whether the wide local excision should be converted to a mastectomy is unknown. One study has reported an increased frequency of BRCA1 and BRCA2 carriers in women who subsequently developed local relapse after breast conserving surgery, compared to a similar group who do not develop local relapse, but the numbers of patients in each group is small [22]. The risk of ovarian cancer in gene carriers starts to rise from the age of 40 [23], suggesting that prophylactic oophorectomy after the age of 40 is a reasonable management option in gene carriers whether they have previously developed breast cancer or not. Whether a 32 year old gene carrier who develops breast cancer should be offered prophylactic oophorectomy at the time of her definitive breast surgery again remains unknown.

There is an urgent need to collect robust treatment and outcome data on gene carriers.
The management of women who have completed their primary breast cancer treatment before they are identified as gene carriers is difficult.

4. Options available to unaffected gene carriers

There are several options available to gene carriers. Individuals can only make a properly informed choice if they are given accurate information on their personal cancer risk. Penetrance data from the Breast Cancer Linkage Consortium based on large families with multiple cases of breast and ovarian cancer, estimated risk of breast cancer to BRCA1 mutation carriers to be 50% by age 50, and 85% by age 70 with similar high age dependant penetrances for BRCA2 carriers [23,24]. However several studies in Ashkenazi Jewish populations find lower penetrances of 33% breast cancer risk by age 50 and 56% by age 70 [11]. In the Icelandic population one of the founder BRCA2 mutations confers a cumulative breast cancer risk of 37% by age 70 [15] — less than half the risk calculated by the BCLC. It is not surprising that population based studies report a lower cumulative risk, as the 237 BCLC families have been specifically recognised and ascertained for the study because of the large number of affected relatives. However, all the population studies so far published have only looked at a small number of founder mutations, and it is possible that different mutations have different breast cancer risks, similar to different ovarian cancer risks reported for BRCA1 and BRCA2 [25,26].

An accurate estimate of an individual's risk status probably lies between the BCLC estimate and the population based founder mutation study estimates [27]. It is important to indicate to patients the relatively wide confidence limits on these estimates.

The available options to gene carriers or high risk untested women are:

4.1. Surveillance

Regular mammography to detect early breast cancer in high risk women has been advised by enthusiasts for years [28–30]. However there are no data available to assess the efficacy of this practice. The concept that doing something is better than doing nothing has been accepted in an uncritical fashion. Several lines of recent laboratory investigation have suggested that both BRCA1 [31–36] and BRCA2 [37,38] are involved in cellular mechanisms of DNA repair, possibly also involving another cellular protein called ATM [39]. Ionising radiation damages DNA in a number of ways [40], and it is theoretically possible that regular radiation in the form of annual mammography may be detrimental in individuals carrying a mutated BRCA1 or 2 gene, and therefore deficient in at least one DNA repair mechanism. The clinical relevance of these laboratory findings to normal tissue sensitivity requires elucidation [41,42].

There are several on-going European studies comparing the screening performance of regular MRI scanning with regular mammography [43]. Advantages of MRI scanning over mammography include high sensitivity and the absence of radiation, whilst disadvantages include higher cost and the high false positive rate. Research to clarify the value of different surveillance strategies should be encouraged.

> *The value of regular surveillance in gene carriers is unknown.*

4.2. Chemoprevention

Several randomised studies have examined the utility of the anti-oestrogen tamoxifen as a chemopreventive agent. The largest study, NSABP I, was halted early on the advice of the data monitoring committee because of a significant reduction in the incidence of breast cancer in the treatment group [44]. Two smaller studies [45,46] have failed to corroborate this result. A further study examining the use of raloxifene, a newer selective oestrogen receptor modulator (SERM) in prevention of osteoporosis in post menopausal women reports a 56% reduction in invasive breast cancer in the treatment group [47].

None of these studies have examined the efficacy of tamoxifen specifically in gene carriers or high risk individuals.

The use of reversible chemical ovarian suppression with the gonadotrophin releasing hormone agonist, goserelin acetate (Zoladex®) [48] to reduce breast cancer incidence in high risk premenopausal women is being examined in a series of European pilot studies [49]. The short and long term side effects of this drug are important, and therefore a variety of drug combinations are being tested for acceptability and tolerability within these pilot studies [50].

Chemoprevention should only be offered to high risk women within research studies.

4.3. Prophylactic surgery

Bilateral prophylactic mastectomy using a variety of surgical techniques is another possible management option for high risk women. As with other available options, the evidence base is poor. Several retrospective studies have indicated a high failure rate, although the most modern and largest retrospective study quotes a success rate of over 90% [51–54]. A prospective randomised study examining prophylactic mastectomy may well not be feasible, but the collection of prospective data on current practice and outcome remains a high priority [55]. The psychological effects of prophylactic mastectomy remains an area of active research interest, and the results of several ongoing studies are awaited. Bilateral prophylactic oophorectomy is another available management option. As mentioned previously, the risk of ovarian cancer starts to increase from around the age of 40 in gene carriers [23]. A number of cases of intra-abdominal carcinomatosis, indistinguishable from primary ovarian cancer, after the removal of histologically normal ovaries have been reported [56–58]. A recent study of decision analysis suggests that prophylactic oophorectomy gives limited gain in life expectancy [59]. As with prophylactic mastectomy, a prospective collection of data on current practice and outcome will help to clarify the position.

The limited studies available on prophylactic surgery suggest that this reduces the rates of breast cancer by 90%.

5. Conclusions

Genetic testing in breast cancer patients is a rapidly evolving area of clinical practice. A lack of good research evidence makes the management of patients with inherited breast cancer and their families difficult. There are a number of options available to affected and unaffected gene carriers, many of which may appear unattractive. Almost all are unproven.

Research into treatment outcomes in affected gene carriers, and effective prophylactic strategies in unaffected high risk women should be a high priority over the next decade for all professionals involved in treating patients with breast cancer.

Acknowledgements

Dr James Mackay is funded by the CRC.

References

1. Miki Y, Swevson J, Shattuck-Eidens D et al. A strong candidate for the breast and ovarian cancer susceptibility gene BRCA1. Science 1994; 266: 66–71.
2. Wooster R, Bignell G, Swift S et al. Identification of the BRCA2 gene. Nature 1995; 378: 789–792.
3. Futreal PA, Liu Q, Schattuck-Eidens D et al. BRCA1 mutations in primary breast and ovarian carcinomas. Science 1994; 266: 120–122.
4. Shattuck-Eidens D, McClure M, Simard J et al. A collaborative survey of 80 mutations in the BRCA1 breast and ovarian cancer susceptibility gene. JAMA 1995; 273: 535–541.
5. Wooster R, Neuhausen SL, Mangion J et al. Localisation of a breast cancer susceptibility gene, BRCA2 to chromosome 13q12-13. Science 1994; 265: 2088–2090.

6. Phelan CM, Lancaster JM, Tonin P et al. Mutation analysis of the BRCA2 gene in 49 site-specific breast cancer families. Nat Genet 1996; 13: 120–122.
7. Mackay J. The role of genetic testing in breast cancer by the year 2000. Cancer Treat Rev 1997; 23: S13–S22.
8. Gayther SA, Harrington P, Russell P et al. Rapid detection of regionally clustered germ-line BRCA1 mutations by multiplex heteroduplex analysis. Am J Hum Genet 1996; 58: 451–456.
9. Collins F. BRCA1 - lots of mutations, lots of dilemmas. N Engl J Med 1996; 334: 186–188.
10. Struewing J, Abeliovich D, Peretz T et al. The carrier frequency of the BRCA1 185delAG mutation is approximately 1 percent in Ashkenazi Jewish individuals. Nat Genet 1995; 11: 198–200.
11. Struewing J, Hartge P, Wacholder S et al. The risk of cancer associated with specific mutations of BRCA1 and BRCA2 among Ashkenazi Jews. N Engl J Med 1997; 336: 1401–1408.
12. Oddoux C, Struewing J, Clayton C et al. The carrier frequency of the BRCA2 6147delT mutation among Ashkenazi Jewish individuals is approximately 1 percent. Nat Genet 1998; 14: 188–190.
13. Fodor F, Weston A, Bleiweiss I et al. Frequency and carrier risk associated with common BRCA1 and BRCA2 mutations in Ashkenazi Jewish breast cancer patients. Am J Hum Genet 1998; 63: 45–51.
14. Johannesdottir G, Gudmundsson J, Bergthorsson J et al. High prevalence of the 999del5 mutation in Icelandic breast and ovarian cancer patients. Cancer Res 1996; 56: 3663–3665.
15. Thorlacius S, Sigurdsson S, Bjarnadottir H et al. Study of a single BRCA2 mutation with high carrier frequency in a small population. Am J Hum Genet 1997; 60: 1079–1084.
16. Hartge P, Struewing P, Wacholder S et al. The prevalence of common BRCA1 and BRCA2 mutations among Ashkenazi Jews. Am J Hum Genet 1999; 64: 963–970.
17. EORTC Hereditary Breast Cancer Task Force. Chairman: Dr R A E M Tollenaar MD, PhD, Head of Section Surgical Oncology, Leiden University Medical Center, Leiden, The Netherlands. Secretary: the Author.
18. Early Breast Cancer Trialists Collaborative Group. Tamoxifen for early breast cancer: an overview of the randomised trials. *Lancet* 1998;351:1451-1467.
19. Marcus J, Watson P, Page D et al. Hereditary breast cancer: Pathobiology, prognosis, and BRCA1 and BRCA2 gene linkage. Cancer 1996; 77: 697–709.
20. Robson M, Gilewski T, Haas B et al. BRCA-associated breast cancer in young women. J Clin Oncol 1998; 6: 642–649.
21. Johannsson OT, Ranstam J, Borg A et al. Survival of BRCA1 breast and ovarian cancer patients: a population-based study from southern Sweden. J Clin Oncol 1998; 6: 397–404.
22. Turner BC, Harrold E, Matloff E et al. BRCA1/BRCA2 germline mutations in locally recurrent breast cancer patients after lumpectomy and radiation therapy: Implications for breast-conserving management in patients with BRCA1/BRCA2 mutations. J Clin Oncol 1999; 17: 3017–3024.
23. Ford D, Easton DF, Bishop DT et al. Risks of cancer in BRCA1 mutation carriers. Lancet 1994; 343: 692–695.
24. Ford D, Easton D, Peto J. Estimates of the gene frequency of BRCA1 and its contribution to breast and ovarian cancer incidence. Am J Hum Genet 1995; 57: 1457–1462.
25. Gayther SA, Warren W, Mazoyer S et al. Germline mutations of the BRCA1 gene in breast and ovarian cancer families provide evidence for a genotype-phenotype correlation. Nat Genet 1995; 11: 428–433.
26. Gayther SA, Mangion J, Russell P et al. Variation of risks of breast and ovarian cancer associated with different germline mutations of the BRCA2 gene. Nat Genet 1997; 15: 103–105.
27. Devilee P. BRCA1 and BRCA2 testing: weighting the demand against the benefits. Am J Hum Genet 1999; 64: 943–948.
28. Burke W, Daly M, Garber J et al. Recommendation for follow-up care of individuals with an inherited predisposition to cancer. II. BRCA1 and BRCA2. JAMA 1997; 277: 997–1003.
29. Hoskins JF, Stopfer JE, Calzone CA. Assessment and counseling for women with a family history of breast cancer: a guide for clinicians. JAMA 1995; 273: 577–585.
30. Vasen HFA. Screening in breast cancer families: is it useful? Ann Med 1994; 26: 185–190.
31. Zhong Q, Chen CF, Li S et al. Association of BRCA1 with the hRad50-hMre11-p95 complex and the DNA damage response. Science 1999; 285: 747–750.
32. Chen J, Silver DP, Walpity D et al. Stable interaction between the products of the BRCA1 and BRCA2 tumor suppressor genes in mitotic and meiotic cells. Mol Cell 1998; 2: 317–328.
33. Thomas JE, Smith M, Tonkinson JL et al. Induction of phosphorylation on BRCA1 during the cell cycle and after DNA damage. Cell Growth Differ 1997; 8: 801–809.
34. Scully R, Chen J, Plug A et al. Association of BRCA1 with Rad51 in mitotic and meiotic cells. Cell 1997; 88: 265–275.
35. Zhang H, Tombline G, Weber BL. BRCA1, BRCA2 and DNA damage response: collision or collusion? Cell 1998; 92: 433–436.
36. Moynahan ME, Chiu JW, Koller BH et al. BRCA1 controls homology-directed DNA repair. Mol Cell 1999; 4: 511–518.

37. Yuan SS, Lee SY, Chen G et al. BRCA2 is required for ionizing radiation-induced assembly of Rad51 complex in vivo. Cancer Res 1999; 59: 3547–3551.
38. Patel KJ, Vu VP, Lee H et al. Involvement of BRCA2 in DNA repair. Mol Cell 1998; 1: 347–357.
39. Cortez D, Wang Y, Qin J et al. Requirement of ATM-dependent phosphorylation of BRCA1 in the DNA damage response to double-strand breaks. Science 1999; 286: 1162–1165.
40. McMillan TJ, Steel GG. DNA damage and cell killing. In *Basic Clinical Radiobiology*, 2nd edition, 1997; Steel GG (ed): pp. 58-69.
41. Carlomagno F, Burnet NG, Turesson I, et al. Comparison of DNA repair protein expression and activities between human fibroblast cell lines with different radiosensitivities. *Int J Cancer*. In press.
42. Burnet NG, Johansen J, Turesson I et al. Describing patients' normal tissue reactions: concerning the possibility of individualising radiotherapy dose prescriptions based on potential predictive assays of normal tissue radiosensitivity. Steering Committee of the BioMed2 European Union Concerted Action Programme on the Development of Predictive Tests of Normal tissue Response to Radiation Therapy. Int J Cancer 1998; 79: 606–613.
43. UK MRC/NHS R & D study of MRI scanning and mammography in high risk women. Contact: Linda Pointon, Institute of Cancer Research, The Royal Marsden NHS Trust, Downs Road, Sutton, Surrey SM2 5PT. Tel: 0181 661 3720. E-mail: lindap@icr.ac.uk.
44. Fisher B, Joseph PC, Lawrence Wickerham D et al. Tamoxifen for prevention of breast cancer: report of the national surgical adjuvant breast and bowel project P-1 study. J Nat Cancer Inst 1998; 90: 1371–1388.
45. Powles T, Eeles R, Ashley S et al. Interim analysis of the incidence of breast cancer in the Royal Marsden Hospital tamoxifen randomised chemoprevention trial. Lancet 1998; 352: 98–101.
46. Veronesi U, Maisonneuve P, Costa A et al. Prevention of breast cancer with tamoxifen: preliminary findings from the Italian randomised trial among hysterectomised women. Lancet 1998; 352: 93–97.
47. Cummings SR, Eckert S, Krueger KA et al. The effect of Raloxifene on risk of breast cancer in postmenopausal women. Results from the MORE randomized trial. JAMA 1999; 281: 2189–2197.
48. West CP, Baird DT. Suppression of ovarian activity by Zoladex depot (ICI 118630), a long-acting luteinizing hormone releasing hormone agonist analogue. Clin Endocrinol 1987; 26: 213–220.
49. Dowsett M, Cuzick J. IBIS-RAZOR Study. Raloxifene and Zoladex Research Study. Protocol for a randomised trial of zoladex plus raloxifene plus screening versus screening alone for the prevention of breast cancer in premenopausal women at high genetic risk. Oct 1999.
50. IBIS. The International Breast Cancer Intervention Studies. Chairman: Dr J Cuzick, ICRF, P O box 123, Lincoln's Inn Fields, London W2 1NY. Tel: 1071 269 3006. E-mail: cuzick@icrf.icnet.uk.
51. Goodnight Jr. JE, Quagliani JM, Morton DL. Failure of subcutaneous mastectomy to prevent the development of breast cancer. J Surg Oncol 1984; 26: 198–201.
52. Eldar S, Meguid M, Beatty JD. Cancer of the breast after prophylactic subcutaneous mastectomy. Am J Surg 1984; 148: 692–693.
53. Ziegler L, Kroll S. Primary breast cancer after prophylactic mastectomy. Am J Clin Oncol 1994; 14: 451–454.
54. Harmann LC, Schaid DJ, Woods JE et al. Efficacy of bilateral prophylactic mastectomy in women with a family history of breast cancer. N Engl J Med 1999; 340: 77–84.
55. Fentiman IS. Prophylactic mastectomy: deliverance or delusion? We don't know so we need to start registering all cases now. BMJ 1998; 317: 1402–1403.
56. Tabacman JK, Tucker MA, Kase R et al. Intra-abdominal carcinomatosis after prophylactic oophorectomy in ovarian cancer-prone families. Lancet 1992; ii: 795–797.
57. Kemp GM, Hsiu JG, Andrews MC. Papillary peritoneal carcinomatosis after prophylactic oophorectomy. Gynecol Oncol 1993; 47: 395–397.
58. Piver MS, Jishi MF, Tsukada Y et al. Primary peritoneal carcinoma after prophylactic oophorectomy in women with a family history of ovarian cancer. A report of the Gilda Radner Familial Ovarian Cancer Registry. Cancer 1993; 71: 2751–2755.
59. Schrag D, Kuntz KM, Garber JE et al. Decision analysis-effects of prophylactic mastectomy and oophorectomy o life expectancy among women with BRCA1 or BRCA2 mutations. N Engl J Med 1997; 336: 1465–1471.

Breast Cancer: Diagnosis and Management
J.M. Dixon (Ed.)

CHAPTER 12

Management of the contralateral breast in patients with hereditary breast cancer

Diana M. Eccles and D. Gareth Evans

1. Introduction

A number of genes have been identified in the last 10 years which, when inherited in a mutant form, confer a high risk of early onset breast cancer and often a spectrum of other cancers. These genes are relatively uncommon (together estimated to occur in about 1 in 300 individuals) [1–3] in the general population and to account for about 5% of all breast cancers. The proportion of young breast cancers accounted for by these high risk genes is however considerably higher [4–6]. In addition to these high risk susceptibility genes there are also likely to be a number of lower penetrance more commonly occurring genetic polymorphisms which increase breast cancer risk and which are likely to interact significantly with epidemiological risk factors [7]. Not many such genes have been identified as yet. In broad terms we will refer to this 'weaker' genetic susceptibility as familial breast cancer.

2. The BRCA genes

BRCA1 was mapped to chromosome 17q in 1990 [8] and the genetic sequence was finally published in 1994 [9] along with reports of the location of a second major susceptibility gene BRCA2 [10]. The sequence of BRCA2 was published in 1995 [11]. These genes are both large and mutation analysis is expensive and time consuming. However, in families with a high chance of a genetic predisposition genetic testing is offered in most UK Regional Genetics Centres. Thus an increasing number of young women with a strong family history of breast and ovarian cancer may have the opportunity of undergoing pre-symptomatic genetic testing.

TP53 is a tumour suppressor gene which plays an integral role in maintaining the integrity of DNA — it has been described as the 'guardian of the genome' [12]. Mutations in the TP53 gene are extremely common in all types of cancer however inherited mutations are rare. The Li Fraumeni syndrome is the striking pattern of childhood malignancy (typically soft tissue and osteosarcomas, gliomas or adrenocortical carcinoma) and very early onset breast cancer (50% of female gene carriers have developed breast cancer by 30 years of age) which results from inherited TP53 mutations [13]. There is good in vitro evidence to suggest an abnormal response to low dose radiation with defective apoptosis [14]. Recognition of this syndrome is therefore important not least because it has implications for breast screening methods. Current practice is to avoid ionising radiation for screening purposes where possible.

Other recently discovered genes which confer an increase in risk of breast cancer and are associated with bilateral benign and malignant breast disease are: Cowden's disease (due to mutations in the PTEN gene) [15] and Peutz Jegher syndrome (PJS) due to mutations in CDNK4 [16]. Both are rare but the diagnostic features for PJS are hamartomatous gastrointestinal polyps and typical skin and buccal mucosal pigmentation: fibroadenosis and carcinoma of the breast are both increased in frequency. Cowden's disease is associated with macrocephaly, benign and malignant disease of the breasts and thyroid with hamartomas of the gut also present in some patients.

For families in which BRCA1, BRCA2 or TP53 mutations segregate, bilaterality is relatively common and some use this as a criterion alone in an individual for inferring high genetic risk. The contralateral risk could be as high as 60% for BRCA1/2 mutation carriers [8,17] but these estimates are based on families ascertained for a strong likelihood of segregating a highly penetrant dominant gene, ascertainment bias will enhance the risks estimated. Population based studies of high risk gene mutations give lower estimates for breast cancer risk (penetrance) than other methods [18]. Bilateral disease in an isolated case of later onset is much less likely to be an indicator of BRCA1 or 2 mutation carriers [4,19]. However for a young onset breast cancer, in the context of either a known or suspected genetic predisposition, options for primary breast cancer management and management of the contralateral breast must be carefully considered and discussed with the patient in the light of currently available information.

Approximately 5% of all breast cancers arise on a background of one of the high risk breast cancer genes (hereditary breast cancer and hereditary breast and ovarian cancer).

An estimated 20% of cases arise in the presence of a less striking family history with later average age at onset and a lower penetrance.

3. Breast cancer treatment

Since the days of Halsted's radical mastectomy, and even forequarter amputations, breast cancer treatment has come a long way. There are now good data to show that treatment of early breast cancer with wide excision followed up with adjuvant radiotherapy to the breast is as effective at achieving good local control and long term survival as is simple mastectomy [20–22]. The use of other adjuvant therapies can also independently and in combination improve survival [23–25]. In a modern multidisciplinary approach to breast cancer treatment breast conservation is now an option presented to and chosen by many women with early breast cancer in preference to mastectomy. For women in whom mastectomy is deemed necessary, reconstructive surgery has become popular, in many cases this has been traditionally offered a few years from diagnosis and treatment once prognosis is easier to judge, but in recent years, combined mastectomy and reconstruction has been increasingly offered in many centres [26].

3.1. Treatment of hereditary breast cancer

Once breast cancer develops in an individual, appropriate management of that cancer is the primary consideration. Since many of these patients are young and present with early cancers, breast conservation is in many cases technically possible. Wide local excision and axillary node dissection or sampling with adjuvant radiotherapy might be expected to produce equivalent results to simple mastectomy if this disease is similar in all respects to sporadic breast cancer.

For hereditary breast cancer there are some interesting biological differences compared with apparently sporadic cancers. Firstly for BRCA1 there is a greater proportion which are high grade and histologically medullary or atypical medullary in type [27,28]. These tumours are also more likely to be oestrogen receptor negative [29] and less likely to be associated with an in situ component (and usually comedo or high grade when found) [30]. Overall survival has been variously reported for hereditary cancer as worse [31] better [17] and the same [29,32] when compared with sporadic cancers. All of these features may influence breast cancer management.

For TP53 mutation carriers response to low dose radiation is abnormal in vitro — and although there is no evidence of excessive acute toxicity from high dose radiation (radiotherapy) data are sparse as this is a rare condition. Nonetheless data are emerging indicating a very high risk of sarcoma in the radiation field [33].

3.2. Breast conserving treatment

The issue of whether breast conserving surgery is appropriate should consider the prognostic factors for the disease itself, the feasibility of breast conservation and the wishes of the woman being treated. In addition for a woman with either a proven or suspected genetic susceptibility the chance of recurrence must take into account the background susceptibility of the breast tissue as a whole which includes the risk of a new primary in the contralateral breast. In order to discuss this rationally some idea of the risk involved is required. As familial cancers are more likely to be multifocal and bilateral the risk of a new primary on the treated side is likely to be high without adjuvant therapy. We have experience of one BRCA1 carrier developing five primary tumours in the same breast over a five year period from 29 years of age. Radiotherapy may significantly reduce the number of viable breast epithelial cells primed for transformation however any surviving cells could be more likely to become malignant due to unrepaired DNA damage from radiation. Again we have evidence for two BRCA1 mutation carriers who have developed a new ipsilateral primary 3 and 10 years after irradiation. Long term (10–20 years) follow up should provide answers not only to recurrence rates after radiotherapy but also to the risk of ipsilateral new primary.

Following a report on the outcome of breast conservation in a small number of hereditary versus sporadic early age breast cancers in an American cohort [34], we have completed a retrospective review of 304 breast cancer patients. The patients were classified according to genetic status into 142 hereditary breast cancers cases (75 known gene carriers, the remainder with a significant family history in addition to the index case) and 162 sporadic controls. The hereditary and sporadic groups were well matched for age at diagnosis, tumour size and stage and length of follow up. There was no difference in overall survival and no difference in chance of ipsilateral recurrence in the hereditary compared with the sporadic group over a median follow up period of 7 years [35,36]. Another study [37] implied a greater risk for gene carriers for ipsilateral breast cancer recurrence with a 7.8 year median time to this event, this group suggested that the tumour characteristics in these cases were likely to imply new primary tumours. Thus the evidence is conflicting and at present although there is no clear contraindication to breast conservation for the affected breast the risk for ipsilateral recurrence is unclear.

3.3. Management of the contralateral breast

There are substantial data pointing to an increase in risk of bilateral breast cancer in women with a hereditary predisposition. The overall lifetime risk to the contralateral breast for a woman with her first primary breast cancer and a hereditary predisposition has been estimated to be as high as 60% [38]. In general the greatest chance of recurrence of breast cancer, either locoregional or metastatic, is in the first two years after diagnosis. In our own series the cumulative risk of contralateral breast cancer at two years from diagnosis was 10% for hereditary cases compared to 2% in the sporadic group rising to 36% compared with 11% at 10 years [35]. Thus contralateral breast cancer risk is high and at the very least close surveillance is imperative.

For hereditary breast cancer, bilateral is a recognised feature. But bilateral breast cancer alone is not necessarily a strong indicator of hereditary breast cancer.

3.4. Surveillance

Of course for young women with an increased genetic risk, screening for early breast cancer is of uncertain benefit in terms of a clear reduction in mortality [39,40] although early cancers can undoubtedly be detected [41–43]. Conventional mammographic screening may be less sensitive in the younger breast [39] although the position remains unclear. There is an increase in the rate of false positive results in younger women undergoing regular breast screening [44]. The efficacy of other methods including magnetic resonance imaging and ultrasound scanning also at present remain unproven. Clinical follow up in this context is also of unproven benefit as it has not been formally evaluated.

3.5. Hormonal therapy

Oophorectomy was one of the earliest adjuvant treatments for premenopausal breast cancer and is still an option presented to patients with premenopausal ER positive breast tumours today [25]. It makes sense for a breast cancer patient with a family history of breast and ovarian cancer and a proven mutation in BRCA1 or BRCA2 to consider an oophorectomy particularly for an ER positive tumour. This may not only improve her chance of disease free survival but also reduce her risk of subsequent ovarian cancer. A radiation induced menopause would be less appropriate because of the potential risk of future ovarian malignancy. The position for an early onset breast cancer in the context of a family history of breast only cancer and an ER negative tumour is less clear. Some of these will be due to BRCA1 gene mutations (for more than three young breast cancers in close relatives an estimated 21–28% [45]) but the majority will be due to other genes. The later the average age at onset of the cancers, the less likely is the cluster to be due to a high risk dominant gene. Data are not available to inform decisions in the less clear cut situation and management should be based on best practise in terms of treating the primary cancer.

The use of Tamoxifen as a primary preventive agent seems to be effective in reducing the incidence of ER positive tumours in the short term [46]. However, ER negative tumours may be unaffected by oestrogen receptor blocking agents [47,48]. Nonetheless primary prevention of breast cancer by suppression of cell proliferation and thus accumulation of mutations remains a possibility. Although for BRCA related tumours where 50% of gene carriers have developed breast cancer by 50 years of age, intervention at an earlier age than 35 years may be necessary for any reduction in risk to ensue. Other agents are likely to be tried as chemoprevention for this very high risk group and may be best explored initially in trials of adjuvant therapy for primary breast cancers by observing the effect on the contralateral breast in clearly genetically defined groups. Recent evidence of an effect of tamoxifen in improving disease free survival for patients undergoing treatment for DCIS [49] is encouraging but again may be less relevant for BRCA1 gene carriers in particular.

Data from the NSABP prevention trial suggest that tamoxifen reduces the risk of estrogen receptor positive breast cancers.

3.6. Breast surgery

Scientific and media attention has recently focused on the option of prophylactic mastectomy which is now becoming a more acceptable option in some countries (notably the UK and USA) [50] but still culturally unacceptable to most women in countries such as Italy and France [51]. For the first time this year data have been published which indicate a substantial reduction in breast cancer risk from this option [52]. However, operative techniques differ widely and presumably the residual risk will relate to a large extent to the amount of breast tissue left in situ. In addition of course there has been controversy about breast implants and a possible adverse effect on health. Mastectomy without reconstruction as a primary preventive procedure is chosen much less frequently in centres able to offer reconstruction [53].

The situation is complicated for a woman undergoing breast cancer treatment because the prognosis of the presenting disease has to be taken into consideration in decisions about radical treatment. This may be an argument for delaying preventive options for a year or two. Also the logic of conserving the affected breast whilst removing the unaffected breast would be difficult to understand for most women. Women who are able to have pre-symptomatic genetic testing because there is a known BRCA1 or 2 mutation within their family, are increasingly opting for bilateral mastectomy as prevention; to date 12/24 (50%) asymptomatic gene carriers in Manchester have chosen this option. Given the need for a fairly rapid decision as to the type of initial surgery that is to be performed there may be a case for a fast track genetic test for some women keen on the idea of determining whether contralateral breast cancer is reasonable after diagnosis. However, in the context of a clearly hereditary pattern of breast cancer in a family a negative test could still be falsely reassuring. The health service may also be unlikely to pay for commercial testing at $2,400 per test, most private health insurers are also reluctant to pay for genetic tests in the UK.

Breast conserving treatment appears to be as effective in gene carriers as in matched controls although this evidence is from retrospective studies.

4. Conclusion

Where a genetic predisposition to breast cancer is known or suspected there is a high risk of contralateral invasive breast cancer over time. Breast conserving treatment appears to be as effective in gene carriers as in matched controls but this evidence is retrospective. Bilateral mastectomy at the time of diagnosis might be viewed by some as a fairly radical measure but it is one which some women cogniscent of their risks and informed about their genetic status and primary prognosis may welcome as a treatment option. This option could be presented at the time of diagnosis (and in certain circumstances should be). Many BRCA1 gene carriers will have high grade ER negative tumours, for these women chemotherapy is almost inevitable. Four to six months of treatment allows time during which the definitive surgical options can be more rationally reviewed. For women who choose bilateral mastectomies, some may prefer immediate reconstruction if this is possible. Data about contralateral breast cancer risk and ipsilateral recurrence risks must be derived from good long term prospective studies before risks can be further clarified. On the current imperfect data all treatment choices for newly diagnosed primary breast cancer may still be valid. The patient's choice based on contemporary data provided by a multidisciplinary team should underpin management decisions and should ensure that a satisfactory decision is reached in each individual case.

References

1. Claus EB, Risch N, Thompson WD. Autosomal dominant inheritance of early onset breast cancer. Cancer 1994; 73: 643–651.
2. Eccles DM, Marlow A, Royle GT, Collins A, Morton NE. Genetic epidemiology of early onset breast cancer. J Med Genet 1994; 31: 944–949.
3. Ford D, Easton D, Peto J. Estimates of the gene frequency of BRCA1 and its contribution to breast and ovarian cancer incidence. Am J Hum Genet 1995; 57: 1457–1462.
4. Eccles DM, Engelfield P, Soulby MA, Campbell IG.

BRCA1 mutations in Southern England. Br J Cancer 1998; 77: 2199–2203.

5. Langston AA, Malone KE, Thompson JD, Daling J, Ostrander EA. BRCA1 mutations in a population-based sample of young women with breast cancer. N Engl J Med 1996; 334: 137–142.
6. Struewing J, Abeliovich D, Peretz T et al. The carrier frequency of the BRCA1 185delAG mutation is approximately 1 percent in Ashkenazi Jewish individuals. Nat Genet 1995; 11: 198–200.
7. Easton D. Breast cancer genes - what are the real risks? Nat Genet 1997; 16: 210–211.
8. Hall JM, Lee MK, Newman B et al. Linkage of early-onset familial breast cancer to chromosome 17q21. Science 1990; 250: 1684–1689.
9. Miki Y, Swensen J, Shattuck-Eidens D et al. A strong candidate gene for the breast and ovarian cancer susceptibility gene BRCA1. Science 1994; 266: 66–71.
10. Wooster R et al. Localisation of a breast cancer susceptibility gene BRCA2 to chromosome 13q12-13. Science 1994; 265: 2088–2090.
11. Wooster R, Bignell G, Lancaster J et al. Identification of the breast cancer susceptibility gene BRCA2. Nature 1995; 378: 789–792.
12. Lane D. Awakening angels. Nature 1998; 394: 616–617.
13. Varley JM, Evans DGR, Birch JM. Li Fraumeni syndrome - a molecular and clinical review. Br J Cancer 1997; 76: 1–14.
14. Boyle JM, Greaves MJ, Camplejohn RS, Birch JM, Roberts SA, Varley JM. Radiation induced G(1) arrest is not defective in fibroblasts from Li-Fraumeni families without TP53 mutations. Br J Cancer 1999; 79: 1657–1664.
15. Marsh DJ, Coulon V, Lunetta KL et al. Mutation spectrum and genotype-phenotype analyses in Cowden disease and Bannayan-Zonana syndrome, two hamartoma syndromes with germline PTEN mutations. Hum Mol Genet 1998; 7: 507–516.
16. Hemminki A, Markie D, Tomlinson IPM et al. A serine/threonine kinase gene defective in Peutz-Jeghers syndrome. Nature 1998; 391: 184–187.
17. Porter DE, Cohen BB, Wallace MR et al. Breast cancer incidence, penetrance and survival in probable carriers of BRCA1 gene mutations in families linked to BRCA1 on chromosome 17q12-21. Br J Surg 1994; 81: 1512–1515.
18. Struewing J, Hartge P, Wacholder S et al. The risk of cancer associated with specific mutations of BRCA1 and BRCA2 amongst Ashkenazi Jews. New Engl J Med 1997; 336: 1401–1408.
19. Robinson E, Gershoni Baruch R, Dagan E, Kepten I, Fried G. BRCA1 and BRCA2 founder mutations in patients with bilateral breast cancer. ASCO 1999; abstract 2359:
20. Fisher B, Anderson S, Redmond CK et al. Reanalysis and results after 12 years of follow-up in a randomised clinical trial comparing total mastectomy with lumpectomy with and without irradiation in the treatment of breast cancer. N Engl J Med 1995; 333: 1456–1461.
21. Jacobson JA, Danforth DN, Cowan KH et al. 10-Year results of a comparison of conservation with mastectomy in the treatment of stage I and stage II breast cancer. N Engl J Med 1995; 332: 907–911.
22. Veronesi U, Banfi A, Salvadori B et al. Breast conservation is the treatment of choice in small breast cancer - long term results of a randomised trial. Eur J Cancer 1990; 26: 668–670.
23. Abe O, Abe R, Enomoto K et al. Polychemotherapy for early breast cancer: an overview of the randomised trials. Lancet 1998; 352: 930–942.
24. Clarke M, Collins R, Davies C, Godwin J, Gray R, Peto R. Tamoxifen for early breast cancer: An overview of the randomised trials. Lancet 1999; 351: 1451–1467.
25. Early Breast Cancer Trialists Group. Ovarian ablation in early breast cancer: overview of the randomised trials. Lancet 1996; 348: 1189-1196.
26. Gershenwald JE, Hunt KK, Kroll SS et al. Synchronous elective contralateral mastectomy and immediate bilateral breast reconstruction in women with early-stage breast cancer. Ann Surg Oncol 1998; 5: 529–538.
27. Armes JE, Egan AJM, Southey MC et al. The histologic phenotypes of breast carcinoma occurring before age 40 years in women with and without BRCA1 and BRCA2 germline mutations. Cancer 1998; 83: 2335–2345.
28. Lakhani S et al. Multifactorial analysis of differences between sporadic breast cancers and cancers involving BRCA1 and BRCA2 mutations. JNCI 1998; 90: 1138–1145.
29. Verhoog LC, Brekelmans CTM, Seynaeve C et al. Survival and tumour characteristics of breast-cancer patients with germ-line mutations of BRCA1. Lancet 1998; 351: 316–321.
30. Wood ME, Mullineaux LG, Sedlacek SM. Ductal carcinoma in situ (DCIS) may be a feature of hereditary breast cancer (HBC). ASCO 1999; abstract 2364: www.asco.org
31. Foulkes W, Wong N, Brunet JS et al. Germ-line BRCA1 mutation is an adverse prognostic factor in Ashkenazi Jewish women with breast cancer. Clin Cancer Res 1997; 3: 2465–2469.
32. Marcus JN, Watson P, Page DL et al. Hereditary Breast Cancer. Pathobiology, prognosis and BRCA1 and BRCA2 gene linkage. Cancer 1996; 77: 697–709.
33. Varley JM, McGowan G, Thorncroft M, Evans DGR, Kelsey AM, Birch JM. Analysis of a panel of patients with childhood adrenocortical tumours for germline TP53 mutations. Am J Hum Genet 1999; in press.

34. Chabner E, Nixon A, Gelman R et al. Family history and treatment outcomes in young women after breast-conserving surgery and radiation therapy for early-stage breast cancer. J Clin Oncol 1998; 16: 2045–2051.
35. Eccles DM, Simmonds P, Goddard JG, et al. Management of hereditary breast cancer. Dis Markers 1999; 15 (1–3): 187–189.
36. Simmonds P, Eccles DM, Goddard JG, et al. Is breast conservation appropriate for women with a family history of breast cancer? Proc ASCO 1999; 18: abs 2363.
37. Turner BC, Harrold E, Matloff E, Smith T, Gumbs AA, Beinfield M, Ward B, Skolnick M, Glazer PM, Thomas A, Haffy B. BRCA1/BRCA2 germline mutations in locally recurrent breast cancer patients after lumpectomy and radiation therapy: implications for breast-conserving management in patients with BRCA1/BRCA2 mutations. J Clin Oncol 1999; 17(10): 3017–3024.
38. Easton D, Ford D, Bishop DT, and Breast Cancer Linkage Consortium. Breast and ovarian cancer incidence in BRCA1 carriers. Am J Hum Genet 1995; 56: 265-271.
39. Dickersin K. Breast screening in women aged 40-49 years: what next? Lancet 1999; 353: 1896–1897.
40. Tabar L, Larsson LG, Anderson I et al. Breast-cancer screening with mammography in women aged 40-49 years. Int J Cancer 1996; 68: 693–699.
41. Kollias J, Sibbering DM, Blamey RW et al. Screening women aged less than 50 years with a family history of breast cancer. Eur J Cancer 1998; 34: 878–883.
42. Lalloo F, Boggis CRM, Evans DGR, Shenton A, Threlfall AG, Howell A. Screening by mammography, women with a family history of breast cancer. Eur J Cancer 1998; 34: 937–940.
43. Moller P, Maehle L, Heimdal K et al. Prospective findings in breast cancer kindreds: annual incidence rates according to age, stage at diagnosis, mean sojourn time, and incidence rates for contralateral cancer. Breast 1998; 7: 55–59.
44. Elmore JG, Barton MB, Moceri VM, Polk S, Arena PJ, Fletcher SW. Ten-year risk of false positive screening mammograms and clinical breast examinations. N Engl J Med 1998; 338: 1089–1096.
45. Ford D, Easton DF, Stratton M et al. Genetic heterogeneity and penetrance analysis of the BRCA1 and BRCA2 genes in breast cancer families. Am J Hum Genet 1998; 62: 676–689.
46. Fisher B, Constantino JP, Wickerham DL et al. Tamoxifen for prevention of breast cancer: Report of the National Surgical Adjuvant Breast and Bowel Project P-1 study. JNCI 1998; 90: 1371–1388.
47. Powles TJ. Status of antiestrogen breast cancer prevention trials. Oncology (New York) 1998; 12: 28–31.
48. Pritchard KI. Is tamoxifen effective in prevention of breast cancer. Lancet 1998; 352: 80–81.
49. Fisher B, Dignam J, Wolmark N et al. Tamoxifen in treatment of intraductal breast cancer: National Surgical Adjuvant Breast and Bowel Project B-24 randomised controlled trial. Lancet 1999; 353: 1993–2000.
50. Eisinger F, Geller G, Burke W, Holtzman NA. Cultural basis for differences between US and clinical recommendations for women at increased risk of breast and ovarian cancer. Lancet 1999; 353: 919–920.
51. Julien-Reynier C, Evans G, Bouchard L et al. Attitudes towards preventive options for hereditary breast/ovarian cancer: cultural differences between Marseille, Manchester and Montreal. Eur J Hum Genet 1998; 391: 184–187.
52. Hartmann LC, Schaid DJ, Woods JE et al. Efficacy of bilateral prophylactic mastectomy in women with a family history of breast cancer. N Engl J Med 1999; 340: 77–84.
53. Evans DGR, Anderson E, Lalloo F, et al. Utilisation of prophylactic mastectomy in 10 European centres. Dis Markers 1999; 15 (1–3): 159–165.

Breast Cancer: Diagnosis and Management
J.M. Dixon (Ed.)

CHAPTER 13

DCIS and LCIS — surgical options

Virgilio Sacchini, Fabio Bassi and Wolfgang Gatzemeier

1. Introduction

Paralleling the widespread use of mammographic screening, the detection of clinically non-palpable intraductal carcinoma in situ (DCIS), without an invasive component has increased significantly by a factor of 15 times over the last 10 years. In the past, DCIS was infrequently diagnosed, accounting for only 1–5% of all breast cancers. It was usually detected as a palpable lesion, Paget's disease or bloody nipple discharge and mastectomy — with or without axillary dissection — was the standard treatment with cure rates of up to 98% [1].

DCIS now accounts for 20% or more of mammographically detected carcinomas [2–4] and 12% of all newly diagnosed breast cancers. It is most commonly diagnosed after finding clustered microcalcifications on mammography. DCIS detected by screening has a peak incidence in the age range 45–50 years followed by a steady decline [5,6]. Histopathology also shows that the incidence of DCIS declines in mastectomy specimens after the menopause [7]. The incidence of DCIS declines in frequency in the breast after the menopause [7]. Studies comparing risk factors for DCIS and invasive cancer have shown that the risk factors are similar for both (family history, nulliparity, and age at birth of first child, previous breast biopsies) [8]. Although the discrepancy between the high prevalence of DCIS found in some post mortem series and the cumulative incidence of infiltrating cancers suggests that not all DCIS have the potential to progress to invasive cancers within a woman's lifetime [9–11], the variation in prevalence of DCIS between post mortem series indicate that some of what is reported as DCIS in these publications may be a combination of hyperplasia and post mortem cellular changes due to autolysis rather than true DCIS. The important question is whether the detection of DCIS contribute to a reduction in breast cancer mortality. The ability to detect early DCIS has resulted in more attention being given to define both its natural history and optimal treatment. Mastectomy, once accepted as the standard treatment of DCIS when it presented as a palpable or symptomatic lesion seems to be inappropriate for all DCIS, especially when one considers the acceptance of breast-conserving therapy (BCT) for invasive cancers.

A major challenge for the clinician when treating DCIS is selecting a group of patients in whom breast conservation therapy is appropriate. This requires suitable and reproducible guidelines to ensure the optimal therapeutic approach for each individual patient. Several classification systems have been developed to help identify the optimal treatment for each lesion. Unfortunately, none of the classification systems has been unanimously accepted as being clinically useful. The search for reliable prognostic indicators which can be used as a basis for treatment options continues.

2. Natural history of the disease

There is limited knowledge on the natural course of DCIS, i.e. the rate of progression to invasive carcinoma. DCIS presented initially as a gross palpable mass and was treated with mastectomy. Today, DCIS is detected most commonly following mammography and these screen detected DCIS lesions may be biologically different to those presenting symptomatically. Well differentiated DCIS appears to have a limited risk of progressing to invasive cancer, and when it develops, the invasive cancer is more likely to have a better prognosis than those developing from poorly or intermediately differentiated DCIS [12–14].

The time needed for the evolution from DCIS to an infiltrating cancer appears to be different for poorly and well-differentiated subtypes [15]. Long term follow up after biopsy alone comes from series of lesions classified as benign but identified as DCIS on review many years later. In three series with follow up times between 3 and 17.5 years invasive carcinomas developed in between 11 and 28% of patients with DCIS [13,15–17].

3. Pathohistological classification

DCIS is characterised by proliferation of malignant epithelial cells within the mammary ductal–lobular system, without evidence of invasion into surrounding stroma (by conventional light microscopy). DCIS encompasses a pathologically heterogeneous group of lesions that differ both in their growth pattern and cytological features. Traditionally DCIS has been classified on the architectural pattern of the lesion. The most common types are comedo, cribriform, micropapillary/papillary and solid.

4. Prognostic indicators and predictive variables related to treatment selection

In recent years several classification systems [12] have been proposed to assist selection of optimal treatment for the individual patient with the diagnosis of DCIS. Among these are an architectural classification [18], cytonuclear classification [19], Van Nuys classification [20], Holland classification [21], Nottingham classification [22] and classification based on extent of necrosis [23]. To date no commonly accepted classification system exists. Some forms of DCIS express biological markers which are associated with more aggressive clinical behaviour in invasive breast cancer and some subtypes of DCIS have been shown to be more likely to recur following excision alone [24–27].

The search for dependable prognostic and predictive factors to assist in treatment selection has produced some answers but has also raised a large number of questions.

5. Clinical versus mammographically detected DCIS

Most clinicians distinguish between clinically apparent (gross) and microscopic DCIS. Symptomatic DCIS is more likely to be characterised by large size with a significant risk of occult invasion and is associated with a significant risk of in situ and invasive recurrence following breast conservation.

6. Histological and molecular biological patterns

Much emphasis has been placed on histological classification. A commonly used classification is whether a lesion is comedo or non-comedo. Comedo DCIS has been shown to have a poor prognosis, is often poorly differentiated, has high tumour labelling indices with thymidine and overexpression of the neu protein [4,28–30]. It is usually larger than other types of DCIS, is most frequently seen (74%) mammographically. Lagios found comedonecrosis and high grade nuclei in 7 out of 9 of his patients who developed local recurrence [31]. Studies have found that comedocarcinoma is more commonly associated with microinvasion than other types and represents a high percentage (85%) of all lesions described as high grade [32]. Although comedo DCIS accounts for a large portion of DCIS lesions which recur, not all comedo DCIS will recur following breast conservation treatment. Nuclear morphology may be the best predictor of recurrence [33]. Patchefsky's analysis of nuclear grade shows a direct relationship between increasing nuclear grade, the amount of disease in the breast and increased microinvasion. This study concluded that histological type and nuclear grade are interrelated [32]. Finally in a paper by Moriya, factors suggesting more aggressive DCIS behaviour were a solid intraductal growth pattern and high nuclear grade. Central necrosis was also associated with aggressiveness but the association was not as strong as the other two factors [34].

Oestrogen receptor expression in invasive cancer is associated with lower tumour grade, lower degree of biological tumour aggressiveness, possibly a small survival advantage and a greater probability of response to endocrine therapy. Oestrogen receptor has been found in 30% of DCIS compared with 60% in invasive cancers. Studies have shown that a lower frequency in comedo DCIS of oestrogen receptors than non-comedo types. Differences in the actual values between series have been explained by differences in case selection and pathologic techniques. C-erbB2 overexpression has been suggested as a prognostic marker of poorer prognosis in invasive cancer. Poller found that comedo DCIS shows greater c-erbB2 overexpression than the non-comedo type. Oestrogen receptor negative DCIS is more likely to have c-erbB2 overexpression and may be a group of lesions more likely to progress to invasive disease [35,36].

DCIS is a heterogeneous group of lesions with different biological and malignant potential. The prognostic significance of different markers remains unclear.

7. Margin status

Results from early studies of DCIS are difficult to interpret and their findings are probably not relevant to the type of DCIS now diagnosed. Many lesions were palpable and there was no consideration of pathologic margin status and follow-up mammograms were not used. In a series of mastectomy specimens, Patchefsky found 31% of mastectomy specimens which contained residual DCIS following biopsy [32]. Silverstein and others have concluded that inadequate excision of the primary lesion is the most important cause of local failure after conservation treatment. In their large series, 68% of mastectomy specimens had residual DCIS at the biopsy site and 31% of patients treated with breast conservation treatment and radiotherapy had initial involved margins as assessed by re-excision. This indicates that these DCIS lesions were much larger than initially assessed [37]. The NSABP B-17 study reported margin status to be the most important independent prognostic variable for ipsilateral local relapse (2.33 relative risk, 95% confidence interval 1.32–4.12, $P = 0.004$) [38]. Important studies by Holland [39] correlated radiology and pathology and showed that poorly differentiated DCIS develops usually in the terminal duct and extends by continuous growth, while well-differentiated DCIS develops usually in the lobule and has a discontinuous multifocal growth. For this reason, margin evaluation may have a different prognostic significance in these two types of DCIS. In conclusion, an uncertain or involved margin is an independent predictor of relapse although negative margins do not exclude residual disease.

Prognostic indicators for local recurrence were not considered in decision-making of the surgical treatment of DCIS in early published series.

Although individual studies identified single factors as important it was only with the Van Nuys Prognostic Index that different factors were combined to assist treatment decisions [4]. The Index is based on three significant predictors for local recurrence: tumour size, margin width and pathologic characterisation DCIS (high grade or non-high grade ± necrosis). By giving a numerical value from 1 to 3 for each factor these were added to give a total score. Three groups with scores of 3, 4, 5–7 and 8, 9 were identified. When the total score was studied in a series of 333 patients undergoing breast conservation there was a significant correlation between local control and the three groups. DCIS patients with a score of 3 or 4 had small tumours, wide free margins and non-comedo DCIS and had low recurrence rates following local excision alone. Intermediate scores 5–7 (larger tumours, narrow margins, comedo DCIS) benefited from radiotherapy after wide excision. Mastectomy was recommended for scores of 8 or 9 (tumours larger than 2.5 cm, comedo type, large area of DCIS, involved margins at subsequent re-excisions) because of unacceptably high local recurrence rates after breast conservation with or without radiotherapy. This prognostic index provides a scientific approach for selecting treatment but may be too complicated for clinical use, especially when tumour size is difficult to assess. In a further evaluation of their series [41] it became clear margin width was the most important predictor of local recurrence, being more important than size or pathologic type. In patients with margin widths of 10 mm or more in every direction there appeared to be no benefit from postoperative radiation therapy and these women had a very low risk of local relapse. There was also no statistically significant benefit from postoperative radiation therapy among patients with margin width between 1 to <10 mm. In the patients in whom the margin width was less than 1 mm there was a statistically significant benefit from radiation. These data are not from a randomised series and other publications have not found the same importance of width of normal tissue removed around DCIS. Likewise, not all studies which have assessed the value of the Van Nuys prognostic index have found that it predicts for recurrence. Furthermore, the groups of patients treated by wide excision and radiotherapy and wide excision were not treated during the same time period and there were significant differences in size and histological types of DCIS between patients who did and did not have radiotherapy. While the data from Van Nuys suggest that certain subgroups of patients may be treated successfully by very wide excision alone (1 cm clear margins) they require confirmation before wide excision alone can be considered an acceptable treatment for localised DCIS.

Excision alone may be an appropriate procedure for a selected patient population of women with small (up to 2.5 cm) lesions which are low grade.

8. Treatment options

8.1. Mastectomy

This was considered the most appropriate treatment for DCIS for several decades and yet it has a limited role today. The rationale supporting the use of mastectomy included the incidence of multicentricity and the possibility of an occult invasive carcinoma associated with DCIS. These have been shown not to be important with most DCIS having a unicentric rather than a multicentric distribution [42]. There are no clinical trials comparing mastectomy to breast conservation in DCIS. Kinne's series from Memorial Hospital reports on 101 patients with DCIS treated by mastectomy with a median follow up of 11.5 years with only one relapse and subsequent death [43]. Although the rate of local recurrence for this non-invasive disease should be 0%, combined data from seven series of women with DCIS treated with mastectomy demonstrated a local relapse rate of 3.1% and a mortality of 2.3% [44]. Vezerides' review

Table 1. Local breast recurrence after wide local excision alone

Author, year	Patients (*n*)	Follow up (month)	Recurrences *n* (%)	Invasive *n* (%)
Arnesson et al., 1989 [47]	38	60	51 (3)	2 (40)
Schwartz et al., 1992 [33]	72	49	11 (15)	3 (27)
Price et al., 1990 [48]	35	108	22 (63)	12 (55)
Baird et al., 1990 [49]	30	39	4 (13)	1 (25)
Lagios et al., 1989 [31]	79	44	8 (10)	4 (50)
Carpenter et al., 1989 [50]	28	38	5 (18)	1 (20)

found the overall local relapse ranged from 0 to 4% and mortality from 0 to 8% during follow up over 8 years [45]. These data suggest that foci of invasion were missed at histologic examination thus explaining the risk of local recurrence and metastasis. Another possibility is that the mastectomies were sub-optimal leaving residual breast tissue and even DCIS behind with a subsequent risk of invasive breast relapse. The missed foci of invasion explain the finding of occasional lymph node metastasis found in DCIS (1%) [46].

Total mastectomy for DCIS is associated with a more than 98% cure for all types of DCIS.

8.2. Breast conserving surgery

Several retrospective studies have evaluated the outcomes of patients treated with conservative surgery only (Table 1). Differences in case selection, accuracy of pathologic diagnosis of DCIS, type of operation and margin assessment are probably responsible for the wide range of local recurrence rates. A constant finding in all these studies was that almost all relapses were in the area of the primary lesion. This suggests that local recurrence is due to inadequate excision of DCIS rather than due to multicentricity of the disease. Retrospective studies of wide excision and radiotherapy for the treatment of DCIS have likewise shown the same wide range of local failure rates (Table 2). The role of radiotherapy has been investigated in three randomised clinical trials of DCIS; the NSABP B-17 study, the EORTC and UK studies. The NSABP trial was designed to evaluate the role of radiotherapy in the treatment of DCIS. It included women with DCIS detected as a lump or by mammography. A group of 818 women with histologically proven DCIS was randomly assigned to have either a lumpectomy or lumpectomy plus radiotherapy (56 Gy to the residual breast). Patients in whom tumour free margins were unattainable, or who had residual disease at

Table 2. Local breast recurrence after wide local excision and radiotherapy

Author, year	Patients (*n*)	Follow up (months)	Recurrences *n* (%)	Invasive *n* (%)
Solin et al., 1993 [51]	172	84	16 (9)	7 (44)
Cutuli et al., 1992 [52]	34	56	3 (9)	1 (33)
Silverstein et al., 1992 [37]	103	63	10 (10)	5 (50)
Bornstein et al., 1991 [53]	38	81	8 (21)	5 (63)
Hafty et al., 1990 [54]	60	43	4 (7)	1 (25)
McCormick et al., 1991 [55]	54	36	10 (18)	3 (30)
Kurtz et al., 1994 [56]	43	61	3 (7)	3 (100)
Zafrani et al., 1986 [57]	55	55	3 (6)	1 (33)

Table 3. Annual hazard rates per 100 patients according to pathological characteristics and treatment (from Ref. [59])

Feature	Local recurrence rates Expressed as % per year		Relative risk	*P* value
	WLE	WLE + XRT		
Comedo necrosis:				
Absent/slight	3.5	1.8	1.0 [a]	
Moderate/marked	7.5	2.1	1.72	0.0002
Margins:				
Free	4.7	1.9	1.0	
Uncertain/involved	7.2	2.5	1.48	0.06
Nuclear grade:				
Good	4.4	1.7	1.0	
Poor	6.1	2.3	1.36	0.07
Focality:				
Unifocal	4.0	1.2	1.0	
Multifocal	5.8	2.5	1.55	0.02
Histologic type				
Cribriform	4.4	0.6	1.0	
Solid	6.6	3.6	2.41	
Other	4.7	2.1	1.64	0.006
Lymphoid infiltration:				
Absent/slight	4.7	1.7	1.0	
Moderate/marked	7.6	3.1	1.59	0.02

[a] Risk relative to baseline, e.g. absent/slight necrosis, margin features.

follow up mammography, were supposed to be excluded. As noted earlier, some patients with involved margins were included in the study. Five year event-free survival was 84.4% for the radiation treated group and 73.8% for the group treated by lumpectomy alone ($p = 0.001$). The improvement was due to a reduction in the recurrence of ipsilateral breast cancers: 16.4% in the lumpectomy alone group vs 7% in the group receiving radiotherapy. In addition, this reduction was most apparent for invasive carcinoma. Fifty per cent of local relapses in the non-irradiated patients were invasive compared to only 28% in the irradiated group [58]. Difficulties in interpreting the results of this study include the fact that 42–45% of the tumours were less than 0.1 cm, 30–31% were 0.01–1.0 cm and only 8% were greater than 2 cm, and that this study makes no reference to prognostic indicators such as histologic type or nuclear grade. This study was recently updated considering a pathologic subset: 73% of the cohort group was evaluated with 21% of cases being excluded due to inadequate pathologic material or different diagnosis (atypical dysplasia or invasive cancer on re-evaluation of the slides). The results confirmed the protective role of radiotherapy with a 3 times greater risk of local recurrence in the surgery alone group, and a marked reduction in invasive relapses. Criticism of a lack of pathologic correlation in the first published NSABP B-17 study was addressed by this update in which the authors found that comedo necrosis and margin status being the the most important independent predictors of ipsilateral breast relapse [38]. In the eight year update for this study the degree of comedo necrosis continued to discriminate for in breast recurrence (IBR) following lumpectomy for DCIS. Unlike the previous report, margin

Table 4. Results of the EORTC DCIS trial (Ref. [60])

	4 year No radiotherapy	Recurrence free rates Radiotherapy	*P* value
All local recurrences	84%	91%	0.005
DCIS recurrence	92%	95%	0.06
Invasive recurrence	92%	96%	0.04
Distant metastases	98%	99%	0.96
Death	99%	99%	0.94
Contralateral breast cancer	99%	97%	0.01
Event free survival	82%	86%	0.20

status was found to have only borderline influence on the frequency of IBR although the authors advise excision with free margins (Table 3) [59]. This multicentre trial provides a pragmatic answer on the effectiveness of radiotherapy in DCIS, but no sub-group in which radiotherapy could be avoided was identified by the NSABP trial. For this reason the Van Nuys prognostic index [40] has gained acceptance in an effort to individualise treatment of DCIS.

The EORTC trial also demonstrated that radiotherapy reduced local relapse following excision of DCIS but reported an increase in contralateral cancers probably related to the radiotherapy technique used in this study (Table 4) [60]. The UK Trial has only reported in abstract form and shows again a significant reduction in recurrences with radiotherapy.

For the majority of cases of localised DCIS, radiation should be given to the whole breast following complete excision (clear margins).

The recent publication of the NSABP B-24 study [61], a randomised double blinded study of adjuvant tamoxifen versus placebo after lumpectomy and radiation therapy in patients with DCIS shows a benefit for tamoxifen in reducing the local relapse and contralateral tumour risk. After a median follow-up of 74 months (range 57–93) the benefit of tamoxifen was greater in high risk sub-groups (less the 50 years old patients, comedonecrosis, positive margins) (Table 5). The side effects of tamoxifen in this trial included a 1% incidence of deep vein thrombosis vs 0.2% in placebo, a 0.2% incidence of pulmonary embolism and a 0.15% incidence of endometrial cancer vs 0.45 in placebo, which are acceptable and the benefits in reducing local failure and contralateral cancer development were greater than drug related morbidity even in low risk DCIS. In this trial patients did not require free margins to enter and the risk of local failure in this subgroup of patients with involved margins who took tamoxifen was quite low (17%) with a marked

Table 5. Local recurrence rate after adjuvant tamoxifen versus placebo in patients with DCIS treated by lumpectomy and radiation therapy (from Ref. [61])

	Placebo No. of pts, 902	Local recurrence Rate % per year	Tamoxifen No. of pts, 902	Local recurrence Rate % per year
< = 49 yrs	48	3.3	32	2.1
> = 50 yrs	39	1.3	31	1.0
Negative margins	54	1.6	42	1.2
Positive margins	33	3.1	21	1.7
No comedo necrosis	29	1.3	24	1.0
Comedo necrosis	56	2.7	39	1.9

reduction in invasive relapse. The overall conclusion was that triple treatment (conservation surgery, radiotherapy and tamoxifen) is an alternative to mastectomy in a subgroup of patients without clear margins.

> *Following excision in a subgroup of patients with involved margins, radiotherapy followed by tamoxifen has been proposed as an alternative to mastectomy.*

In this trial there was no stratification using hormonal receptor and c-erbB2 overexpression, two factors which may influence response to tamoxifen [61]. The use of triple therapy in all women with DCIS may result in over-treatment of some patients with small, well-differentiated DCIS with clear margins.

9. Diagnostic biopsy

DCIS nowadays is usually diagnosed mammographically as a non-palpable lesion with microcalcifications or may be an incidental finding in a breast tissue resection performed for another reason. Core needle biopsy or a vacuum assisted mammotome biopsy is the diagnostic approach of choice for lesions considered likely to be DCIS [62]. If this fails to establish a diagnosis or if DCIS is identified and the lesion is to be excised, a stereotactic localisation procedure is required. Options for localising the calcification include the use of a needle or hook-wire or localisation using dye or carbon and the new radioguided excision, using radiolabelled albumin and a gamma-probe. Each technique has its own particular advantages and disadvantages to assist the surgeon in resecting non-palpable lesions [63–65]. After complete removal the specimen should be orientated with surgical clips on three different margins. Specimen radiography should be performed to verify that the entire lesion has been removed and re-excision of any potentially involved margin should be performed. Intraoperative histological examination by frozen section is not recommended for several reasons. First, the identification of DCIS on frozen section is not always easy and second, margin assessment and exclusion of microinvasion have too low a sensitivity to be clinically useful. Post-operative mammography should be performed to confirm adequate removal of the lesion and to obtain a baseline for future comparison.

> *A careful mammographic and pathological evaluation of excisions performed for DCIS is necessary to confirm the localised nature of the DCIS and to assess the completeness of resection.*

10. Role of axillary dissection

In localised pure DCIS, axillary dissection is not indicated. In large area of microcalcification in which histology shows high grade DCIS there is a distinct possibility of invasion, and so a level I or lower axillary dissection may be appropriate in patients undergoing mastectomy to avoid a second operation if invasion is verified [38]. In a recent paper Zavotsky demonstrated that it was feasible to perform a sentinel node biopsy to detect lymph node micrometastases in patients with DCIS with microinvasion [66].

> *There is no indication for axillary dissection in pure DICS.*

> *In patients with extensive microcalcification where histology shows high grade DCIS and a mastectomy is being performed a lower axillary dissection or alternatively a sentinel node biopsy of the axilla may be appropriate.*

11. Summary

Pure DCIS is a local, non invasive cancer. Total mastectomy is associated with a more than 98%

cure for all types of DCIS. (Furthermore the advantage of total mastectomy is the identification of occult microinvasion in a high percentage.) A breast conserving approach should be selected for patients with localised DCIS. Excision alone may be an appropriate procedure only for a high selected patient-population with low-grade small lesion (1–2.5 cm). [67,68] In all other cases of localised DCIS a the combination with irradiation should be taken into consideration. Nevertheless for all breast-conserving surgery a conscientious mammographic evaluation as well as a meticulous pathological investigation to confirm the localised nature of the DCIS and to assess the completeness of resection has to be done. In DCIS with diffuse suspicious microcalcifications or positive margins after local (re-) resection total mastectomy – with or without simultaneous reconstruction – is the treatment of choice. There is no indication for axillary dissection in pure DCIS. In case with large high-grade lesion in which a mastectomy has to be performed a lower axillary dissection or alternatively a sentinel node biopsy of the axilla has to be taken into consideration, to avoid a second operation if invasion is identified. Triple treatment (conservative surgery, radiotherapy and tamoxifen) may be an alternative to mastectomy in subgroup of patients without clear margins. DCIS represents a heterogeneous group of lesions with different biological and malignant potential. Until now the prognostic significance of the various predictive and prognostic markers remains unclear. As a consequence these markers can only be enlisted restrictively for the treatment selection. After "informed consent" the patient should given the opportunity to take part in the decision-making process concerning the various treatment options.

12. Lobular carcinoma in situ (LCIS)

12.1. Incidence

The true incidence of LCIS in the general population is unknown because of a lack of frequent clinical or mammographic features and it is usually an incidental microscopic finding in breast tissue removed for another reason. LCIS is nowadays considered to be a risk factor for the development of invasive breast cancer with the risk being approximately 7–10 times higher than in the general population [69]. There is a low incidence of synchronous invasive cancer being approximately 5%. Most carcinomas which develop in women with LCIS are invasive ductal carcinomas but there is a higher incidence of invasive lobular cancers than that in the general population. The incidence of bilaterality in LCIS is up to 70%.

12.2. Pathology

Histological features of LCIS show little variation in individual cells in contrast to DCIS. LCIS arises from the epithelial cells lining the breast lobules.

12.3. Treatment options

LCIS requires no treatment in itself but careful clinical and mammographic follow up is mandatory because of the increased risk of developing invasive breast cancer. Wide resection and negative surgical margins after the diagnosis of LCIS are not necessary when careful follow up is being performed. There is no role for radiation or systemic chemotherapy in patients with LCIS. Bilateral prophylactic mastectomy with simultaneous reconstruction might be an option for patients with LCIS who feel this is the appropriate and best treatment for them.

Another option is chemoprevention. Studies have shown an approximately 50% reduction in the incidence of both infiltrating cancer and intraductal carcinoma in situ in patients taking tamoxifen, 20 mg/day for five years vs placebo [70]. Considering the risk/benefit ratio, this treatment may be offered to LCIS patients.

References

1. Kinne DW, Petrek JA, Osborne MP et al. (1989) Breast carcinoma in situ. Arch Surg, 124, 1303.
2. Rebner M, Raju U (1994) Noninvasive breast cancer. Radiology, 190, 623–631.
3. Lagios MD (1990) Duct carcinoma in situ, pathology and treatment. Surg Clin N Am, 70/4, 853–871.
4. Schnitt SJ, Silen W, Sadowsky NL et al. (1988) Ductal carcinoma in situ. N Engl J Med, 318, 898–902.
5. Gibbs NM (1998) Topographical and histological presentation of mammographic pathology in breast cancer. J Clin Pathol, 41, 3–11.
6. Wazer DE, Gage J, Homer M et al. (1996) Age-related differences in patients with non-palpable breast carcinomas. Cancer, 78, 1432–1437.
7. Nielsen M, Thomsen JN, Primdahl S et al. (1987) Breast cancer and atypia among young and middle-aged women: a study of 110 medicolegal autopsies. Br J Cancer, 56, 814–819.
8. Kerlikowske K, Barclay J, Grady D, Sickles EA, Ernster V (1997) Comparison of risk factors for ductal carcinoma in situ and invasive breast cancer. J Natl Cancer Inst, 89, 76–82.
9. Alpers C, Wellings S. (1985) The prevalence of carcinoma in situ in normal and cancer associated breast. Hum Pathol, 16, 796.
10. Bartow S, Pathak D, Black W et al. (1987) Prevalence of benign, atypical, and malignant breast lesions in population at different risk for breast cancer. Cancer, 60, 2751.
11. Andersen J, Nielsen M, Christensen L (1985) New aspects of the natural history of in situ and invasive carcinoma in the female breast: results from autopsy investigation. Verh Dtsch Ges Pathol, 69, 88.
12. Douglas-Jones AG, Gupta SK, Attanoos R et al. (1996) A critical appraisal of six modem classifications of ductal carcinoma in situ of the breast: correlation with grade of associated invasive carcinoma. Histopatology, 29, 397–409.
13. Eusebi B, Feudale E, Foschini et al. (1994) Long-term follow-up of in situ carcinoma of the breast. Semin Diagn Pathol, 11, 223–35.
14. Holland R, Peterse JL, Millis RR et al. (1994) Ductal carcinoma in situ: a proposal for a new classification. Semin Diagn Pathol, 11, 167–180.
15. Page DL, Dupont WD, Rogers et al. (1995) Continued local recurrence of carcinoma 15 to 25 years after a diagnosis of low-grade ductal carcinoma in situ of the breast treated by biopsy only. Cancer, 76, 1197–200.
16. Lewkowitz M, Lewkowitz W, Wargotz ES (1994) Intraductal (intacystic) papillary carcinomas of the breast and its variants: a clinico-pathological study of 77 cases. Hum Pathol, 25, 802.
17. Rosen PP, Braun D, Kinne D (1980) The clinical significance of preinvasive breast carcinoma. Cancer, 46, 919.
18. Bellamy CO, Mc Donald C, Salter DM et al. (1993) Noninvasive ductal carcinoma of the breast: the relevance of histologic categorization. Hum Pathol, 24, 16–23.
19. National Coordinating Group for Breast Screening Pathology (1995) Pathology Reporting in Breast Cancer Screening. 2nd ed., 23–27.
20. Silverstein MJ, Poller DN, Waisman JR et al. (1995) Prognostic classification of breast ductal carcinoma in situ. Lancet, 345, 1154–1157.
21. Holland R, Peterse JL, Millis RR et al. (1994) Ductal carcinoma in situ: a proposal for a new classification. Semin Diagn Pathol, 11, 167–180.
22. Poller DN, Silverstein MJ, Galea M et al. (1994) Ductal carcinoma in situ of the breast: a proposal for a new simplified histological classification association between cellular proliferation and c-erbB-2 protein expression. Mod Pathol, 7, 257–262.
23. Douglas-Jones AG, Schmid HW, Bier B et al. (1995) Metallothionein expression in duct carcinoma in situ of the breast. Hum Pathol, 26, 217–222.
24. Lagios MD (1995) Heterogeneity of duct carcinoma in situ (DCIS): relationship of grade and subtype analysis to local recurrence and risk of invasive transformation. Cancer Lett, 90, 97–102.
25. Bobrow LG, Happerfield LC, Gregory WM et al. (1994) The classification of ductal carcinoma in situ and its association with biological markers. Semin Diagn Pathol, 11, 199–207.
26. Zafrani B, Leroyer A, Forquet A et al. (1994) Mammographical detected ductal carcinoma in situ of the breast analysed with a new classification. A study of 127 cases: correlation with estrogen and progesterone receptors, p53 and c-erbB-2 protein and proliferative activity. Semin Diagn Pathol, 11, 208–214.
27. Leal CB, Schmitt FC, Bento ML et al. (1995) Ductal carcinoma in situ of the breast Histologic categorisation and its relationship to ploidy and immunohistochemical expression of hormone receptors, p53 and c-erbB-2 protein. Cancer, 75, 2123–2131.
28. Vezeridis MP, Bland KI (1994) Management of ductal carcinoma in situ. Surg Oncol, 3, 309–325.
29. Fisher B, Costantino J, Redmond C et al. (1993) Lumpectomy compared with lumpectomy and radiation therapy for the treatment of intraductal breast cancer. N Engl J Med, 328, 1581–1586.
30. Gump FE, Jicha DL, Ozzello L (1987) Ductal carcinoma in situ [DCIS]: a revised concept. Surgery, 102, 790–795.
31. Lagios M, Margolin FR, Westdahl PR et al. (1989) Mammographically detected duct carcinoma in situ frequency of local recurrence following tylectomy and prognostic effect of nuclear grade on local recurrence. Cancer, 63, 618–624.

32. Patchefsky AS, Schwartz GF, Finkelstein SD et al. (1989) Heterogeneity of intraductal carcinoma of the breast. Cancer, 63, 731–741.
33. Schwartz GF, Finkel GC, Garcia JC et al. (1992) Subclinical ductal carcinoma of the breast-treatment by local excision alone. Cancer, 70, 2468–2474.
34. Moriya T, Silverberg SG (1994) Intraductal carcinoma [ductal carcinoma in situ] of the breast. Cancer, 74, 2972–2978.
35. Poller DN, Snead DRJ et al. (1993) Oestrogen receptor expression in ductal carcinoma in situ of the breast relationship to flow cytometric analysis of DNA and expression of the c-erbB-2 oncoprotein. Br J Cancer, 68, 156–161.
36. Barnes DM et al. (1992) Overexpression of the c-erbB-2 oncoprotein: why does this occur more frequently in ductal carcinoma in situ than invasive mammary carcinoma and is this of prognostic significance? Eur J Cancer, 28, 644–648.
37. Silverstein MJ, Cohlan BF, Gierson E et al. (1992) Duct carcinoma in situ: 227 cases without microinvasion. Eur J Cancer, 28, 630–634.
38. Fisher ER, Costantino J, Fisher B, Palekar AS, Redmond C, Mamounas E (1995) Pathologic findings from the national surgical adjuvant breast project (NSABP) protocol B-17. Cancer, 75, 1310–1319.
39. Holland R, Hendricks JHCL (1994) Microcalcifications associated with ductal carcinoma in situ: mammographic–pathologic correlation. Semin Diagn Pathol, 11, 181–192.
40. Silverstein MJ, Lagios D, Craig PH et al. (1996) A prognostic index for ductal carcinoma in situ of the breast. Cancer, 77, 2267–2274.
41. Silverstein MJ, Lagios MD, Groshen S, Waisman JR, Lewinsky BS, Martino S, Gamagami P, Colburn WJ (1999) The influence of margin width on local control of ductal carcinoma in situ of the breast. NEJM, 340, 1455–61.
42. Holland R, Hendricks JHCL, Verbeek ALM, Mravunac M, Schuurmans Stekhoven JH (1990) Extent, distribution, and mammographic/histological correlations of breast ductal carcinoma in situ. Lancet, 335, 519–522.
43. Kinne D, Petrek JA, Osborne MP, Fraccchia AA, DePalo AA, Rosen PP (1989) Breast carcinoma in situ. Arch Surg, 124, 33.
44. Balch CM, Singletary SE, Bland KI (1993) Clinical decision-making in early breast cancer. Ann Surg, 217, 207–225.
45. Vezeridis MP, Bland KI (1994) Management of ductal carcinoma in situ. Surg Oncol, 3, 309–325.
46. Silverstein MJ, Gierson ED, Colburn WJ et al. (1991) Axillary lymphadenectomy for intraductal carcinoma of the breast. SGO, 72, 211–214.
47. Arnesson LG, Smeds S, Fagerberg G et al. (1989) Follow-up of two treatment modalities for ductal cancer in situ of the breast. Br J Surg, 76, 672–675.
48. Price P, Sinnet HD, Gusterson B et al. (1990) Ductal carcinoma in situ: predictors of local recurrence and progression in patients treated by surgery alone. Br J Cancer, 61, 869–72.
49. Baird RM, Worth A, Hislop G (1990) Recurrence after lumpectomy for comedotype intraductal carcinoma of the breast. Am J Surg, 159, 479–81.
50. Carpenter R, Boulter PS, Cooke T et al. (1989) Management of screen detected ductal carcinoma in situ of the female breast. Br J Surg, 76, 564–7.
51. Solin LJ, Yeh I-T, Kurtz J et al. (1993) Ductal carcinoma in situ (intraductal carcinoma of the breast treated with breast conservation surgery and definitive irradiation). Cancer, 71, 2523–42.
52. Cutuli B, Teissier E, Pait J-M et al. (1992) Radical surgery and conservative treatment of ductal carcinoma in situ of the breast. Eur J Cancer, 18, 649.
53. Bornstein BA, Recht A, Connolly JL et al. (1991) Results of treating ductal carcinoma of the breast with conservative surgery and radiation therapy. Cancer, 67, 7–13.
54. Haffty BG, Peschel RE, Papadopoulos D et al. (1990) Radiation therapy for ductal carcinoma in situ. Conn Med, 54, 482–4.
55. Mc Cormick B, Rosen PP, Kinne D et al. (1991) Duct carcinoma of the breast: an analysis of local control after conservative surgery and radiotherapy. Int J Radiat Oncol Biol Phys, 21, 289–92.
56. Kurtz J, Solin L, McNeese, Forquet A, McCormick B, Recht A, Schultz D, Barret W, Fowble B et al. (1994) Importance of invasive recurrence after breast–conserving treatment of ductal carcinoma in situ. Proc Annu Meet Am Soc Clin Oncol, 13, A210.
57. Zafrani B, Fourquet A, Vilcoq JR, Legal M, Calle R (1986) Conservative management of intraductal breast carcinoma with tumorectomy and radiation therapy. Cancer, 301, 1299.
58. Fisher B, Constantino J, Redmond C et al. (1993) Lumpectomy compared with lumpectomy and radiation therapy for the treatment of intraductal breast cancer. N Engl J Med, 328, 1581.
59. Fisher ER, Dignam J, Tan-Chiu, E et al. (1999) Pathological findings from the National Surgical Adjuvant Breast Project (NSAPB) Eight year update of Protocol B-17. Cancer, 86, 429–38.
60. Julien J-P, Bijker N, Fentiman IS, Peterse JL, Delledonne V, Rouanet P, Avril A, Sylvester R, Mignolet F, Bartelink H, Van Dongen JA on behalf of the EORTC Breast Cancer Cooperative Group and EORTC Radiotherapy Group (2000). Radiotherapy in breast-conserving treatment for ductal carcinoma in situ: first results of the EORTC randomised phase III trial 10853. Lancet, 355, 528–533.

61. Fisher B, Dignam J, Wolmark N, Wickerham DL, Fisher ER, Mamounas E, Smith R, Begovic M, Dimitrov NV, Margolese RG, Kardinal CG, Kavanah MT, Fehrenbacher L, Oishi R (1999) Tamoxifen in treatment of intraductal breast cancer: National Surgical Adjuvant Breast and Bowel Project B-24 randomised controlled trial. Lancet, 353, 1993–2000.
62. Morrow M (1995) When can stereotactic core biopsy replace excisional biopsy? A clinical perspective. Breast Cancer Res Treat, 36(1), 1–9.
63. Velanovic V, Lewis FR Jr., Nathanson SD et al. (1999) Comparison of mammographically guided breast biopsy techniques. Ann Surg, 5, 625–633.
64. Zurrida S, Galimberti V, Monti S et al. (1998) Radioguided localisation of occult breast lesions. Breast, 7, 11–13.
65. Luini A, Zurrida S, Paganelli G et al. (1999) Comparison of radioguided excision with wire localisation of occult breast lesion. Br J Surg, 86, 522–525.
66. Zavotsky J, Hansen N, Brennan MB et al. (1999) Lymph node metastasis from ductal carcinoma in situ with microinvasion. Cancer, 85, 2439–43.
67. Page DL, Lagios MD (1994) Pathology and clinical evaluation of ductal carcinoma in situ (DCIS) of the breast. Cancer Lett, 86, 1–4.
68. Lagios MD (1995) Heterogeneity of duct carcinoma in situ (DCIS): relationship of grade and subtype analysis to local recurrence and risk of invasive transformation. Cancer Lett, 90, 97–102.
69. Page DL, Kitt DT Jr., Dupont WD (1991) Lobular neoplasia of the breast: higher risk for subsequent invasive cancer predicted by more extensive disease. Hum Pathol, 22, 11232.
70. Fisher B, Costantino JP, Lawrence D et al. (1998) Tamoxifen for prevention of breast cancer: report of the National Surgical Adjuvant Breast and Bowel Project P-11 study. J Natl Cancer Institute, 1371–88.

Breast Cancer: Diagnosis and Management
J.M. Dixon (Ed.)

CHAPTER 14

Radiotherapy and in situ breast cancer

John M. Kurtz

1. Introduction

When breast-conserving surgery with radiotherapy came to be introduced for invasive breast cancer in scattered institutions in Europe and North America during the 1960's and 1970's, some of the rarer non-invasive ductal carcinoma in situ lesions also started to be managed in the same fashion. As DCIS has come under increasing scrutiny over the past 15 years, reports of small series of patients treated with local excision and radiotherapy have been published by these institutions [1]. As local control in these studies appears to be similar to that observed in the management of invasive breast cancers, and few data were available regarding the results of local excision alone, breast-conserving surgery and radiotherapy came to be considered by many as standard treatment for localised DCIS lesions [1,2]. More recently, the need for routine post-operative radiotherapy has been questioned. Newer data suggest that DCIS is often an unicentric, segmental disease and that with optimal collaboration between radiologists, surgeons, and pathologists, some DCIS lesions can be 'completely excised' and adjuvant treatment rendered unnecessary [3–5].

2. How is radiotherapy administered in DCIS?

Treatment techniques for DCIS do not differ substantially from those used in invasive breast cancers [6]. Although DCIS is usually a segmental disease, it can sometimes be extensive [3]. Radiotherapy is thus generally delivered to the entire breast, and there is no published experience with more localised techniques. There is no reason to irradiate lymph node draining areas. Although skin and chest wall are not formally included in the target volume, for technical and anatomical reasons they are incidentally irradiated. There is no evidence that doses lower than those used in invasive breast cancers are indicated in DCIS. Typically 45–50 Gy in 18 to 25 fractions are administered over 4.5–5.5 weeks using opposed tangential fields with megavoltage X-rays or telecobalt. As most recurrences occur in the vicinity of the index lesion, it may be justified to give a localised boost of 10 to 20 Gy to the site of the lesion, most often using an external electron beam or an interstitial radioactive implant. Although the value of boost irradiation has been prospectively studied in invasive breast cancers, this role of boost for DCIS lesions is unlikely to be submitted to the scrutiny of a randomised trial.

- *Breast irradiation techniques and doses: should be the same as those for invasive cancer.*
- *There is no indication for irradiation of lymph node areas.*

Table 1. Eight-year results of the NSABP B-17 Trial, in which patients were randomised after 'complete excision' to receive 50 Gy breast irradiation (RT) or no further therapy [8]

	Without RT $N = 403$	With RT $N = 411$	
Number of invasive local recurrences	53	17	$P < 0.000005$
8-year rate	13.4%	3.9%	
Number of intraductal local recurrences	51	30	$P = 0.007$
8-year rate	13.4%	8.2%	
Number of mastectomies for recurrences	50	29	

3. Is radiotherapy effective in DCIS?

In DCIS radiotherapy may prevent progression by affecting residual DCIS, occult foci of invasive carcinoma, or precancerous changes within the ductal system surrounding the index lesion. The effectiveness of an adjuvant treatment can be conclusively demonstrated by prospective controlled trials randomising patients to receive or not to receive the treatment under test. In invasive breast cancers the efficacy of breast irradiation has been shown by multiple trials to reduce risk of recurrence by a factor of about 4 compared with surgery alone [7]. In DCIS there are fewer prospective data to rely on. In the single published trial on this topic 818 patients with localised DCIS were randomised following 'complete' excision to have 50 Gy breast radiotherapy or no further treatment (Table 1) [8]. At 8 years the cumulative incidence of intramammary cancer recurrence was 26.8% in patients without radiotherapy, compared with 12.1% after radiotherapy. Interestingly, the efficacy of radiotherapy was greater in preventing invasive recurrence (relative risk 0.29) than for non-invasive recurrence (relative risk 0.53). In the above trial, no significant difference was noted between the two arms regarding contralateral breast cancer incidence, distant failure or survival. Although breast-conserving surgery was favoured in many cases for treatment of local failures, more patients in the arm without radiotherapy required mastectomy for salvage of recurrence. Approximately 90% of lesions in this trial were smaller than 1 cm in size.

- *There are few published randomised trials of adjuvant therapy in DCIS.*
- *Irradiation seems somewhat less effective in DCIS than in invasive cancers.*
- *50 Gy breast irradiation reduces recurrence risk by 2–3 fold.*

4. Are there predictive factors for response to radiotherapy?

Selection of patients to receive or not to receive adjuvant radiotherapy is currently based on estimation of recurrence risk, under the assumption that all lesions will respond in a similar fashion to radiotherapy. Although this is unlikely to be the case, no data currently allow prediction of the degree of radiation responsiveness. Because of lower proliferative activity, low grade lesions might be expected to be less radio-responsive, as might be the case for lesions associated with extensive necrosis (implying a degree if hypoxia and hence radioresistance). However, clinical data to support these views are lacking. In the NSABP B-17 trial no patient subgroups could be identified using clinical or pathological features, which did not appear to benefit from administration of radiotherapy [9]. The study's authors concluded that radiotherapy is appropriate treatment for all patients with localised DCIS [8]. 'Biological' factors, including hormone receptors, proliferation markers, and oncogene or tumour suppressor gene expression are currently being investigated with respect to radiation response in invasive breast cancers [10]. Such predictive markers may ultimately prove useful in the selection of patients for radiotherapy after surgery for DCIS.

- *All subtypes of DCIS seem to be influenced favourably by breast irradiation.*
- *There are thus far no known factors predictive of radiocurability.*

5. What are the disadvantages of breast radiotherapy?

The disadvantages of breast radiotherapy include its cost and inconvenience, acute side effects (fatigue, skin reactions), late complications (including cosmetic ones), and the potential interference with subsequent follow-up [11,12]. Although in invasive cancers the acute and late tolerance are generally viewed favourably in the light of the benefits of radiotherapy, a reassessment of treatment-related morbidity may be appropriate in the case of non-invasive tumours, where disease-related mortality is small. As radiotherapy in DCIS is limited to the breast, symptomatic pulmonary reactions should be uncommon and without long term consequences. Although a portion of the anterior aspect of the heart may be irradiated in some patients with left-sided cancers, no serious cardiac morbidity has to date been associated with breast irradiation in the absence of nodal irradiation or chemotherapy. Secondary cancers potentially associated with the use of radiotherapy include a possible increase in contralateral breast cancers, especially in patients treated below the age of 40. Whilst such an effect has not been conclusively shown in breast cancer patients, an effort should nonetheless be made to limit radiation scatter to the contralateral breast. Secondary sarcomas of the skin or parenchyma of the breast are observed in about 1 to 2 cases per 10,000 patient-years, starting about 5 years after radiotherapy. There is thus far no convincing evidence linking breast irradiation with secondary leukaemia, lung cancer or other secondary malignancies, so that such risks are presumed to be extremely small.

Radiotherapy after conservative surgery for DCIS is generally associated with satisfactory long-term cosmetic results [6,12]. The proportion of patients experiencing unacceptable normal tissue reactions (fibrosis, retraction) should not exceed 5%. As most patients will not have had axillary dissection, breast oedema in DCIS patients should not be a significant clinical problem. Nonetheless the irradiated breast can be more difficult to examine both clinically and mammographically, leading potentially to a delay in diagnosis of recurrences, especially if a zone of fibrosis develops as a consequence of boost irradiation [13].

Patients having breast irradiation will not usually be able to have additional radiotherapy should local recurrence occur. Recurrence in irradiated patients will probably tend to be treated more often by mastectomy, whereas recurrence in unirradiated patients might be more amenable to local excision and irradiation. However, there are almost no clinical data to support the effectiveness of the latter strategy. Although recurrences in irradiated breasts tend to be diagnosed later, it is not known whether such recurrences are more extensive or more difficult to treat [13,14].

- *Breast irradiation is costly, inconvenient, and has (minor) acute side effects.*
- *Poor cosmetic results due to radiotherapy should be seen in < 5% of patients.*
- *Other than (rare) sarcomas there are no life-threatening complications associated with radiotherapy limited to the breast.*

6. Which DCIS patients should not have breast radiotherapy?

Since radiotherapy has been shown to be effective in reducing local failure, especially invasive recurrence, many consider that this treatment should be given routinely after conservation surgery for

DCIS [2,8]. However, compared with the treatment of invasive cancers, the absolute benefit of breast irradiation seems smaller, and the consequences of local failure less threatening to the patient's future health. It is thus desirable to restrict the use of breast radiotherapy to patients expected to have a rather substantial risk of local failure, particularly of invasive disease, after conservative excision alone. Future research will define what is to be considered an acceptable risk and what factors will be useful in defining this risk. Lesion size, pathological features, and width of resection margins currently appear to be of use in this regard [4,5]. Small low grade lesions that are widely excised are likely to be adequately managed without radiotherapy. Breast irradiation may find its major role in the treatment of more extensive and/or intermediate and high grade lesions [5].

- *Currently it is not clear which DCIS patients should be selected for treatment without breast irradiation.*
- *This question remains the object of current and future clinical trials.*

References

1. Morrow M, Schnitt SJ, Harris JR. Ductal carcinoma in situ. In: Harris JR, Lippman ME, Morrow M, Hellman S, eds. Diseases of the Breast, Philadelphia/New York, Lippincott-Raven 1996; pp. 355–368.
2. Solin LJ, Kurtz J, Fourquet A et al. Fifteen-year results of breast-conserving surgery and definitive breast irradiation for the treatment of ductal carcinoma in situ of the breast. J Clin Oncol 1996; 14: 754–763.
3. Holland R, Hendriks JHCL, Verbeek ALM, Mravunac M, Schuurmans Stekhoven JH. Extent, distribution, and mammographic/histologic correlations of breast ductal carcinoma in situ. Lancet 1992; 335: 519–522.
4. Silverstein M, Lagios MD, Groshen S et al. The influence of margin width on local control of ductal carcinoma in situ of the breast. N Engl J Med 1999; 340: 1455–1461.
5. Recht A, Rutgers EHT, Fentiman IS, Kurtz JM, Mansel RE, Sloane JP. The fourth EORTC DCIS Consensus Meeting. Eur J Cancer 1998; 11: 1664–1669.
6. Mills JM, Schultz DJ, Solin LJ. Preservation of cosmesis with low complication risk after conservative surgery and radiotherapy for ductal carcinoma in situ of the breast. Int J Radiat Oncol Biol Phys 1997; 39: 637–641.
7. Forrest AP, Stewart HJ, Everington D et al. Randomised controlled trial of conservation therapy for breast cancer: 6-year analysis of the Scottish trial. Lancet 1996; 348: 708–713.
8. Fisher B, Dignam J, Wolmark N et al. Lumpectomy and radiation therapy for the treatment of intraductal breast cancer: Findings from the National Surgical Adjuvant Breast and Bowel Project B-17. J Clin Oncol 1998; 16: 441–452.
9. Fisher ER. Pathobiological considerations relating to the treatment of intraductal carcinoma (ductal carcinoma in situ) of the breast. CA Cancer J Clin 1996; 47: 52–64.
10. Bergh J. Time for integration of predictive factors for selection of breast cancer patients who need postoperative radiation therapy? J Natl Cancer Inst 1997; 89: 605–607.
11. Kurtz JM, Miralbell R. Radiation therapy and breast conservation: cosmetic results and complications. Sem Radiat Oncol 1992; 2: 125–131.
12. Recht A. Side effects of radiation therapy. In: Silverstein MJ, ed. Ductal Carcinoma in Situ of the Breast. Baltimore, Williams and Wilkins, 1997: pp. 347-350.
13. Silverstein MJ, Lagios MD, Martino S et al. Outcome after invasive local recurrence in patients with ductal carcinoma in situ of the breast. J Clin Oncol 1998; 16: 1367–1373.
14. Solin LJ, Fourquet A, McCormick B et al. Salvage treatment for local recurrence following breast conserving surgery and definitive irradiation for ductal carcinoma in situ (intraductal carcinoma) of the breast. Int J Radiat Oncol Biol Phys 1994; 30: 3–10.

Breast Cancer: Diagnosis and Management
J.M. Dixon (Ed.)

CHAPTER 15

Prognostic indices and current consensus management of ductal carcinoma in situ of the breast

Melvin J. Silverstein

1. Current consensus management

DCIS is a heterogeneous group of lesions with diverse malignant potential and it is unlikely that there will be a single treatment in the near future for this wide range of lesions. As information regarding DCIS has accumulated during the last 10 years, the treatment selection process has become more complex and extremely controversial. For most of this century, the treatment for DCIS was mastectomy. Even as breast preservation for invasive breast cancer began to be accepted in the 1980s, paradoxically the treatment for DCIS, an earlier and more favorable lesion than invasive breast cancer, continued to be mastectomy. The reason was straightforward. During the 1970s, there were many patients worldwide with invasive breast cancer being prospectively randomized into mastectomy versus breast preservation protocols; there were no ongoing prospective randomized studies for patients with DCIS and hence, there were no data upon which to base conservative treatment for DCIS patients.

With the increase of new DCIS cases, a number of prospective randomized trials were started in the mid to late 1980s. Two of these have been published. One performed by the National Surgical Adjuvant Breast Project (NSABP) (protocol B-17) [1] and one performed by the European Organization for Research and Treatment of Cancer (EORTC) [2]. The results of the NSABP trial were updated in 1995 [3], 1998 [4], and 1999 [5].

At 8 years, 27% of patients treated with excision only had recurred locally, whereas, only 12% of those treated with excision plus irradiation had recurred. There was a significant decrease in local recurrence rates of both DCIS and invasive breast cancer for irradiated patients. The 8-year data led the NSABP to stand by their 1993 position and to continue to recommend post-operative radiation therapy for all patients with DCIS who chose to save their breast.

The early results of B-17, in favor of radiation therapy for patients with DCIS, led the NSABP to perform protocol B-24. In this trial, more than 1800 patients with DCIS were treated with excision and radiation therapy and then they were randomized to receive either tamoxifen or placebo. At 5 years, 8.6% of patients treated with placebo had recurred locally, whereas, only 6.4% of those treated with tamoxifen had recurred [6]. The difference, while small, was statistically significant for invasive local recurrence but not for non-invasive (DCIS) recurrence. The results of B-17, B-24 and the NSABP Breast cancer Prevention Trial [7] have led the NSABP to recommend both radiation therapy and tamoxifen for all patients with DCIS treated with breast preservation [8].

More recently, the EORTC published the results of its prospective randomized DCIS study

[2], a trial with a similar randomization to B-17. This trial (EORTC protocol 10853) included 1010 patients: at 4 years, 9% of patients treated with excision plus radiation therapy had recurred locally compared with 16% of patients treated with excision alone. The results were similar to the NSABP's at 4 years and the difference in the two treatment arms was statistically significant.

The current standard for patients with DCIS treated with breast preservation requires postoperative radiation therapy.

However, there may be some subgroups of DCIS patients who benefit so little (a few percent) from postoperative radiation therapy (for example, small, well-excised, low-grade lesions), that consideration can be given to excision only for these patients. In an attempt to select patients who are likely to benefit from additional therapy and conversely, those who are not likely to benefit, the Van Nuys Prognostic Index [9,10] was developed.

There may be some subgroups of DCIS patients who benefit so little from postoperative radiation therapy that consideration can be given to excision only for these patients.

2. The Van Nuys prognostic index (VNPI)

The VNPI is a numerical algorithm based on tumor features and recurrence data from the Van Nuys series of DCIS patients. The VNPI quantifies measurable prognostic factors, separating DCIS patients into three clearly defined risk groups. It was designed to be usable with the resources of any hospital and to permit a more rational approach to the treatment of DCIS. The VNPI was designed to be used in conjunction with and not instead of, clinical experience and prospective randomized data. As with all such aids to treatment planning, the VNPI will need to be independently validated.

The VNPI is a numerical algorithm based on tumor features and recurrence data and should be used in conjunction with clinical experience and prospective randomized data.

A histologic, biologically based classification by itself does not yield enough information to determine proper treatment. Two additional factors, tumor size and margin width have also been shown to be independent predictors of local recurrence in conservatively treated patients with DCIS [11–13]. It may be possible, by using a combination of these factors, to select subgroups of patients who do not require irradiation, if breast conservation is elected, or to select patients whose recurrence rate is so high, even with breast irradiation, that mastectomy is preferable.

Nuclear grade and comedo-type necrosis were used to develop the Van Nuys Pathologic Classification [14]. Although, nuclear grade and comedo-type necrosis reflect the biology of the lesion, they are inadequate as sole guidelines in the treatment selection process. Tumor size and margin width reflect the anatomical distribution of disease and the surgeons ability to adequately excise the disease. The VNPI was developed by combining these three factors. Table 1 shows the VNPI scoring system. Scores from 1 to 3 were given for each of the three different predictors of local breast recurrence (tumor size, margin width, and pathologic classification). The scores for all three predictors for each individual patient are totaled to yield a VNPI score ranging from a low of 3 to a high of 9 for a group of 461 patients with DCIS treated with breast preservation (the Van Nuys series through 1997). Fig. 1 shows all 461 patients divided into 3 subgroups by score (3 or 4 versus 5, 6 or 7 versus 8 or 9). The probability of local recurrence is significantly different for each subgroup. More importantly, patients with a low VNPI scores (3 or 4) showed no difference in local recurrence-free survival at 10 years regardless of whether or not they received radiation therapy (Fig. 2) and can be considered for treatment with excision only. Patients with intermediate scores

Table 1. The Van Nuys Prognostic Index scoring system

Score	1	2	3
Size (mm)	≤15	16–40	≥41
Margins (mm)	≥10	1–9	<1
Pathologic classification	Non-High Grade without Necrosis (Nuclear grades 1 and 2)	Non-High Grade with Necrosis (Nuclear grades 1 and 2)	High Grade with or without Necrosis (Nuclear grade 3)

One to three points are awarded for each of three different predictors of local breast recurrence (size, margin width, and pathologic classification). Scores for each of the predictors are totaled to yield a VNPI score ranging from a low of 3 to a high of 9. Reprinted with permission. Silverstein MJ, Lagios MD, Craig PH, et al. A prognostic index for ductal carcinoma in situ of the breast. Cancer 1996; 77: 2267–2274.

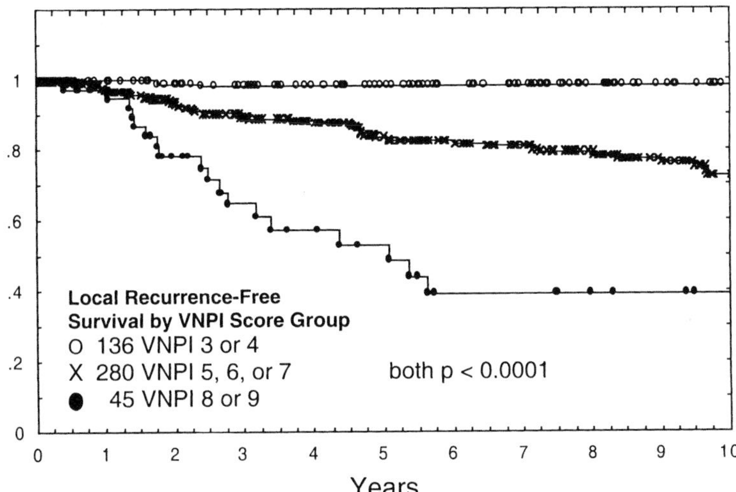

Fig. 1. Probability of local recurrence-free survival for 461 breast conservation patients grouped by Van Nuys Prognostic Index score (3 or 4 versus 5, 6 or 7 versus 8 or 9) (all $p < 0.0001$). Reprinted with permission. Silverstein MJ. Ductal Carcinoma in Situ of the Breast: Controversial Issues. The Oncologist 1998; 3: 94–103.

(5, 6, or 7) showed a statistically significant decrease in local recurrence rates with radiation therapy (Fig. 3) and should be considered for treatment with radiation therapy. Conservatively treated patients with VNPI scores of 8 or 9 had unacceptably high local recurrence rates, regardless of irradiation (Fig. 4), and mastectomy is the procedure of choice for these patients.

3. Margin width as the sole predictor of local recurrence

Margin width is the distance between DCIS and the closest inked margin and reflects the completeness of excision. Although the multivariate analysis used to derive the VNPI suggests approximately equal importance for the three significant factors (margin width, tumor size and biologic classification), the fact that DCIS can be thought of in Halstedian terms (it is a local disease and complete excision should cure it) suggests that margin width should be the single most important factor. Currently, the best way to evaluate complete excision is by determining margin width (Table 2). Serial subgross evaluation of more than 100 breasts after mastectomy for DCIS suggests that when margin widths exceed 10 mm, the likelihood of residual disease is relatively small, in the range of 10–15%.

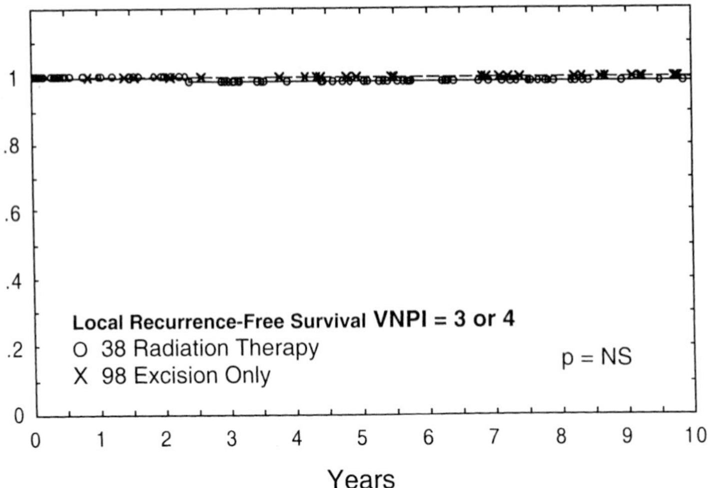

Fig. 2. Probability of local recurrence-free survival by treatment for 136 breast conservation patients with Van Nuys Prognostic Index scores of 3 or 4) (p = NS). Silverstein MJ. Ductal Carcinoma in Situ of the Breast: Controversial Issues. Reprinted with permission. Silverstein MJ. Ductal Carcinoma in Situ of the Breast: Controversial Issues. The Oncologist 1998; 3: 94–103.

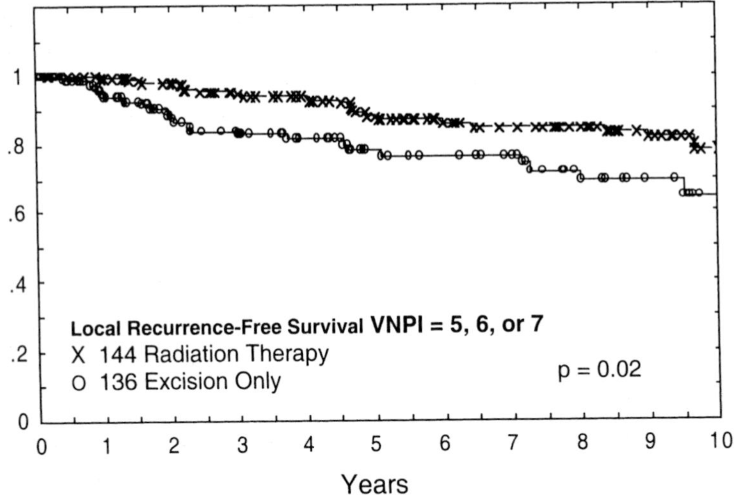

Fig. 3. Probability of local recurrence-free survival by treatment for 280 breast conservation patients with Van Nuys Prognostic Index scores of 5, 6 or 7 ($p = 0.02$). Silverstein MJ. Ductal Carcinoma in Situ of the Breast: Controversial Issues. Reprinted with permission. Silverstein MJ. Ductal Carcinoma in Situ of the Breast: Controversial Issues. The Oncologist 1998; 3: 94–103.

Supporting data from The Van Nuys series suggest that there is little to be gained from post-operative radiation therapy if all margins are greater than 10 mm, regardless of nuclear grade or the presence of comedo-type necrosis [12].

> *There is some evidence that post-operative radiation therapy may not be necessary if all margins are greater than 10 mm clear of disease.*

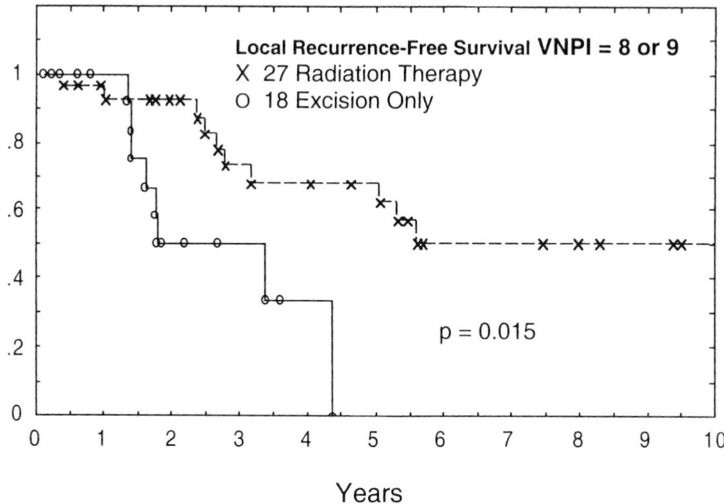

Fig. 4. Probability of local recurrence-free survival by treatment for 45 breast conservation patients with Van Nuys Prognostic Index scores of 8 or 9 ($p = 0.015$). Reprinted with permission. Silverstein MJ. Ductal Carcinoma in Situ of the Breast: Controversial Issues. The Oncologist 1998; 3: 94–103.

4. The axilla in patients with DCIS

There is now uniform agreement that for patients with DCIS, the axilla does not need treatment [15, 16]. In the Van Nuys series, a total of 364 node dissections or node samplings were performed. Only two patients had axillary metastases without evidence of invasion in the breast primary. For patients treated with excision plus post-operative radiation therapy, the lower axilla is included by the tangential fields to the breast.

> *There is now uniform agreement that for patients with DCIS, the axilla does not need treatment.*

For patients with DCIS lesions large enough to merit mastectomy, an axillary staging procedure such as a sentinel node biopsy [17–19] using a vital blue dye, radioactive tracer or both at the time of mastectomy is being evaluated in many centers. This is done because in the event that permanent sections of the mastectomy specimen reveal one or more foci of invasion, axillary lymph node status will have been assessed. If invasion is documented, no matter how small, the lesion is no longer considered DCIS but rather, it is an invasive breast cancer. The sentinel node is evaluated by hematoxylin and eosin (H and E) staining followed by immunohistochemistry for cytokeratin when routine H and E stains are negative.

5. My personal approach to patients with DCIS

With the development of high-quality screening mammography, it has become common to see an asymptomatic patient in whom routine mammography has revealed an area of microcalcifications. During the 1980s, this patient would have had a wire or dye-directed breast biopsy to make a diagnosis. Approximately 70% to 75% of biopsies at that time for microcalcifications yielded benign lesions. In addition, surgeons did not fully appreciate the segmental distribution of most DCIS lesions nor the profound importance of clear margins. During the 1980s, all conservatively treated patients in my unit received post-operative radiotherapy. I was not anxious to perform a wide segmental-type resection initially when the majority of lesions were benign, and I often accepted

Table 2. 8-year probability of local recurrence by treatment and then further subdivided by margin width and additionally by the presence of comedo-type necrosis

	Excision + Radiation	Excision only	*P* value
Number of patients ($n = 461$)	209	252	
Local recurrence rate (all patients)	16%	22%	0.04
Margins $\geq$ 10 mm ($n = 131$)	4%	5%	NS
Margins = 1–9 mm ($n = 223$)	12%	19%	0.05
Margins < 1 mm ($n = 107$)	29%	63%	0.002
8-year actuarial local recurrence rate by nuclear grade and margin width:			
Nuclear Grade 1 (low nuclear grade) ($n = 100$)			
Margins $\geq$ 10 mm ($n = 33$)	0%	0%	NS
Margins = 1–9 mm ($n = 59$)	6%	7%	NS
Margins < 1 mm ($n = 8$)	25%	50%	NS
Nuclear Grade 2 (intermediate nuclear grade) ($n = 176$)			
Margins $\geq$ 10 mm ($n = 42$)	10%	0%	NS
Margins = 1–9 mm ($n = 93$)	7%	11%	NS
Margins < 1 mm ($n = 41$)	23%	44%	NS
Nuclear Grade 3 (high nuclear grade) ($n = 185$)			
Margins $\geq$ 10 mm ($n = 56$)	0%	6%	NS
Margins = 1–9 mm ($n = 71$)	25%	39%	NS
Margins < 1 mm ($n = 58$)	36%	73%	0.01
8-year actuarial local recurrence rate by comedonecrosis and margin width:			
Comedonecrosis present ($n = 286$)			
Margins $\geq$ 10 mm ($n = 78$)	7%	3%	NS
Margins = 1–9 mm ($n = 124$)	16%	30%	0.04
Margins < 1 mm ($n = 84$)	31%	68%	0.003
Comedonecrosis absent ($n = 175$)			
Margins $\geq$ 10 mm ($n = 53$)	0%	7%	NS
Margins = 1–9 mm ($n = 99$)	9%	10%	NS
Margins < 1 mm ($n = 23$)	20%	33%	NS

Reprinted with permission. Silverstein MJ. Ductal Carcinoma in Situ of the Breast: Controversial Issues. The Oncologist 1998; 3: 94–103.

close or focally involved margins without re-excision. My view was that radiation therapy would deal with any residual cancer cells.

My approach changed in the early 1990s. I had a greater appreciation of the extent and distribution of DCIS and I was much more concerned with clear margins and I lost my enthusiasm for radiation therapy for DCIS. The development of stereotactic core biopsy and a specially designed table, with the patient in the prone position, allowed a preoperative diagnosis using a 14 gauge needle. This allowed preoperative consultation and planning. For most patients it meant only one trip to the operating theater for definitive treatment. The main problem with the 14 gauge core biopsy was that because of the relatively small sample size, the final diagnosis was invasive cancer in approximately 20% of the time, following definitive surgery. In other words, one patient in five, in whom the 14 gauge core diagnosis was DCIS, actually had invasive breast cancer. This generally forced us back to the operating theater on a separate occasion to dissect the axilla. We had the same problem with a 14 gauge stereotactic biopsy that yielded a diagnosis of atypical ductal hyperplasia (ADH). In over 20% of cases at definitive surgery these lesions turned out to be DCIS. Because of this, I routinely perform open biopsy following 14 gauge core biopsy reported as showing atypical hyperplasia.

By the late 1990s, this problem was partly remedied with the development of a number of new larger core tissue acquisition systems for percutaneous minimally invasive breast biopsy. We have experience with one of these, the 11 gauge vacuum assisted Mammotome probe (Ethicon Endo-Surgery, Cincinnati, OH). This tool takes significantly larger cores of tissue when compared with the 14 gauge needle and affords the ability to sample tissue contiguously. Consequently, upgrading or changing the diagnosis following definitive surgery is far less frequent, occurring in only about 5% in large series.

Currently, I manage patients with suspicious non-palpable mammographic lesions in the following manner. My first step is to get an 11 gauge Mammotome biopsy. If the diagnosis of DCIS is made, I counsel the patient thoroughly about the nature of the disease, paying particular attention to the size and distribution of her disease as seen mammographically. If she is a good candidate for breast preservation (an area of DCIS that I think I can remove completely with clear margins without dramatically deforming the breast) and she is anxious to preserve her breast, I generally perform a 4-wire directed segmental resection and I commonly use a radial incision because of the radial distribution of some DCIS lesions. I often remove a small amount of skin and I dissect the entire segment down to and including the pectoralis major muscle fascia. This guarantees that the anterior and posterior margins will be clear. If widely clear margins, 10 mm or more in the other four directions (superior, inferior, medial, and lateral) are obtained, I do not recommend postoperative radiation therapy. If the margins are between 1 and 9 mm, I consider re-excision or adding radiation therapy.

In patients whose lesions are too large mammographically to yield clear margins and an acceptable cosmetic result, I prefer to go directly to skin-sparing mastectomy and autologous reconstruction, generally with a free TRAM flap. Having performed only a percutaneous minimally invasive breast biopsy in these patients, I am seldom faced with a skin incision in the wrong place or a biopsy scar that needs re-excision.

Some DCIS lesions extend well beyond their mammographic features and may be extremely difficult to excise completely. These patients are usually best served with mastectomy and reconstruction.

Patients with DCIS treated with breast preservation should be followed closely. At the USC/Norris Breast Center, they are examined physically every six months forever. Mammography is performed every six months on the ipsilateral breast with annual mammography of the contralateral breast.

References

1. Fisher B, Costantino J, Redmond C, et al. Lumpectomy compared with lumpectomy and radiation therapy for the treatment of intraductal breast cancer. N Engl J Med 1993; 328: 1581–1586.
2. Julien JP, Bijker N, Fentiman I, et al. Radiotherapy in breast conserving treatment for ductal carcinoma in situ: First results of EORTC randomized phase III trial 10853. Lancet 2000; 355: 528–533; 1999; 340: 1455–1461.
3. Fisher ER, Constantino J, Fisher B, et al. Pathologic Finding from the National Surgical Adjuvant Breast Project (NSABP) Protocol B-17: Intraductal Carcinoma (Ductal Carcinoma In Situ). Cancer 1995; 75: 1310–1319.
4. Fisher B, Dignam J, Wolmark N, et al. Lumpectomy and radiation therapy for the treatment of intraductal breast cancer: Findings from National Surgical Adjuvant Breast and Bowel Project B-17. J Clin Oncol 1998; 16: 441–452.
5. Fisher ER, Dignam J, Tan-Chiu E, et al. Pathologic findings from the National Surgical Adjuvant Breast Project (NSABP) eight-year update of Protocol B-17: Intraductal Carcinoma. Cancer 1999; 86: 429–438.
6. Fisher B, Dignam J, Wolmark N, et al. Tamoxifen in treatment of intraductal breast cancer: National Surgical Adjuvant Breast and Bowel Project B-24 randomized controlled trial. Lancet 1999; 353: 1993–2000.
7. Fisher B, Costantino JP, Wickerham DL, et al. Tamoxifen for Prevention of Breast Cancer: Report of the National Surgical Adjuvant Breast and Bowel Project P-1 Study. J Natl Cancer Inst 1998; 90: 1371–1388.
8. Wolmark N. Tamoxifen after surgery/RT decreases local recurrence risk in DCIS patients. Oncology News International February 1999; 8(2): 12 (Suppl 2).

9. Silverstein MJ, Lagios MD, Craig PH, et al. A prognostic index for ductal carcinoma in situ of the breast. Cancer 1996; 77: 2267–2274.
10. Silverstein MJ. Van Nuys Prognostic Index for DCIS. In: Silverstein MJ (ed). Ductal Carcinoma In Situ of the Breast. Baltimore, Williams and Wilkins, 1997: 491–504.
11. Silverstein MJ. Prognostic factors and local recurrence in patient with ductal carcinoma in situ of the Breast. The Breast J 1998; 4: 349–362.
12. Silverstein MJ, Lagios MD, Groshen S, et al. The influence of margin width on local control in patients with ductal carcinoma in situ (DCIS) of the breast. New Engl J Med 1999; 340: 1455–1461.
13. Schwartz GF. The role of excision and surveillance alone in subclinical DCIS of the breast. Oncology 1994; 8(2): 21–26.
14. Silverstein MJ, Poller DN, Waisman JR, et al. Prognostic classification of breast ductal carcinoma in situ. Lancet 1995; 345: 1154–1157.
15. Hansen N, Giuliano A. Axillary dissection for ductal carcinoma in situ. In: Silverstein MJ (ed). Ductal Carcinoma In Situ of the Breast. Baltimore, Williams and Wilkins, 1997: 577–584.
16. Silverstein MJ, Rosser RJ, Gierson ED, et al. Axillary dissection for intraductal breast carcinoma — Is it indicated? Cancer 1987; 59: 1819–1824.
17. Krag DN, Weaver DL, Alex JC, et al. Surgical resection and radiolocalization of sentinel lymph node in breast cancer using a gamma probe. Surg Oncol 1993; 2: 335–340.
18. Giuliano AE, Dale PS, Turner RR, et al. Improved axillary staging of breast cancer with sentinel lymphadenectomy. Ann Surg 1995; 222: 394–401.
19. Albertini JJ, Lyman GH, Cox C, et al. Lymphatic mapping and sentinel node biopsy in the patient with breast cancer. JAMA 1996; 276: 1818–1822.

Breast Cancer: Diagnosis and Management
J.M. Dixon (Ed.)

CHAPTER 16

Classification and staging of breast cancer: operable, locally advanced and metastatic

K.C. Chan and N.J. Bundred

1. Introduction

Staging of a breast cancer defines the extent of anatomic spread of the tumour. This is an important process because it determines options for therapy and defines the patient's treatment choices and gives an indication of prognosis (Fig. 1). It also assists in the evaluation of results of treatment and facilitates exchange of information between centres.

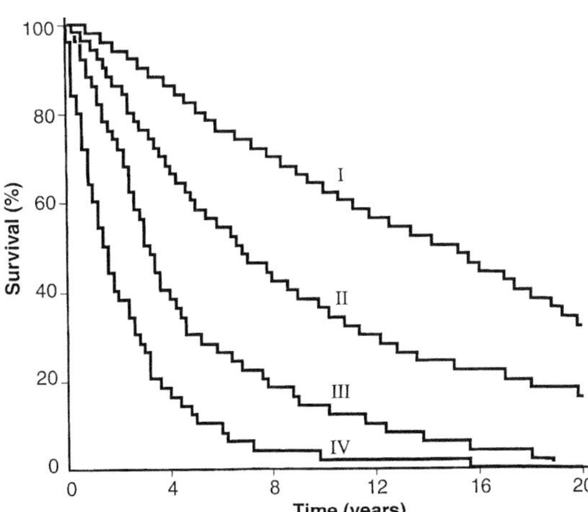

Fig. 1. Survival by TNM Stage of 5430 cases of breast cancer from the Manchester Breast Unit.

> *Staging is absolutely vital for appropriate management of patients.*

2. Histological classification of breast cancer

Invasive breast cancer has been traditionally classified into ductal and lobular types, however, both invasive ductal and lobular cancers both arise from the terminal ductal lobular unit, so this classification is not related to the site of origin of these cancers. A current classification based on patterns of growth and cellular morphology dividing invasive cancers into special and no special types is therefore preferred [1–3]. This classification has clinical relevance in that certain special type tumours (e.g. tubular) have a much better prognosis than tumours that are of no special type. Invasive lobular carcinomas are classified as separate entities because they have a different biological behaviour to other special types with a higher rate of contralateral disease.

> *Invasive breast cancers with favourable prognosis (special types)*
> - *Cribriform*
> - *Tubular*
> - *Papillary*
> - *Mucoid*
> - *Medullary*

Table 1. Tumour Node Metastases (TNM) System

TNM Clinical Classification (c TNM)		TNM Pathology Classification (pTNM)
T (Primary Tumour)		
Tx:	Primary tumour cannot be assessed	Same as clinical classification except for pN1
To:	No evidence of primary tumour	
Tis:	Ductal or lobular carcinoma in situ, Paget's disease with no palpable tumour	
T1:	Tumour 2 cm in greatest dimension T1a: 0.5 cm T1b: >0.5 to 1 cm T1c: >1 to 2 cm	
T2:	>2 to 5 cm	
T3:	Tumour >2 to 5 cm in greatest dimension	
T3:	Tumour >5 cm in greatest dimension	
T4:	Tumour of any size with chest wall or skin involvement T4a: chest wall involvement T4b: skin oedema/ulceration, satellite skin nodules T4c: T4a and T4b T4d: inflammatory cancer	
N (Regional Lymph Nodes)		
Nx:	Lymph nodes (LN) cannot be assessed	
N0:	No LN palpable	
N1:	LN palpable and mobile	pN1: pN1a: Micrometastasis 0.2 cm pN1b: Gross metastasis pN1bi: 1–3 nodes and >0.2 to 2 cm pN1bii: 4 nodes and >0.2 to 2 cm pN1biii: through capsule and <2 cm pN1biv: 2 cm
N2:	LN palpable and fixed	
N3:	Metastasis to ipsilateral internal mammary LN	
M (Distant Metastasis)		
MX:	Cannot be assessed	
M1:	No distant metastasis	
M2:	Distant metastasis (includes metastasis to ipsilateral supraclavicular lymph node(s))	

3. Staging classification of breast cancer

3.1. Classification system

Many staging classifications have been developed for breast cancer [4–8]. The only one that is still in general use is the Tumour Node Metastases (TNM) classification (Table 1). Both the American Joint Committee on Cancer (AJCC), and International Union Against Cancer (UICC) incorporate the TNM classification in their staging system (Table 2). TNM staging has 2 components: clinical (cTNM/TNM) and pathological (pTNM).

Clinical staging is based on information available prior to first definitive treatment and includes findings on physical examination, imaging studies, and diagnostic biopsy (fine needle aspiration cytology, core-cut biopsy). Clinical measurement of tumour size and assessment of axillary lymph node status is inaccurate. Tumour size has been shown to be more accurately determined by imaging than by palpation [9]. A combination of clin-

Table 2. Correlation of UICC, TNM, and Pragmatic Staging

Pragmatic Staging	TNM	UICC
Operable	T_{is-3}, N_{0-1}, M_0	I–III
Locally Advanced	any T, N_{2-3}, M_0; T_4, any N, M_0	III
Metastatic	any T, any N, M_1	IV

ical and radiological assessment of tumour size is used to decide the most appropriate initial surgery. To improve the TNM system, a separate pathological classification (pTNM) has been added.

pTNM is based on information acquired from histopathological examination of resected specimens (tumour and axillary lymph nodes), and from data of clinical staging. The pathological system because of its ability to more precisely define extent of the disease, is more important in predicting prognosis and planning subsequent adjuvant therapy following surgery.

4. Staging investigations

Following initial confirmation of breast cancer, staging of the cancer into three categories, operable, locally advanced, or metastatic is performed and defines how the cancer can be appropriately managed. The TNM staging classification should be documented as there is no better system at present which permits for valid comparison of results from different centres. A suggested correlation of TNM with pragmatic staging of operable, locally advanced, or metastatic is described in Table 2.

Depending on whether a tumour is classified as operable, locally advanced or metastatic, the number of staging investigations will differ as the yield of positive results for the investigation varies depending on stage of disease. A full blood count and serum liver function test should be performed for all patients diagnosed with invasive cancer as these tests are relatively inexpensive and give some indication of whether to proceed to other staging investigations to determine the presence or absence of metastases. A chest X-ray is commonly requested as a screening investigation for pulmonary metastases even though the yield of abnormal X-rays suggestive of pulmonary metastases is low, especially in stage I and II patients where less than 1% of patients have pulmonary metastases detectable on chest X-ray [10]; several studies in patients with invasive breast cancer have shown that approximately 40–50% of solitary pulmonary lesions seen on chest X-ray are metastases from the breast cancer and 50–55% are due to a primary lung cancer [11,12]. Patients with operable cancers (stages I and II) have a low incidence of detectable metastatic disease, and in the absence of abnormal liver function tests or specific signs or symptoms they do not need to undergo a liver ultrasound or bone scan [10,13]. Patients with locally advanced (stage III) and metastatic disease (stage IV) should normally have a liver and bone scan [10]. Pre-operative diagnosis using a core-cut biopsy technique provides valuable information in staging. If the diagnosis is pure ductal carcinoma in situ, patients should not undergo axillary surgery [14], and if it is invasive then an axillary clearance or sampling with a minimum of four nodes is indicated [15]. Knowledge of the patient's oestrogen and progesterone receptor status plays a key role in the management with locally advanced particularly in the elderly patient (see Ch. 6 by J.M. Dixon) and in the treatment planning of patients with metastatic disease (see Ch. 1 by R.E. Coleman).

5. Operable breast cancers

Factors predictive of outcome which are valuable for assessing optimal treatment include tumour size, nodal status and the presence or absence of chest wall or skin involvement, and metastases. Stages I and II and some stage III cancers are operable. The majority of stage I and II cancers (<4 cm in size and unifocal) can be treated with breast conserving surgery.

6. Locally advanced breast cancers

T4 cancers can be frequently rendered operable by a combination of endocrine, chemotherapy, and radiotherapy.

7. Prognostic indices

Various Prognostic Indices have been developed to aid post-surgical selection for adjuvant therapy and estimate prognosis. These indices, which incorporate biological factors, have been prospectively validated to relate to survival, and address deficiencies in the TNM system. The Nottingham Prognostic Index (NPI) utilises tumour size, lymph node stage, and histological grade [16]. The Manchester Prognostic Index takes into account the lymph node positive ratio, the menopausal status, tumour grade and size.

Overexpression of tumour biological factors such as erb-B2, EGFR, nm23, p53, Ki-67, S-phase fraction, and cathepsin D have been associated with poor prognosis [14–16], however, level of overexpression has not been shown to correlate with stage of disease [20].

8. Evolving staging investigations

Investigations which may improve the staging process are sentinel node biopsy of the axilla (see Ch. 13 by V. Galimberti), dynamic contrast-enhanced 3D Magnetic Resonance Imaging (MRI) and Positron Emission Tomography (PET). MRI has been shown to be highly sensitive and specific in assessing tumour size and identifying the presence of multicentric disease [20]. Detection of skeletal metastases has similarly been reported to be accurate [22,23], however, its accuracy in detecting metastases elsewhere, especially the axilla, remains unclear [24]. PET has been used to evaluate primary lesions, regional and systemic metastases by use of tracers such as (^{11}C)L-methionine, and (^{18}F)fluoro-17-oestradiol. Various degrees of sensitivity and specificity in detecting axillary lymph nodes have been reported [25,26]. The role of PET in the diagnosis and management of breast cancer is covered in Ch. 4 by F. Gilbert.

References

1. Scarff RW, Torloni H. Histological typing of breast tumours. International histological Classification of tumours, no 2. Geneva: 1968 (WHO).
2. Page DL, Anderson TJ, Sakamoto G. Infiltrating carcinoma: major histological types. In: Page DL, Anderson TJ, eds. Diagnostic Histopathology of the Breast. London: WB Saunders, 1987; 193–235.
3. Rosen PP. The pathological classification of human mammary carcinoma: past, present, and future. Ann Clin Lab Sci 1979; 9: 144–156.
4. Paterson R. The Treatment of Malignant Disease by Radium and X-Rays. London: Edward Arnold, 1948.
5. Portmann UV. Clinical and pathological criteria as a basis for classifying cases of primary breast cancer. Cleveland Clin Q 1943; 10: 41–47.
6. Haagensen CD. Clinical classification of the stage of advancement of breast carcinoma. In: Diseases of the Breast. Philadelphia: WB Saunders, 1986.
7. Hermanek P and Sobin LH. UICC TNM classification of malignant tumours, 4th edn, 2nd revision. Berlin: Springer, 1992.
8. Beahrs OH, Henson DE, Hutter RVP, Kennedy BJ. AJCC Manual for Staging of Cancer, 4th edn. Philadelphia: Lippincott, 1992.
9. Davis PL, McCarty KS Jr. Technologic considerations for breast tumour size assessment. Magn Reson Imaging Clin N Am 1994; 2(4): 623–31.
10. Ciatto S, Pacini P, Azzini V, et al. Preoperative staging of primary breast cancer. A multicentric study. Cancer 1988; 61: 1038–1040.
11. Cahan WG, Castro EB. Significance of a solitary lung shadow in patients with breast cancer. Ann Surg 1975; 181: 137–143.
12. Casey JJ, Stempel BG, Scanlon EF, Fry WA. The solitary pulmonary nodule in the patient with breast cancer. Surgery 1984; 96: 801–805.
13. Khansur T, Haick A, Patel B, Balducci L, Vance R, Thigpen T. Evaluation of bone scan as a screening work-up in primary and local-regional recurrence of breast cancer. Am J Clin Oncol 1987; 10: 167–170.
14. Hansen N, Giuilano A. Axillary dissection for Ductal carcinoma in situ. In: Silverstein MJ, ed. Ductal carcinoma in situ of the breast Baltimore: Williams and Wilkins, 1997; 577–584.
15. Chetty U, Jack W, Dillon P, Tyler C, Prescott R. Axillary surgery in patients with breast cancer being treated by breast conservation: a randomised trial

of node sampling and axillary clearance. The Breast 1997; 6: 226.

16. Galea MH, Blamey RW, Elston CE, Ellis IO. The Nottingham Prognostic Index in primary breast cancer. Breast Cancer Res Treat 1992; 22: 207–219.
17. Regidor PA, Callies R, Schindler AE. Level of c-erbB-2 oncoprotein in the homogenate of malignant and benign breast tumour samples. Eur J Gynaecol Oncol 1995; 6(2): 130–137.
18. Marks JR, Humphrey PA, Wu K, Berry D, Banderenko N, Kerns BJ, Iglehart JD. Overexpression of p53 and HER-2/neu proteins as prognostic markers in early stage breast cancer. Ann. Surg 1994; 219(4): 332–241.
19. Tandon AK, Clark GM, Chamness GC, Ullrich A, McGuire WL. HER-2/neu oncogene protein and prognosis in breast cancer. J Clin Oncol 1989; 7: 1120–1128.
20. Burke HB, Hoang A, Iglehart JD, Marks JR. Predicting response to adjuvant and radiation therapy in patients with early stage breast carcinoma. Cancer 1998; 82(5): 874–877.
21. Davis PL, McCarty-KS J. Magnetic resonance imaging in breast cancer staging. Top Magn Reson Imaging 1998; 9: 60–75.
22. Downey SE, Wilson M, Boggis C, Baildam AD, Howell A, Bundred NJ. Magnetic resonance imaging of bone metastases: a diagnostic and screening technique. Br J Surg 1997; 84: 1093–1094.
23. Chan Y, Chan K, Lam W, Metreweli C. Comparison of whole body MRI and radioisotope bone scintigram for skeletal metastases detection. Chin Med J Engl 1997; 110(6): 485–489.
24. Orel SG. High resolution MR Imaging of the Breast. Semin Ultrasound CT MR 1996; 17(5): 476–493.
25. Wahl RL. Overview of the current status of PET in breast cancer imaging. Q J Nucl Med 1998; 42: 1–7.
26. Utech CI, Young CS, Winter PF. Prospective evaluation of fluorine-18 fluorodeoxyclucose positron emission tomography in breast cancer for staging of the axilla related to surgery and immunocytochemistry. Eur J Nucl Med 1996; 23: 1588–1593.

Breast Cancer: Diagnosis and Management
J.M. Dixon (Ed.)

CHAPTER 17

Breast surgery: a historical perspective and new technique for the future

U. Veronesi and S. Zurrida

1. Introduction

One major area of development and of controversy in the next decade will concern breast cancer. Breast cancer is the leading cause of cancer death in women aged 35–65 years and developments in the epidemiology and molecular biology of the disease are producing revolutionary changes in our understanding. These are likely to lead to new and more effective diagnostic and therapeutic improvements.

2. Risk factors

One of the key issues concerns genetically determined breast cancer. The discovery of BRCA1 and BRCA2 germ-line mutations as predisposing factors for the development of breast and ovarian cancer opens the question of how the disease can be prevented in such high-risk patients. The presence of a mutation in BRCA1 or BRCA2 site increases the risk of breast cancer at a younger age with a more malignant phenotype, even though the prognosis of BRCA1 and BRCA2 mutation-positive breast cancer patients is not any worse than women with sporadic breast cancer.

The subset of women who should be tested for mutations of BRCA1 and BRCA2 mutation is not yet clear, but a family with more than two close relatives affected has been suggested as being the minimum criteria [1].

Some consider that surveillance may be sufficient to safeguard survival in women with BRCA1 and BRCA2 mutation and newer surveillance methods such as breast MRI are currently being evaluated. However, the most effective prevention method seems to be subcutaneous bilateral mastectomy, although one must consider the psychological aspects of such radical surgery. Subcutaneous bilateral mastectomy is complicated by the problem of performing the operation in many women who do not need it, the difficulty of the operation itself, and the risk of leaving 5–15% of residual breast tissue which could nullify the effort of trying to prevent breast cancer. Chemoprevention is another alternative but even at best will reduce the risk only by 50%.

3. Chemoprevention

Chemoprevention is a specific pharmacological intervention aimed at inhibiting the development of a malignancy by blocking DNA damage or reversing malignant cell progression. Fenretinide, a synthetic vitamin A derivative, has been shown in recent years to be active in preclinical models of breast, bladder, lung, ovarian, and endometrial cancer and also in neuroblastoma, leukaemia and prostate cancer. This agent has now been demonstrated to reduce the risk of breast cancer in young women by about 35% [2].

Tamoxifen administered for five years reduces

the incidence of breast cancer by about 50%; this effect is more evident in women older than 50 years of age, but it has also been shown to be effective in younger women [3]. It appears likely that a reduced dose, lower than that present 20 mg utilised in women with breast cancer may have an equal protective potential.

Other drugs are currently being tested with encouraging results. One promising agent is raloxifene, a derivative of tamoxifen. Raloxifene has been shown to be effective in increasing bone density, lowering blood total and LDL cholesterol levels and having little or no effect on the endometrium [4]. Recent data have shown inhibition of breast cancer in women treated for osteoporosis with raloxifene. To confirm the efficacy of raloxifene a randomised study of breast cancer prevention using raloxifene or tamoxifen is underway in the USA.

4. Innovations in breast conservative surgery

In the field of breast surgery, many innovative procedures have been developed in the recent years with encouraging results for the future. One of the major aims in breast cancer surgery has been to reduce the extent of surgical and subsequent treatment, as the understanding of the natural history of breast cancer has increased and both presentation and type of disease now diagnosed has changed. The objectives are to minimise surgery, and maximise cosmesis while achieving effective local control.

5. ROLL

At the beginning of the century, breast cancer was usually diagnosed when locally advanced: when the neoplastic mass was large and the skin was involved. Today, small, palpable lesions are normal in symptomatic breast clinics and with screening non-palpable lesions without lymph node involvement are commonly identified. The current proportion of non-palpable breast lesions is approximately 30%. This poses important new challenges for breast surgeons. One of the key questions faced by surgeons today is whether surgery can be simplified — and preferably minimised — when the cancer is impalpable. Microcalcifications, for example, are often the first sign of neoplastic proliferation and if localised their presence could indicate the need for a very limited resection providing clear margins are obtained.

Options for localising impalpable lesions include the use of a hooked wire, skin marking or injecting carbon or large molecular weight colloids labelled with radioisotope around the cancer. With radioactive colloid the surgeon is guided during surgery by the use of a hand held gamma radiation detector which picks up signals from the radioactivity injected around the mass lesion or microcalcification and allows a resection to be performed easily and the suspicious area to be removed together with an adequate and uniform margin of healthy tissue [5]. If the surgeon is able to remove a sufficient margin of normal tissue around the 'hot spot', then, even if a diagnosis of invasive carcinoma is made on pathology the margin can be sufficiently clear so that no further tissue needs to be removed from the breast.

6. Sentinel node biopsy

Current research in the area of conservative breast cancer surgery has been concentrated in developing methods that will replace removal of all axillary lymph nodes when there is a high probability that they are disease-free. The sentinel node is the first node to receive the lymph flow from an area of breast, and it is therefore expected that if a cancer has spread then the sentinel node will contain malignant cells. The hypothesis is that if the sentinel node is clear of disease, then others draining nodes will also be disease-free. If, however, metastatic growth is detected in this node, others may also be affected by the disease, and in such cases a full axillary clearance or radiotherapy is necessary. More than 10,000 cases of sentinel node biopsy are currently archived in the world-wide literature, and the method has been shown to be a reliable for predicting the real status of axillary nodes.

The technique used in Milan for sentinel node biopsy, in patients with tumours up to 2.0 cm in size (determined mammographically and sonographically), is to inject 5–10 MBq of ^{99m}Tc-labelled human albumin colloidal particles, in 0.2 ml of saline, close to the tumour. The injection is subdermal if the tumour is superficial and peritumoural if the tumour is deeper within the breast. This is followed by lymphoscintigraphy. Anterior and anterior–oblique projections of the breast and axilla are obtained to determine the exact location of any sentinel node. We employ a gamma-detecting probe throughout the operation to locate the radioactive node precisely and assist in its removal. We have found the combined use of a radioactive tracer and the gamma-detecting probe to be more accurate and reliable than the blue-dye method.

Our accumulated data show that in small-size tumours, an uninvolved sentinel node correlates almost perfectly with a completely clear axilla as determined by subsequent dissection and histological examination. The positive predictive value in large series of 371 cases was close to 99% [6]. The presence of extensive multifocality, as determined by histological investigation of the resected specimen, has emerged as a limiting factor of the reliability of this method.

7. Menstrual cycle

Many parameters have been studied in relation to the outcome of breast cancer in different populations of patients. The timing of the surgical operation for breast cancer in relation to the menstrual phase has been retrospectively studied by some researchers in the past few years. Some studies have suggested that when surgery is performed in the follicular phase of the cycle patient's prognosis is worse than in luteal phase. This difference is significant especially in case of axillary involvement by the disease, and axillary dissection seems to represent an important variable in this field.

Randomisation has been a 'natural' one on the base of the phase of the menstrual cycle. The detection of an 'ideal' menstrual phase to perform surgery for breast cancer in premenopausal women could be of importance. Ongoing prospective studies are evaluating the effects of operations performed in different parts of the menstrual cycle and the results of these large studies are awaited with interest. Until these publications there remains conflict in the literature and few surgeons have changed their practice and timing of surgery in relation to the patient's menstrual cycle.

8. Intraoperative radiotherapy (IORT)

Intraoperative radiotherapy may become an important area in the management of early breast cancer. Intraoperative radiotherapy is the delivery of radiation directly to the tumour bed as determined at surgery. It can be used as a boost to external beam radiotherapy or as a stand alone treatment, at present with palliative intent in aggressive forms of cancer (e.g. pancreatic cancer) and can be delivered immediately after resection of the tumour mass to the open tumour bed or to the tumour mass itself if it is unresectable. In breast cancer, reports of the use of IORT are few. The theoretical gain in the use of IORT in the treatment breast cancer is delivery of a high dose of radiotherapy to a very limited area sparing surrounding normal tissue and surrounding organs. The incidence of local relapse in breast cancer is higher around the site of tumour resection, with a much lower probability of relapse in the other quadrants of the same breast. Shortening the course of external beam radiotherapy after conservative surgery is one argument for using IORT.

At the European Institute of Oncology we have recently started to test IORT as a substitute for external radiation therapy boost in early breast cancer. We deliver 10 Gy IORT in a dedicated operating theatre using an Olympus linac immediately after the surgical removal of the affected breast quadrant, using 3-5-7-9 MeV electrons, in patients over 50 years of age. Our aim is to verify the early and late toxicity of this approach and to escalate IORT dose up to 20–22 Gy so that the entire course of radiation treatment could soon be substituted by a single dose of IORT. The use of IORT in the treatment of early breast cancer could become an integral part of the conservative treatment of breast cancer. Reports of its efficacy are awaited with interest.

> *Advances in the management of breast cancer include a better understanding of the genetics of inheritance, chemoprevention, the widespread use of breast conserving surgery, the use of radioisotopes to localise impalpable lesions and to detect the sentinel node. Controversy surrounds the outcome of surgery performed in different phases of the menstrual cycle. The prospect of using intraoperative radiotherapy to limit the radiotherapy to the tumour bed is being investigated.*

References

1. Burke W, Daly M, Garber J et al. Recommendations for follow-up care of individuals with an inherited predisposition to cancer. JAMA 1997; 277: 997–1003.
2. Veronesi U, De Palo G, Marubini E et al. Randomized trial of fenretinide to prevent second breast malignancy in women with early breast cancer. J Natl Cancer Inst 1999; 91(21): 1847–1856.
3. Veronesi U, Maisonneuve P, Costa A, et al. Drop-outs in tamoxifen prevention trials. Lancet 1999, Jan 16:244.
4. Delmas PD, Bjarnason NH, Mitlak BH et al. Effects of raloxifene on bone mineral density, serum cholesterol concentrations, and uterine endometrium in postmenopausal women. Engl J Med 1997; 337(23): 1641–1647.
5. Luini A, Zurrida S, Paganelli G et al. Comparison of radioguided excision with wire localization of occult breast lesions. Br J Surg 1999; 86(4): 522–525.
6. Veronesi U, Paganelli G, Viale G et al. Sentinel lymph node biopsy and axillary dissection in breast cancer: results in a large series. J Natl Cancer Inst 1999; 91(4): 368–373.

Breast Cancer: Diagnosis and Management
J.M. Dixon (Ed.)

CHAPTER 18

Breast conservation: quadrantectomy: its current role and technical aspects

Stefano Zurrida and Giovanna Gatti

1. Introduction

Conserving the breast is one of the main objectives in treating patients affected by breast carcinoma. This objective must be compatible with good local control of disease with the aim being to keep the risk of local failure as low as possible.

2. Historical note

During the 1970s the concept of surgical radicality in breast cancer, as defined by Halsted at the beginning of this century underwent a major conceptual change. Breast cancer came to be viewed at least in its initial phase as a disease involving only a part of the breast and not affecting the whole gland. Many terms have been used to define removal of part of the breast containing the cancer including wide excision, segmental excision, lumpectomy, tumourectomy, quadrantectomy and partial mastectomy. The first accepted approach for breast preservation was described by Veronesi in Milan [1] in the early 1970s and was called quadrantectomy. This involved excision of a breast cancer with an ample portion of surrounding healthy normal tissue varying from 2–3 cm. The view that 2–3 cm needed to be excised was based on the histological findings of examining mastectomy specimens removed for breast cancer by Holland and colleagues [2]. Long-term follow up of patients involved in large scale randomised trials has shown that quadrantectomy is as safe as more extensive surgery both in terms of overall survival and local failure rates [3].

Quadrantectomy, axillary dissection and radiotherapy produce local control rates and survival equivalent to radical mastectomy.

3. Indications

Although quadrantectomy can be used for tumours in all quadrants, many surgeons prefer mastectomy for centrally located tumours, including even non-invasive disease such as Paget's disease. In a large breast conservation is possible even if the tumour measures greater than 2.5 cm in maximum dimension.

Quadrantectomy can be used for single cancers situated anywhere in the breast measuring less than 2.5 cm or for larger 'cancers' in large breasts.

4. Surgical technique

4.1. Quadrantectomy

The term quadrantectomy should be used only if the classical procedure described by Veronesi in the first Milan trial is performed, i.e. local radical excision of the cancer combined with a complete axillary dissection and adequate post-operative radiotherapy. Some other less extensive local surgical techniques such as tumourectomy [4] or quadrantic excision without radiation [5]. It has been demonstrated in trials that both extensive surgery and radiotherapy are necessary if low local failure rates are to be obtained although studies to date have failed to show that both lesser surgical procedures and the addition of radiotherapy does not influence survival [6].

A lozenge-shaped cutaneous incision with the long axis radiating from the nipple is the most suitable incision in the majority of cases, particularly since it facilitates removal of a large portion of the ductal tree that drains from the tumour. This excision includes any extra-ductal spread that may be present. For some tumour sites particular incisions and techniques can be adopted which while ensuring oncological radicality produce a better aesthetic result or provide easier access.

50% of breast cancers occur in the upper outer quadrant. This position allows the best cosmetic outcome and permits the most convenient access to the axilla for lymph node clearance. The incision generally begins at the areola margin including any biopsy scar and incorporates at its widest margin skin directly over the tumour and it continues to the axilla (Fig. 1). The width of the incision varies form patient to patient but is never less than the major axis of the tumour. Whether the cutaneous incision includes a portion of the areola depends on how close the tumour is to the nipple [7]. The areola is spared when the tumour is peripheral.

The operation continues by deepening the skin incision on one side down to the pectoral fascia but incorporating 2–3 cm of adjacent healthy breast tissue. The breast tissue is then detached from the pectoral fascia and unless the tumour is close to the pectoralis major muscle, the muscle is not disturbed. If there is direct muscle involvement, then a portion of underlying muscle should be removed. Having mobilised the breast

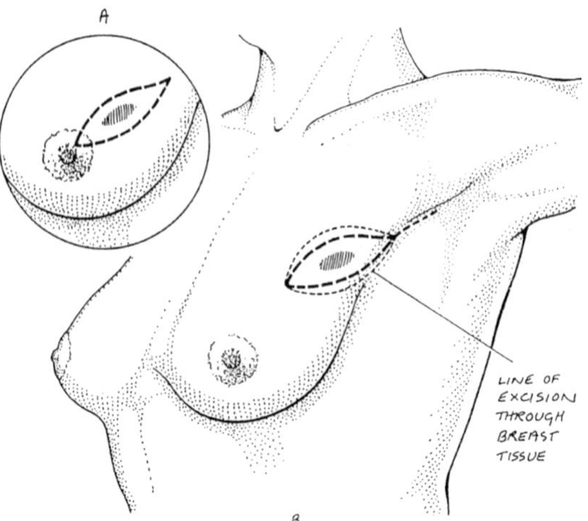

Fig. 1. Typical incision for Veronesi's quadrantectomy in upper–outer breast cancer close to nipple (a) or with axillary dissection in continuity (b).

tissue. From the pectoral fascia the tumour can be palpated between the finger and thumb and the quadrantectomy is completed. Once removed, the excised tissue is bisected by the pathologist along the major axis of the lesion to verify that the tumour has been completed excised and to verify the extent of the carcinoma. Failure to identify sufficient tissue at each lateral margin or concern by the pathologist that the tissue beyond the edge of the palpable mass is abnormal is an indication for removal of extra tissue from the margins of concern. Histopathological assessment of margins is mandatory.

Quadrantectomy consists of excision of skin overlying the cancer and 2–3 cm of normal surrounding breast tissue.

If axillary dissection is being performed in continuity with the quadrantectomy, the closure of the defect in the breast is postponed until the axillary dissection is completed. Closure of the quadrantectomy includes three distinct phases — first haemostasis, second reconstruction and third closure of the skin. If any of these is performed with insufficient care then the aesthetic outcome can be poor and the aim of breast conservation cannot be achieved. Although not usually required, a drain should be inserted if bleeding cannot be controlled effectively by electrocoagulation as bleeding and haematoma can compromise the aesthetic outcome. Any drain inserted should be removed within 48 hours to avoid development of a permanent skin depression.

Breast reconstruction is achieved by mobilising the breast tissue off the skin and subcutaneous fascia superficially and the pectoral muscle posteriorally and advancing breast tissue across the defect. The two cut edges of the breast tissue are then approximated with absorbable sutures. In some instances, loss of breast tissue can be made good by advancing a flap of breast tissue which is detached from the muscular fascia and rotated in to fill the defect. Closure of the skin is by continuous intradermal absorbable monofilament suture.

The defect in the breast left by quadrantectomy should be closed following careful attention to haemostasis by mobilising breast tissue from the overlying skin and subcutaneous fat and the pectoral muscle and approximating these with sutures.

35% of breast tumours are located in the lower half of the breast. For these quadrantectomy usually begins with a radial incision and axillary dissection is performed through a separate incision. Quadrantectomy performed in the lower half of the breast often produces aesthetically unsatisfactory results because of loss of substances from the lower half of the breast and distorts and lowers the nipple. This problem can be corrected by performing remoulding of the breast through a reduction mammoplasty type incision with an inferior based cutaneous pedicle. For tumours located immediately medial to or lateral to the nipple equal portions of breast tissue from the superior and inferior parts of the breast are removed with axillary clearance being performed through a separate incision. Central quadrantectomies are possible with the central defect being filled with a rotation flap.

Radial incisions are used for upper and outer quadrant cancers and the axillary dissection is performed in continuity through the same incision. For tumours in the lower half of the breast consideration should be given to performing a reduction type pattern incision.

5. Axillary dissection

An axillary lymph node dissection is performed in continuity with the quadrantectomy when the tumour is situated in the upper outer quadrant, otherwise a separate incision is normally used. Dissection should be complete and nodes from all three levels excised.

6. Radiotherapy

Patients treated by quadrantectomy should receive radiotherapy starting four to six weeks after surgery. Radiotherapy is delivered using two opposing tangential fields to a dose of 40–50 Gy usually given over a four to five week period (20–25 fractions) with a boost to the tumour bed using electrons or reduce photon fields in a dose of 10–16 Gy.

All patients should have adequate radiotherapy after quadrantectomy.

7. Complications

Major bleeding is unusual and is almost always due to insufficient care with haemostasis. Rarely persistent bleeding is a problem and blood may escape from the wound or build up as a haematoma in the breast or axillary region. If it is not possible to control the blood loss by using local means, re-operation may be necessary to secure haemostasis and/or drain a haematoma. Infection affecting the quadrantectomy wound occurs in between 3 and 4% of patients.

References

1. Veronesi U, Saccozzi R, Del Vecchio M et al. Comparing radical mastectomy with quadrantectomy, axillary dissection, and radiotherapy in patients with small cancers of the breast. N Engl J Med 1981; 305(1): 6–11.
2. Holland R, Veling SHJ, Mravunac M et al. Histologic multifocality of Tis, T1-2 breast carcinomas. Implications for clinical trials of breast-conserving surgery. Cancer 1985; 56(5): 979–990.
3. Veronesi U, Salvadori B, Luini A et al. Breast conservation is a safe method in patients with small cancer of the breast. Long-term results of three randomised trials on 1,973 patients [see comments]. Eur J Cancer 1995; 31A(10): 1574–1579.
4. Veronesi U, Volterrani F, Luini A et al. Quadrantectomy versus lumpectomy for small size breast cancer. Eur J Cancer 1990; 26(6): 671–673.
5. Veronesi U, Luini A, Del Vecchio M et al. Radiotherapy after breast-preserving surgery in women with localized cancer of the breast [see comments]. N Engl J Med 1993; 328(22): 1587–1591.
6. Zurrida S., Costa A., Luini A., Galimberti V., Sacchini V., Intra, M. The Veronesi quadrantectomy: an established procedure for the conservation treatment of early breast cancer. Int J Surg Inv 2000; in press.
7. Galimberti V, Zurrida S, Zanini V et al. Central small size breast cancer: How to overcome the problem of nipple and areola involvement. Eur J Cancer 1993; 8(29): 1093–1096.

Breast Cancer: Diagnosis and Management
J.M. Dixon (Ed.)

CHAPTER 19

Breast conservation: wide local excision: current results and technical aspects

D.M. Sibbering

1. Introduction

Breast conservation is an alternative to mastectomy for the treatment of primary operable breast cancer. A number of studies have now shown that although local recurrence may be slightly more common after breast conservation than mastectomy, disease-free survival and overall survival are the same [1]. The main advantage of breast conservation surgery is that the majority of women should achieve an acceptable cosmetic result, and in comparison to those treated by mastectomy this results in an improvement in body image and allows increased freedom of dress [2,3]. However, high rates of local recurrence need to be avoided, even though this may have little impact on survival, it can cause considerable psychological morbidity.

The main aims of breast conservation therapy are:
- *a local recurrence rate comparable to that after mastectomy;*
- *an acceptable cosmetic result.*

In order to achieve these aims, good patient selection for breast conservation is essential. If an unselected group of breast cancer patients with tumours up to 5 cm diameter are treated with macroscopic excision of their tumour (but no margin of normal breast tissue) followed by radiotherapy, local recurrence rates as high as 21% at 3 years median follow up have been reported [4]. Studies from Milan have demonstrated that by selecting patients with smaller tumours (≤ 2 cm) and taking a 2–3 cm macroscopic margin of excision (quadrantectomy) followed by radiotherapy, low rates of local recurrence can be achieved comparable to those after mastectomy (2.6% at median 6 years follow up) [5]. The Milan II Trial compared quadrantectomy and tumourectomy (≤ 1 cm macroscopic margin of normal breast tissue), both followed by radiotherapy, as treatments for tumours ≤ 2.5 cm. An improved cosmetic result was achieved in the tumourectomy group [6], and this has subsequently been confirmed by another Italian study [7]. However, the improved cosmesis was at the expense of a marked increase in local recurrence in the tumourectomy group (18.6% versus 7.4% 10 year crude cumulative incidence) [8]. This is almost certainly explained by the increased rate of involvement of excision margins in the tumourectomy group (16% vs 4% in quadrantectomy group where margins were assessed), with no re-excision procedures being carried out in this trial [9]. It is now clear that the presence of invasive or in situ cancer at the microscopic margins of excision is an important risk factor for local recurrence [10]. Histological assessment of excision margins and the presence of other risk factors for local recurrence (see Chapter 4) such as lympho-vascular invasion [4] are important in selecting patients for breast conservation therapy.

2. Pre-operative selection of patients for wide local excision

When a diagnosis of breast cancer has been made as many patients as possible should be given the choice of conservation therapy, although not all patients are suitable [11] (Table 1). If a patient prefers treatment by mastectomy to breast conservation, then after appropriate counselling her wishes should be adhered to. It is important to identify patients with multifocal or multicentric disease as treatment by breast conservation is associated with a high incidence of local recurrence [12,13]. Pre-operative mammography is essential to detect those patients with extensive impalpable disease [14].

The size and site of the tumour relative to the size of the patient's breast are important factors to consider. Wide local excision of tumours over 4 cm in diameter usually produces an unacceptable cosmetic result except in patients with very large breasts. In such cases primary chemotherapy may be considered to shrink the tumour to allow subsequent local surgery (see Chapter 24). Patients with smaller tumours that are centrally placed may require removal of the nipple–areolar complex, and those with small breasts are often best advised to have a mastectomy with or without breast reconstruction.

Table 1. Indications and contraindications for selection of patients for breast conservation (NIH Consensus Conference Statement 1991) [11]

Indications:	T1, T2 (< 4 cm), N0, N1, M0 T2 > 4 cm in large breasts
Contraindications:	Large or central tumours in small breasts Multifocal/multicentric disease Collagen vascular disease
Relative contraindications:	An extensive in situ component Young age (under 35–39 years) Widespread lymphovascular invasion

Patients with bilateral disease can be treated by bilateral breast conserving surgery and radiotherapy. Patients of all ages are potentially suitable for conservation surgery, provided they are fit for an anaesthetic.

3. Operative technique

The skin incision should be carefully planned taking into account the direction and orientation of Langer's lines (largely circumferential) and the resting skin tension lines (predominantly transverse) in the breast [15]. Curvilinear incisions are generally associated with the best cosmetic results. The incision should be placed directly over the tumour. The use of circumareolar incisions for tumours some distance from the nipple should be avoided as this can cause difficulty for the surgeon if a subsequent re-excision procedure is required, and for the radiotherapist in accurately identifying the tumour site. It is unnecessary to routinely excise skin overlying the tumour and the removal of a large amount of skin is often associated with a poor cosmetic outcome. Skin excision is only required if the tumour is causing visible skin tethering or if the tumour lies very superficially. It is also advisable to excise the scar when performing a re-excision procedure.

Initially skin flaps are raised over and around the tumour by dissecting in the plane between the breast tissue and the subcutaneous fat. It is important to avoid cutting these skin flaps too thin as this can result in a poor final cosmetic outcome. The aim of wide local excision is to remove the palpable lesion with a 1 cm margin of normal surrounding breast tissue. Using the fingers of the non-dominant hand as a guide, an incision is made circumferentially around the tumour dissecting a good 'finger's breadth' away from the palpable tumour edge. At one margin of the proposed excision the dissection is carried down posteriorly through the breast tissue until the pectoral fascia is reached. Care must be taken at this point

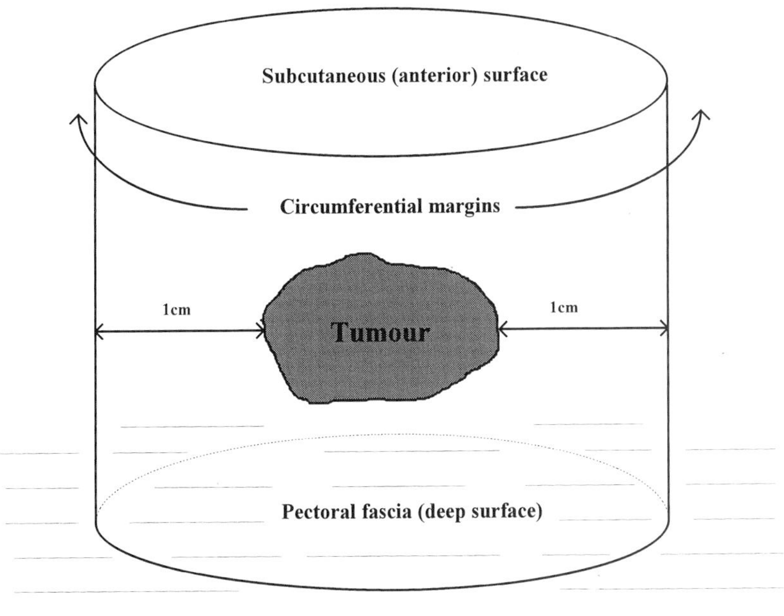

Fig. 1. The aim is to excise a cylinder of breast tissue around the tumour. The anterior surface is directly subcutaneous; the posterior surface is on or including pectoral fascia; the circumferential margins are then examined histologically to ensure complete excision.

to carry the plane of dissection perpendicular to the chest wall to prevent inadvertently removing more breast tissue than planned. The plane is then developed deep to the tumour, no attempt being made to excise the pectoral fascia unless it is tethered to the tumour or the tumour directly infiltrates the fascia and/or the underlying pectoral muscle. If muscle is involved a rim of muscle should be excised deep to the tumour to achieve the necessary margin of clearance. Once the deep plane has been developed the area of breast tissue to be excised can be gripped between the thumb placed subcutaneously and a finger placed deeply and excision completed at the other margins. A complete cylinder of tissue is thus excised around the tumour, removing all the tissue between the subcutaneous plane and the pectoral fascia with a clear margin depth around the circumference (Fig. 1). It may not be necessary to excise a full thickness portion of breast tissue down to pectoral fascia for superficial tumours, but in this case it will also be necessary to obtain a clear histological margin of normal breast tissue at the deep as well as circumferential margins.

> *The aim of wide local excision is to remove the palpable lesion with a 1 cm margin of normal surrounding breast tissue.*

Screen-detected tumours are often impalpable and require pre-operative radiological localisation. For tumours that are well visualised on an ultrasound scan marking of the position on the skin by the radiologist may suffice. It is important that the skin is marked with the patient lying flat with the ipsilateral arm abducted ie, in the same position to that on the operating table. It is useful for the radiologist to note the size of the tumour and the distance it lies from the skin surface. This technique is best reserved for tumours in the upper and medial aspects of the breast where the breast tissue is relatively fixed, and is best avoided in women with large breasts. The skin incision is placed directly over the marked tumour site and the technique used is otherwise identical to that for a palpable tumour. More commonly impalpable lesions are localised by placement of a hooked wire close to the lesion using either stereotactic or ultrasound guidance. Following insertion of the wire, craniocaudal and lateral mammograms are taken and these are discussed by the surgeon and radiologist prior to surgery. The surgeon aims to locate the wire in the breast tissue before it enters the mammographic lesion and uses this as a guide to excise the tumour with the necessary margin.

The excised specimen should be weighed. The specimen should be orientated by marking with sutures or ligaclips. Specimen radiography should be performed at the time of surgery, and this is especially important for impalpable lesions. The appropriately orientated specimen is compressed between two plastic plates and a radiograph taken in the antero-posterior plane using a dedicated specimen X-ray device situated in or close to the operating theatre complex. If the margin of clearance at the circumferential edge appears on specimen X-ray to be less than 1 cm, re-excision of the relevant margin can be carried out at the same operation [16]. Any re-excision specimen is also carefully orientated with sutures or ligaclips to assist the pathologist in assessing the depth of margin clearance. Some surgeons perform routine excision of the cavity margins for histological assessment in the belief that this is a more accurate method of assessing completeness of excision [17]. All excised specimens should be submitted to the pathologist either fresh or in formalin according to local protocols. Dissection of the specimen by the surgeon should be avoided as this causes difficulty in accurately assessing excision margins.

The excised specimen should be:

- *weighed;*
- *orientated with sutures or ligaclips;*
- *X-rayed;*
- *submitted fresh or in formalin to the pathologist.*

Meticulous haemostasis is secured with diathermy. Studies have shown savlon (dilute chlorhexidine) to be tumouricidal [18], and many surgeons advocate routine lavage of the wound cavity with a dilute savlon solution left in situ for two minutes. Apposition of the cut edges of breast parenchyma with absorbable sutures may be appropriate, but is best avoided after a larger resections as it may lead to distortion of breast shape and nipple position. A drain is rarely required. The deep dermis is approximated with interrupted absorbable sutures, followed by a continuous subcuticular (intradermal) absorbable suture such as Monocryl (Ethicon Limited UK). If this suture enters and exits the skin at least 1 cm from the wound ends then knots are unnecessary and the suture may be trimmed at the level of the skin. Steristrips may be applied and an occlusive dressing covers the wound.

4. Post-operative pathological assessment

Histological assessment of excision margins is essential following wide local excision. The surfaces of the surgical specimen are painted with ink. Blocks are taken from the margins of the surgical specimen to allow examination of the entire circumferential excision margin. Examination of four radial blocks allows the accurate measurement of the microscopic circumferential margin of normal breast tissue achieved around the tumour (Fig. 2). The superficial (subcutaneous) and deep excision margins are less important as tissue has already been taken as far as possible in these two directions. If either invasive or in situ cancer is seen at a circumferential excision margin, then a further surgical procedure (either re-excision or mastectomy) is required to obtain clear margins. Some surgeons advocate a 5 mm clear margin of normal breast tissue around the tumour, and will advise further surgery if this is not achieved [19]. If the technique of cavity shavings is used after a wide local excision, if tumour is seen in these shavings a further surgical procedure is indicated [17].

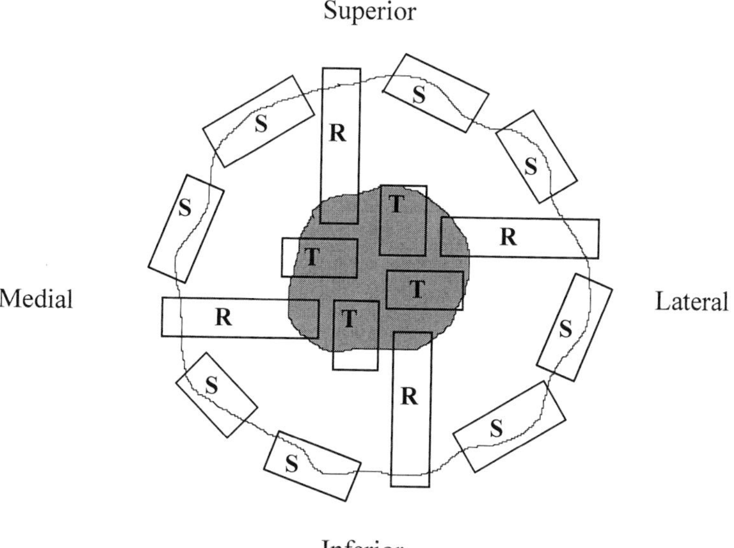

Fig. 2. Histopathological assessment of excision margins. Peripheral shave excision margin blocks (S) are taken to examine the entire cicumferential surgical excision margin. Four radial blocks (R) enable accurate measurement of microscopic excision margins. T = tumour blocks.

The presence of extensive ductal carcinoma in situ associated with the invasive tumour (EIC) has been used as a relative contraindication for breast conservation [11], but is now thought to be less significant if histological excision margins are clear [10]. The combination of the presence of lymphovascular invasion in and around the tumour in younger women (< 50 years) is regarded as an indication for conversion to a mastectomy by some surgeons due to the increased risk of local recurrence [19].

- *Post-operative histological assessment of excision margins is essential following wide local excision.*
- *If clear histological excision margins are not achieved then re-excision or mastectomy is indicated.*

5. Post-operative radiotherapy

Radiotherapy to the whole breast is indicated after wide local excision of the tumour is achieved with clear excision margins (see Chapter 21). To date, no group of patients has been identified in whom radiotherapy can be safely omitted after wide local excision. An ongoing randomised trial run by the British Association of Surgical Oncology is assessing the need for post-operative radiotherapy in patients with small ($\leq$ 2 cm), grade 1, node negative tumours with clear excision margins.

6. Outcome of treatment

A large number of studies and randomised trials have published results of treatment by breast conservation, and there is wide variation in the rates of local recurrence reported. Such different results, in part reflect varied patient selection (particularly relating to tumour size), the extent of surgical clearance, differing post-operative radiotherapy regimes, the inclusion/exclusion of local recurrence developing after the emergence of other systemic metastases, differing definitions of 'local recurrence', varying length of follow up and differing use of adjuvant systemic therapies.

References

1. Early Breast Cancer Trialists' Collaborative Group. Effects of radiotherapy and surgery in early breast cancer an overview of the randomised trials. N Engl J Med 1995; 333: 1444–1455.
2. Kiebert GM, de Haes JCJM, van der Velde CJH. The impact of breast conserving treatment and mastectomy on the quality of life of early breast cancer patients; a review. J Clin Oncol 1991; 9: 1059–1070.
3. Lee MS, Love SB, Mitchell JB et al. Mastectomy or conservation for early breast cancer: psychological morbidity. Eur J Cancer 1992; 28A(89): 1340–1344.
4. Locker AP, Ellis IO, Morgan DAL et al. Factors influencing local recurrence after excision and radiotherapy for primary breast cancer. Br J Surg 1989; 76: 890–894.
5. Veronesi U, Salvadori B, Luimi A et al. Conservative treatment of early breast cancer: long-term results of 1232 cases treated with quadrantectomy, axillary dissection, and radiotherapy. Ann Surg 1990; 211: 250–259.
6. Veronesi U, Voilterrani F, Luini A et al. Quadrantectomy versus lumpectomy for small size breast cancer. Eur J Cancer 1990; 26: 670–673.
7. Fagundes MA, Fagundes HM, Brito CS et al. Breast-conserving surgery and definitive radiation: a comparison between quadrantectomy and local excision with special focus on local regional control and cosmesis. Int J Radiat Oncol Biol Phys 1993; 27: 553–560.
8. Mariani L, Salvadori B, Marubini E et al. Ten year results of a randomised trial comparing two conservative treatment strategies for small size breast cancer. Eur J Cancer 1998; 34: 1156–1162.
9. Veronesi U, Salvadori B, Luini A et al. Breast conservation is a safe method in patients with small cancer of the breast. Long-term results of three randomised trials on 1,973 patients. Eur J Cancer 1995; 31A: 1574–1579.
10. Gage I, Schnitt SJ, Nixon AJ et al. Pathologic margin involvement and the risk of recurrence in patients treated with breast-conserving therapy. Cancer 1996; 78: 1921–1928.
11. NIH Consensus Conference. Treatment of early-stage breast cancer. J Am Med Assoc 1991; 265: 391-395.
12. Fisher ER, Sass R, Fisher B et al. Pathologic findings from the National Surgical Adjuvant Breast Project (protocol 6): relation of breast local recurrence to multicentricity. Cancer 1986; 57: 1717–1724.
13. Kurtz JM, Jacquemier G, Amalric R et al. Breast-conserving therapy for macroscopically multiple cancers. Ann Surg 1990; 212: 38–44.
14. Dixon JM, Chetty U. Mammography in the management of patients with small breast cancer. Br J Surg 1991; 78: 218–219.
15. Matory Jr. WE, Wertheimer M, Love S et al. Partial masectomy: technical considerations in achieving cosmesis. Breast Dis 1992; 5: 225–233.
16. Dixon JM, RaviSekar O, Walsh J et al. Specimen-orientated radiography helps define excision margins of malignant lesions detected by breast screening. Br J Surg 1993; 80: 1001–1002.
17. MacMillan RD, Purushotham AD, Mallon E et al. Tumour bed positivity predicts outcome after breast conserving surgery. Br J Surg 1997; 84: 1559–1562.
18. Park KGM, Chetty U, Scott WN et al. The activity of locally applied cytotoxics to breast cancer cells in vitro. Ann R Coll Surg Engl 1991; 73: 96–99.
19. Sibbering DM, Galea MH, Morgan DAL et al. Safe selection criteria for breast conservation without radical excision in primary operable breast cancer. Eur J Cancer 1995; 31A: 2191–2195.

Breast Cancer: Diagnosis and Management
J.M. Dixon (Ed.)

CHAPTER 20

Factors affecting local recurrence after breast conservation for invasive carcinoma

John M. Kurtz

1. Introduction

Breast cancer usually begins as a unicentric or segmental disease and spreads within the breast by interstitial invasion, lymphatic space involvement, or intraductal extension. After gross excision of an apparently unifocal tumour, about 40% will have no or minimal residual cancer foci limited to within 2 cm of the margins, about 40% will have limited extensions beyond 2 cm, and 20% will have more extensive local disease, often at considerable distance from the index lesion [1]. Thus, even an apparently 'complete' local excision, in the absence of breast irradiation, will not infrequently be followed by tumour recurrence, most often near the site of the primary lesion. The risk of such a 'true' recurrence depends upon the intensity of treatment directed to the involved breast quadrant, the characteristics of the tumour, and certain patient-related factors [2]. Moreover, systemic therapy may also influence local recurrence risk. Very little is known about parameters correlating with risk of cancer growth in areas at some distance from the index lesion ('new tumours'). The present chapter will discuss the principal factors thought to be related to recurrent cancer within the anatomical confines of the conserved breast (termed 'ipsilateral breast tumour recurrence', IBTR), making little distinction between true recurrences, new tumours, skin recurrences or diffuse recurrences.

Ipsilateral breast tumour recurrence (IBTR) in the treated breast following breast conserving surgery and radiotherapy most commonly occurs near the primary lesion.

Most information on risk factors for IBTR are derived from series of patients treated with radiotherapy, and there are only limited data concerning patients treated with breast-conserving surgery alone. After surgery alone, the risk of IBTR depends essentially upon whether or not residual cancer has been left behind, whereas when radiotherapy is given recurrence risk depends additionally on the number of residual clonogenic cancer cells and their particular radiosensitivity. However, there are no reliable predictive tests for the radiocurability of a given breast tumour, and further research in this area is warranted [3]. It is generally assumed, as it will be for the purposes of this chapter, that the same risk factors are operative both in the presence and in the absence of radiotherapy.

2. Factors that are not generally useful in estimating IBTR risk

Many patient-related and tumour-related features appear to correlate with IBTR risk [2]. This chapter will discuss those whose significance has been most consistently demonstrated, and those that appear to be most useful in practice. Unlike local–regional failure after mastectomy, IBTR risk is not markedly influenced by tumour size or lymph node status [2], at least when radiotherapy is given, and neither histological subtype (e.g., lobular [4]), nor tumour location within the breast (e.g., subareolar [5]), are risk factors for local recurrence.

Although some studies have found that high grade cancers show a greater tendency to recur locally [2], other large series do not show any influence of histological grade on IBTR rate [4,6]. The limited usefulness of tumour size, nodal status and grade in predicting IBTR risk may reflect the more aggressive therapy generally received by patients with unfavourable tumours, thereby compensating for the inherently increased risk of local failure.

The presence of multiple masses or widespread malignant calcifications usually signifies more diffuse involvement and represents a contraindication to breast conservation. However, the pre- or peri-operative finding of more than one discrete tumour mass, even within separate quadrants, may not necessarily be an expression of widespread malignant change within the breast. Although these patients are usually treated with mastectomy, available data suggest that the ability to achieve negative resection margins may serve to distinguish between localised and diffuse involvement, with the results of breast conservation being satisfactory in the subgroup with clear margins [7].

- *IBTR risk seems independent of major histological subtype and tumour location.*
- *Tumour size, lymph node status, and histological grade are of limited value in predicting IBTR risk.*

3. Effect of treatment on IBTR risk

Local failure is the expression of tumour-host factors that are operative in the setting of a specific treatment strategy. In a particular patient, the absolute risk of IBTR is profoundly influenced by treatment. The specific effect of a given treatment can be quantified by randomised trials. The relative risk of recurrence is affected by the volume of breast tissue resected, the administration of radiotherapy, and by both chemotherapy and tamoxifen. Quadrantectomy reduces IBTR risk by a factor of 2–3 compared with excisional biopsy [8]. This presumably reflects wider excision margins which are generally obtainable with the larger operation. Similar results might be achieved with wide excision (lumpectomy), including re-excision in case of microscopically positive margins (see discussion of margins below). Breast irradiation reduces IBTR risk by about four-fold [9]. Boost irradiation to the tumour bed may further reduce this risk [10], and results of a large European study will shed light on this point. Current tamoxifen schedules reduce IBTR risk by two- to three-fold in receptor-positive tumours [11,12]. Similar reductions have been reported for combination chemotherapy (Table 1), at least when administered in association with breast irradiation [13]. It is unclear under what circumstances the interval between surgery and radiotherapy influences IBTR risk significantly, and little is known

Table 1. Data from controlled, randomised trials of the National Surgical Adjuvant Breast and Bowel Project demonstrating the effect of systemic therapy on the risk of local recurrence in node-negative patients after conservation surgery and 50 Gy breast irradiation. Patients received systemic treatment during radiotherapy

Agents	Number	IBTR rate	Follow-up	*p*-value
Tamoxifen[a] [12]				
without Tam	532	10.3%	10 years	0.0001
with Tam	530	3.4%		
Chemotherapy[b] [13]				
without M-F	119	12.9%	8 years	0.001
with M-F	116	2.6%		

[a] Oestrogen receptor positive; tamoxifen 20 mg daily for at least 5 years.
[b] Oestrogen receptor negative; sequential methotrexate (M) and 5-fluorouracil (F) for 12 cycles.

about the effect of treatment sequence upon local control [14].

IBTR risk is strongly affected by treatment: and relates to volume of excised tissue, the use of breast irradiation, tamoxifen, and chemotherapy.

4. Young age

Although the reasons for this are not well understood, the risk of IBTR is a decreasing function of age, a phenomenon that is particularly apparent in pre-menopausal patients (Table 2) [4,15]. The higher risk associated with young age, especially in the subgroup younger than 35 or 40 years, does not seem to be entirely explained by a higher prevalence of unfavourable prognostic factors, e.g., tumour grade and lymph vessel invasion in these women [4,15]. A demonstrated tendency to use narrower excisions in younger patients, perhaps for cosmetic reasons, may partially explain the higher recurrence risk observed [16]. However, an age effect is also seen in patients treated by very wide excisions such as quadrantectomy [4]. Although 35 years is often used as a cut-off to define the high-risk subgroup, some have found that patients aged 35–40 [15], or even up to age 45 [4] have similar risks of IBTR. However, 35 is a convenient cut-off, as patients in this subgroup have a poorer prognosis regardless of type of local therapy, and these patients consequently require more aggressive overall treatment [4]. At the other end of the spectrum, over the age of about 55 years the risk of IBTR is generally low (Table 2).

- *IBTR risk is increased in younger women, particularly those aged less than 35 years.*
- *The reason for the high IBTR risk in very young patients is unclear.*
- *IBTR risk tends to be much lower in patients older than 55.*

Table 2. Crude IBTR rates in patients treated with quadrantectomy and breast irradiation, according to the presence or absence of risk factors [4]. The Milan quadrantectomy series was chosen to minimise the potential confounding impact of resection margin status. 27% of the 2233 patients were known to have received adjuvant systemic therapy. Median follow-up was 8.5 years. Differences between the highest and lowest risk categories are all highly significant

Risk factor	IBTR (%)
Patient age	
< 36	22/168 (13)
36–45	76/690 (11)
46–55	32/723 (4)
56–65	13/454 (3)
> 65	8/198 (4)
Extensive intraductal component	
ductal cancer with EIC	21/150 (14)
ductal cancer without EIC	98/1487 (7)
Lymphatic vascular invasion [a]	
with LVI	11/59 (19)
without LVI	48/850 (6)

[a] Reported in node-negative patients only.

5. Extensive intraductal component (EIC)

As intraductal extension is an important mechanism of spread within the breast, it is logical that tumours demonstrating EIC are more commonly excised with positive margins, and often have residual intraductal carcinoma, sometimes extensive, in re-excision or mastectomy specimens [17]. As EIC was originally defined in studies of small excisional biopsies, the definition necessarily emphasised the morphology of the primary tumour. The Harvard group diagnosed EIC when at least 25% of the tumour mass consisted of ductal carcinoma in situ (DCIS), in the presence of unquantified DCIS in the surrounding breast tissue [17]. More recent studies of wide excision specimens have used alternative definitions. The Amsterdam definition of EIC, based on the number of involved peripheral ductulo-lobular units, may prove to be a more reliable measure of residual DCIS than that of the Harvard group, as the former definition more clearly reflects cancer extension outside the tumour mass [18]. Lesions that are predominantly DCIS with a small invasive component are included within all definitions of EIC.

As EIC is confounded with positive excision margins, some have contested any influence of EIC on IBTR risk in the presence of clear margins [9]. It has been suggested that local control in the presence of EIC is satisfactory if excision margins are negative or only focally involved [19]. However, even using quadrantectomy, tumours with EIC recur locally more often than those without EIC (Table 2) [4]. Two large recent studies, using different definitions of EIC, have shown that EIC was an independent risk factor in multivariate models including resection margin status [20,21]. The presence of EIC seems to increase IBTR risk by about two fold. It has been suggested that the association of EIC with high nuclear grade defines a particularly high risk group (relative risk four fold [20]), whereas another study found that the increased risk associated with EIC was limited to tumours with comedo-type (high-grade) intraductal component [21].

- *Cancers with EIC tend to have a higher residual tumour burden after local excision.*
- *EIC may lose significance as a risk factor if excision margins are microscopically clear.*
- *The association of high grade and EIC may predict higher IBTR risk, independently of resection margin status.*

6. Lymphatic vessel invasion (LVI)

Most, but not all, studies show a somewhat increased risk of IBTR (generally less than two fold) in patients with LVI (Table 2) [4,18,22]. However, LVI also increases the risk of chest wall recurrence after mastectomy, and subgroup analysis of data from two randomised trials suggests that local control in these patients may not be improved by mastectomy alone compared with conservative surgery and radiotherapy [23]. Nonetheless, it is possible that LVI has special significance, as it may be associated with extensive recurrences [22,24]. In a large case-control study, the association of LVI and positive margins correlated strongly with recurrences that were diffuse or involved the skin of the breast [20]. This may represent a special situation justifying more aggressive multimodality therapy.

LVI may be a risk factor for local recurrences that are diffuse or involve the skin of the breast, especially if LVI is present at resection margins.

7. Excision margins

Microscopic evaluation of the inked margins of an excision specimen provides significant information regarding IBTR risk. Both the positivity of margins and possibly also the width of the negative margin correlate with the likelihood of residual cancer (either DCIS or invasive disease) remaining in the breast following local excision [25]. Because radiotherapy typically reduces IBTR risk by a factor of 4 [9], in a population of patients who have microscopic residual cancer, breast irradiation will at best result in a 75% local control rate. Conversely, if cancer cells are not found at inked specimen margins, approximately 40% of patients will develop IBTR, even in the absence of radiotherapy [9]. Not all studies have shown a significant correlation between IBTR and margin status [20,21,26], especially in multivariate analyses, perhaps reflecting the methodology of margin assessment [27], the confounding of margin status with other morphological risk factors [19,20], or the use of higher radiotherapy doses in patients with positive margins [26,28]. How patients with positive margins should be managed is controversial, although most surgeons advocate re-excision or mastectomy.

In an effort to 'improve' on the principle of clear inked margins, some have proposed the concept of 'close' margins, i.e., those where tumour cells extend to within 1 or 2 mm of the edge of the specimen [19,26]. Although it is likely that residual tumour burden decreases with margin width, it is unclear what the consequences of 'close' margins should be, at least if radiotherapy is to be given. By the same token, positive margins have also been subjected to further refinement, by 'quantifying' margin involvement as single versus multiple [29], or focal versus diffuse [19]. The purpose of these latter distinctions is to define margin-positive situations that do not necessarily require re-excision prior to breast irradiation, thus sparing patients the negative consequences, cosmetic or otherwise, of further surgery.

- *Microscopic study of inked margins is the best marker of residual tumour burden.*
- *There is no proven value in subclassifying negative margins according to width.*
- *Subclassifying positive margins as focal or diffuse may be useful in judging the potential value of re-excision.*

8. How should risk factors be used in the current multidisciplinary clinical setting?

Clear histological margins provide optimal conditions for breast conservation, as very few patients will have a residual tumour burden than cannot be effectively dealt with by radiotherapy. At present it is unclear whether any of the other risk factors mentioned above result in an unacceptable rate of IBTR in the presence of negative margins. However, it seems prudent to insist on wider margins in very young patients, as the results of quadrantectomy [4] appear superior to those generally associated with narrower excision in this age group [2]. Although there is some evidence that EIC loses its prognostic significance in the face of negative margins [9,19], new data suggest that high-grade EIC might confer a high IBTR risk independently of margin status [20,21].

The main usefulness of risk factors is in patients whose resection margins are not unequivocally clear. Although obtaining negative margins is desirable even when breast irradiation is to be given, the benefit expected from re-operation should be evaluated in light of the risks associated with a given situation. Certain margin-positive patients are at high-risk (e.g. involved margins in the presence of LVI [20]), whereas others may be low risk and not justify re-operation (e.g., focally positive margins in the absence of other risk factors [19]). Moreover, concerns about IBTR risk need to be tempered by considerations of metastatic risk. In patients at high risk for distant spread, obtaining a small improvement in the rate of local control may not be a clinical priority.

These considerations are made more pertinent in the light of the increasingly widespread use of systemic treatment. Prospective studies in which all patients received appropriate systemic management (Table 3) show IBTR rates well below 1% per year [11–13], with a rate below 0.3% per year reported for node negative, oestrogen receptor-positive patients receiving both tamoxifen and CMF chemotherapy [30]. In the face of such low IBTR rates the question of risk factors in this setting may be less important. The low risks cited above from prospective, randomised trials concern patients who have received systemic treatment simultaneously with breast irradiation. As an interaction with radiotherapy may contribute to the excellent local control observed, it is possible that IBTR rates might be higher

Table 3. Five-year crude IBTR rates in 338 patients treated by excisional biopsy and breast irradiation as a function of microscopic evaluation of inked resection margins [19]. Focally positive was defined as 3 or less low-power microscopic fields using a 4× objective and 10× ocular

Margin status	IBTR (%)	*p*-value
Negative, > 1 mm	3/107 (3)	0.87
Negative, < 1 mm	1/54 (2)	
Negative, width unknown	0/48 (0)	
Focally positive	7/79 (9)	0.003
> Focally positive	14/50 (28)	

when systemic treatments are administered sequentially with breast radiotherapy. The relevance of risk factors for local failure, including excision margins, will require additional study in patients receiving optimal systemic treatment. It is possible that future concerns about IBTR risk will focus primarily on those favourable-prognosis patients not requiring systemic treatment.

One of the goals of current and future research is to define highly favourable risk situations in which breast irradiation is unlikely to add significant benefit. Such a putative low-risk group will probably comprise older patients with small, widely excised tumours having favourable morphological features. Low IBTR rates have been reported using quadrantectomy without radiotherapy in patients older than 55 years, but follow-up was short [31]. However, another prospective study based on putative low-risk criteria was closed prematurely because of an unexpectedly high IBTR rate [32].

- *After conservation surgery and radiotherapy IBTR rates are very low in patients receiving systemic therapy.*
- *It is unclear whether IBTR risk factors will influence treatment decisions in this setting.*
- *Risk factors for IBTR may retain their usefulness in patients not receiving systemic treatment, or in establishing subgroups appropriately treated without breast irradiation.*

References

1. Holland R, Veling SHJ, Mravunac M, Hendriks JCL. Histologic multifocality of Tis, T1-2 breast carcinomas: implications for clinical trials in breast-conserving surgery. Cancer 1985; 56: 979–990.
2. Kurtz JM. Factors which predict breast relapse. Recent Results Cancer Res 1993; 127: 137–150.
3. Bergh J. Time for integration of predictive factors for selection of breast cancer patients who need postoperative radiotherapy. J Natl Cancer Inst 1997; 89: 605–607.
4. Veronesi U, Marubini E, DelVecchio M et al. Local recurrences and distant metastases after conservative breast cancer treatments: partly independent events. J Natl Cancer Inst 1995; 87: 19–27.
5. Haffty BG, Wilson LD, Smith R, Fischer D, Beinfield M, Ward B, McKhann C. Subareolar breast cancer: long-term results with conservative surgery and radiation therapy. Int J Radiat Oncol Biol Phys 1995; 33: 53–57.
6. Nixon AJ, Schnitt SJ, Gelman R et al. Relationship of tumor grade to other pathologic features and to treatment outcome of patients with early stage breast carcinoma treated with breast-conserving therapy. Cancer 1996; 78: 1426–1431.
7. Kurtz JM, Jacquemier J, Amalric R et al. Breast-conserving therapy for macroscopically multiple cancers. Ann Surg 1990; 212: 38–44.
8. Mariani L, Salvadori B, Marubini E et al. Ten year results of a randomised trial comparing two conservative treatment strategies for small size breast cancer. Eur J Cancer 1998; 34: 1143–1144.
9. Fisher B, Wickerham DL, Deutsch M, Anderson S, Redmond C, Fisher ER. Breast tumor recurrence following lumpectomy with and without breast irradiation: an overview of recent NSABP findings. Sem Surg Oncol 1992; 8: 153–160.
10. Romestaing P, Lehingue Y, Carrie C et al. Role of a 10-Gy boost in the conservative treatment of early breast cancer: Results of a randomized trial in Lyon, France. J Clin Oncol 1997; 15: 963–968.
11. Dalberg K, Johansson H, Johansson U, Rutqvist LE. A randomized trial of long term adjuvant tamoxifen plus postoperative radiation therapy versus radiation therapy alone for patients with early stage breast carcinoma treated with breast-conserving surgery. Cancer 1998; 82: 2204–2211.
12. Fisher B, Dignam J, Bryant J et al. Five versus more than five years of tamoxifen for breast cancer patients with negative lymph nodes and estrogen receptor-positive tumors. J Natl Cancer Inst 1996; 88: 1529–1542.
13. Fisher B, Dignam J, Mamounas EP et al. Sequential methotrexate and fluorouracil for the treatment of node-negative breast cancer patients with estrogen receptor-negative tumors: eight-year results from National Surgical Adjuvant Breast and Bowel Project (NSABP) B-13 and first report of findings from NSABP B-19 comparing methotrexate and fluorouracil with conventional cyclophosphamide, methotrexate, and fluorouracil. J Clin Oncol 1996; 14: 1982–1992.
14. Dubey AK, Recht A, Come S, Shulman L, Harris J. Why and how to combine chemotherapy and radiation therapy in breast cancer patients. Recent Results Cancer Res 1998; 152: 247–254.
15. Kurtz JM, Jaquemier J, Amalric R et al. Why are local recurrences after breast-conserving therapy more frequent in younger patients? J Clin Oncol 1990; 8: 591–598.

16. Vrieling C, Collette L, Fourquet A et al. The higher local recurrence rate after breast conserving therapy in young patients explained by larger tumor size and incomplete excision at first attempt? Int J Radiat Oncol Biol Phys 1998; 42(Suppl 1): 125.
17. Holland R, Connolly JL, Gelman R et al. The presence of an extensive intraductal component following a limited excision correlates with prominent residual disease in the remainder of the breast. J Clin Oncol 1990; 8: 113–118.
18. Borger J, Kemperman H, Hart A et al. Risk factors in breast-conservation therapy. J Clin Oncol 1994; 12: 653–660.
19. Gage I, Schnitt SJ, Nixon AJ et al. Pathologic margin involvement and the risk of recurrence in patients treated with breast-conserving therapy. Cancer 1996; 78: 1921–1928.
20. Voogd AC, Peterse JL, Crommelin MA et al. Histologic determinants for different types of local recurrence after breast-conserving therapy of invasive breast cancer. Eur J Cancer 1999; 35: 1828–1837.
21. Sinn HP, Anton HW, Magener A, von Fournier D, Bastert G, Otto HF. Extensive and predominant in situ component in breast carcinoma:their influence on treatment results after breast-conserving therapy. Eur J Cancer 1998; 34: 646–653.
22. Locker AP, Ellis IO, Morgan DAL, Elston CW, Mitchell A, Blamey RW. Factors influencing local recurrence after excision and radiotherapy for primary breast cancer. Br J Surg 1989; 76: 890–894.
23. Voogd AC, Nielsen JL, Peterse JL, et al. Are risk factors for local and distant recurrence after breast-conserving therapy for stage I and II breast cancer similar to those after mastectomy? In: Voogd AC, ed. Breast-conserving Treatment of Operable Mammary Cancer: Evaluation of Patient Selection and Treatment Outcome. Thesis, University of Amsterdam, 1998, pp. 88-104.
24. Kurtz JM, Jacquemier J, Brandone H et al. Inoperable recurrence after breast-conserving surgical treatment and radiotherapy. Surg Gynecol Obstet 1991; 172: 357–361.
25. Wazer DE, Schmidt-Ullrich RK, Schmid CH et al. The value of breast lumpectomy margin assessment as a predictor of residual tumor burden. Int J Radiat Oncol Biol Phys 1997; 38: 291–299.
26. Peterson ME, Schultz DJ, Reynolds C, Solin LJ. Outcomes in breast cancer patients relative to margin status after treatment with breast-conserving surgery and radiation therapy: The University of Pennsylvania experience. Int J Radiat Oncol Biol Phys 1999; 43: 1029–1035.
27. Fisher ER. Lumpectomy margins and much more. Cancer 1997; 79: 1453–1458.
28. Wazer DE, Schmidt-Ullrich RK, Ruthhazer R et al. Factors determining outcome for breast-conserving irradiation with margin-directed dose escalation to the tumor bed. Int J Radiat Oncol Biol Phys 1998; 40: 851–858.
29. DiBiase SJ, Komarnicky LT, Schwartz GF, Xie Y, Mansfield CM. The number of positive margins influences the outcome of women treated with breast preservation for early breast carcinoma. Cancer 1998; 82: 2212–2220.
30. Fisher B, Dignam, Wolmark N et al. Tamoxifen and chemotherapy for lymph node-negative, estrogen receptor-positive breast cancer. J Natl Cancer Inst 1997; 89: 1673-1682.
31. Veronesi U, Luini A, Del Vecchio M et al. Radiotherapy after breast-preserving surgery in women with localized cancer of the breast. N Engl J Med 1993; 328: 1587–1591.
32. Schnitt SJ, Hayman J, Gelman R et al. A prospective study of conservative surgery alone in the treatment of selected patients with stage I breast cancer. Cancer 1996; 77: 1094–1100.

Breast Cancer: Diagnosis and Management
J.M. Dixon (Ed.)

CHAPTER 21

Achieving symmetry after breast conservation: the role of surgery to the contralateral breast

J.Y. Petit, A. Marando, V. Donati, C. Garusi and M. Rietjens

1. Introduction

The development of reconstructive surgery as part of breast cancer treatment has lead the plastic surgeon and the cancer surgeon to become experienced in surgical alteration of the contralateral breast to achieve symmetry [1–3].

During breast conserving treatment if a large volume of breast tissue is resected on the involved side then following breast reshaping a surgical procedure may be needed on the healthy side in order to achieve a satisfactory degree of symmetry. Another consideration is removal of suspicious areas in the contralateral breast. Contralateral breast cancers have been reported in between 5 to 10% of cases and occult cancers have been discovered during plastic surgical intervention of the opposite breast in 4% of cases in a series of contralateral procedures performed to achieve symmetry at the Institut Gustave-Roussy [2,3].

Surgery on the contralateral breast provides an excellent opportunity to check the gland and the surgeon should choose an appropriate technique based both on what surgical treatment is being performed on the affected breast and the results of preoperative clinical examination and imaging of the healthy breast [4].

Pre-operative mammography of both breasts should always be performed and any doubtful opacities imaged further or investigated by cytology or core biopsy. The technique chosen for symmetrisation of the contralateral breast should take into account any areas of concern observed preoperatively as well as the location of the cancer in the treated breast, to try and perform a symmetrical resection and produce a good final cosmetic result.

Following very wide excision for breast cancer a contralateral surgical procedure performed on the opposite breast may be needed to achieve symmetry.

2. Techniques

2.1. Breast reduction

2.1.1. Superior pedicle technique (Fig. 1a)

The superior pedicle technique allows wide exploration of the mammary gland and permits excision of glandular tissue from the lower pole of the breast. With the help of prepectoral fixation which is necessary for correction of breast ptosis, good access to the deep part of the breast is obtained and bimanual palpation of the whole gland is possible. This intraoperative examination allows the surgeon to identify small mass lesions which are sometimes not evident clinically or radiologically.

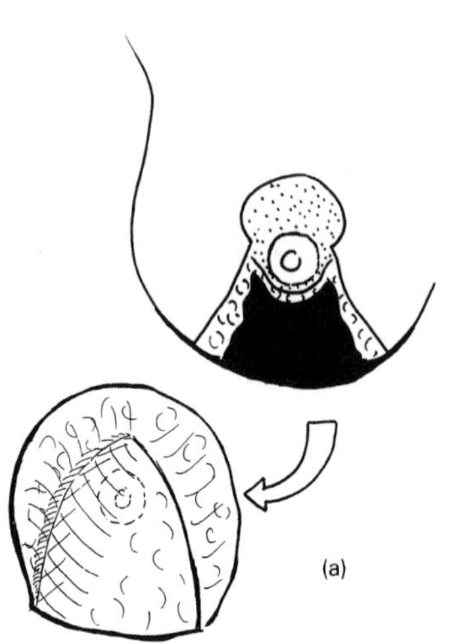
(a)

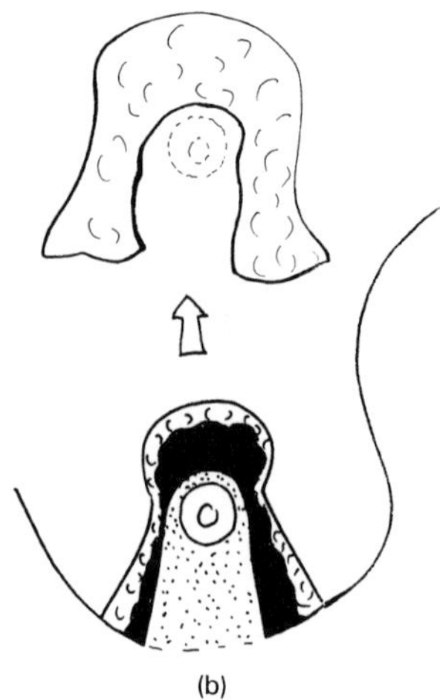
(b)

Fig. 1.

It can also confirm whether a lesion imaged radiologically in the breast is benign. This technique allows a very wide excision of the cancer increasing the chances of getting clear margins and it permits glandular remodelling which produces better aesthetic results.

The superior pedicle technique, because of the large area of deepithelisation, permits lateral variation in choosing the areolar pedicle and produces better and easier remodelling of the breast than other approaches.

The retroareolar area is one of the richest areas of glandular tissue in the breast. It can be explored and biopsied as long as the nipple and areola flap are about 1 cm thick because this will preserve an adequate blood supply.

Fixation of the breast to the underlying pectoralis major muscle and plication of the superior dermo-glandular flap allows remodelling of the superior segment of the breast. It also helps to maintain the position of the breast and prevents the recurrence of ptosis.

2.1.2. Inferior pedicle technique (Fig. 1b)

This technique is most commonly used in mammary hypertrophy. The blood supply to the NAC is maintained by perforating vessels coming from the retroareolar–inferior dermoglandular pedicle, which must be left untouched and cannot be explored. The main indication for using an inferior pedicle technique is a cancer situated in the upper half of the breast. It is possible to perform a quadrantectomy on the affected side and a symmetrisation of the contralateral breast leaving an inverted T scar bilaterally, as following a breast reduction. This procedure is less often used than the superior pedicle technique. This technique is most frequently used in cases of large breast size associated with significant ptosis. The main indication for this technique is exploration of the upper half of the breast because the lesion to be resected is located in the upper half of the breast. The main drawback of this technique is the inability to explore the central area (retroareolar) and the long scar in the inframammary fold.

2.1.3. Periareolar technique (Fig. 2)

In all types of mammoplasty, the main goal is to limit scarring. The scar in the submammary fold is visible, particularly when one is lying down. The ideal result is confining the scar to the periareolar area.

Benelli in 1990 and Goes in 1996 described this technique and their modifications. The key-

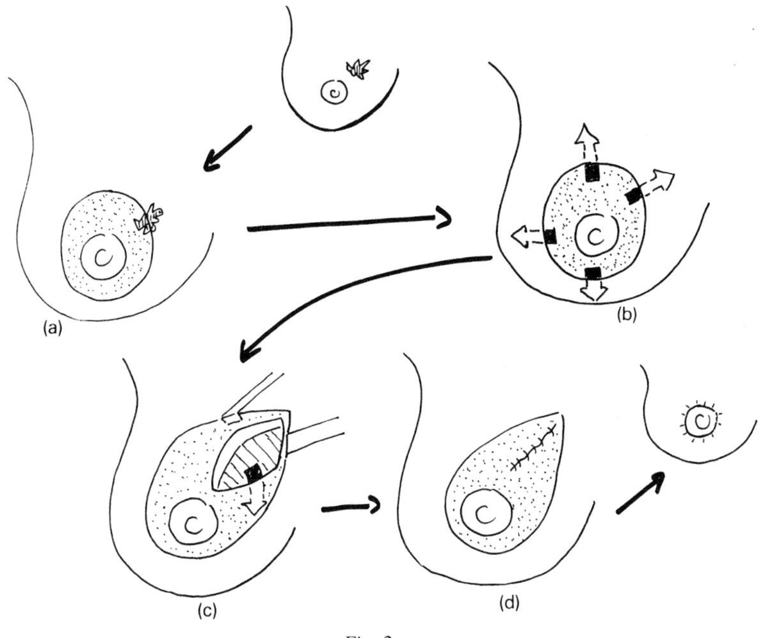

Fig. 2.

stone of this procedure lies in the dermo–glandular retroareolar pedicle which supplies the NAC. It gives to the surgeon access to all quadrants and provides the opportunity of reshaping the mammary gland through a concentric reduction of breast tissue leaving a minimal periareolar scar and a more regular breast contour. By performing the same procedure on the unaffected side, it is possible to reduce or lift the opposite breast, according to the shape desired, leaving bilateral periareolar scars. The blood supply to the NAC comes from the glandular tissue posterior to the NAC.

As part of contralateral breast reduction the nipple areolar complex is kept alive either on a superior or inferior pedicle or on the retroareolar glandular tissue in the periareolar technique. The choice of technique depends on what procedure is being performed on the opposite breast, the breast size and the site of any suspicious or abnormal areas in the 'healthy' breast being reduced.

3. Choice of procedure

The superior pedicle technique is the best choice for exploring the inferior half of the breast and the inferior pedicle technique for exploring the superior half (Fig. 3). Rotation of the flaps means that the zones explored can be modified in individual patients.

The superior pedicle technique allows complete exploration of high risk regions namely the upper outer quadrant and the retroareolar regions. However the periareolar mammoplasty may become more popular in the future especially to remove tumours located in the peripheral area of the gland since it is the technique which produces less scarring. The retroareolar region cannot be evaluated and undermined when using a central or inferior pedicle technique. It is also not possible to use these incisions for axillary dissection, which has to be done through another axillary incision.

The use of different aesthetic surgical techniques as part of the conservative treatment of breast cancers allows large excisions with good

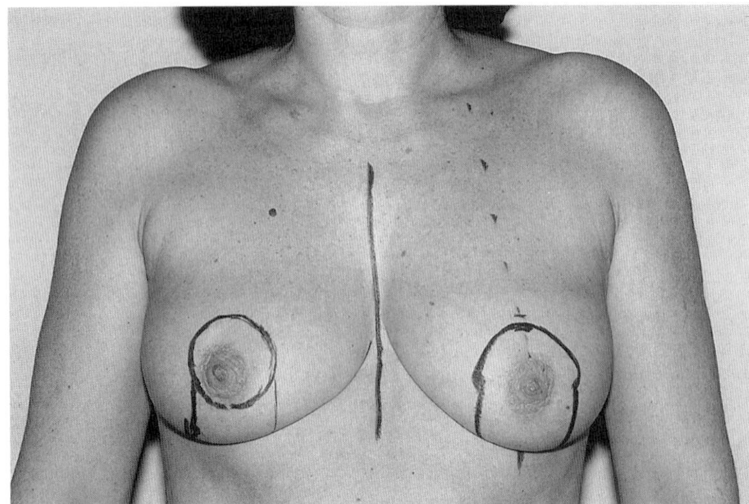

Fig. 3. Pre-operative drawings of the right central quadrantectomy and immediate partial breast reconstruction with an inferior lateral glandular flap and contralateral vertical scar technique breast reduction.

aesthetic results as has been demonstrated in a large number of publications. The major problem remains in organising teams which is not easy to achieve outside specialised centres.

Plastic surgery techniques after conservative surgery allow a reduction of the number of patients who require mastectomy but in 50% of cases a mastoplasty on the opposite side is needed to achieve symmetry. The choice of techniques should be made according to the preoperative evaluation of the glandular tissue using mammograms and the location of the opposite breast cancer. Fig. 4 shows the result after 6 month.

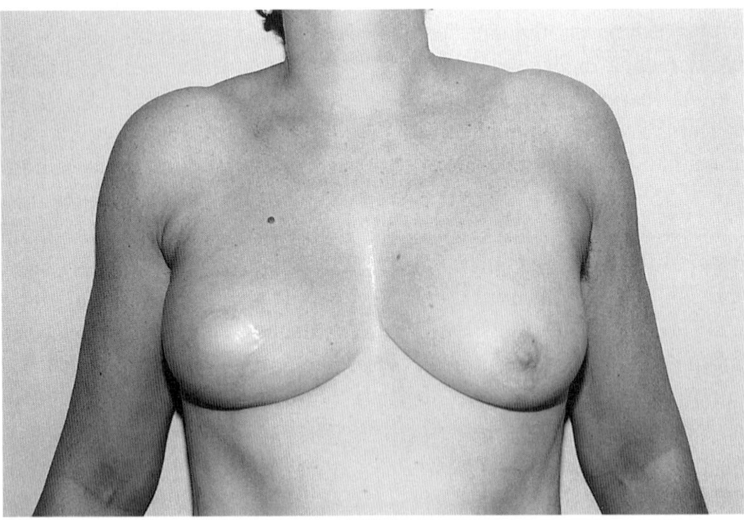

Fig. 4. Same patient 6 months after the bilateral surgical procedure, radiotherapy and before the nipple–areola complex reconstruction.

4. Breast augmentation

Breast augmentation is not commonly performed in patients with breast cancer and should only be performed on the normal breast when an augmentation of the volume of the diseased breast has been performed either by a partial reconstruction with a myocutaneous flap (latissimus dorsi of TRAM flap) or with a total breast reconstruction with a flap or implant.

Partial augmentation with implants of the diseased breast is not recommended where radiotherapy is planned because of capsule formation and the risk of contracture. Latissimus dorsi partial reconstruction can be performed to restore the volume of the breast following quadrantectomy or very wide excision.

References

1. Dixon JM et al. Breast incisions for conservation surgery. Ann R Coll Surg Engl 1997; 79(5): 387–388.
2. Petit JY et al. Integration of plastic surgery in the course of breast-conserving surgery for cancer to improve cosmetic results and radicality of tumor excision. Recent Results Cancer Res 1998; 152: 202–211.
3. Clough KB et al. Plastic surgery and conservative treatment of breast cancer. Indications and results. Ann Chir Plast Esthet 1992; 37(6): 682–692.
4. Petit JY, Rietjens M, Contesso G, Bertin F, Gilles R. Contralateral mastoplasty for breast reconstruction: a good opportunity for glandular exploration and occult carcinomas diagnosis. Ann Surg Oncol 1997; 4(6): 511–515.

Breast Cancer: Diagnosis and Management
J.M. Dixon (Ed.)

CHAPTER 22

The role of mastectomy in the management of breast cancer

R.A. Linforth and N.J. Bundred

1. Introduction

For most of this century, mastectomy was the standard treatment of breast cancer. In the 1970s surgical management evolved to define a balance between therapeutic efficacy, cosmesis and reduced surgical morbidity. The aim of surgical treatment today remains to achieve local control of disease by removing the primary tumour, obtain accurate prognostic information whilst maximising chances for cure preventing recurrence and minimising mortality. A meta-analysis of studies has confirmed that breast conserving surgery (wide local excision combined with radiotherapy and axillary clearance) produces equivalent survival rates to mastectomy with axillary clearance for women with small tumours (<4 cm) [1] (Fig. 1). Large tumours (>4 cm) are usually unsuitable for breast conservative surgery, and approximately one third of screen detected cancers and half of symptomatic cancers require mastectomy [1–4].

Patients with multiple tumours or multifocal disease are also usually treated by mastectomy to ablate all disease (Table 1). Multicentricity can be defined as two areas of cancer separated by normal breast tissue and multifocality as the presence of in situ disease or lymphatic invasion more than 1 cm from an infiltrating margin [4].

Some patients who are suitable for breast conservation opt for mastectomy for fear of local recurrence or anxiety at preserving the breast [5]. It is important for the surgeon to discuss which operation is best for the patient prior to surgery and each woman should be able to choose whether to have breast conserving surgery or mastectomy if either is an option. Those requiring or electing for mastectomy should be offered immediate reconstruction to aid adaptation and improve body image [6].

In a bid to reduce local recurrence following breast conserving surgery, several pathological factors have been identified which predispose to recurrence and are therefore relative indications towards mastectomy [7]. Poorly differentiated (Grade III) tumours with lymphovascular invasion, extensive in situ disease, young age (<35), multicentricity, mutifocality and extensive microcalcification as seen on mammography are all associated with increased rates of local recurrence [7,8] (Table 2).

2. Clinical trials

An overview of the effects of surgery in early breast cancer by the Early Breast Cancer Trialists' collaborative group [1] analysed ten trials comparing radical mastectomy with less extensive mastectomy techniques (Fig. 1). Overall 50.0% of the radical group and 51.6% of the less radical

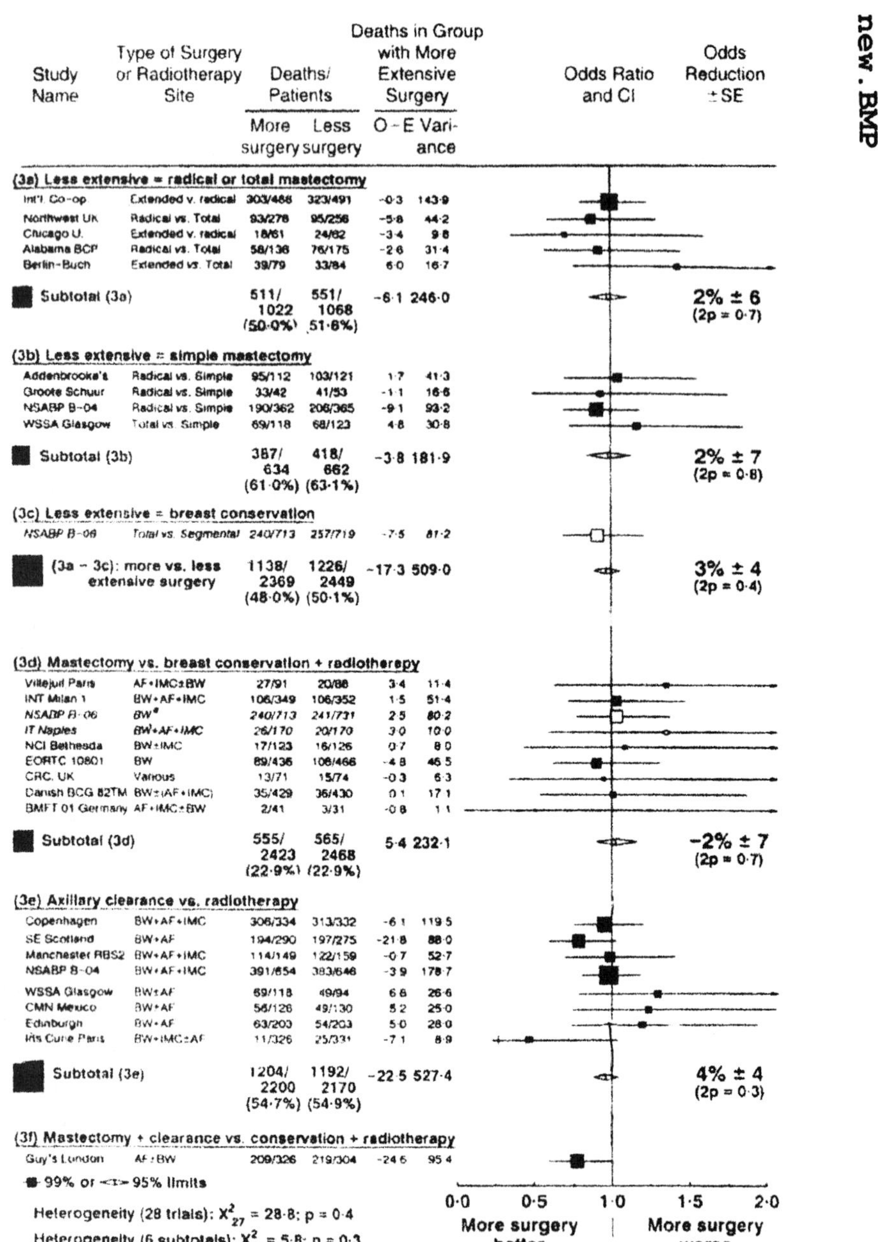

Fig. 1. Breast conserving surgery for women with small tunmours. (Reprinted from N. Eng. J. Med.,1995 [1].)

mastectomy group died at ten years. There was no significant difference in survival among the two groups for either women with node positive or node negative tumours (Fig. 2). Similarly no difference in survival was seen between breast conserving surgery with radiotherapy and mastectomy in the meta-analysis of nine trials (Fig. 1).

Current mastectomy techniques usually remove the whole breast but preserve both the pectoralis major and minor. An axillary clear-

Table 1.

Indications for mastectomy Absolute indications	Relative indications
1. Patient preference	1. Tumour > 4 cm depends on breast size
2. Multifocal disease/ill defined margins	2. Central lesions involving nipple
3. Extensive intraductal disease	3. Occult cancer present with axillary disease
4. Diffuse mammographic calcification	4. Ductal carcinoma in situ
5. Pregnancy (1st 2nd trimester)	5. Failure of neoadjuvant therapy
6. Prior irradiation	
7. Failed conservative surgery	
8. Male patient	

Table 2. Factors associated with increased risk of local recurrence

1. Lymphovascular invasion
2. Axillary node involvement
3. High grade lesion
4. Large cancers >4 cm

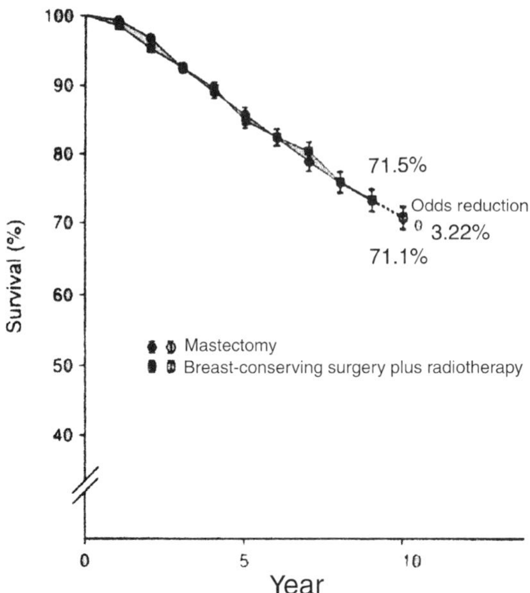

Fig. 2. Survival rate among the two groups for either women with node positive or node negative tumours.

ance removing all the lymphatic tissue of the axilla up to and including the level three apical nodes, is usually performed at the same time. Total mastectomy without axillary dissection should be reserved for ductal carcinoma in situ or for local recurrence after breast conserving surgery in patients who have already had axillary surgery.

Post operative radiotherapy for selected women at high risk of local recurrence is given to skin flaps. Risk factors include pectoral muscle involvement, large (>4 cm) lesions, high grade tumours, lymphovascular invasion within the tumour and heavy (>4) nodal involvement [9].

> *There is no significant survival advantage of radical mastectomy over total mastectomy.*

3. Skin flaps

Halsted originally believed that wide skin excision of 5 cm on each side of the tumour, with skin flaps cut thin to remove the superficial fascia sparing only the dermis provided the lowest risk of local flap recurrence [10]. This he believed removed nests of glandular breast tissue found very close to the dermis, just below the superficial fascia enveloping the breast. Despite the anatomical rationale behind Halsted's dissection, no evidence of improved survival or reduction in local recurrence has been demonstrated by such radical surgery.

In a study of thick verses thin mastectomy skin flaps the formation of ultra thin skin flaps and wide skin margin excision were compared with skin flaps retaining a superficial layer of fat and less skin excision. Ten year survival statistics between the two groups were not significantly different (53% vs 46%) nor were local recurrence rates (13% vs 7%) (thin vs thick). However the more radical thin excision was associated with an increase in wound complications such as skin flap necrosis, and lymphoedema [11]. Flap recurrence is now recognised as a reflection of histopathological features of the primary tumour and not residual disease.

Skin sparing mastectomy is used to aid breast reconstruction and removes only skin overlying or adjacent to the cancer instead of 2–3 cm around the cancer. This leads to an improved cosmetic result compared to much wider excisions when combined with some form of breast reconstruction. In a series of 51 patients with early breast cancer undergoing skin sparing mastectomy defined as a 5 mm margin of skin around the border of the nipple–areola complex, with additional skin flap biopsies of the remaining tissue taken, five patients developed recurrence, two in the wound, two in the axilla and one had distant bone metastases. Histological examination of flap biopsies failed to show any breast ductal tissue in the dermis. Twenty one percent of patients developed a degree of skin edge necrosis [12].

Skin sparing mastectomy and reconstruction has been compared to modified radical mastectomy with reconstruction. Of 435 patients, 327 patients had skin sparing and 188 patients conventional mastectomy. Local recurrence rates were 4.8% and 9.5%, respectively, and overall recurrence rates of 16% and 29.8% after a mean follow up of 37.5 months and 48.2 months; these are not significantly different [13,14]. A review of 104 patients treated by skin sparing mastectomy and immediate reconstruction showed 6.7% developed local recurrence, 12.5% developed distant metastases and 7.75% died of breast disease [15]. Studies suggest no significant increase in local recurrence or systemic disease in patients with early breast cancer when treated with skin sparing mastectomy compared to conventional mastectomy although follow up is as yet short.

There is no evidence to support the use of ultra thin skin flaps.Skin sparing mastectomy appears as safe as a standard mastectomy.

4. Complications after mastectomy

Mastectomy is generally regarded as a clean operation, although the incidence of wound infection varies from 4 to 18% [16] (Table 3). Prophylactic intravenous antibiotics given at induction of anaesthesia can significantly reduce this rate by about 38% [17]. When infections do occur nearly all are due to skin contaminants such as staphylococcus aureus and as such co-amoxyclav is the ideal choice of antibiotic [18]. Infection may not cause pain because skin flaps are denervated by the operation. Erythema of skin edges associated with a slight temperature rise is seen first and if untreated may progress to skin necrosis and wound dehiscence. If this occurs, wounds should be reopened and debrided. Most will heal by secondary intention but split skin grafts are occasionally required.

Haematoma formation occurs if bleeding occurs post-operatively and suction drains fail to evacuate this. Haematoma large enough to elevate the skin flaps results in delayed wound healing and should be evacuated and any bleeding points secured. This is usually possible under local anaesthetic.

Neuropathy following mastectomy can occur but is usually mild and temporary in the form of tingling of the fingers, but occasionally severe motor weakness and dysaethesia of the entire arm in a sleeve distribution is seen. The more severe disability which occurs in approximately 0.7%

Table 3. Complications after mastectomy

1. Wound infection
2. Seroma formation
3. Skin flap necrosis
4. Lymphoedema
5. Nerve damage

probably develops from inadvertent overstretching of the brachial plexus during surgery [19]. Most recover completely within a few weeks and early arm movement with physiotherapy will help maintain range of motion of the limb.

Injury to the long thoracic nerve causes paralysis of the serratus anterior muscle and winging of the scapula. If the nerve is divided, paralysis is permanent. If the nerve is intact most will recover within a few weeks. Injury to the thoracodorsal nerve causes paralysis of latissimus dorsi with a reduction in the patient's ability to reach behind their back. In addition the scapula tip becomes more prominent as the muscle atrophies.

Suction drains are used post operatively to drain the mastectomy bed and axilla to evacuate post-operative bleeding and to limit seroma formation. Usually one is removed around day 2 and the other at day 5. No difference in wound outcome between groups randomised to have drains removed at three or six days is seen [20]. In an attempt to determine whether there is an advantage in using two drains, one in the axilla and one beneath the skin flaps, rather than a single axillary drain after mastectomy, a randomised clinical controlled trial was undertaken in 84 women undergoing modified radical mastectomy, 37 patients had one axillary drain and 47 had two drains one in the axilla and the other beneath the pectoral flaps. No statistically significant difference in volume drained or wound complications was seen, although there was a slightly higher incidence of flap necrosis in the two drain group [21]. A second randomised trial of single versus multiple drains showed no significant advantage in amount drained or duration of drainage for multiple drains [22]. Seroma formation occurs in one third of patients who have undergone mastectomy and this can be treated by needle aspiration if troublesome. Attempts to reduce the incidence of seroma formation following mastectomy include suturing of skin flaps to underlying muscle and application of fibrin glue to cavity walls. Seroma formation is significantly more common when the mastectomy flaps are raised by electrocautery (diathermy).

The effect of suturing skin flaps to underlying muscle in patients who underwent mastectomy, and had 2 closed suction drains removed at 48 h was that seroma formation occurred in only 10% of patients; all were minor and required aspiration only once or twice [23]. Thus closing the dead space by suturing and the use of closed suction drains removed early, may reduce seroma incidence after mastectomy, but remains unproven. Most studies of fibrin glue have not shown any significant improvement in seroma incidence, but one study did show a reduction in effusion and capsular contraction around implants inserted after mastectomy [24]. Symptomatic lymphoedema occurs in less than 5% of patients treated with a mastectomy. Treatment with compression bandaging and physiotherapy may help to control symptoms.

Common complications after mastectomy include seroma formation, infection and haematoma formation.

5. Follow up

Local recurrence after mastectomy is commonest during the first two years and then decreases thereafter with time. Clinical review and examination should be performed annually with all patients having mammography. The incidence of local recurrence after mastectomy is around 1% per annum which is similar to that following breast conservation surgery [25]. Around 75% of local recurrences present between annual clinic visits.

All forms of mastectomy whether radical, modified or skin sparing leave residual breast tissue as microscopic islands within the skin and inframammary fold [26]. Early surgical literature associated locoregional relapse with inadequate surgical technique with recurrences being attributed to residual tumour left behind at the time of surgery. Histological examination of local recurrences in fact rarely show surrounding identifiable breast tissue. Despite mastectomy, the locoregional recurrence rate for breast cancer has remained relatively constant over the years. Factors other than excision margins including the biology of the tumour are predictors of recurrence [6,27].

> *Local recurrence after mastectomy occurs at a rate of 1% per year for the first two years then reduces.*

6. Mastectomy after failed conservation surgery

After optimal breast conserving surgery and radiotherapy there is a 1% annual risk of breast relapse [28]. Following staging to exclude distant metastatic disease, such women are usually best treated by mastectomy with or without reconstruction. For those women who remain node negative, survival results are as good as at primary surgery [29]. For those who are node positive survival is poor. Tissue expansion is rarely used after radiotherapy due to fibrosis of chest wall musculature, but latissimus dorsi flap and TRAM flap reconstruction are safe options.

7. Treatment of elderly patients

As many as 40% of cancers occur in women over the age of 70 [30]. The grade of these tumours are similar to those in younger patients. However mortality in these women has not fallen. This is because of the tendency to give hormonal therapy, e.g. tamoxifen, as first line therapy and reserve surgery for relapse. Even when hormonal treatment is given to oestrogen sensitive tumours only, as many as 40% will not gain long term control [31]. Trials have shown that elderly women have no greater morbidity or mortality from mastectomy and relapses rates are lower after such local therapy [32].

Therefore these patients should undergo the same surgical procedures as those offered to younger patients. Few patients are not fit for any surgery, and mastectomy can even be performed under local anaesthesia only [33].

Table 4. Contraindications to mastectomy

1. Inflammatory breast cancer
2. Chest wall fixation of primary tumour
3. Distant metastatic disease
4. Concurrent medical contraindications to general anaesthesia
5. Supraclavicular lymph node metastases.

8. Contraindications to mastectomy

Women with locally advanced or metastatic breast cancer are usually best treated by systemic therapy at the onset. Mastectomy is generally not indicated for tumours which are locally advanced (Table 4).

References

1. Early Breast Cancer Trialists' Collaborative Group (1995) Effects of Radiotherapy and surgery in Early Breast Cancer. N. Eng. J. Med., 333, 1444–55.
2. Cailais G, Berger C et al. (1994) Conservative treatment feasibility with induction chemotherapy, surgery and radiotherapy for patients with breast carcinoma larger than 3 cm. Cancer, 74, 1283–8.
3. Collins J (1994) The role of the surgeon. Cancer Forum, 18, 92–95.
4. Danoff BF, Haller DG, Glick JH, Goodman RL (1985) Conservative surgery and Irradiation in the treatment of early breast cancer. Ann. Intl. Med., 102, 634–642.
5. Moyer A, Salovey P (1998) Patient participation in treatment decision making and the psychological consequences of breast cancer surgery. Womens-Health, Summer, 4(2), 103–16.
6. Dean C, Chetty U, Forrest APM (1983) Effect of immediate breast reconstruction on psychosocial morbidity after mastectomy. Lancet, I, 459–61.
7. O'Rouke S, Galea MH, Morgan D, Euhus D, Prider S, Ellis IO, Elston CW, Blamey RW (1994) Local recurrence after simple mastectomy. BJS, 81, 386–389.
8. Harris JR, Connolly JL, Schnitt SJ (1984) The use of pathological features in selecting the extent of surgical resection necessary for breast cancer patients treated by primary radiation therapy. Ann. Surg., 201, 164.

9. Cuzick J, Stewart H, Peto R et al. (1987) Overview of randomised trials of post-operative adjuvant radiotherapy in breast cancer. Cancer Treat. Rep., 71, 15–29.
10. Halsted WS (1894) The results of operations for the cure of cancer of the breast performed at the John Hopkins Hospital from June 1889 to Jan 1894. Arch. Surg., 20, 497–501.
11. Krohn IT, Cooper DR, Basset JG (1982) Radical mastectomy. Arch. Surg., 117, 6.
12. Slavin SA, Schnitt SJ, Duda RB, Houlihan MJ, Koufman CN, Morris DJ, Troyan SL, Goldwyn RM (1998) Skin sparing mastectomy and immediate reconstruction. Plast. Reconstr. Surg., 102(1), 49–62.
13. Carlson GW, Bostwich J, Styblo TM, Moore B, Bried JT, Murray DR, Wood WC. Skin sparing mastectomy. Ann. Surg., 225, 5, 570–578.
14. Carlson GW (1998) Local recurrence after skin sparing mastectomy. Ann. Surg., 5(7), 571–572.
15. Kroll SS, Schusterman MA, Tadjalli HE, Singletary SE, Ames FC (1997) Risk of recurrence after treatment of early breast cancer with skin sparing mastectomy. Ann. Surg., 4(3), 193–7.
16. Hayes JA, Bryan RM (1984) Wound infection following mastectomy. Aust. N.Z. J. Surg., 54, 25–7.
17. Platt R, Zucker JR, Zaleznik DF (1993) Peri-operative antibiotic prophylaxis and wound infection following breast surgery. J. Antimicrob. Chemother., 31, 43–8.
18. Chen J, Gutkin Z, Bawnik J (1991) Postoperative infections in breast surgery. J. Hosp. Infection, 17, 61–5.
19. Budd DC, Cochran RC, Sturtz DL, Fouty WJ Jr. (1978) Surgical morbidity after mastectomy operations. Am. J. Surg., 135(2), 218–20.
20. Parikh HK, Badwe RA, Ash CM, Hamed H, Freitas R Jr., Chaudary MA, Fentiman IS (1992) Early drain removal following modified radical mastectomy: a randomised trial. J. Surg. Oncol., 51(4), 266–9.
21. Terrell GS, Singer JA (1992) Axillary versus combined axillary and pectoral drainage after modified radical mastectomy. Surg. Gynecol. Obstet., 175(5), 437–40.
22. Petrek JA, Peters MM, Cirrincione C, Thaler HT (1992) A prospective randomised trial of single versus multiple drains in the axilla after lymphadenectomy. Surg. Gynecol. Obstet., 175(5), 405–9.
23. O'Dywer PJ, O'Higgins NJ, James AG (1991) Effect of closing dead space on incidence of seroma after mastectomy. Surg. Gynecol. Obstet., 172(1), 55–6.
24. Patrizi I, Maffia L, Vitali CM, Boccoli G, La Rocca R (1993) Immediate reconstruction after radical mastectomy for breast carcinoma with a Becker-type prosthesis. Minerva Chir., 48(9), 453–8.
25. Fisher B, Redmond C, Fisher ER (1985) Ten year results of a randomised clinical trial comparing radical mastectomy with or without radiation. N. Eng. J. Med., 312, 674–81.
26. Carlson GW, Grassl N, Lewis MM et al. (1996) Preservation of the inframammary fold. Plastic Reconstr. Surg., 98, 203–10.
27. Gilliland MD, Barton RM, Copeland EM (1983) The implications of local recurrence of breast cancer. Ann. Surg., 197, 284–7.
28. Sarrazin D, Dewar JA, Arriaganda R (1986) Conservative management of breast cancer. Br. J. Surg., 73, 604–6.
29. Van Donegan JA, Bartelink H, Fentiman IS (1992) EORTC trial 10801. Eur. J. Cancer, 28A, 801–5.
30. Chen J, Gutkin Z, Bawnik (1991). Post operative infection in breast surgery. J. Hosp. Infection, 17, 61–5.
31. CRC Br. J. Surg. 1991, 78, 591–4.
32. Gaskell DJ, Hawkins RA, Sangster K, Chetty U, Forrest APM (1989) Lancet, I, 1044–6.
33. Hunt KE, Fry DE, Bland KI (1990) Breast carcinoma in the elderly patient. Am. J. Surg., 140, 339–342.

Breast Cancer: Diagnosis and Management
J.M. Dixon (Ed.)

CHAPTER 23

Selection of patients for chest wall radiotherapy after mastectomy

David A.L. Morgan

1. Introduction

In 1994, Kurtz [1] published the findings of a questionnaire he had circulated to thirteen internationally acknowledged experts in radiotherapy in breast cancer, asking them about their current indications for post-mastectomy irradiation. The diversity of opinion expressed was striking. Yet it is half a century since Paterson in Manchester initiated one of the very first randomised trials in cancer medicine [2], to address this very issue! Many further trials have followed but as Kurtz's survey shows, consensus has been difficult to achieve. Why is this, and what does it imply for evidence-based medicine in this area?

2. The evidence

2.1. Radiotherapy — benefit or harm

Paterson's seminal trial has been followed over subsequent years and decades by many essentially-similar studies, and these have been combined in meta-analysis [3], regularly updated by the Early Breast Cancer Trialists Collaborative Group.

From the meta-analyses two clear messages emerge:
Whatever the surgical procedure, and whatever the characteristics of the tumour, post-mastectomy radiotherapy reduces local and regional recurrences to about a third of that seen after surgery alone; this remains true even when systemic therapy (either hormonal or chemotherapy) is given.
Patients given radiotherapy died less often from breast cancer, but more often from other diseases, notably cardiovascular events, although these effects take several years to manifest (particularly deaths from other causes).

A number of important general points emerge from the meta-analysis. Firstly, the impact of radiotherapy on reducing risk of local recurrence, and of risk of death from breast cancer, and the increased risk of cardiovascular death is almost constant if expressed as a proportional increase or decrease of the risk in unirradiated patients. This tells us that if we can identify accurately the various risk factors, we can predict for individual patients whether the net effect of radiotherapy is likely to be beneficial or detrimental. If radiotherapy reduces local and regional recurrence but also carries a fixed risk of increasing mortality, then the benefit of reduced loco-regional recurrence can only translate into a survival benefit for patients with the highest risk of recurrence, while in those with a low risk, the chances of a benefit from radiotherapy are exceeded by the increased mortality from other causes. Many early studies involved no quality-assurance programmes for radiotherapy, so there is a greater likelihood of treatment related morbidity and mortality than would be the case with modern, optimally applied radiotherapy, assuming that the harmful effects of radiotherapy can be minimised by the careful use of modern technology. While it is assumed that this is true, it cannot be proven as yet from currently available data.

The consistency of the proportional effect on risk seen across all studies has another important implication. The impact of radiotherapy, expressed in this way, is the same (or to be precise falls within the same band of confidence intervals) for patients in trials where no systemic treatment was given as in the more recent studies where most patients have received adjuvant systemic therapy regardless of whether they have received adjuvant endocrine or adjuvant chemotherapy. This answers, by implication, the question of whether risk factors are the same in patients receiving systemic therapy as in those not doing so and suggest it is likely they are.

Analysis of the relatively recent work of the Danish Breast Cancer Group (DBCG) emphasises these points. This Group has performed [4] a study worthy of detailed attention and they report a reduction in risk of recurrence and breast cancer death in irradiated patients in line with those reported in other papers although it is still too early to know if the impact of radiotherapy on other causes of death is increased as the overview has suggested. This study is particularly interesting because it confirms the hypothesis that when carefully given to patients with high-risk breast cancer, the benefit from radiotherapy in terms of reduction of local recurrence and reduced breast cancer death risk exceeds the harm done by radiotherapy, and results in a significant improvement in overall survival.

In the DBCG trial (Trial No. 82b), pre-menopausal patients with 'high risk' breast cancer (see below for definition of high risk) who underwent mastectomy and axillary sampling and received standard adjuvant chemotherapy, were randomised to either receive radiotherapy or not to the chest wall and axilla. At 10 years of follow-up, a highly statistically significant improvement in survival was seen for the patients who received radiotherapy.

As well as targeting patients with a high risk of breast cancer recurrence, the technique of radiotherapy used in this trial is of interest. The internal mammary and medial supraclavicular nodes were irradiated in all patients having radiotherapy and by using an electron beam for the internal mammary chain, the cardiac dose was minimised. There has been much debate as to the value of giving radiotherapy to these nodal areas, and the question can only be resolved by randomised trials. Fortunately, one such trial is currently running under the auspices of the EORTC (Trial 22962), and recruiting well, although it will be many years before it is mature enough to produce an answer. The issue of internal mammary node irradiation, is part of a more general, unresolved, issue — to what extent the target volume should encompass draining lymph nodes. The wide variation in practice, both surgical and radiotherapeutic in terms of lymph node treatment means that it is impossible to use meta-analyses to clarify this complex issue.

The radiotherapy technique for the chest wall used by the DBCG employed an electron beam. This form of radiation, where all the energy deposited in the tissues is within a few centimetres at most of the skin surface, ensures that only a small amount of radiation is received by the heart and in particular the dose to the major coronary vessels is small even when patients with a left sided tumour are being treated. The excess cardiovascular mortality identified by meta-analysis did not clearly emerge until the second decade of follow-up. This means we cannot be sure at present that the careful radiotherapy technique used by the Danish group, which results in only a minimal dose to the heart, avoids the problem of cardiovascular mortality seen in earlier radiotherapy trials. It would seem likely on the basis of our understanding that this should follow, but the history of clinical trials in breast cancer have taught us to be wary about drawing conclusions on the basis of what seems sensible, rather than on the evidence from controlled trials! This trial does suggest that potentially by minimising cardiac dose, radiotherapy may confer a survival benefit to patients whose risk of breast cancer death is the same or even less than the 'high risk' group included in the Danish studies. If deaths related to radiotherapy can be minimised, one might expect a survival advantage for most groups of patients, although for those in the very lowest risk group any survival advantage would be minimal. This is comparable to the current situation with adjuvant systemic treatment. At the present time it is not clear that chest wall radiotherapy following mastectomy can be given in such a way as to avoid cardiac mortality, so it should be administered only to patients at high risk of local recurrence.

> *If non-breast cancer deaths can be minimised postoperative radiotherapy in high-risk women following mastectomy would be expected on the basis of currently available data to produce improvement in survival.*

2.2. Identification of risk factors

2.2.1. Risk factors for local recurrence

It is not possible from historical data to determine whether factors which indicate a high risk of local recurrence, are influenced by radiotherapy, or are the same as those related to an increased risk of breast cancer death. The DBCG trials produced unexpected results, in that patients with a small number of involved nodes (1–3 positive nodes) had a greater survival benefit than those with greater nodal involvement and likewise patients with tumours less than 5 cm in diameter gained greater benefit than those with tumours over 5 cm [5]. A biological explanation for these observations is difficult but as the data are derived from a retrospective sub-set analysis they may not be correct.

Identification of patients at high risk of chest wall recurrence after mastectomy has not attracted a great deal of interest. Multivariate analyses have rarely been applied with univariate comparisons forming the basis of most reports. Some of what is generally accepted and practised is based more on traditional beliefs than on high-quality evidence. Rarely do authors distinguish between chest wall and axillary recurrences, simply reporting loco-regional failure rates. The wide variability in surgical approach to the axilla compounds this difficulty.

Systemic treatments reduce overall risk of local recurrence, but using available evidence, the factors that predict increased risk remain the same as those identified prior to the widespread use of systemic therapy. The observation of a constant proportional reduction by radiotherapy on the risk of recurrence in trials where systemic treatment has been used, supports this view [6].

A consistent feature predicting a higher risk of chest wall recurrence following mastectomy is involvement of axillary nodes with the extent of nodal involvement (number of nodes involved) being important, with the risk of recurrence rising as the number of nodes involved increases. The evidence that node positivity is an important risk factor has been reviewed by Fowble [6]. Much of the data are derived from studies where a complete axillary clearance was routinely performed. In a large series where node sampling rather than axillary clearance was employed, any node positivity emerged as the highest risk factor for chest wall recurrence [7].

The second factor where there is widespread agreement is that the risk of local recurrence rises with increasing size of the primary tumour [6].

Involvement, or fixation to underlying muscle or fascia, are viewed as features indicating a high risk of local recurrence after mastectomy, although data to support these views is not abundant [6].

Age is another factor which has been consistently reported to be associated with local recurrence risk, with younger patients found in most but not all studies to be at higher risk [6].

Grading of tumours, an established indicator of prognosis, is also related to risk of local recurrence [7]. Lympho-vascular invasion also appears as a significant risk factor [7], although the number of reports connecting this with a recurrence after mastectomy are relatively few.

Another factor thought to increase the risk of local recurrence is disease up to and involving a mastectomy margin (particularly the deep margin). One small study of only 105 patients has addressed this question [8]. Although no statistical significance was found (as might be expected with the small numbers), eight of nine local recurrences occurred when the tumour was within 5 mm of the deep margin.

Tumour size, fixation to underlying structures, extent of axillary lymph node involvement, histological grade and histological evidence of vascular invasion are risk factors for local recurrence after mastectomy. Age may also be a risk factor.

2.2.2. Risk of being harmed by radiotherapy

The meta-analysis produced striking findings on the risks of improved survival associated with radiotherapy. By the very nature of meta-analysis, the conclusions that can be drawn are rather general, but some clear points emerge.

Studies which have been 'pooled' for the meta-analysis are consistent and show an increased risk of death from causes other than breast cancer in patients who receive chest wall radiotherapy. This increased risk is not apparent until the second decade after treatment, presumably reflecting the time scale of the late effects of radiation on certain tissues. Deaths from heart disease appears to be the major (if not sole) contributing factor. The proportionally-constant increase in cardiac risk caused by radiotherapy means that young women, whose absolute cardiac risk is small, show a negligible increase in cardiac mortality, whereas older women, with a bigger absolute risk, show a proportionally comparable increase in that risk.

The dose of radiotherapy received by the heart is usually much less for patients having right sided chest wall irradiation than for those having left (although the dose to the heart received by an internal mammary node irradiation field even for right sided tumours may be significant, depending upon the precise technique used). One might expect therefore that patients with left sided tumours would be more likely to be harmed than those with right sided ones. This is borne out by evidence from Sweden [9,10]. Unfortunately, laterality of tumour was not an item of information collected on an individual basis for the patients analysed in the published meta-analysis.

Radiotherapy does have other local effects that can vary from the very minor to the devastating, such as severe brachial plexus damage. In considering the pros and cons of giving radiotherapy to patients after mastectomy, these must be considered together with the assessment of impact on survival and local recurrence.

Radiotherapy is usually detrimental to cosmetic outcome following mastectomy. However, in many cases, any detrimental impact is small, and is insufficient to influence the decision whether or not radiotherapy is indicated. This would certainly be the case in patients who had undergone breast reconstruction using a vascularised flap. Distortion consequent upon fibrosis around a prosthesis is more of a problem following radiotherapy.

3. Conclusion

The decision as to whether or not to give radiotherapy to a patient after mastectomy remains an individual decision based on potential risks and benefits. Certain patients at high risk of breast cancer recurrence may survive longer if given radiotherapy, yet others will gain no benefit and may suffer harm. Improvements in radiotherapy technique should shift the balance towards the use of radiation, as long as it is delivered in an optimal fashion [11].

References

1. Kurtz JM (1994) Radiotherapy in the curative treatment of breast cancer: current status and future trends. An opinion sample of radiation oncologists active in breast cancer research. Radiother Oncol, 32(1), 21–8.
2. Paterson R, Russell MH (1959) Clinical trials in malignant disease. Part III — breast cancer. J Fac Radiol (London), 10, 175–180.
3. Early Breast Cancer Trialists Collaborative Group (2000) Favourable and unfavourable effects on long-term survival of radiotherapy for early breast cancer: an overview of the randomised trials. Lancet, 355: 1757–1770.
   Early Breast Cancer Trialists' Collaborative Group. Favourable and unfavourable effects on long-term survival of radiotherapy for early breast cancer: an overview of the randomised trials (in preparation).
4. Overgaard M, Hansen PS, Overgaard J (1997) Post-operative radiotherapy in high-risk pre-menopausal patients who receive adjuvant chemotherapy. N Engl J Med, 337, 949–955.
5. Harris JR, Halpin-Murphy P, McNeese M, Mendenhall NP, Morrow M, Robert NJ (1999) Consensus statement on post-mastectomy radiation therapy. Int J Radiat Oncol Biol Phys, 44, 989–990.
6. Fowble B (1997) Postmastectomy irradiation: then and now. Oncology, 11, 213–139.
7. O'Rourke S, Galea MH, Morgan DAL et al. (1994) Local recurrence after simple mastectomy. Br J Surg, 81, 386–389.
8. Mentzen SJ, Osteen RT, Wilson RE (1986) Local recurrence and the deep resection margin in carcinoma of the breast. Surg Gynecol Obstet, 16, 513–517.
9. Rutqvist LE, Lax I, Fornander T, Johansson H (1991) Cardiovascular mortality in a randomised trial of adjuvant radiation therapy versus surgery alone in breast cancer. Int J Radiat Oncol Biol Phys, 22, 887–896.
10. Gyenes G, Fornander T, Carlens P, Rutqvist LE (1993) Morbidity of ischemic heart disease in early breast cancer 15–20 years after adjuvant radiotherapy. Int J Radiat Oncol Biol Phys, 28, 1235–1241.
11. Recht A, Bartelink H, Fourquet A et al. (1998) Post-mastectomy radiotherapy: questions for the twenty-first century. J Clin Oncol, 16, 2886–2889.

Breast Cancer: Diagnosis and Management
J.M. Dixon (Ed.)

CHAPTER 24

Subcutaneous mastectomy: its role in the treatment of breast cancer and its role in high risk women

Andrew D. Baildam

1. Introduction

Whilst there is no formalised definition, the term 'subcutaneous mastectomy' is understood to refer to an operation whereby the glandular tissue of the breast is removed, leaving the skin envelope and nipple areola complex intact, together with immediate glandular volume replacement by means of subcutaneous breast implant. The operation developed in parallel with the development of silicone breast prostheses [1–3].

Indications for subcutaneous mastectomy evolved to encompass women with benign proliferative disease in whom there was deemed to be a higher than average risk of developing breast cancer, and whose breasts were difficult to evaluate by annual surveillance. Criteria for subcutaneous mastectomy soon extended to women deemed at high risk of developing breast cancer by virtue of personal risk factors such as strong family history of the disease [4]. At a time when wide local excision of the breast for cancer treatment with or without radiotherapy was being evaluated in breast cancer management, there were no scientific trials of subcutaneous mastectomy, and hence no rigorous scientific evaluation either of its indication or its outcomes.

What became clear was that the term 'subcutaneous mastectomy' was applied to a number of different operations. There was variablilty in the extent of resection of breast parenchyma: skin flaps left with thick subcutaneous tissue led to the more acceptable cosmetic results but did not remove more than a majority of the breast gland, whereas thin skin flaps and greater gland removal resulted in poor cosmetic results with frequent skin flap and implant loss and poor cosmetic outcome [2,5–7]. Even radical mastectomy however leaves behind some breast tissue [8].

Enthusiasm for subcutaneous mastectomy as a means of preventing breast cancer in otherwise well, but high risk women, was tempered by complications, including nipple loss, skin loss and implant loss, and often modest or poor cosmetic outcomes. Some complication rates could be reduced by attention to specific surgical detail, such as preservation of the vascular plexus deep to the nipple [4]. Notwithstanding, the main indication for subcutaneous mastectomy became that of breast cancer risk reduction for women at high personal risk. Some series did report a very low incidence of breast cancer following this operation [4,9].

The classic subcutaneous mastectomy operation was performed using an inframammary fold incision and removing as much as possible of the glandular tissue from the breast using this lower pole access. The oncological efficacy of this approach has been questioned on two counts: first, the axillary tail and upper outer quadrant of the breast which geographically within the breast has the highest rate of development of breast cancer, is the most inaccessible part of the breast using this approach. Secondly, thick skin flaps have to be maintained under the nipple and in the lower pole to prevent nipple and/or lower pole skin necrosis. For these reasons subcutaneous mastectomy has never had a significant role in the management of women with proven invasive cancer — incomplete glandular excision results in an unacceptably high local recurrence rate, and the addition of radiotherapy in the presence of a subcutaneous prosthesis with variable tissue cover invited cosmetic deterioration, particularly from capsular formation and fibrosis, and implant extrusion.

Subsequently a number of case reports of cancer developing after subcutaneous mastectomy fuelled uncertainties about the operation as a prophylactic procedure [10–13].

Recent developments in risk reducing mastectomy have been spurred by two factors: the ability to identify women at high risk of hereditary breast cancer by identification of BRCA1 or 2 gene mutations or by using Claus data [16], and secondly the awareness that women who carry such mutations and who develop breast cancer have significantly worse prognostic features in their tumours compared to women with sporadic breast cancer [14]. At a time when the science of genetics is in advance of the science of preventative treatment, the aims and techniques of risk reducing mastectomy with or without breast reconstruction have been revisited.

Women with BRCA 1 or 2 mutations carry that genotype in all cells, but those who develop cancer of the breast seldom develop multicentric disease. Like most women with sporadic breast cancer, they are more likely to have a unifocal breast cancer, but are at a much higher risk of bilateral cancers. The objective of surgery is to reduce the incidence of and mortality from breast cancer in women at high risk, and to do so in a way most consistent with quality of life and aesthetic concerns. Breast restorative procedures for women who undergo mastectomy for breast cancer have progressed rapidly, with significantly improved aesthetic results compared to those possible a decade ago. The use of skin-sparing mastectomy with immediate submuscular expander/implant or myocutaneous flap volume replacement is one such advance. Risk reducing mastectomy has been developed using the techniques of skin sparing surgery and volume replacement.

At all stages of operative planning the patient must be involved in the decisions which are made. Women must be told that no operation will remove all risk, but risk reduction may be of the order of 80% [15]. Whether or not to conserve the nipple is controversial. Breast tissue immediately deep to the nipple areola complex (NAC) is uncommonly a site of primary breast cancer, nevertheless preservation of the nipple areola complex must theoretically carry a slight diminishing in risk reduction. With awareness of this, most women who undergo risk reducing mastectomy with immediate reconstruction do request NAC preservation, but are warned that NAC sensory loss is likely and NAC ischaemic loss possible.

The operation described is the procedure developed and now most commonly requested by women from the Manchester Breast Unit Family History Clinic [17]. It comprises a skin-sparing mastectomy with NAC conservation when requested, and immediate breast volume replacement by means of submuscular tissue expansion. At a second procedure some months later after tissue expansion in the clinic, the infra-mammary fold is recreated on each breast and the tissue expanders replaced with permanent implants. This second procedure affords the best chance of adjusting the aesthetic quality of the breast reconstructions such that ideally the woman will look as near-normal as possible not only when wearing a bra but also when undressed. Pre and postoperative photographs are mandatory.

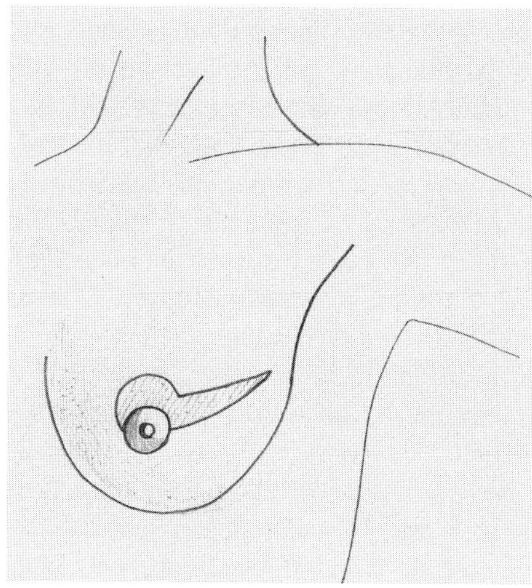

Fig. 1. Mastectomy incision including mastopexy.

2. Operative sequence

(1) Positioning of the patient: the patient lies supine with both hands under her waist with the shoulder and elbow slightly flexed and both arms and wrists well protected and padded. This allows full access to the axillary tail and the patient can be sat up during the procedure to judge asymmetry and shape when indicated.

(2) Skin incisions are made transversely across the outer half of the breast towards the axillary tail, extended around the areola and depending on the size of the breast, medially for 1–2 cm (Fig. 1). A mastopexy pattern is drawn with the patient sitting, to determine the extent of nipple elevation required such that the skin envelope best matches the submuscular expanded mound. Otherwise lower pole skin dropout looks unsightly and is difficult to correct. A second de-epithelialised incision in an elliptical fashion at the inframammary fold can be used to balance the position of the NAC on the expanded mound, if necessary to prevent the nipple from riding too high on the breast. Postoperative position of a nipple is extremely difficult to correct.

(3) With removal of the skin in the mastopexy shape, a paper template can be made to orientate and mark the incision on the contralateral breast. De-epithelialised skin bridges are left in place around the upper half of the NAC, to preserve the subdermal vascular plexus. Transverse scars are used to enable direct access to all quadrants of the breast, including the peripheral upper outer quadrant and axillary tail.

(4) Breast parenchyma removal: the plane of dissection continues leaving just sufficient tissue under the surface of the skin to preserve and support the subdermal vascular plexus across the breast. Wherever possible all glandular tissue is removed. The conical dissection is taken down to the pectoralis fascia and the breast mobilised from the pectoralis major muscle by sharp dissection (Fig. 2). Where possible the perforating vessels from the second intercostal inter-space medially are preserved as this reduces the incidence of skin flap necrosis. The breast is removed en bloc with the axillary tail but the axillary lymph nodes as far as possible are left in situ. The breast is removed laterally to the lateral border of latissimus dorsi. The breast is weighed and the bleeding controlled using bipolar diathermy. Warm saline soaked packs are placed on the skin flaps.

(5) Submuscular expander: an incision is made on the lateral border of pectoralis major in its outer third, and a plane developed underneath pectoralis major superior and medial using finger dissection (Fig. 3). Once the submuscular pocket has been developed as far as possible using this technique, lighted retractors can be inserted under the muscle and the dissection continued on the under surface of the muscle using bipolar haemostatic scissors under direct vision. Medially the deepest fibres of pectoralis major are divided from their origin from the costal cartilages. Inferiorly sharp dissection elevates the upper origins of the serratus anterior

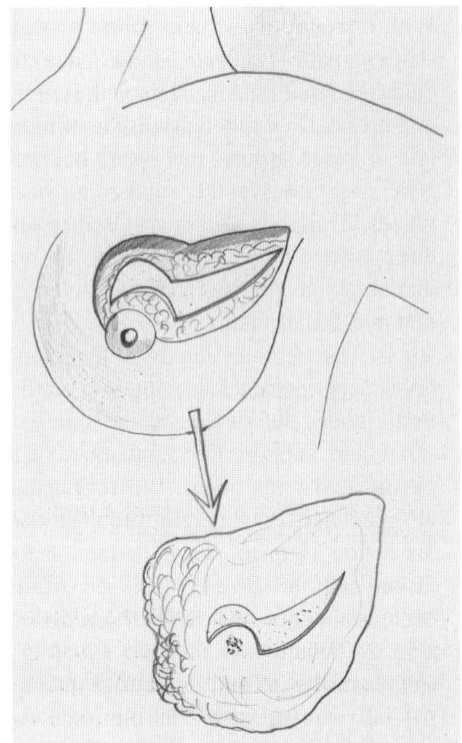

Fig. 2. Mastectomy: breast parenchymal excision shape.

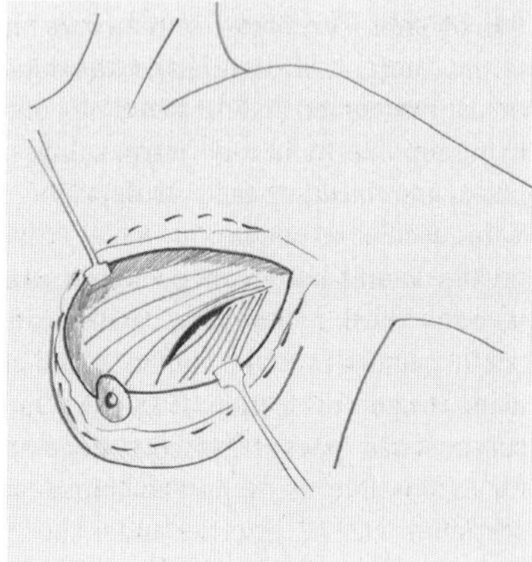

Fig. 3. Development of the submuscular pocket.

muscle, leaving a single sheet in continuity with the lower edge of pectoralis major, with the fascia between the two muscles intact. The lower pole of the pocket is dissected 2 cm below the projected infra-mammary fold, and this may involve entering the anterior rectus sheath medially. Laterally the serratus anterior is elevated as far as the anterior axillary line, and the pectoralis minor muscle is divided at its origin, and moved laterally to increase the muscle cover over the expander. The pocket is packed and then irrigated with betadine soaked swabs.

(6) Insertion of the tissue expander: the tissue expander is selected for size and shape to match the removed breast. Its handling involves utmost precaution to prevent infection. The expander is handled only by the surgeon, who double-gloves and places a clean towel on the operating field. The expander air is evacuated by needle, 3 way tap and syringe and the device steeped in betadine. The expander is rolled and inserted into the submuscular pocket and unrolled. Once the ideal base placement is achieved, the device valve is located through the upper half of the pectoralis major and a 23 or 21 gauge butterfly connected to a three way tap and giving set with 0.9% normal saline on line. The tissue expander is inflated to between 200 and 350 ml of saline (Fig. 4). The access window to the submuscular pocket is closed

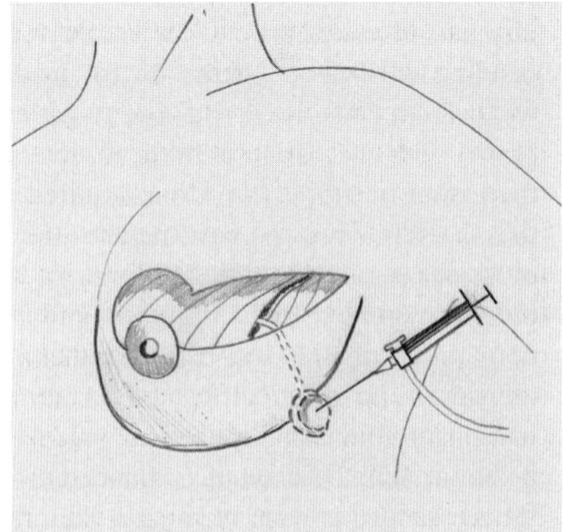

Fig. 4. Placement and inflation of the tissue expander/ implant device.

using 2/0 continuous vicryl approximating the edges of pectoralis major, pectoralis minor and serratus anterior. Any residual blood or betadine solution within the submuscular pocket is aspirated using an aspiration quill. The pocket may be drained by a closed vacuum drainage system.

(7) Closure: the subcutaneous breast space is drained using closed vacuum drains, one to the axilla and one medially, both exiting through the lateral infra-mammary crease. The mastopexy incision is closed using absorbable sutures. The wounds are covered with adhesive tapes.

(8) Postoperative care: intravenous prophylactic antibiotics are employed followed by oral antibiotics for five days (whilst drains are still in situ). A soft supporting sports bra is worn after the first 24 hours and for the next two weeks. Any suspected tissue viability problems may be addressed by hydration, dextran 40 intravenously, and rarely, by glyceryl trinitrate paste on the nipple areola complex. Obvious total NAC necrosis must be excised early in order to avoid an infection spreading to the tissue expander beneath the muscle.

(9) Outpatient care: following discharge the woman is seen in the outpatient clinic and the tissue expander inflated with normal saline using a 23 gauge butterfly needle and a sterile technique. Up to 100 ml may be installed at any time, depending upon the tension in the overlying muscle and skin. For most women two expansions are sufficient but occasionally more are needed. Following optimum expansion, the patient waits for three months so that maximum ptosis can develop. Discussions regarding the definitive implant and any adjustment procedures take place. The patient is subsequently admitted for the second procedure.

(10) The second procedure: the patient is again supine with the planned infra-mammary fold incisions marked. Provided that the original incisions have healed well, the incision is made in the midline of each breast 4 cm long at the midpoint of each infra-mammary fold. The submusclar pocket is entered using diathermy dissection, the tissue expander is aspirated and removed. Where necessary to achieve better shape, an inferior and medial capsulotomy can be performed using bipolar scissors (Fig. 5). It is seldom the case that a lateral capsulotomy is indicated nor a superior capsulotomy. The definitive prosthesis is selected and subjected to stringent insertion precautions. The most commonly requested implant is an anatomically shaped cohesive gel silicone implant. Once in position the patient can be sat up on the operating table to ensure symmetry and optimum shape. Each wound is closed with layers 2/0 vicryl followed by 3/0 or 4/0 monocryl and tapes.

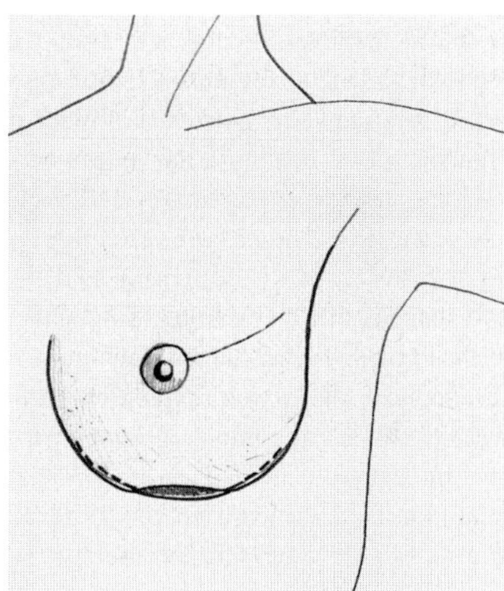

Fig. 5. Second operation: inframammary crease incision, exchange of implant, inferior capsulotomy.

If the NAC has not been conserved the NAC reconstruction followed by NAC tattoo is performed later under local anaesthetic.

3. Outcomes

The concept of a single operation to include mastectomy and reconstruction is an attractive ideal, and to try to achieve this the first four patients referred to the Manchester Breast Unit for surgery underwent subcutaneous mastectomy with immediate placement of submuscular permanent implants. The cosmetic outcome was satisfactory in two cases and in the other two cases there was a mismatch between ptosis correction and the volume and shape achieved by immediate placement. One of these patients had her implants removed.

Subsequently the tissue expander technique has been used and the idea of immediate permanent implant placement abandoned. This new technique allows significant cosmetic advantage, and allows full development of the medial and inferior poles of the reconstructed breasts, together with the opportunity for accurate nipple placement. The aesthetic results of the two stage process for most women are a significant improvement over a one stage operation. The procedure has evolved by attention to detail to correct possible cosmetic inadequacies.

In the Manchester Unit less than 10% of women in the Family History Clinic considered at high risk of breast cancer and counselled regarding surgery, ultimately undergo the operation. Of these only one third are confirmed BRCA1 or 2 mutation carriers: in the remaining two thirds the higher risk is identified by family history and reproductive history, but cannot be verified by genetic testing.

Patient details are shown in Table 1.

In two patients invasive cancers were diagnosed preoperatively following clinical examination and needle biopsy: in neither case was malignancy diagnosed on mammography. Both women proceeded with bilateral mastectomy and reconstruction, and one underwent postoperative adjuvant chemotherapy. There were no cases of invasive cancer diagnosed from the pathology following surgery.

Table 1. Profile of women undergoing bilateral risk reducing mastectomy with breast reconstruction (to end 1999)

	n = 43
BRCA 1 or BRCA 2	12
Fixed volume implants	4
Tissue expander/implants	37
Bilateral TRAM flaps	2
Nipple conservation	35
Ischaemic nipple loss	1

Age: median, 40 years; range, 26–61 years.

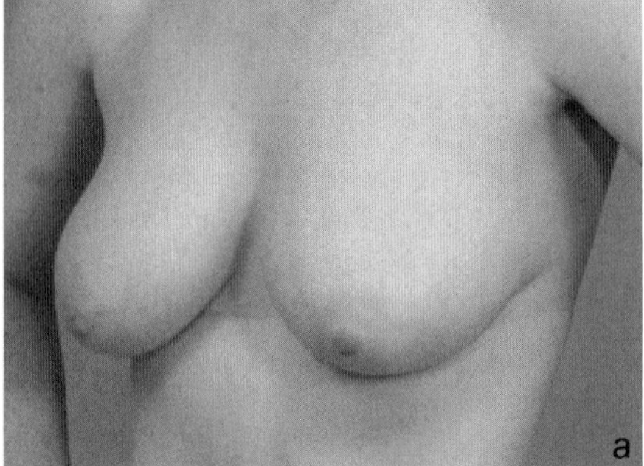

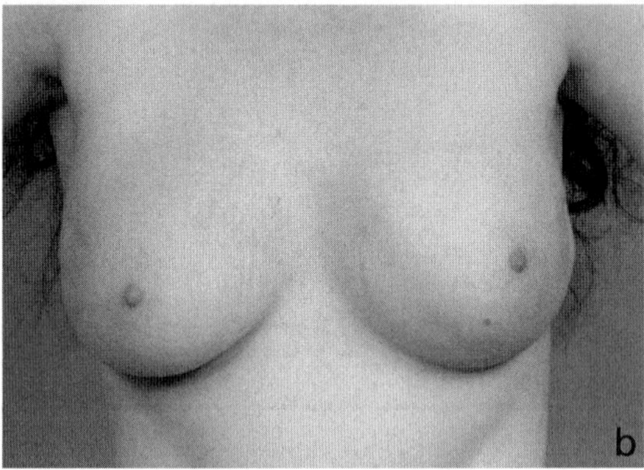

Fig. 6. A patient (a) before and (b) after bilateral risk reducing mastectomies and reconstructions.

Cosmetically the aim has been to achieve the results of high aesthetic quality. Most women undergoing this procedure express considerable relief of anxiety, but they should not have to face a constant physical reminder that they have undergone bilateral mastectomy. It is easy to demonstrate a patient with a good cosmetic result, nevertheless the 'before' and 'after' surgery photographs shown in Fig. 6 are typical of the majority of women in this series.

The cosmetic key is to match the skin envelope surface area to that achievable by the expanded muscle pocket which constitutes the neo-breast mound. In any breast with natural, minor or moderate ptosis, a good match can be achieved if breast volume is not much larger than 500 cc. If there is major ptosis then inframammary fold de-epithelialisation and shortening of the nipple to inframammary fold distance is essential if both the nipple position is to be accurate whilst at the same time avoiding redundant inferior pole skin.

In a natural breast of greater than 700 cc in size or with gross ptosis, nipple elevation using a mastopexy technique is not possible, and in these cases the nipple should be removed and either grafted or reconstructed at a later date. The position of the nipple is crucial. A nipple placed too high on the reconstructed breast will never look satisfactory and will be very difficult to correct.

Complications have been uncommon in our series. One patient had ischaemic NAC loss followed by infection of both tissue expanders. These were removed, but delayed reconstruction was successful four months later. In two partial de-pigmentation of the natural areola was corrected by tattoo.

There were a number of complications related to tissue expander device failure. These were mechanical problems associated with the port or spontaneous expander deflation unrelated to surgery or to saline installation. All were corrected but did require surgery.

This series has only short follow up: nevertheless there have been no women so far diagnosed with any breast problem following surgery. There are potential psycho-social morbidities associated with this procedure, and these are the subject of an ongoing multicentre study in the United Kingdom to which many of these women have contributed.

4. Summary

Risk reducing mastectomy with reconstruction has been developed to address the need of women assessed for personal risk in the family history clinics. The place of risk reducing surgery has been confirmed. Only a small proportion of women who might consider this operation actually pursue this path, but a strict protocol is in place to ensure that each woman makes the correct decision for herself. This process is dependent upon good communication between the Geneticist, Psychiatrist and specialist Surgeon. The decision to proceed with surgery is not a light one, and ultimately only the individual woman can make that choice for herself.

An operation has been developed to balance oncological needs and aesthetic outcome. This process involves at least two stages, and each stage is planned individually with each woman. Some women have concerns about the use of long term breast implants, and two women have undergone immediate reconstruction with bilateral bi-pedicled TRAM flaps. For the women who underwent these procedures, the quality of the reconstruction was very important. For some women, having to live with a poor cosmetic result may be as equally tormenting as living with an elevated breast cancer risk. It is essential that the highest quality of reconstruction is achieved for individual women, and in turn that they do not have unrealistic expectations of what the operation comprises and what the outcomes are likely to be.

Risk reducing mastectomy with reconstruction is likely to be a temporary phenomenon, an imperfect solution to the problem of how to manage women at high risk in whom no other treatment is as effective or acceptable. Doubtless some women will ultimately present with cancer of the breast having previously undergone this procedure, but a risk reduction of a gene mutation carrier from 80 to 10% is a highly significant personal benefit for the majority. Chemoprevention or gene therapy will likely surpass risk reducing mastectomy. Until that time it is important that this operation be carried out to the highest oncological and cosmetic standards and that women are offered the surgery in a controlled protocol-driven setting, and that treatment is entirely at the specialist level. Furthermore, the consistency of technique and meticulous follow up data are essential.

References

1. Pennisi VR, Capozzi A, Perez FM. Subcutaneous mastectomy data. Breast 1979; 5: 18.
2. Goldman ID, Goldwin RM. Some anatomic considerations of subcutaneous mastectomy. Plast Recon Surg 1972; 50: 211–215.
3. Pennisi VR, Capozzi A, Perez FM. Subcutaneous mastectomy data: a preliminary report. Plast Recon Surg 1977; 59: 53–56.
4. Pennisi VR, Capozzi A. Subcutaneous mastectomy data: a final statistical analysis of 1,500 patients. Aesth Plast Surg 1989; 13: 15–21.
5. Pennisi VR, Lozado G, Capozzi A. Minimising the complications of subcutaneous mastectomy. Breast 1980; 6: 22–25.
6. Pennisi VR. Redefined indication for subcutaneous mastectomy in patients with benign breast diseases. Aesth Plast Surg 1986; 10: 101–104.
7. Pennisi VR, Capozzi A. Treatment of chronic cystic mastitis by subcutaneous mastectomy. Plast Recon Surg 1973; 52: 520–524.
8. Hickin NF. Mastectomy: a clinical pathological study demonstrating why most mastectomies result in incomplete removal of the mammary gland. Arch Surg 1940; 40: 6–14.
9. Holzgreve W, Beller FK, Niedner W, Nienhaus H. Bilateral subcutaneous mastectomy as a prophylactic operation to prevent breast cancer. Breast Disease 1989; 2: 27–33.
10. Ziegler LD, Kroll SS. Primary breast cancer after prophylactic mastectomy. Am J Clin Oncol 1981; 14(5): 451–454.
11. Willemsen HW, Kaas R, Peterse JH, Rutgers EJTH. Breast carcinoma in residual breast tissue after prophylactic bilateral subcutaneous mastectomy. Eur J Surg Oncol 1998; 24: 331–338.
12. Goodnight JE, Quagliana JM, Morton DL. Failure of subcutaneous mastectomy to prevent the development of breast cancer. J Surg Oncol 1984; 26: 198–201.
13. Eldar S, Meguid MM, Beaty JD. Cancer of the breast after prophylactic subcutaneous mastectomy. Am J Surg 1984; 148: 693.
14. Watson P, Marcus JN, Lynch HT. Prognosis of BRCAI hereditary breast cancer. Lancet 1998; 351: 304–305.
15. Hartman LC, Schaid DJ, Woods JE et al. Efficacy of bilateral prophylactic mastectomy in women with a family history of breast cancer. New Engl J Med 1999; 340(2): 77–84.
16. Claus EB, Risch N, Thompson WD. Autosomal dominant inheritance of early-onset breast cancer. Cancer 1994; 73(3): 643–651.
17. Baildam AD. The role of bilateral prophylactic mastectomy (BPMX) in women at high risk of breast cancer. Disease Markers 1999; 15: 197–198.

Breast Cancer: Diagnosis and Management
J.M. Dixon (Ed.)

CHAPTER 25

The role of hormones in the aetiology and evolution of breast cancer

W.R. Miller

1. Introduction

1.1. Hormones and the aetiology and evolution of breast cancer

That the normal breast is a target for hormones is evident from the simple observations that major development changes occur at puberty, during pregnancy and following the menopause [1]. These are all times of major endocrinological upheaval involving both protein and steroidal hormones but the influences of the latter, in particular oestrogens, appear critical.

- *hormones control breast development*
- *major changes occur at puberty, during pregnancy and following the menopause*

It is perhaps not surprising that the processes associated with the development or progression of malignancies within the breast should also be influenced by the same hormones. The evidence for this is as follows.

2. Hormones and risk

Epidemiological and endocrinological studies provide support for the contention that hormones influence the risk for breast cancer [2].

Epidemiological data relate to (i) aetiological associations between reproductive/menstrual history and breast cancers and (ii) the effects of exogenous administration/intake of hormones and incidence of breast cancer.

The aetiology of breast cancer has a strong hormonal component (Table 1). The disease is predominantly a disease of females in whom it does not appear before puberty [3]; women who have extended exposure to menstrual activity either by an early menarche or late menopause or nulliparity have increased risk [4]. Conversely risk is decreased by a premature menopause whether this be natural or artificially induced [5]; there is also a quantitative relationship between the age at which ovarian function ceases and increased likelihood of protection, such that castration at 35 years is calculated to reduce the risk to one third that experienced by women who undergo a normal menopause [6]. Other factors which superficially do not have an obvious endocrinological influence may also be mediated by hormones. For example body weight, a risk factor, in postmenopausal women (heavier individuals being more susceptible than lighter counterparts) may be mediated through oestrogens [7]. Heavy women are more likely to be obese and adipose tissue is the major site of oestrogen biosynthesis in postmenopausal women [8] in whom there is a direct correlation between body weight/degree of obesity and levels of circulating oestrogens [9]. Similarly, it has

Table 1. Risk factors for breast cancer

Factor	High risk	Low risk	Relative excess
Gender	Female	Male	100×
Age	Elderly	Young	>10×
Geography	USA/UK	Japan	5×
Family History	2 1st degree relatives	None	4–6×
Age at menopause	>50 years	<35 years	3×
Age at menarche	<12 years	>13 years	2×
Age at 1st birth	>41 years	<20 years	2×
Parity	Parous	Nulliparous	1.5×
Body weight	Highest percentile	Lowest percentile (postmenopausal)	1.5×
Height	Highest percentile	Lowest percentile	1.3×

been suggested that since postmenopausal women in Western societies tend to be more overweight than those in Oriental countries, obesity might be a factor largely accounting for geographic differences in the incidence of breast cancer in these women [10].

If endocrine factors influence the risk of breast cancer it might be expected that women given exogenous hormones would have a higher incidence of cancer. There are three situations in which exogenous hormones have been administered to women on a relatively wide scale: (i) during child-bearing years as contraceptives [11]; (ii) during pregnancy to avoid spontaneous abortion [12]; and (iii) at and after the menopause to relieve symptoms associated with oestrogen deficiency [13]. In each case there is evidence that exogenous administration of hormones increased risk although for oral contraceptives and replacement oestrogens, the effects are relatively small, such that meta analyses or subgroup analyses have been required to demonstrate significant interactions. The most convincing case for hormones increasing susceptibility to breast cancer relates to the practice in the 1950s and 1960s of giving very high doses of diethyl stibestrol to pregnant women in the US in an attempt to prevent gynaecological complications and abortions. Extensive follow-up suggests that the practice increased breast cancer risk by about 35% although there could be a substantial latency time between oestrogen administration and appearance of cancer [12].

- *aetiological factors for breast cancer have a strong endocrine component*
- *exogenous administration of hormones increases risk (although effects may be difficult to detect unless (i) cumulative doses are high or given at susceptible times and (ii) follow up is prolonged)*

Considerable research has been directed to demonstrate that in attempting to demonstrate that women at high risk of breast cancer or those who subsequently develop the disease have abnormal endocrine profiles. However these investigations have not yielded consistent results although individual studies have produced some interesting observations and recent meta-analyses are now revealing significant trends [14,15]. Of particular interest is the prospective study initiated by Bulbrook in 1961 in the Island of Guernsey which recruited and followed up 5,000 ostensibly normal women. When cases of breast cancers were subsequently diagnosed they were matched with controls who were still free from the disease. Amongst the more provocative results were the findings that: (i) urinary androgen excretion (aetiocholanolone and androsterone) were lower in cases compared with controls (particularly in premenopausal women) [16]; and (ii) cases had a higher proportion of circulating oestrogen in nonprotein bound form [17]. However these differences tended to disappear as the study matured, provoking the suggestion that abnormalities reflected time to diagnosis rather than absolute risk, ie were associated with rapidly growing tumours which appeared in the early years of the study.

Recently, prospective studies have demonstrated increased plasma levels of oestradiol in women who later went on to develop breast cancer (values being about 20% higher than those who remained disease free) [18]. Whilst these studies relate mainly to postmenopausal women (Fig. 1), similar data are emerging for premenopausal cases [14,19]. The results are therefore compatible with the concept that relatively high oestradiol concentrations increase breast cancer risk. Conversely populations of women from countries with reduced risk have low serum oestradiol concentrations both before and after the menopause [20]. These findings have revealed such correlations given the limitations that: (i) many are based on a single blood sample; (ii) local levels of hormones within the breast may be different from those in the circulation (particularly in postmenopausal women); (iii) effects of hormones may be dependent upon concentrations of others; (iv) cumulative exposure may be more important than levels at a particular time point; and (v) cyclicity may be equally influential as absolute hormone concentration. It should be noted

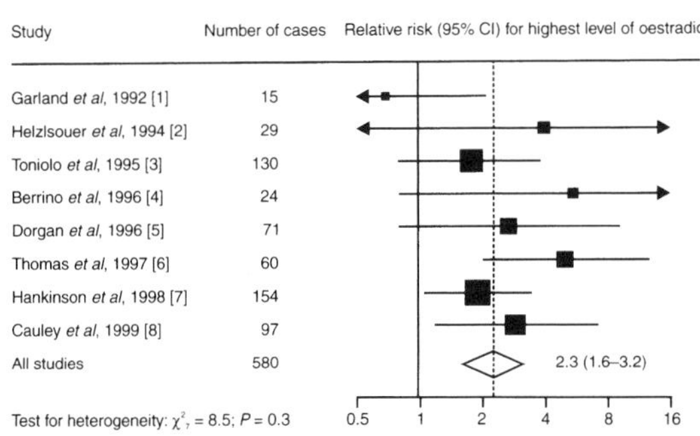

Fig. 1. Prospective studies of oestradiol and breast cancer risk in postmenopausal women. For each study (full list of references in Key and Verkasalo [34]) the relative risk plotted is for women with the highest oestradiol concentration (tertile or quartile) compared with women with the lowest concentration. The 'all studies' estimate was calculated by weighting the individual relative risks by the inverse of their estimated variances, on a logarithmic scale.

that these differences in hormones which have been observed have resulted from comparisons of groups of women and absolute differences are small. This means that hormone assays are unlikely to be accurate predictions of risk to cancer.

- *it has been difficult to show that women at high risk of cancer or those who subsequently develop the disease have abnormal circulating levels of hormones*
- *abnormalities in urinary androgens in women who develop cancer may reflect differences in tumour growth rates rather than absolute risks*
- *prospective studies and meta-analyses suggest that both pre- and postmenopausal women may have raised levels of circulating oestrogens; conversely women from populations with low risk may have lower levels*
- *circulating hormones are unlikely to be predictive of subsequent risk in individual women*

3. Mechanism of hormone-induction of cancer

Classically, the induction of cancer has been subdivided into two processes — 'initiation' or the transformation from the normal to the transformed malignant phenotype and 'promotion' whereby the population of transformed cells are selectively expanded until they appear clinically as tumours (Fig. 2). Since the evidence that hormones stimulate the growth of both normal and malignant cells within the breast is substantial (as will be discussed below), the belief has been that major influences on tumour induction are mediated through promotional effects. However, insofar as proliferating cells may be more prone to genetic errors which lead to oncogenesis, hormones could be regarded as co-initiators. Whether they are full initiators is more debatable. In standard assays for mutagens, most naturally occurring hormones produced negative results although synthetic steroids may test positive in

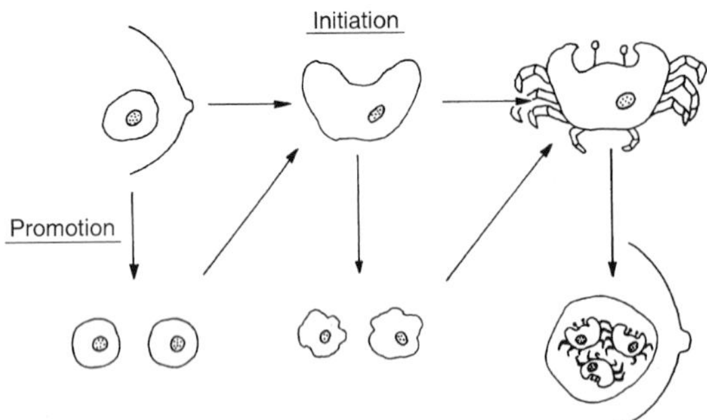

Fig. 2. The classical two-step process of carcinogenesis whereby normal cells are transformed into those with a malignant phenotype (initiation) which also involves promotional events, either the expansion of cells susceptible to transformation or the expansion of occult disease to clinically detectable tumours.

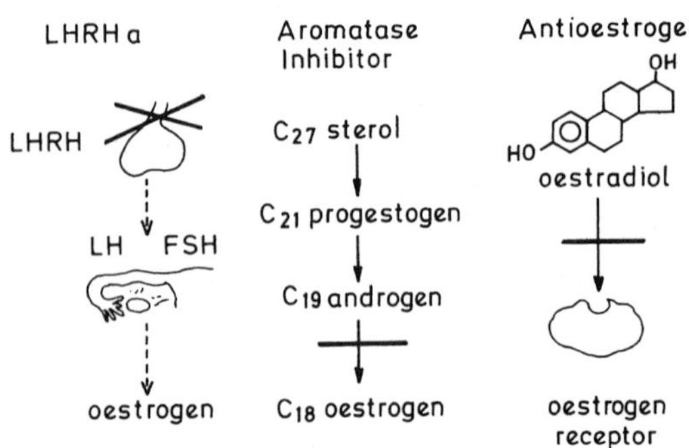

Fig. 3. Strategies underlying the development of drugs designed for oestrogen deprivation. LHRH agonists (LHRHa) prevent release of trophic gonadotrophins, aromatase inhibitor block the synthesis of oestrogen from androgens and antioestrogens to interfere with the interaction of oestrogen with its receptors.

some systems [21]. However, certain steroid hormones may be metabolised to intermediate which are capable of producing free radicals causing DNA damage and adducts. It is unclear whether this genotoxic activity is carcinogenic.

- *unless hormones are metabolised to reactive intermediates, they are unlikely to be primary initiators of breast cancer*
- *hormones promote the growth of transformed cells and sub-clinical cancers*
- *because proliferating cells are susceptible to genetic mistakes, hormones may act as co-initiators*

4. Hormones and disease progression

There is abundant evidence that hormones may maintain the growth of established cancers. The whole basis of endocrine therapy is that hormone deprivation may cause tumour regression. Thus it is well established that oophorectomy or the use of LHRH agonists in premenopausal women and of hypophysectomy, adrenalectomy, antioestrogens and aromatase inhibitors in postmenopausal patients will produce remissions in at least one third of women [22,23]. These treatments have in common the ability to remove sources of hormones, inhibit synthesis and release of hormones or blockade their mechanism of action (Fig. 3). These benefits are also largely restricted to tumours possessing hormone-receptors [24,25]. Conversely there is evidence that administration of steroid hormones may accelerate tumour growth. For example, thymide labelling index may be increased in skin metastasis following treatment with oestrogen and progesterone [26]; similarly urinary calcium excretion can be raised in patients with metastatic disease in bone following administration of oestrogen [27].

In addition to having effects on proliferation, hormones may also promote the spread and dissemination of breast cancer. For example experimental data suggest that hormones may increase: (i) the expression and activity of proteolytic enzymes which degrade basement membrane [28]; (ii) the production and secretion of growth factors which influence cell mobility [29]; and (iii) angiogenesis [30]. In contrast drugs with anti-hormone activity such as tamoxifen may reverse these effects. The latter influences which would be in keeping with the reduced incidence of contralateral breast cancers in women treated adjuvently with tamoxifen [31]. This apart, there is little direct clinical evidence for hormones stimulating tumours spread in vivo. It has been suggested that the poorer prognosis of patients offered surgery in the follicular phase of the menstrual cycle is caused by the action of oestrogen unopposed by progesterone promoting metastatic spread [32]. However this is still highly controversial. Indeed there are data which suggest that with tumour evolution, breast cancers tend to lose hormone sensitivity [33]. Thus more clinically advanced cancers and those of less differentiated phenotype tend to be hormone-receptor negative and more resistant to endocrine therapy. Whether hormonal autonomy is causally related to general aggressive behaviour or whether the phenotypes share common underlying mechanisms is unproven.

- *hormones maintain the growth of some breast cancers*
- *endocrine deprivation is a major treatment modality for breast cancer*
- *hormones may activate the machinery required for tumour metastasis and progression in experimental systems*
- *anti-hormones may delay the appearance of clinically detectable metastatic disease*
- *high grade tumours and clinically advanced stage disease are associated with hormone insensitivity*

References

1. Miller WR, Anderson TJ. Oestrogens, progestogens and the breast. In: Whitehead MI, Studd J, eds. The menopause. Blackwell Scientific Press, 1988: 234–246.
2. Boyle P. Epidemiology of breast cancer. Bailliere's Clin Oncol 1988; 2: 1–57.
3. MacMahon B, Cole P, Brown J. Etiology of human breast cancer: a review. JNCI 1973; 50: 21–42.
4. Henderon BE, Ross RK, Judd HL et al. Do regular ovulatory cycles increase breast cancer risk? Cancer 1985; 56: 1206–1208.
5. Wienfeld AM. The relationship of cancer of female breast to artificial menopause and menstrual status. Cancer 1956; 9: 927–936.
6. Trichopoulos D, MacMahon B, Cole P. Menopause and breast cancer risk. JNCI 1972; 48: 605–613.
7. de Waard F, Baanders-van Halewijn EA. A prospective study in general practice on breast cancer risk in postmenopausal women. Int J Cancer 1974; 14: 153–160.
8. MacDonald PC, Edman CD, Hemsell DL et al. Effect of obesity on conversion of plasma androstenedione to estrone in postmenopausal women with and without endometrial cancer. Am J Obstet Gynecol 1978; 130: 448–455.
9. Vermeulen A, Verdonck L. Sex hormone concentrations in postmenopausal women. Relation to obesity, fat mass, age and years postmenopause. Clin Endocrinol 1978; 9: 59–66.
10. Pike MC, Krailo MD, Henderson BE et al. "Hormonal" risk factors, "breast tissue age" and the age-incidence of breast cancer. Nature 1983; 303: 767–770.
11. La Vecchia C. Oral contraceptives and breast cancer. The Breast 1992; 2: 76–81.
12. Colton T, Greenberg R, Noller K et al. Breast cancers in mothers prescribed diethylstilbestrol in pregnancy. JAMA 1993; 269: 2069–2100.
13. Collaborative Group on Hormonal Factors in Breast Cancer. Breast cancer and hormone replacement therapy: collaborative reanalysis of data from 51 epidemiological studies of 52,705 women with breast cancer and 108,411 women without breast cancer. Lancet 1997; 350: 1047–1059.
14. Key TJ. Serum oestradiol and breast cancer risk. Endocrine Related Cancer 1999; 6: 175–180.
15. Thomas HV, Reeves GK, Key TJA. Endogenous estrogen and postmenopausal breast cancer: a quantitative review. Cancer Causes Control 1997; 8: 922–928.
16. Bulbrook RD, Thomas BS, Wang DY. A retrospective view of androgen and corticoid metabolites in the etiology and clinical course of breast-cancer. Endocrine Related Cancer 1997; 4: 285–288.
17. Bulbrook RD, Moore JW, Clark GMG et al. Relation between risk of breast cancer and bioavailability of estradiol in blood: prospective study in Guernsey. In: Angelli A, Bradlow HL, Dogliotti L, eds. Endocrinology of the breast: basic and clinical aspects. Annals NY Acad Sci 1986; 464: 373–388.
18. Santen RJ, Yue W, Naftolin F et al. The potential of aromatase inhibitors in breast cancer prevention. Endocrine Related Cancer 1999; 6: 235–243.
19. Thomas HV, Key TJ, Allen DS, Moore JW, Dowsett M, Fentiman IS, Wang DY. A prospective study of endogenous serum hormone concentrations and breast cancer risk in premenopausal women on the Island of Guernsey. Br J Cancer 1997; 75: 1075–1079.
20. Key TJA, Chen J, Wang DY et al. Sex hormones in rural China and in Britain. Br J Cancer 1990; 24: 29–43.

21. World Health Organization/International Agency for Research on Cancer: Genetic and related effects: an IARC monograph on the evaluation of carcinogenic risks to humans. 1987; Suppl 250–256; 293–295; 369–371; 426–433; 437–443.
22. Miller WR. Estrogens and endocrine therapy for breast cancer. In: Miller, WR, ed. Estrogen and Breast Cancer. Austin, TX, RG Landes, 1996; 125–150.
23. Wyld DK, Chester JD, Perrell TJ. Endocrine aspects of the clinical management of breast cancer — current issues. Endocrine Related Cancer 1998; 5: 97–110.
24. Hawkins RA, Roberts MM, Forrest APM. Oestrogen receptors in breast cancer: current status. Br J Surg 1980; 67: 153–169.
25. Ferenczy A, Bertrand G, Gelfand MM. Proliferation kinetics of human endometrium during the normal menstrual cycle. Am J Obstet Gynecol 1979; 133: 859–867.
26. Dao TL, Ainha DK, Nemoto T et al. Effect of estrogen and progesterone on cellular replication of human breast tumours. Cancer Res 1982; 42: 359–362.
27. Pearson OH, West CD, Hollander VP, Treves NE. Valuation of endocrine therapy for advanced breast cancer. JAMA 1954; 154; 234–239.
28. Rochefort H, Augereau P. Briozzo P et al. Oestrogen-induced pro-cathepsin D in breast cancer: from biology to clinical applications. Proc Roy Soc Edin 1989; 95B: 107–118.
29. Rochefort H, Platet N, Hayashido Y et al. Estrogen receptor mediated inhibition of cancer cell invasion and motility: an overview. J Steroid Biochem Mol Biol 1998; 65: 163–168.
30. Sypridopoulos I, Sullivan AB, Kearney M et al. Estrogen-receptor-mediated inhibition of human endothelial cell apoptosis. Estradiol as a survival factor. Circulation 1997; 18: 1505–1514.
31. Cuzick J, Baum M. Tamoxifen and contralateral breast cancer. Lancet 1985; ii: 282–282.
32. Badwe RA, Gregory WM, Chaudrey MA et al. Timing of surgery during the menstrual cycle and survival of premenopausal women with operable breast cancer. Lancet 1991; 337: 1261–1264.
33. Blanco G, Alavaikho M, Ojalo A. Estrogen and progesterone receptors in breast cancers: relationships to tumor histopathology and survival of patients. Anticancer Res 1984; 4: 383–389.
34. Key TJ, Verkasalo PK. Endogenous hormones and the aetiology of breast cancer. Breast Cancer Res Treatment 1999; 1: 18–21.

Breast Cancer: Diagnosis and Management
J.M. Dixon (Ed.)

CHAPTER 26

Breast reconstruction after mastectomy

J.M. Dixon

1. Introduction

Breast reconstruction is a safe technique which has been shown to have no influence on recurrence free and overall survival or the detection of local recurrent disease [1,2]. It can be performed immediately following mastectomy [3] or as a delayed procedure. Immediate reconstruction has the benefits of reduced overall costs, better reconstructive outcome and a reduction in patient anxiety about losing a breast [4]. It does not lead to significant delays in the administration of adjuvant chemotherapy or radiation therapy [5]. The costs of a mastectomy with a myocutaneous flap reconstruction is equal to or less than the costs of a wide excision and radiation therapy with the added bonus that mastectomy may be associated with a slightly lower recurrence rate than breast conserving surgery. A potential disadvantage of immediate breast reconstruction is that a patient's expectation following immediate reconstruction may be higher because they have never experienced loss of a breast. Although there are no absolute contraindications to immediate reconstruction, where there is concern about tumour clearance or where post-operative radiotherapy is being planned, it is worth considering whether delayed reconstruction will produce a better final result than an immediate reconstruction which is irradiated. The problem with radiation therapy following immediate breast reconstruction is that it can produce significant fibrosis particularly when implant reconstructions are used and this can adversely affect the long-term cosmetic results [6]. If breast reconstruction is being performed following chest wall radiotherapy, the choices available for reconstruction are limited because the chest wall tissue will usually not allow tissue expansion. The choice of reconstructive procedure for any individual patient depends on several factors [7,8]. The options for reconstruction are outlined in Table 1.

Immediate breast reconstruction is not associated with any increase in the rate of local recurrence nor does it make local recurrence more difficult to detect.

2. Indications

Indications for particular techniques are dependent upon the surgeon's skills, patient preference and the site of the cancer and the size of the breast. There are a number of potential contraindications.

3. Systemic factors

Patients with ischaemic heart disease and patients with diffuse metastatic disease are not usu-

Table 1. Reconstructive options

Implant based techniques:
- Implant alone
- Tissue expander with subsequent implant exchange
- Expander-implant insertion (Becker device)
- Latissimus dorsi with implant or expander insertion

Pedicled autologous techniques:
- Latissimus dorsi without implant insertion
- Transverse rectus abdominis myocutaneous (TRAM) flap (unipedicled/bipedicled/turbo-charged)
- Latissimus dorsi mini-flap for lumpectomy defects
- Tumour specific immediate reconstruction or oncoplastic surgery

Microvascular autologous techniques:
- TRAM flap
- Perforator TRAM flap
- Rubens' flap
- Superior and inferior gluteal flaps
- Ilio-lumbar flap
- Lateral thigh flap

ally candidates for breast reconstruction. Obesity, diabetes or steroid treatment is associated with an increased risk of complications and are relative contraindications to breast reconstruction. Smoking has an impact on the microcirculation throughout the body and a variety of different studies have demonstrated it increases the frequency of complications with the most commonly used reconstructive techniques.

4. Local factors

Breast irradiation increases the rates of complications because of the effects on tissue compliance and vascularity. Blood flow to the latissimus dorsi and rectus abdominis muscles can be reduced by radiation and this increases the rates of flap loss if pedicled flaps are used. Pedicled flaps are used in previously irradiated parients.

Mastectomy usually but not always removes large amounts of skin and this can leave little room for implant alone insertion and obtaining satisfactory ptosis usually requires the use of either a tissue expander or autologous skin. Previous surgery and the resulting scars may influence the ability to use local skin flaps. If the patient has had a previous mastectomy with destruction of the inframammary fold this needs to be redefined at the time of delayed reconstruction.

Local factors need to be taken into account when considering the type of reconstruction that is appropriate for the patient.

5. Implant-based techniques

5.1. Implant reconstruction

Implant insertion alone is rarely used although there has been a resurgence in their use because of the increase in skin-sparing mastectomies which means that tissue expansion is not always necessary when implants are used. Because implants are usually placed underneath the chest wall muscle, even with skin sparing mastectomy some type of expansion is frequently needed to produce a muscular pocket of sufficient dimension to take up the overlying skin [2,9,10]. It is important that the implant has complete musculofascial cover. There is a much higher rate of capsular contraction if implants are placed subcutaneously.

Implant only reconstruction rarely produces a satisfactory breast reconstruction.

5.2. Tissue expander reconstruction

Following Radovan's initial introduction of the technique there has been considerable development of the expander. They now come in smooth or rough textures with integral ports and shapes include oval, teardrop, anatomic, differential and two compartment designs [11,12]. This is covered in the chapter by Khoo on Tissue Expanders and Implants.

Tissue expanders allow small or moderate breast mounds with little ptosis to be recon-

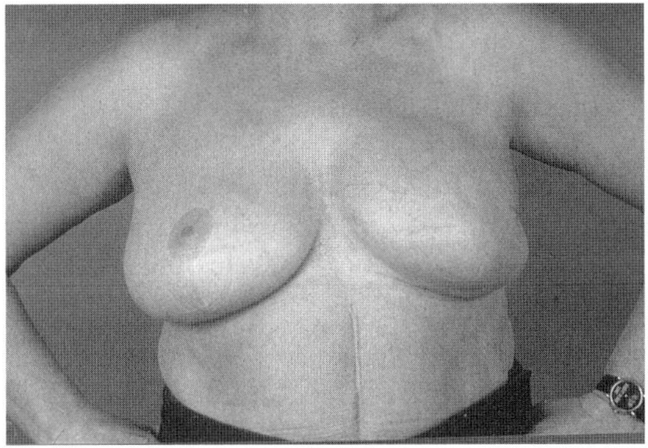

Fig. 1. Results following tissue expansion and subsequent gel filled implant exchange.

structed (Fig. 1). Textured expanders and implants have reduced the rate of capsular contracture [13].

Tissue expanders can be used to reconstruct a breast mound of small to moderate size. Reconstructions using expanders lack ptosis. No more than 7 cm of tissue can be recruited with tissue expansion.

5.3. Expander implant devices

Combined expander implants have been available for some time [14]. The Becker expander implant is a double lumen expander containing a gel-filled lumen surrounding an expandable saline filled lumen with a removable filler tube and injection port. It is inserted in a similar way to remote valve expanders and the post-operative expansion protocol is identical. One manufacturer produces expander/prosthesis with a filler port and tube which is non-removable. The use of these devices is covered in the chapter by Khoo on Tissue Expanders and Implants.

Becker expander/implant devices allow a one stage reconstruction. Unless a device of the correct volume is used, rippling of the device or firmness of the reconstruction can be a problem.

6. Latissimus dorsi myocutaneous flap reconstruction

When using latissimus dorsi to reconstruct the breast, an implant is usually required, unless the patient has substantial adipose tissue overlying the muscle [15]. The muscle is harvested either through a conventional open approach or through an axillary approach with or without endoscopes and lighted retractors if skin is not required. When raising a skin island over the muscle this is usually performed with an elliptical incision placed transversely or diagonally over the muscle [16]. The skin and overlying muscle is transposed anteriorally having divided the muscle from its origins on the spinous processes, lumbar fascia and the iliac crest. An extended latissimus dorsi flap including harvest of considerable fat over the muscle can provide sufficient bulk for small and medium sized breasts. Usually however, the latissimus dorsi flap has to be used in association with a breast implant. The muscle can either be sutured to the free lower border of the pectoralis major with the implant placed underneath the pectoral and latissimus dorsi muscles or the edge of the latissimus dorsi flap can be sutured to subcutaneous tissues of the lower and medial skin flaps with the implant being placed under the latissimus dorsi muscle and lying on the pectoralis major. This can result in part of the implant medially and inferiorally being subcutaneous but this gives a natural inframammary fold and cleavage (Fig. 2). The thoracodorsal nerve is usually left intact to preserve muscle bulk but can be secondarily divided if abnormal or unsightly contractures occur. Fortunately this latter complication is rare. Some surgeons prefer to routinely divide the latissimus dorsi insertion in the humerus to increase ptosis of the reconstructive breast mound.

Latissimus dorsi myocutaneous flap reconstruction is a reliable method of breast reconstruction. It can be used alone to reconstruct small breasts or with an implant to reconstruct moderate and some large breasts.

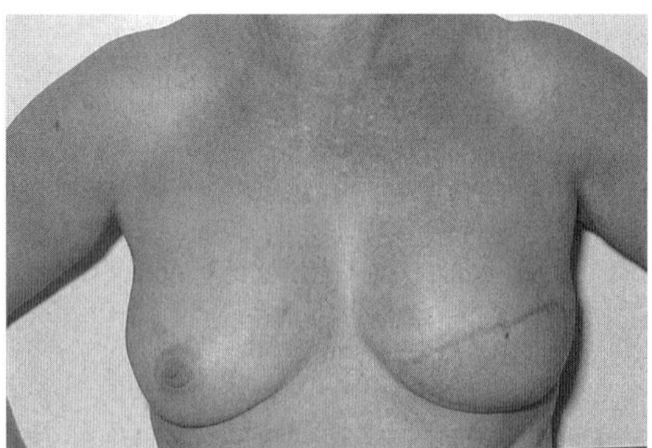

Fig. 2. Final cosmetic result following mastectomy and latissimus dorsi flap reconstruction prior to nipple reconstruction.

7. Transverse rectus abdominis myocutaneous (TRAM) flap

The tissue from the lower abdomen and periumbilical area is supplied in part by perforators from the deep superior epigastric vessels arising from the termination of the internal mammary artery. The other major supply comes from the deep inferior epigastric vessels. The vessels from the deep superior and deep inferior epigastric vessels penetrate the rectus muscle on its deep aspect and travel either as single or duplicated vessels up and down the flap to communicate in the periumbilical region. The skin of the lower abdomen can be kept alive on the perforating branches from the superior or the inferior epigastric vessels. In a pedicled TRAM the skin and subcutaneous tissues are supplied by the deep superior epigastric vessels whereas in a free TRAM flap the deep inferior epigastric vessels are used. A pedicled flap can be based either on a single superior epigastric vessel or on both superior epigastric pedicles. The uni-pedicled TRAM flap can be used when reconstructing a small to moderate sized breast in an unscarred abdomen in a patient with no previous radiation and in somebody who is not overweight. There are four zones recognised over the lower abdomen and only zones 1, 2 and part of 3 have sufficiently reliable blood supply for a unipedicled flap to be used in the new breast reconstruction. Zone four is usually discarded, as is part of zone three. Where there is no skin loss or fat necrosis, then the cosmetic result is excellent.

A bi-pedicled TRAM flap is indicated where a large volume reconstruction is being performed in patients who may have had a previous midline incision or who are smokers, obese or who have had previous radiation to one pedicle. Abdominal wall strength is compromised when compared with uni-pedicled procedures and the bi-pedicled procedure should be performed with caution in young patients.

Free TRAM flaps can be used in any patient with sufficient abdominal pannis but are particularly indicated in whom smoking, large volume requirements, previous radiation therapy and abdominal scars constitute significant risk factors [17]. This procedure is associated with a lower rate of skin necrosis than pedicled procedures but the fat necrosis rate is similar [18,19]. The success of TRAM flaps as a microsurgical technique should be better than 95% for this procedure to be offered as a viable alternative to pedicled TRAM flaps. Muscle and fascial harvest can be minimised by raising a perforator flap on one or two perforators from the deep inferior epigastric vessels, the so-called di-ep flap. The most common site for anastomosis of the deep inferior epigastric vessels is to the thoracodorsal vessels or to the subscapular vessels. The internal mammary vessels can also be utilised.

The transverse rectus abdominis myocutaneous flap provides a very natural feeling breast reconstruction and does not usually require the use of implants. Options include a pedicled flap based on the deep inferior and deep superior epigastric vessels or a free TRAM flap based on the deep inferior epigastric vessels.

8. Other free flaps

Other options for reconstruction include a free flap based on the deep circumflex iliac osteocutaneous artery, the lateral thigh flap based on the transverse branch of the lateral circumflex femoral branch of the profunda femoris artery [20] and a lumbar flap based on the posterior blood supply of the iliac lumbar vessels.

9. Complications

Breast reconstruction techniques are not without complications and some of them are significant. Skin necrosis can occur either as a complication of using thin mastectomy flaps or from pressure necrosis during tissue expansion. Using implants there is the problem of capsular contracture. Around capsular contracture rates vary between 5 and 30% but have been reduced by using textured prostheses. Post-operative radiotherapy significantly increases the rates of capsular contracture. Between 2 and 5% of patients develop infection around the implants which requires the implant to be removed. Patients who develop low grade infection in a prosthesis have a high rate of capsular contracture. Implant fatigue and rupture [21] are a major concern amongst patients who have second generation smooth walled thin-shelled gel implants. About 10–12% of these rupture by 10 years. The newer lower bleed implants have a lower rate of rupture. There is no convincing evidence that leakage of silicone even in patients with complete intracapsular rupture causes problems in other organs [22,23].

The rates of latissimus flap loss should be less than 1%. Seroma formation under the back scar is the most troublesome complication. Visible muscle contractions are rare in innervated flaps but may require late denervation.

TRAM flaps carry significant morbidity. Pedicled TRAM flaps have total loss rates of between 5 and 10%. Risk factors include smoking, obesity, and radiotherapy to the pedicles and multiple abdominal incisions. Skin necrosis is rare with free TRAM flaps but total TRAM flap loss has been reported in between 2 and 6% in most series. Abdominal hernias and bulges occur with a frequency of between 1 and 6%. There is much lower incidence of abdominal problems with de-ep flaps. Deep venous thrombosis and embolism occur with all forms of reconstruction but are rare when adequate prophylaxis is provided.

Complications of implant based reconstruction include implant loss, mastectomy skin loss, infection and capsular contracture. Capsular contracture has been reduced by using textured prostheses. Rates of total loss of myocutaneous flaps should be less than 1% for the latissimus flaps and less than 5% for TRAM flaps.

10. Latissimus dorsi mini-flaps

The first endoscopically harvested latissimus dorsi muscle flap was raised in early 1993 [24] and transferred as a free flap to cover traumatic tissue loss on the leg. The entire muscle can be elevated through a trans-axillary incision using endoscopes or lighted retractors and allows large volumes of breast tissue to be resected and the defect in the breast reconstituted. One of the major oncological objections to this procedure has been insertion of a flap following immediate wide excision without knowledge whether the tumour has been completely excised. For this reason, one option is to perform an initial wide excision to ensure adequate margin clearance and then to follow this a week later by an axillary dissection and latissimus dorsi mini-flap reconstruction. It is possible to excise significant amounts of breast tissue and to reconstruct the breast using the latissimus dorsi muscle with overlying fat (Fig. 3).

11. Oncoplastic surgery

These techniques allow removal of the cancer with a wide margin of surrounding tissue while at the same time reconstructing the breast defect with various forms of creatively fashioned breast pedicles similar to those used for breast reduction surgery [25]. They are particularly useful when re-

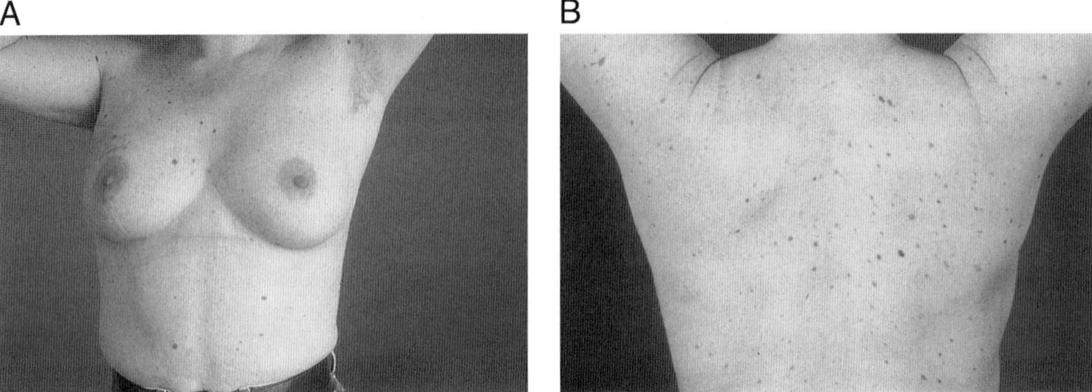

Fig. 3. (a) Anterior and (b) posterior views of a patient having a two stage wide local excision, axillary clearance and latissimus dorsi mini-flap.

constructing medial breast defects following wide excision of medial tumours. When large excision are performed, a contralateral reduction is usually necessary [26]. While innovative and highly successful, these procedures carry the same theoretical objections as one-stage mini-flaps, namely that the breast is reconstituted and reconstructed before histological evidence is obtained of complete excision. The use of oncoplastic procedures in a previously irradiated breast is associated with a high rate of complications and a significant rate of poor cosmetic outcome. Despite these concerns, these techniques have a valuable role in patients with larger breasts.

12. Reconstructing breasts following wide excision

Up to 20% of patients who have wide excisions have poor cosmetic results. This means that the treated breast is not symmetrical with the other breast. Options for achieving symmetry include reducing both breasts or augmenting the size of the treated breast. Although implants can be used, the best results are obtained using myocutaneous flaps. As there is often skin loss as well as tissue loss, it is usually necessary to bring in skin and muscle. Results of a patient following a latissimus dorsi myocutaneous flap reconstruction af-

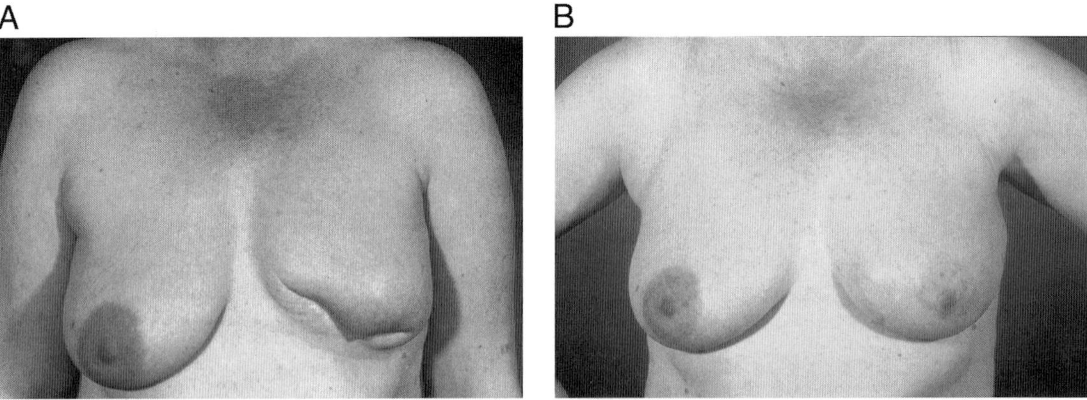

Fig. 4. Patient having a wide local excision with a poor cosmetic result before (a) and after (b) latissimus dorsi flap.

ter breast conservation is shown in Fig. 4a and b [27].

13. Nipple reconstruction

A variety of techniques are available to reconstruct a new nipple/areola complex. The nipple is usually created from skin present on the breast with the areola being created either from transplantation of darker skin from the upper, inner thigh or preferably by tattooing of the skin around the reconstructed nipple. An alternative is to use a stick-on nipple which can be removed and worn by the patient at her will.

References

1. Badellino F et al. The impact of reconstructive surgery in breast cancer. Ann N Y Acad Sci, 1993; 698: 219–226.
2. Clough KB et al. Immediate breast reconstruction by prosthesis: a safe technique for extensive intraductal and microinvasive carcinomas. Ann Surg Oncol, 1996; 3(2): 212–218.
3. Bailey MH et al. Immediate breast reconstruction: reducing the risks [see comments]. Plast Reconstr Surg, 1989; 83(5): 845–851.
4. Khoo A et al. A comparison of resource costs of immediate and delayed breast reconstruction. Plast Reconstr Surg, 1998; 101(4): 964–968.
5. Kroll SS and Marchi M. Immediate reconstruction: current status in cancer management. Tex Med, 1991; 87(9): 67–72.
6. Williams JK et al. TRAM flap breast reconstruction after radiation treatment. Ann Surg, 1995; 221(6): 756–764.
7. Kroll SS et al. Comparison of resource costs between implant-based and TRAM flap breast reconstruction. Plast Reconstr Surg, 1996; 97(2): 364–372.
8. Kroll SS et al. Comparison of resource costs of free and conventional TRAM flap breast reconstruction. Plast Reconstr Surg, 1996; 98(1): 74–77.
9. Francel TJ, Ryan JJ and Manson PN. Breast reconstruction utilizing implants: a local experience and comparison of three techniques. Plast Reconstr Surg, 1993; 92(5): 786–794.
10. Cohen IK and Turner D. Immediate breast reconstruction with tissue expanders. Clin Plast Surg, 1987; 14(3): 491–498.
11. Becker H and Maraist F. Immediate breast reconstruction after mastectomy using a permanent tissue expander. South Med J, 1987; 80(2): 154–160.
12. May JW Jr et al. Smooth versus textured expander implants: a double-blind study of capsule quality and discomfort in simultaneous bilateral breast reconstruction patients [see comments]. Ann Plast Surg, 1994; 32(3): 225–232.
13. Gibney J. The long-term results of tissue expansion for breast reconstruction. Clin Plast Surg, 1987; 14(3): 509–518.
14. Becker H. The permanent tissue expander. Clin Plast Surg, 1987; 14(3): 519–527.
15. De Mey A et al. Late results and current indications of latissimus dorsi breast reconstructions. Br J Plast Surg, 1991; 44(1): 1–4.
16. Hartrampf CR Jr. The transverse abdominal island flap for breast reconstruction. A 7-year experience. Clin Plast Surg, 1988; 15(4): 703–716.
17. Banic A et al. Late results of breast reconstruction with free TRAM flaps: a prospective multicentric study. Plast Reconstr Surg, 1995; 95(7): 1195–1204.
18. Kroll SS et al. Choice of flap and incidence of free flap success. Plast Reconstr Surg, 1996; 98(3): 459–463.
19. Hartrampf CR Jr et al. Ruben's fat pad for breast reconstruction: a peri-iliac soft-tissue free flap [published erratum appears in Plast Reconstr Surg 1995 Jan; 95(1): 217]. Plast Reconstr Surg, 1994; 93(2): 402–407.
20. Elliott LF, Beegle PH and Hartrampf CR Jr. The lateral transverse thigh free flap: an alternative for autogenous-tissue breast reconstruction. Plast Reconstr Surg, 1990; 85(2): 169–178.
21. Brown LS, Silverman BG, Berg WA. Rupture of silicone-gel breast implants: causes, sequelae and diagnosis. Lancet 1997; 350: 1531–1537.
22. Nyren O, Yin L, Josefsson S et al. Risk of connective tissue disease and related disorders among women with breast implants: a nation-wide retrospective cohort study in Sweden. Br Med J 1998; 316: 417–422.
23. Codner MA, Bostwick J, III, Nahi F. Breast reconstruction after mastectomy. The Breast 1995; 4: 4–10.
24. Eaves FF et al. Subcutaneous endoscopic plastic surgery using a retractor mounted endoscopic system. Perspect Plast Surg, 1993; 7(2): 1–22.
25. Petit JY et al. Poor esthetic results after conservative treatment of breast cancer. Techniques of partial breast reconstruction. Ann Chir Plast Esthet, 1989; 34(2): 103–108.
26. Shestak, KC et al. Partial mastectomy and breast reduction as a valuable treatment option for patients with macromastia and carcinoma of the breast. Surg Gynecol Obstet, 1993; 177(1): 54–56.
27. Watson JD, Dixon JM. Breast reconstruction. In: ABC of Breast Diseases. BMJ Publishing Group, London, 2000, 2nd edition, in press.

Breast Cancer: Diagnosis and Management
J.M. Dixon (Ed.)

CHAPTER 27

Tissue expanders and implants

Christopher Khoo

1. Introduction

Adequate postmastectomy reconstruction of the breast requires the restoration of all missing anatomical components. Unless an immediate reconstruction is to be undertaken, and the skin of the breast is intentionally conserved, a "mastectomy" procedure is usually a dermo-mastectomy, so that both the breast mound and the overlying skin envelope must subsequently be recreated.

The simplest way to achieve breast reconstruction is to use an implant to provide the shape and substance of the breast mound. However, aesthetic appearance also depends on having adequate skin cover, which must be sufficient to allow ptosis, the hallmark of the mature breast. It is seldom possible to achieve a satisfactory reconstruction merely by placing an implant under the skin remaining following mastectomy, and additional skin is almost always necessary. Local cutaneous flaps have been used, but only give a thin layer of cover to the implant. Musculocutaneous flaps such as the latissimus dorsi musculocutaneous flap have added soft tissue to cover and protect the implant, and enhance its feel and appearance. This is particularly important with modern textured implants which adhere to soft tissue and as they have surface ripples these may show through a thin flap.

The technique of skin expansion enables the creation of additional skin in the site of the breast. In the same way that the pregnant abdomen is able to stretch to its full-term size, the flat postmastectomy chest wall can be stretched by an implanted skin expander, or an expander-implant, to achieve sufficient skin to accommodate an implant and to achieve breast ptosis.

2. Silicone and breast implants

The gel-filled silicone implant was introduced by Cronin and Gerrow in 1964 [1]. All current implants and expanders are made of a rubber-like "Silicone" elastomer outer envelope containing a filler, which is commonly silicone gel, saline (or a combination of both, in different chambers within the implant). Other fillers have been tried but have yet to establish a place in routine use. The outer shell may be made sufficiently rigid to give the implant a specific shape, and multiple-layer construction is used to minimise "bleeding", or diffusion of tiny amounts of silicone through the shell.

"Silicone" (*polydimethylsiloxane*, PDMS) is a polymer with an average molecular weight of 24,000. It is insoluble in body fluids. Medical grade silicone is widely used in both solid and liquid forms, for a wide range of medical implants, as well as for lubrication (in syringes and intravenous tubing). The cohesiveness and solidity of the different physical forms depends on the extent of

Table 1. The structure of "Silicone" (polydimethylsiloxane, PDMS) (physical cohesiveness depends on the extent of the cross linkage between the PDMS chains, resulting in different forms ranging from fluid and gel, to solid elastomer)

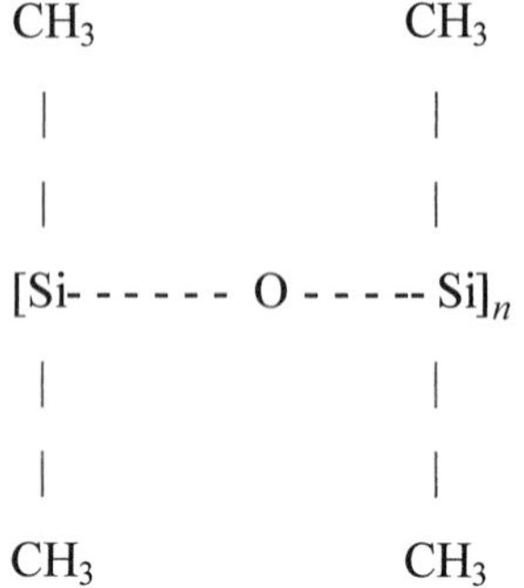

cross linkage between the PDMS chains (Table 1). Silicones are widely encountered in daily life, being present in cosmetics, medications, food processing, and in many domestic applications.

In 1992 the United States Food and Drug Administration (FDA) called for a voluntary moratorium on the use of silicone gel breast implants. A new body, the Independent Expert Advisory Group was established in he United Kingdom to review information on connective tissue disease. It found no evidence of any connection with breast implants [2]. The United Kingdom Independent Review Group (IRG) was set up in 1998 to carry out an extensive scientific review of all available evidence, and concluded that there is no histopathological or conclusive immunological evidence for an abnormal immune response to silicone from breast implants in tissue [3]. Further, there is no epidemiological evidence for a link between silicone gel breast implants and any established connected tissue disease. This view has been consistently supported by a number of large-scale epidemiological studies [4–6].

The IRG concluded, "the overall biological response to silicone is consistent with conventional forms of response to foreign materials". Even though there is no convincing evidence for adverse systemic effects, it is recognised that there may be local effects related to the presence of the implant as a foreign body within living tissue. These complications include the formation of capsular contracture, infection, gel bleeding and implant rupture. If gel were to leak from an implant there might not be any perceptible difference in the shape of the breast because the gel would be most likely to remain within the fibrous capsule. At a later stage, firmness may develop in the reconstructed breast.

The decision to use a silicone implant to achieve a breast reconstruction should be discussed fully with the patient when surgery is being planned, so that appropriate counselling can be given.

> *Silicone breast implants have been subjected to a number of scientific investigations and have not been found to be associated with any connective tissue or other systemic disease.*

3. Reconstructive options with implants and expanders

The techniques of implant and expander reconstruction are appropriate to both immediate and delayed reconstruction. The reconstruction may be undertaken as a one-stage or two-stage procedure. It is relatively unusual to be able to achieve a one-stage reconstruction with an implant alone, though it may be possible when matching a small, contralateral breast with good supple skin. It is more usual to need additional soft tissue cover.

Two-stage reconstruction is undertaken by means of a first-stage placement of a skin expander, and substitution with a definitive implant at a second stage. As an alternative to this, reconstruction may be achieved with a "permanent-expander", or adjustable implant. The expander/implant when inserted remains as the permanent breast prosthesis. With some designs, a second minor operation is needed to remove the valve, though with other designs the valve is integrated into the wall of the device. All expanders and expander-implants incorporate an injection port/valve. It is located either by palpation, or by means of a magnetic location device, and needled percutaneously so that saline can be introduced or removed to alter the volume of the expander.

Whist the concept of a single-stage reconstruction is attractive, there are few implant reconstructions which do not benefit from a subsequent adjustment. A second operative procedure allows the surgeon to refine the reconstruction, and improve the final result. Even when an adequate breast mound is achieved in one surgical stage, the shape and volume of the reconstructed breast may still need to be adjusted, and a nipple and areolar reconstruction undertaken.

A further *contralateral* operation may be needed to achieve symmetry matching the normal breast to the reconstructed side, by means of a mastopexy, reduction, or an augmentation on the opposite side.

4. Implant-only reconstruction in a single stage

This is only appropriate in small-breasted patients with minimal ptosis. If immediate reconstruction is to be undertaken, skin flaps can be preserved for immediate use. The implant should be placed under muscle as far as possible. Jackson and van Heerden [7] point out that a large enough submuscular pocket can only be created if the pocket also extends under the fascia of serratus anterior. Access to the pocket is either through a muscle splitting incision in pectoralis major, or between pectoralis and serratus. Fascial integrity may be compromised by the mastectomy dissection, and muscle fascia tears should be repaired because of the risk of herniation of the implant. If direct repair is not possible, local fascial or myofascial flaps may be used.

If it is not possible to place the implant in a complete submuscular pocket, it may be acceptable to release the lower part of the sternal insertion of the pectoralis major muscle, so that it is free to lie over the implant without causing flattening or compression. This means that part of the implant does not have the benefit of complete muscle cover. As an alternative, it may be decided to place a skin expander in the muscle pocket, which can be then be closed without tension. The inflation may be undertaken after initial healing has occurred.

Delayed implant reconstruction carries fewer concerns than immediate reconstruction. Tissues are well healed, and the muscle, fascia and skin flaps have a more robust blood supply. A shaped "anatomical implant" may give a better match in this situation, in the absence of excess skin to generate ptosis; so the reconstructed breast will take its shape from the implant.

The infra-mammary crease should be placed at the same level as the existing crease, to maintain symmetry with the opposite side. Should volume symmetry not be achieved, because a large enough implant cannot be inserted, it may be necessary either to insert a larger implant at a later stage when some soft tissue stretching has occurred, or to consider a contralateral reduction mammaplasty. In immediate reconstruction, an implant is commonly used with a musculocutaneous flap, to avoid the problems associated with tension in the soft tissue layers from direct wound closure, and to bring in additional soft tissue to achieve aesthetic ptosis.

> *Implants alone rarely give a satisfactory cosmetic result in breast reconstruction.*

5. Soft tissue expansion

Living tissue responds to mechanical deformation. The skin and soft tissues of the body stretch to accommodate growth, or physiologically enlargement. The stretching can be rapid, as in the swelling associated with acute inflammation. The first clinical soft tissue skin expansion was undertaken in 1956 by Neumann [8], who stretched an area of scalp using a home-made device in order to reconstruct a traumatic ear defect.

The precedent already existed in aesthetic breast surgery, where initially, the saline inflatable breast prosthesis, and later the double lumen saline/gel breast prosthesis were in use for augmentation mammaplasty. These implants were used for breast enlargement, being placed in an existing skin pocket to achieve an immediate increase in size by taking advantage of laxity in the skin, which was already present through ageing or physiological stretching.

In 1976, Radovan described the inflatable skin expander for reconstructive surgery [9]. He subsequently applied the concept to breast reconstruction [10] where the area of skin deficiency was intentionally stretched to create the fullness and form of a breast, in order to accommodate a prosthesis to restore the entire breast volume.

Apart from the simplicity of the operative procedure, there are local advantages associated with skin expander reconstruction of the breast. Uniquely, no additional scarring is created, either on the chest wall (as part of the mastectomy scar can be reopened for access), or in a donor site elsewhere. The reconstruction is achieved using local skin which has the best possible colour and texture match, and with preservation of cutaneous sensation.

An adequate thickness of soft tissue is important during skin expansion: the expander should be placed in a submuscular plane. The overlying soft tissue is thinned by the expansion process, and muscle gives additional soft tissue thickness and protection for the implant, whilst allowing better tolerance of inflation pressures.

Submuscular expanders provide a simple method of breast reconstruction with minimal scarring and can produce a match for small and medium breasts which have minimal ptosis.

6. Reconstruction with a tissue expander, followed by an implant

A skin expander may be placed at the time of mastectomy or as a delayed procedure. The diameter of the expander should match the width of the breast. "Anatomical", shaped expanders with differential lower pole fullness (as opposed to round expanders) may be chosen to give more expansion inferiorly. These are thinner superiorly, and are fuller below, the shape resembling a pear sliced in half vertically. Total muscle cover is preferred, and if the expander is placed at the time of mastectomy, inflation is undertaken progressively in order not to disrupt the surgical wound. The viability of the overlying flaps is crucial, and complications such as haematoma, infection or ischaemia of the wound edges must be actively managed to allow expansion to progress safely.

Current breast expanders, and implants, have a textured surface. This helps to fix the surface of the device in position against the soft tissues to prevent movement. Surface texturing also reduces capsular contracture during the expansion phase. The nature of the texturing varies between manufacturing processes: in some implants the adhesion between the outer surface of the implant and the soft tissue is such that the two surfaces are closely attached and only come apart with some force, rather like peeling apart the two surfaces of a Velcro fastening. This degree of adhesion will transmit visible rippling to the surface contour of the implant through an overlying skin flap, particularly if the implant contains low-viscosity filler, such as saline.

Expansion needs to continue until the reconstructed breast achieves slightly more fullness and projection than the contralateral breast, so that there is enough skin to accommodate the final prosthesis. When adequate size and shape are achieved, an "exchange" procedure is performed to remove the expander and insert the permanent prosthesis.

At the time of exchange, the level of the infra- mammary crease can be adjusted to equalise it with that on the contralateral side. Buried non-absorbable sutures are inserted between the chest wall (as far deeply as the rib periosteum), and the inner surface of the expanded skin flap, if necessary taking bites of the dermis for secure fixation.

> *Two stage reconstructions where tissue expanders are replaced by implants allow important adjustments which help achieve symmetry and allow the formation of a definite inframammary crease.*

7. The "Permanent Expander" concept

Skin expansion was initially thought of as being a temporary process, at the conclusion of which the skin expander was removed and discarded in favour of a permanent implant. However, in 1984, Sasaki [11] described the prolonged implantation of a skin expander for serial expansion in the treatment of breast hypoplasia in a growing child with Poland's syndrome. The device was gradually expanded over a period of years to match growth on the normal side.

Becker in 1984 [12] introduced the concept of the 'Permanent expander/prosthesis'. The expansion device was intended to be left in place as a permanent prosthesis. He described a double lumen device, which acted initially as a skin expander, and then could be adjusted to the desired final volume, by the addition or removal of saline via the implanted valve.

Subsequent concerns relating to silicone gel prompted the development of single lumen expander prosthesis. The outer gel chamber had been intentionally introduced to facilitate valve closure, improve the feel of the implant and to decrease the chances of failure of the shell of the implant due to creasing and rupture of the envelope. The single chamber saline-only device gives a similar final result to the use of a saline filled prosthesis, without the benefit of the added weight and texture of the gel.

> *Permanent expander/prostheses devices are now available for a one stage tissue expansion and following deflation they then become permanent prostheses.*

8. The creation of ptosis during expansion reconstruction

There are two different philosophies regarding the extent of expansion needed to gain a satisfactory aesthetic appearance. On the one hand the use of a shaped "anatomical" expander, and substitution with an exactly matched, shaped "anatomical" prosthesis, requires the exact stretching of soft tissue to precisely accommodate the specific implant. The shape of the expander, and the prosthesis, gives the final form of the reconstructed breast. This depends on the manufactured shape of the implant, which has a sufficient degree of firmness to maintain its form and contour, and therefore, the shape of the reconstructed breast.

An alternative view is that ptosis is best simulated by creating skin excess, so that the implant sits in a larger pocket than its exact diameter. The implant is free to move within this loose skin pocket, simulating the behaviour of normal breast during changes of posture. This can be regarded as a "dynamic ptosis" as the reconstructed breast is capable of movement in relation to the chest wall, with the breast mound being able to respond to gravity in a natural manner. Over-expansion is necessary to generate adequate skin cover over the implant to achieve this form of ptosis.

A common criticism of skin expansion reconstructions is that ptosis is not achieved, and that the reconstruction does not look natural. This situation arises most commonly when a round implant has been used, and there is insufficient skin to allow movement of the implant on the chest wall in response to gravity.

During over expansion, the expander or the expander-implant enlarges spherically, but because of resistance against the chest wall the expansion is most prominent circumferentially, and outwards against the skin. At this stage, the expander-implant appears to be too large, and in the wrong position. Over a period of months however, the soft tissues soften and stretch, creating drooping, in response to gravity.

Excess saline is now removed from the implant, and subsequently, some degree of soft tissue tightening, or contracture occurs in the lax capsule around the implant. The base circumference of the implant (its "footprint" against the chest wall) reduces, so that the inferior margin of the pocket rises slightly. As the skin envelope is attached to the chest wall at the inferior pole of the breast, this slight contracture is sufficient to create an infra- mammary crease, and to give the appearance of ptosis.

The principle of over-expansion in order to create ptosis has also been proven in aesthetic surgical practice. Persoff [13] found that over expansion during cosmetic augmentation mammaplasty was effective in enhancing ptosis, and creating a more aesthetic appearance when larger volume augmentation was being undertaken. Overexpansion has also been found to decrease pain and shorten the duration of expander placement under skin flaps [14].

A temporary "Stove-in" rib deformity is seen after the over-inflated implant is reduced in size, and is visible as a slight para-sternal depression. This will correct spontaneously, and within a short period of time as normal lung expansion pushes the ribs out to a normal position. However, hollowing may be permanent after ill-advised attempts to carry out expansion in patients who have received chest wall irradiation.

Some degree of ptosis can be achieved with tissue expansion using either shaped expanders or by over-expansion.

9. The choice of implant or expander: correct size and volume

The final size of the reconstructed breast should match not only the volume but also contour of the remaining breast. The implant or expander must therefore be chosen to allow this final symmetry to be achieved. It must also be decided how ptosis will be achieved-whether by means of a contoured implant, or through overexpansion. If reconstruction is to be undertaken at the time of mastectomy, the final size of implant will match the amount of tissue resected, provided that the size of the opposite breast is satisfactory. Some patients may wish to take the opportunity to have the opposite breast adjusted, either by a reduction or augmentation, and the implant or expander should be chosen with this in mind.

When the patient presents for delayed reconstruction it is helpful to note the bra size, and to see whether the external prosthesis (if one is being worn) achieves good symmetry in the bra. The volume of the external prosthesis gives a good guide to the size of the implant expander, which will be needed.

The surgeon needs to assess the approximate weight of the opposite breast. This estimation is initially difficult, but with experience it becomes reliable. The weight of the breast may be available at the time of mastectomy when it is usually weighed. The patient can also be asked to help with volume matching, even if an external prosthesis is not available. Wearing the normal bra, and guided by the surgeon's estimate, the patient inserts sizing prostheses or plastic bags filled with increasing volumes of water until a good match is obtained.

In addition to volume, it is important to be aware of the dimensions of the breast to be matched. The base width of the chosen implant has to be as close to the width of the remaining breast as possible. An implant reconstruction will not look natural if too small a device has been chosen so that its base width is much less than the normal breast. It is much better to choose a larger implant and to under-fill it to achieve this.

The base width and projection are especially important when a contoured, "anatomical" implant is to be used. Careful measurement (rather than volume assessment) is used as the basis for implant selection using the Biodimensional system, as described by Maxwell [15,16]. In this system, the base width and the height are measured with calipers, noting the normal projection of the lateral part of the breast over the anterior axillary fold. A template is used to choose the appropriately sized implant and to help to position the inframammary fold. The choice of expander and subsequent implant are therefore fixed prior to surgery.

When other expanders or "permanent-expanders" are being used, one final technical manoeuvre may be used intra-operatively. Whilst the surgeon may have a estimated the final breast volume preoperatively, he should fill the surgical pocket at the time of dissection either using a silicone sizer of known volume, or using moist swabs.

The volume of a single swab can be simply assessed by putting it into the barrel of a large volume syringe (e.g. a standard 60 ml syringe). The swab is pushed down under moderate pressure into the bottom of the syringe, and the volume it occupies can be easily determined. It follows that if ten swabs of approximately 50 cm^3 volume each are inserted into the pocket and can be moulded into a reasonable shape to match the other breast, an implant of 500 ml final notional volume can be confidently selected.

> *There are a number of different methods available to assess the volume of the implant which will give the best volume match. The shape and base width of the implant also needs to be selected carefully.*

10. "Permanent-Expander" breast reconstruction

10.1. Description of a typical device

A typical "Permanent-Expander" device has a double lumen, with an internal saline-filled chamber and outer gel-filled chamber and a rough textured surface. The valve tube passes through the silicone gel, and into the inner chamber where it runs through a 'pig-tail' self sealing valve: the outer envelope gel surrounds and cushions the inner saline chamber (an important factor during over-inflation), and also acts as sealant.

The low-bleed multi-laminated silicone envelope protects against gel bleeding during the high pressures generated during over-expansion. Single chamber saline-only and 50 : 50 gel–saline devices are also available, but have disadvantages of "feel" (saline alone implants do not feel as good), and the ability to over expand (50 : 50 implants do not allow much over expansion).

Contoured or "anatomical" devices are available, and the surgeon needs to decide which device is to be used for reconstruction, as this will affect the postoperative management of the expander volume, and also the need for temporary overexpansion.

10.2. Indications

Indications for breast reconstruction using a "Permanent Expander" are similar to those for a two stage expander/implant reconstruction, and include the following.

(1) Unilateral or bilateral postmastectomy reconstruction: which may be immediate, or delayed.
(2) Salvage surgery following previously unsuccessful postmastectomy subcutaneous implant reconstruction (after extrusion, contracture, or infection). The permanent expander is placed in the submuscular surgical plane, and expansion reconstruction is begun when the overlying skin wound and tissues have healed sufficiently to tolerate expansion.
(3) In some patients, contralateral augmentation mammaplasty is requested following ipsilateral breast reconstruction. The placement of a second device on the opposite side for a cosmetic augmentation enables symmetry to be achieved with enhancement of volume on both sides. The use of an expander implant for contralateral augmentation allows for continuous variation in volume so that the contralateral side can stay in balance during the evolving expansion reconstruction (Fig. 1).

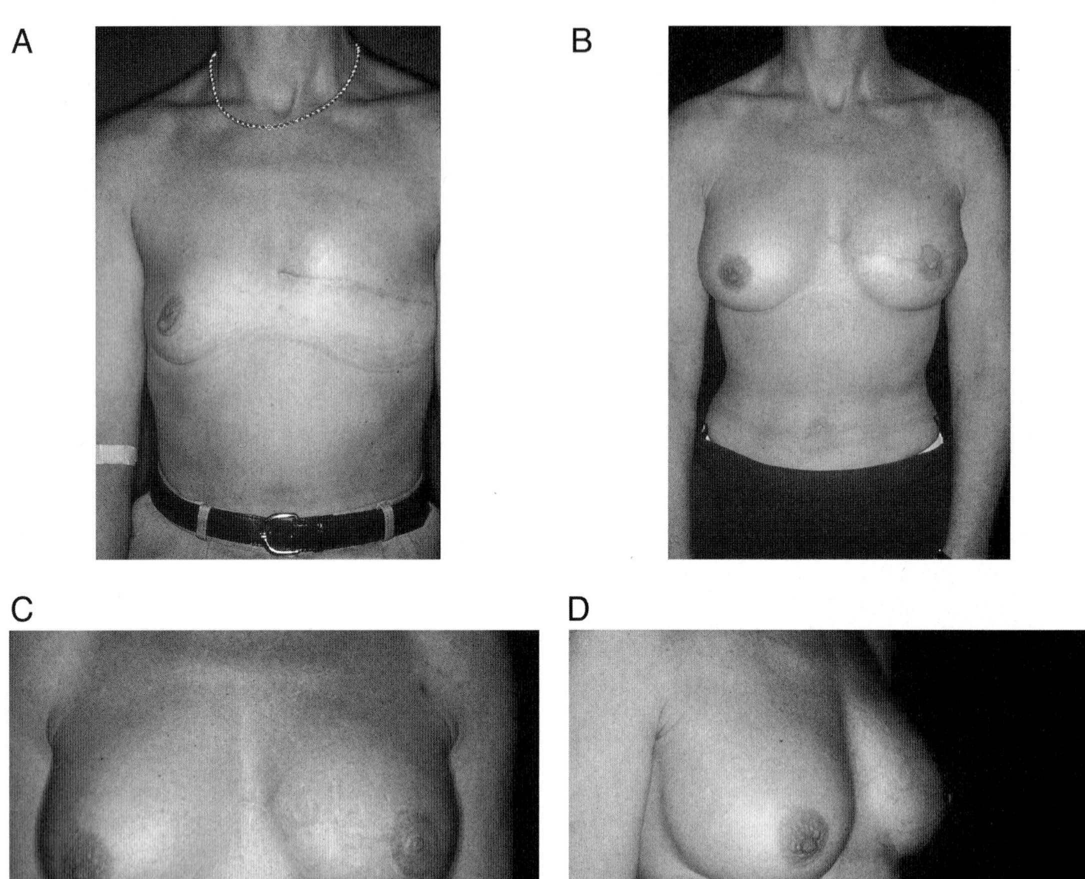

Fig. 1. *Patient 1.* (a) Pre-reconstruction. (b) Post-reconstruction and contralateral augmentation. (c) Close-up view postoperatively. (d) Profile view postoperatively to show profile of reconstructed breast.

(4) Subcutaneous mastectomy can be combined with immediate reconstruction, and the procedure may be undertaken bilaterally with the promise of good symmetry (Fig. 2).

10.3. Contraindications

These are absolute and relative. The presence of a physical problem on the chest wall, which mitigates against eventual success (e.g. the presence of radionecrosis), is a significant and absolute contraindication.

Recent, or active infections elsewhere in the body are significant factors because of the risk of metastatic infection to the implant. Implant reconstruction should be delayed until the infection has been eliminated. Implant reconstruction is usually undertaken under systemic antibiotic cover, and with additional local antiseptic application (e.g. with aqueous povidone iodine irrigation of the implant cavity).

It is also important to ensure that the patient has a full understanding of the expansion process, emphasising that there will inevitably be a wait over a period of months waiting for skin stretching to occur. Patients who are unable to accept the

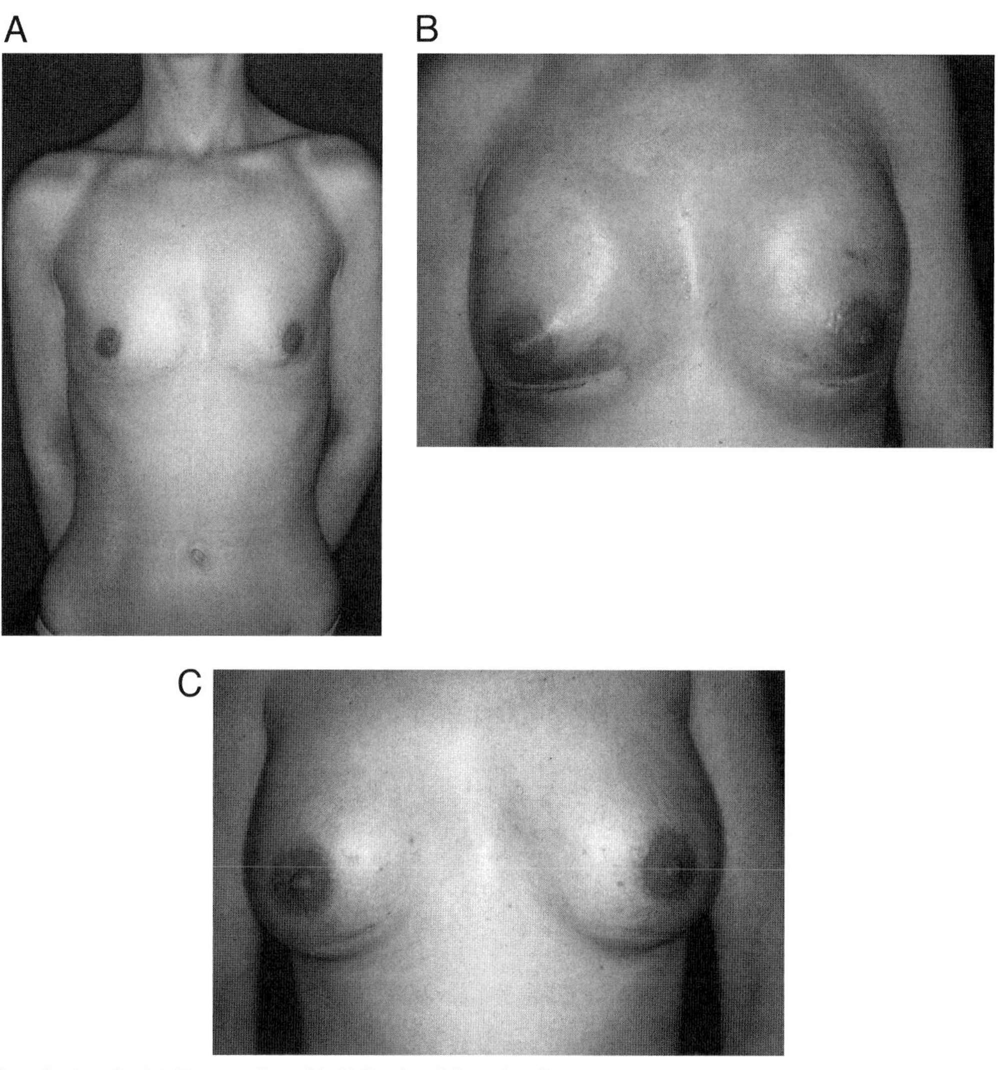

Fig. 2. *Patient 2.* (a) Preoperative. (b) Following bilateral subcutaneous mastectomy — overexpansion. (c) Bilateral augmentation/reconstruction at 10 years.

concept of discomfort, or the extended duration of surgical treatment are not good candidates for skin expansion reconstruction.

10.4. Skin expansion following radiotherapy

There is much controversy surrounding skin expansion reconstruction in patients who have undergone irradiation. In general, irradiated tissues respond poorly to skin expansion and autogenous tissue reconstruction is preferred. The muscle and skin will usually become tight and unyielding, and the underlying costo-chondral junctions may have softened, especially when the internal thoracic chain has been targeted. Any attempt to expand the overlying skin will push the ribs inwards, causing a permanent "stove-in" chest deformity, and with little gain in outward contour. Exceptionally, and only in carefully selected patients with adequate, supple skin, postmastectomy

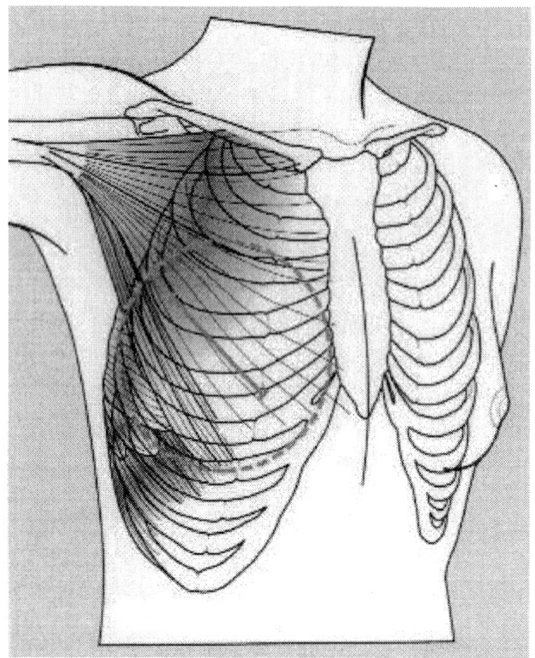

Fig. 3. Surface markings of subpectoral pocket.

reconstruction has been achieved following irradiation using a permanent expander. Techniques involving local flaps have been described by several authors [17–19] and may be used to achieve implant reconstruction in irradiated patients.

> *Tissue expansion following chest wall radiotherapy rarely achieves a satisfactory outcome.*

10.5. Operative technique: expander and implant reconstruction

The surgical techniques for creation of a submuscular pocket for insertion of an initial expander (in a two-stage reconstruction), or a permanent-expander, are essentially similar. Immediate and delayed reconstructions with implants and expanders are also similar, except that the expansion regime in immediate reconstructions is of necessity much slower, whilst for delayed reconstruction a much more rapid expansion is possible.

10.5.1. Surgical approach

The device is inserted into a complete submuscular envelope, access being gained through a small skin incision (usually through the original mastectomy scar so that no fresh scars are created). Dissection is undertaken under the skin flaps to expose a small area of underlying muscle surface. There is usually residual scarring, and any excessive fibrous tissue in the original plane of the dissection is excised to facilitate expansion of the prosthesis and to allow the muscle layer to stretch. It is best to avoid directly overlapping skin and muscle incisions (Fig. 3).

10.5.2. Creation of a complete submuscular pocket

After initial muscle splitting along the line of the fibres, the submuscular plane is developed by blunt fingertip dissection and with the aid of a blunt dissecting instrument, dissection (e.g. with a Hegar's gynaecological dilator), or under direct vision with diathermy and scissors. Superiorly, the submuscular pocket extends under pectoralis major to the level of the clavicle. Medially it is limited by the sternal attachment of the muscle. Inferiorly the pocket extends beyond the normal border of pectoralis, passing under the fascia and continuing under the anterior rectus sheath. The muscle fibres inserting onto the fifth rib are divided under direct vision, and by sharp dissection.

10.5.3. Positioning of device and valve on chest wall

The device must be placed *lower* than the normal position of the inframammary crease, usually by 2–3 cm. This is to facilitate the final correct positioning of the inframammary crease, following over-expansion. If the device has a remote valve connected by tubing, the valve is placed in an adjacent superficial subcutaneous pocket and secured to prevent it rotating or retracting (Fig. 4).

10.5.4. Expansion regime

Immediate expansion to the largest possible volume is desirable: multiple low-volume injec-

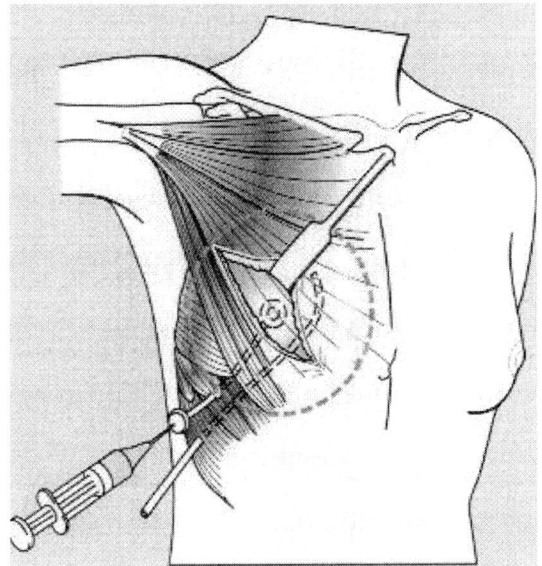

Fig. 4. Subpectoral positioning of partially inflated expander before wound closure.

tion expansion achieves volume expansion more slowly, and causes more discomfort. In delayed reconstruction, 80%–90% of the desired over expanded final volume is inserted immediately, with provision being made for adequate analgesia postoperatively, ideally using a PCA pump.

The end point of on-table expansion is visible blanching in the skin flap. The inflation tolerances of permanent-expander prostheses are wide: volumes of +200% of the eventual volume can be inserted, with no loss of elasticity of the silicone envelope. When reconstruction is undertaken at the time of mastectomy, expansion volumes need to increase much more cautiously for fear of disrupting the wound.

10.5.5. Postoperative management

Outpatient inflation injections, if necessary, are straightforward. Over-expansion is important for the creation of ptosis, and adequate skin stretching may reduce the incidence of capsular contracture. Skin and muscle stretching occurs rapidly, and sequential expansions may be undertaken within a few days for further volume increase. Over-expansion is maintained (depending on skin elasticity) for 3–6 months, and the implant is then deflated to final size, achieving ptosis when the implant lies within a lax soft tissue envelope.

10.5.6. Secondary surgery

A contralateral reduction mammaplasty (Fig. 5), or mastopexy, may be performed as a second stage, although this can also be done at the same time as the mastopexy. To complete the reconstruction a nipple/areola is created and any valve, if present, removed. This final procedure may be carried out under local anaesthetic.

A

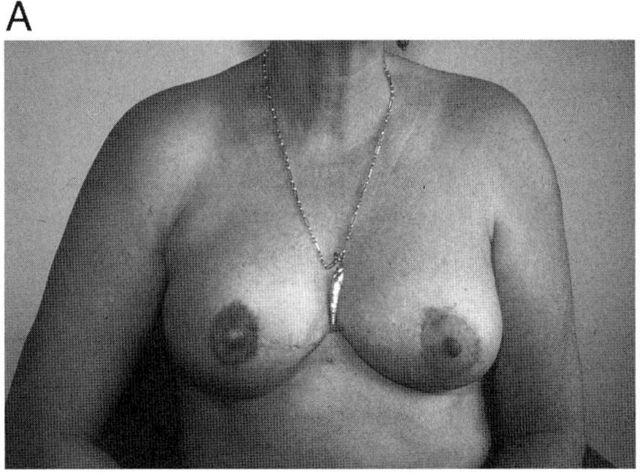

B

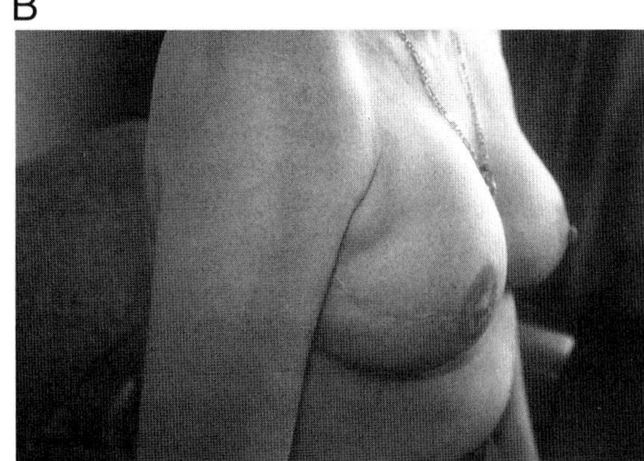

Fig. 5. *Patient 3.* (a) Postoperative result. right reconstruction with nipple and areolar reconstruction and left reduction. (b) Postoperative view to show profile of reconstructed breast.

10.6. Complications

10.6.1. Technical problems and complications of expanders and implants

Complications may arise from faulty surgical technique, incorrect management of expansion, and rarely, through technical failure of an implant device. Problems will be compounded by failure to detect and manage complications at an early stage, as subsequent development of wound dehiscence, infection and implant extrusion are usually beyond salvage.

10.6.2. Capsular contracture

This is due either to a pocket which is too small, the choice of a prosthesis which is too small, or a delay in beginning or progressing expansion. The recruitment of tissue during expansion depends on stretching soft tissues over a wide area. An implant which is too small (i.e. with too-narrow a base diameter), which is sitting in a very small pocket, may not allow adequate soft tissue recruitment because the initial area in contact with the expander is smaller than ideal.

If the commencement of expansion has been delayed, capsular contracture may have occurred so that there may be difficulty in generating adequate pressure to overcome fibrosis. This is a particular problem with immediate reconstruction, when the surgeon may be concerned that inflation will cause disruption of the wound. The problem may be compounded by other causes of fibrosis: for example, following irradiation.

Should irradiation be necessary, it is preferable for this to be administered once the expander/implant has been sufficiently overexpanded. Markings for radiotherapy are made when the overexpanded volume is achieved. This is then maintained after the course of radiotherapy treatments until the tightness in the soft tissue has reduced with resolution of the initial post-irradiation reaction. The incidence of capsular contracture is higher than in the non-irradiated reconstruction.

> *If giving chest wall radiotherapy following expander insertion, achieve full expansion if possible prior to the radiotherapy.*

10.6.3. The correction of capsular contracture

Established capsular contracture is difficult to manage and cannot be overcome by over-expansion alone. Recent experience suggests that a possible solution is the repositioning of the implant in a fresh tissue pocket anterior to the fibrous capsule. An extra-capsular dissection is undertaken over the anterior surface of the encapsulated implant, and when an adequate space has been created under soft tissue, the implant is repositioned in a fresh tissue plane. This is usually above muscle, and under a relatively thin skin flap.

There is reduced soft tissue thickness overlying the implant, but this will often remain soft, allowing correction of capsular contracture. However, there is less soft tissue thickness overlying the implant, with reduced protection, so that rippling in the implant shell can sometimes be seen through the flap. The capsule can be excised and another implant inserted or the capsule is incised and extended (capsulotomy). Both these techniques are sometimes successful at correcting capsular contracture.

10.7. Infection

Early postoperative infection is less common in delayed reconstructions. Antibiotic prophylaxis should be considered, together with topical antiseptic application (e.g. povidone iodine powder spray) to the wound cavity and the skin edges when implants or expanders are inserted. *Staphylococcus epidermidis* is an opportunistic agent which may be transferred into the cavity from the patient's skin, and is responsible for prolonged serous exudation around the implant and a persistent low grade infection. However, with *S. epidermidis* (or coagulase negative staphylococcus) implant salvage is possible, whereas infections with *S. aureus* always necessitate removal of the implant [20].

Infection in the postoperative period will also occur when there is dehiscence in the surgical wound, even when this is of very minor degree. Skin pathogens, and especially *S. epidermidis* gain entry and can reach the implant itself if there is any discontinuity in the underlying muscle layer. Delayed infections may be metastatic, when there is a focus of infection elsewhere in the body.

Minor degrees of infection will sometimes respond to conservative management. A small bore drain can be inserted into the fluid collection under imaging control, allowing the aspiration of fluid for culture and sensitivities, and the instillation of antibiotics. As the agent is most commonly a *Staphylococcus*, a bolus dose of a potent anti-staphylococcal antibiotic such as flucloxacillin, or teicoplanin can be administered in conjunction with systemic antibiotic treatment. In most cases however, the presence of infection requires removal of the implant or expander. The presence of frank pus indicates a *S. aureus* infection. The cavity may need to be packed with iodine soaked swabs, and left to heal by secondary intention. If the exudate is serous, the implant is retrieved, and may be replaced following thorough cleansing of the cavity and implant. The space around the implant is irrigated with antibiotics.

10.8. Valve-related complications

These are seen in implants with a remote valve. Observed complications have included the following.

- Movement of the valve if the subcutaneous pocket is too large to retain the valve in position (including valve rotation or twisting).
- Local chest wall discomfort from inappropriate siting of the valve causing rubbing against the inner arm, or chafing against clothing (e.g. bra straps).
- If the valve is sited too high in the axilla, it may be difficulty in to palpate or to needle. Should the needle inadvertently puncture or cut the valve tubing, a slow leak may occur, leading to deflation of the implant.

Common complications of using breast implants include capsular contracture. Infection, valve related problems and a poor aesthetic result.

10.9. Technical faults

The position of the device may be aesthetically unsatisfactory if placed too high or too lateral. This is commonly due to the submuscular pocket being too small, or the implant being positioned too high on the chest wall. Problems with exposure may also arise when the implant is placed in an unfavourable surgical plane (e.g. under a soft tissue flap which is too thin, rather than in a submuscular pocket).

References

1. Cronin T, Gerow F. Augmentation mammoplasty: a new ‘natural feel’ prosthesis. In Broadbent TR (ed) Transactions Of The Third International Congress Of Plastic Surgery. Amsterdam, Excerpta Medica Foundation 1964.
2. Tinkler JJB, Campbell HJ, Senior JM, Ludgate SM. Evidence For An Association Between The Implantation Of Silicones And Connective Tissue Disease. UK Department of Health, Medical Devices Directorate 1993.
3. Silicone Gel Breast Implants. Report of The Independent Review Group 1998.
4. Deapen DM, Pike PHMC, Casagrande JT, Brody GS The relationship between breast cancer and augmentation mammaplasty: an epidemiologic study. Plastic and Reconstructive Surgery 1986; 77: 361.
5. Nyren O, Yin L, Josefsson S, et al. Risk of connective tissue disease and related disorders among women with breast implants: a nation-wide retrospective cohort study in Sweden. British Medical Journal 1988; 316: 417.
6. Janowsky EC, Kupper LL, Hulka BF Meta-analyses of the relation between Silicone Breast Implants and the risk of Connective Tissue Diseases. New England Journal of Medicine 2000; 342: 781–790.
7. Jackson IT, van Heerden JA. Modified Radical Mas-

tectomy with Immediate Reconstruction versus Conservative Surgery with Radiation Therapy. In Bohmert HH, Leis HP, Jackson IT ed, Breast Cancer, Conservative and Reconstructive Surgery. Georg Thieme Verlag, Stuttgart, p. 135, 1989.

8. Neumann CG. The expansion of an area of skin by progressive distention of a subcutaneous balloon. Plastic and Reconstructive Surgery 1957 19: 124.
9. Radovan C. Adjacent Flap Development Using Expandable Silastic Implants. *Presented at* The American Society of Plastic and Reconstructive Surgery Surgical Forum Boston Massachusetts September 30th 1976.
10. Radovan C. Breast Reconstruction After Mastectomy Using The Temporary Expander. Plastic and Reconstructive Surgery 1982; 69: 195.
11. Sasaki GH. Presented at The Symposium On Tissue Expansion In Reconstructive Surgery, Radcliffe Infirmary, Oxford, February 11th 1984.
12. Becker H. Breast reconstruction using an inflatable breast implant with detachable reservoir. Plastic and Reconstructive Surgery 1984; 73: 678.
13. Persoff MH. Expansion augmentation of the breast. Plastic and Reconstructive Surgery 1993; 91: 393.
14. Isahira Y, Maruyama Y. Combined tissue expansion: Clinical attempt to decrease pain and shorten placement time. Plastic and Reconstructive Surgery 1993; 92: 1052.
15. Maxwell GP. Two stage breast reconstruction using Biospan textured surface skin expanders. McGhan Medical Corporation 1990.
16. Maxwell GP, Spear SL. Two stage breast reconstruction using the saline Biodimensional system. McGhan Medical Corporation 1994.
17. Höhler H, Lemperle G. Der Wideraufbau der weiblichen Brust nach radikaler Mastektomie. Langenbecks Arch Klin Chir 1975; 339: 756.
18. Ryan JJ. A lower thoracic advancement flap in breast reconstruction after mastectomy. Plastic and Reconstructive Surgery 1982; 70: 153.
19. Bohmert H, Gabka CJ. Creation of ptosis with an abdominal advancement flap. In Bohmert H and Gabka CJ, ed, Plastic and Reconstructive Surgery of the Breast. Georg Thieme, Stuttgart, pp. 170–177, 1997.
20. Wong PTL, Nield DV, Khoo CTK. The pathogenicity of coagulase negative staphylococcus in the presence of silicone rubber implants. British Journal of Plastic Surgery 1987; 40: 94.

Breast Cancer: Diagnosis and Management
J.M. Dixon (Ed.)

CHAPTER 28

Latissimus dorsi flap

R.M. Rainsbury

1. Introduction

Latissimus dorsi (LD) breast reconstruction (BR) combines the principles of prosthetic and myocutaneous flap reconstruction in a technique which has stood the test of time. First described by Tanzini in 1896 [1] and rediscovered by Muhlbauer in 1977 [2], LD flaps have been used widely for reconstruction in different anatomical sites. When using LD for breast reconstruction, the advantages of tissue expansion including simplicity, choice and adjustability are coupled with the life-like shape, appearance and consistency which can be achieved with myocutaneous flaps. Moreover thoughtful selection of an expander or implant and careful positioning of the LD flap will ensure that the reconstructed breast is ptotic, with a naturally convex inferior pole.

With careful patient selection, it is possible to achieve some of these features using subpectoral tissue expansion alone. Ptosis is however much easier to achieve with LD reconstruction, and the reconstructed breast tends to age with the patient. These features, coupled with the reliability, durability, and adaptability of LD flaps, accounts for their popularity. Case selection is all important, and LD reconstruction is often the most appropriate procedure for those patients who want to avoid the more significant complications of other techniques. These include the risks of donor site morbidity and flap failure associated with Transverse Rectus Abdominis Myocutaneous (TRAM)-flaps [3], and the relatively high complication rates associated with subpectoral tissue expansion [4].

LD breast reconstruction combines the advantages of tissue expansion with the aesthetic qualities of myocutaneous flaps.

2. Indications for LD reconstruction

The versatility of LD flaps has established their role in three main areas of reconstructive surgery:

- immediate reconstruction
- delayed reconstruction
- salvage procedures

2.1. Immediate reconstruction

The ability to achieve life-like breast replacement at the time of mastectomy is a major feature of LD reconstruction. Combined with tissue expansion, it is often possible to reproduce a facsimile of the native breast with little need for subsequent adjustment. The ugly "patch" effect of donor skin in the reconstructed breast mound can now be minimised by performing skin-sparing mastectomy (SSM), which reduces the size of the skin paddle to that of the areola. Subsequent nipple reconstruction, based on this "neoareola" conceals the scar completely [5,6].

Life-like breast replacement can be achieved by LD reconstruction at the time of conventional or skin-sparing mastectomy.

Immediate LD reconstruction is especially useful in those situations where subpectoral reconstruction produces sub-optimal results. These include reconstruction in patients with large ptotic breasts, and in those requiring postoperative radiotherapy. Conversely, in those patients with small breasts and sufficient soft tissue bulk, implants can be avoided by using the increasingly popular autogenous LD techniques [7]. Reconstruction of resection defects resulting from partial mastectomy with myosubcutaneous or myocutaneous LD flaps is another recent development in breast surgery [8,9].

2.2. Delayed reconstruction

Most patients requesting delayed reconstruction have lost skin or muscle or both. The quality of tissues may be further compromised by pectoral nerve damage, muscle atrophy, and thin irradiated mastectomy flaps. Transposition of a healthy LD flap into this kind of defect allows the reconstruction of damaged or resected structures, including the anterior axillary fold and the breast skin envelope. This can be achieved without having to stretch or compromise the native tissues. Careful positioning of the flap just above the inframammary fold will ensure a less visible donor "patch", lower pole fullness and a more natural breast shape. Extended flap harvest can be used to correct and reconstruct the few patients with extreme "washboard" deformity following classical radical mastectomy.

Careful flap design can help to correct unsightly sequelae of previous surgery and radiotherapy.

2.3. Salvage procedures

Surgeons familiar with LD flaps will appreciate their clinical utility in two further situations demanding salvage surgery:

- loco-regional recurrence
- complications of treatment

Immediate reconstruction following mastectomy for failed breast conservation or following segmental chest wall resection for recurrence demands the reliability and extent of tissue cover provided by LD flaps. Furthermore, iatrogenic problems such as failed subpectoral reconstruction, total TRAM-flap loss and radionecrosis of the chest wall are situations which can be salvaged successfully by the judicious use of LD flaps.

3. Patient selection

Women need adequate information and advice about the different reconstruction options so they can make an informed choice. Books, photographs and "buddy" patients who have experienced similar procedures can help the patient come to an informed decision. Careful counselling and advice will prevent ill-informed choices and the disappointment and resentment which may result. Patients considering LD reconstruction must be fit for a procedure which takes 3–4 hours when combined with mastectomy. Smoking, obesity and diabetes are relative contra-indications, particularly when associated with co-existent cardiovascular disease. Previous use of part of the LD muscle for partial breast reconstruction, and total division of the pedicle during radical axillary dissection or of the LD muscle during thoracotomy prevent the subsequent harvest of a viable flap (Table 1). LD reconstruction results in little functional disability, but some patients are aware of weakness at the extremes of shoulder extension. This may be experienced while pushing up backwards when getting out of a bath, or when swimming or skiing.

Table 1. Criteria for LD breast reconstruction

Indications	Contraindications
IBR	Co-morbidity
DBR	Previous thoracotomy
Large breast	Transected pedicle
Ptotic breast	Previous 'miniflap'
Previous RT	Silicone concerns
Radical mastectomy	Uncertainty
Failed BCS	

IBR = immediate breast reconstruction.
DBR = delayed breast reconstruction.
RT = radiotherapy.
BCS = breast conserving surgery.

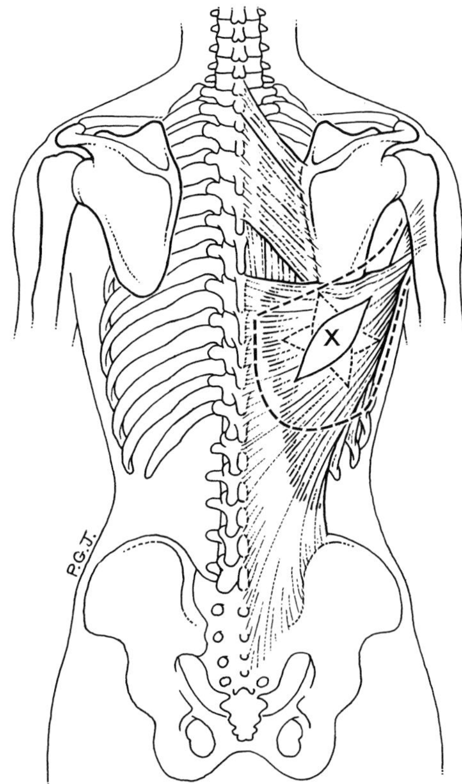

Fig. 1. LD surface anatomy, dissection limits and flap design (p5, under "Anatomy", line 21).

4. Anatomy

Understanding the surface anatomy of LD is fundamental to the design and elevation of the flap (Fig. 1). The large triangular muscle covers most of the lower posterior thoracic and lumbar regions. It takes a wide origin from the thoracolumbar fascia posteriorly and inferiorly, and the lowest three ribs anteriorly. It thickens as it passes towards the insertion into the floor of the bicipital groove. Deeply, fascial attachments bind it to serratus anterior (SA) and terres major (TM), and these attachments need to be divided during mobilisation.

> *LD is a large triangular muscle and successful flap design depends on a clear understanding of the surface anatomy.*

Blood reaches LD via the thoradorsal branch of the subscapular artery (SSA), which enters the muscle about 10 cm below the axillary artery (Fig. 2). The artery breaks up into a number of deep intermuscular branches, which supply the skin over the entire muscle and over a territory 3–5 cm wide of the anterior border. This allows the safe harvest of a skin island with a tip which extends as far as 5 cm beyond the anterior border of the muscle. One or two serratus anterior branches of the SSA cross the intermuscular space between SA and LD. These anastomose freely with the perforating branches of the intercostal and lumbar arteries. Prior division of the SSA during radical mastectomy reverses the flow in these SA vessels, allowing elevation of the entire flap on this pedicle.

Venous return is via a single thoracodorsal vein draining into the axillary vein. The flap is supplied by the thoracodorsal nerve which may be sacrificed to prevent occasional and unsightly flap contraction which can develop spontaneously. Nerve division will lead inevitably to flap atrophy.

> *When the subscapular artery has been divided, the flap can be elevated on the serratus anterior branches.*

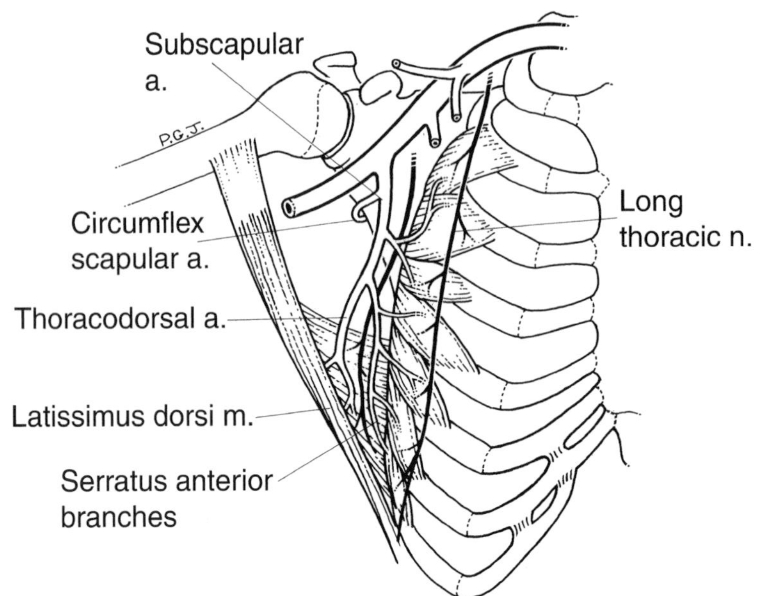

Fig. 2. Regional anatomy (p6, under "pedicle", line 15).

Breast reconstruction using LD can be divided into four equally important steps:

- preoperative planning
- dissection of the breast pocket and axilla
- harvesting the LD flap
- reconstruction of the breast

5. Preoperative planning

The outcome of BR is closely related to the accuracy of the preoperative mark-up of the incisions and the limits of dissection. The procedure must be planned, working out the exact dimensions of the flap and the size of the tissue expander to be used in the reconstruction. Manufacturers templates can help to select the most appropriate expander and to define limits of dissection of the breast pocket and flap. The breast should be reconstructed to the size desired by the patient, which may be smaller or larger than the remaining breast. Subsequent contralateral reduction or augmentation may be necessary to achieve symmetry. Marking-up should always be done on the ward and never in theatre.

Careful preoperative planning of incisions simplifies the surgery and optimises the final result.

5.1. Breast mark-up

To mark-up the breast pocket for delayed BR

- the base of the reconstructed breast should match exactly that of the remaining breast;
- the width of the skin paddle (z) should equal the difference between the base height (y) and the distance from the superior to the inferior border of the remaining breast (x). (Fig. 3); this paddle is usually 12–14 cm long, and mimics the ellipse of skin removed during the mastectomy.

The line of incision which is used to raise the mastectomy flaps will decide the final position of the LD flap. High mastectomy scars are best ignored, placing the incision so that the flap will augment the convexity of the lower pole of the reconstructed breast. Similar principles apply to immediate BR. In this situation, the pocket is marked carefully around the perimeter of the

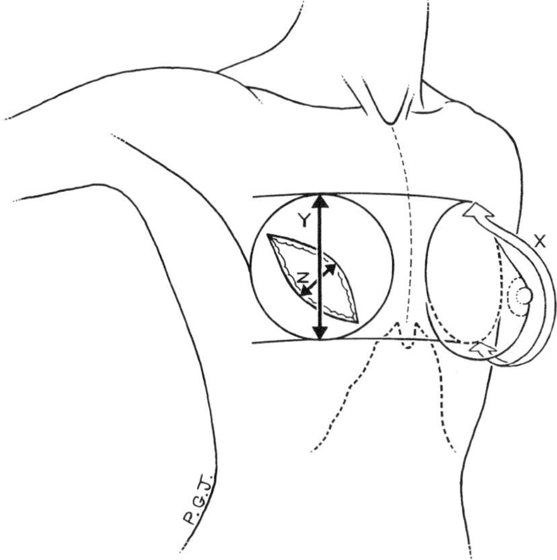

Fig. 3. Mark-up of breast pocket and dimensions of donor skin paddle ($x - y = z$) (p7, under "Breast mark-up", line 18).

breast, and the mastectomy incision is sited as low as possible in the breast envelope to ensure a partly concealed skin island positioned in the inferior pole.

5.2. Flap mark-up

Ideally the donor scar should be concealed under the bra strap. This can be achieved by drawing a vertical line from the tip of the scapula to point x (Fig. 1) which lies under the bra strap. This point is 8–10 cm caudal to the scapula, and is the centrepoint of the elliptical skin island. The orientation of the flap around this point will dictate the orientation of the donor scar. It should be remembered that the flap will rotate through 90°–120° during its transposition into the mastectomy site. The long axis of the mastectomy aperture will therefore decide to a great extent the orientation of the donor incision. An elliptical incision centred on x is marked out, based on the exact dimensions calculated from the Fig. 3. Obtuse angulation of the tips of this flap will help to avoid unsightly "dogears" following closure. The tip of the scapula, spinous processes and anterior border of LD are now marked out to delineate the limits of the muscle, and the extent of dissection and muscle harvest are clearly defined.

The orientation of the donor site skin paddle should take into account the orientation of the mastectomy scar.

5.3. Preparation and equipment

Good lighting, careful positioning, and the use of "state of the art" equipment help to optimise the procedure. A broad spectrum antibiotic is commenced intravenously with the pre-medication, and continued for two days. The patient is "preloaded" with intravenous crystalloid solution to maximise flap perfusion. The procedure can be foreshortened by two surgeons working simultaneously, with the patient lying in the lateral position. One surgeon performs the mastectomy and axillary dissection, while the other raises the flap. Alternatively, the mastectomy is performed with the patient supine, the flap is raised in the lateral position, and the patient is returned to the supine position for the reconstruction. This approach has some distinct advantages. Axillary access is optimal in the supine patient, facilitating dissection and preparation of the pedicle. Moreover, dissection of uniformly thin mastectomy flaps is much easier when the breast is lying flat on the chest wall. By contrast, harvesting of the LD flap is simplified in the lateral position, but achieving a symmetrical reconstruction requires a supine patient to enable a comparison with the remaining breast.

Turning the patient twice during the procedure is time-consuming but can improve access to operating sites. Patients should be in the supine position for placement of a prosthesis or tissue expander.

Haemostasis and thin flaps are greatly facilitated by the injection of 1 : 300,000 adrenaline: saline solution into the subcutaneous tissues overlying the breast and flaps. By artificially increasing the thickness of the subcutaneous tissues, total glandular removal of the breast is simplified and tissue desiccation is prevented. Infiltration of the tissues overlying the LD flap facilitates the harvest of a useful layer of fat on the surface of the muscle, which increases the overall flap volume and thickness.

A high quality headlight system coupled with the use of Argon-enhanced electrosurgery, bipolar diathermy scissor dissection and ultrasonic cutting and coagulation may speed up dissection and help reduce blood loss. Gentle handling of the mastectomy flaps is vital in order to avoid damage and subsequent ischaemic necrosis, particularly when performing SSM.

6. Dissection of the breast pocket and axilla

For delayed BR, the mastectomy flaps are elevated to the previously marked limits of the new breast pocket. When the original scar is not being excised, underlying fibrotic bands may need to be released to prevent unsightly tethering and distortion of the reconstructed breast mound. This problem is not encountered during immediate breast reconstruction. The flaps are raised superiorly to the second intercostal space, medially to the lateral sternal edge, and inferiorly to the level of the contralateral inframammary fold. Laterally, the dissection is continued to the mid-axillary line, stopping short of the lateral border of LD.

The extent of axillary dissection depends on the reason for the mastectomy, but there is a minimum requirement to identify and prepare the thoracodorsal trunk and to preserve the intercostobrachial nerve, if at all possible. This step is simplified by commencing the dissection immediately below the axillary vein, proceeding in a caudal direction. Here, the SSA and vein are large and easily identified, lying deep in the lateral aspect of the dissection field. By lifting the overlying contents out of the axilla, caudal dissection exposes the thoracodorsal nerve and 2 or 3 small anterior tributaries of the SS vein. These require separate ligation and division, to avoid inadvertent avulsion and haemorrhage. During this part of the dissection, the lateral thoracic veins will be identified crossing the intercostobrachial nerve. They are divided taking care not to damage the nerve.

The subscapular trunk is most easily identified lying deep to the axillary vein in the lateral aspect of the axilla, medial to LD.

In a previously dissected axilla, the TD trunk is often plastered to SA on the medial wall of the axilla. Careful identification and dissection of the pedicle is vital in this situation to avoid damage. Once identified, the SA branches are divided for three reasons:

- to increase the blood flow to the LD flap
- to avoid inadvertent damage to these vessels during subsequent elevation of the flap
- to increase the mobility and rotation of the flap.

The patency of the SSA must always be confirmed before division of the branches (see above). The axillary dissection is completed and the anterior border of LD running up to the tendon is identified and dissected free from the surrounding fat. The empty breast pocket is sealed with a clear adhesive dressing and the patient is turned into the lateral position and secured by strapping with the shoulder adducted and flexed.

7. Harvesting the LD flap

An ipsilateral paravertebral block using 30 ml of 0.5% plain Bupivicaine in divided doses at T4, T8 and T12 reduces postoperative discomfort. After further infiltration of subcutaneous tissues of the donor site with an adrenaline: saline solution, the LD flap is mobilised through the previously marked transverse elliptical incision. A layer of fat is harvested on the surface of the flap by developing a deep subcutaneous pocket underneath

Scarpa's fascia. The musculofascial attachments of LD are divided around the perimeter of this pocket, starting first with the superior border. This is identified 1–2 cm above the tip of the scapula. A strong fascial layer binds LD to TM, and this is divided sharply along the superior border (Fig. 1).

> *Harvesting a layer of fat on the surface of LD increases the volume of the flap, providing additional soft tissue cover.*

Next, the posterior border is mobilised by making a vertical window in the thoracolumbar fascia immediately lateral to the spinous processes. This window is extended caudally to the inferior limit of the dissection pocket. At this level, division of the muscle continues anteriorly, level with the costal margin until the anterior border is reached. Finally, the deep surface of the muscle is mobilised by dividing the two posterior layers of the thoracolumbar fascia and perforating branches of the lumbar and intercostal arteries. This allows identification of the intermuscular space between LD and SA at the tip of the scapula. This space is developed caudally, dividing fibrous attachments between the two muscles, and finally the origin of LD from ribs 10, 11 and 12.

Lastly, mobilisation is completed by further division of the fascia between LD and TM under direct vision. Care must be taken to avoid damage to the TD vessels which lie immediately deep to the fascia as LD becomes tendinous. Mobilisation of the anterior border is completed and the flap is tucked through the axilla into the mastectomy pocket (Fig. 4).

8. Reconstruction of the breast

For this final step, the patient is returned to the supine position and re-towelled, exposing both the mastectomy site and the remaining breast. This allows a direct comparison between the reconstructed breast and the contralateral breast, and helps to ensure a symmetrical result. Three steps complete the reconstruction:

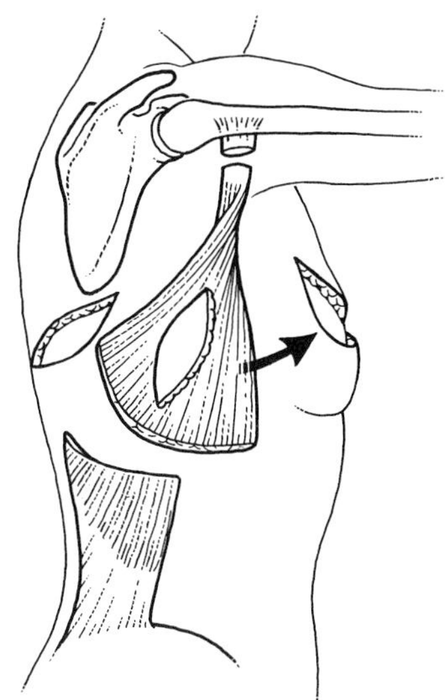

Fig. 4. Transposition of flap (p12, under "ribs 10, 11 and 12", line 22).

- preparation of the flap
- formation of the breast pocket
- selection and placement of the expander/prosthesis

8.1. Preparation of the flap

The remaining fascia between TM and LD is divided, taking care not to damage the pedicle which is closely related to its deep surface. Further dissection leaves the flap attached by the tendon and the pedicle. Division of the tendon at this stage is optional, and allows greater transposition, rotation and mobility of the flap. The ugly bulge produced by the tendon in the axilla is avoided and the flap tends to fall naturally into the lower pole of the breast, adding to its convexity. The pedicle must be protected during division of the tendon. The shape of the correctly orientated flap is now compared with that of a mastectomy pocket before the muscle edges are trimmed to match the surface markings.

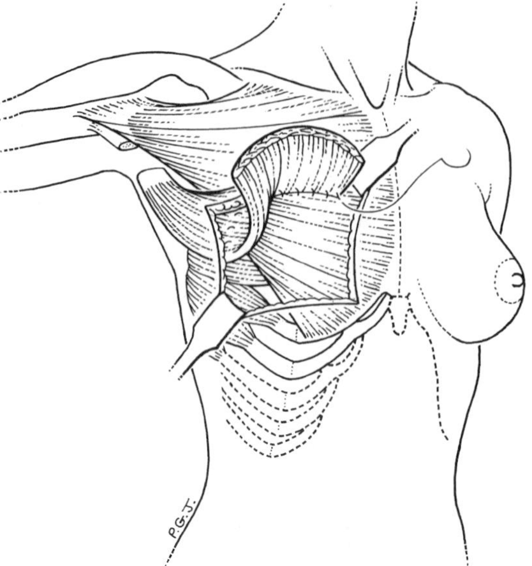

Fig. 5. Suture of flap into mastectomy pocket (p14, under "Formation of the breast pocket", line 1).

8.2. Formation of the breast pocket

The borders of the flap are now sutured to the perimeter of the mastectomy pocket after checking orientation again. Using an absorbable suture, the flap is sutured in turn to SA, the lateral border of PM, and the superior and medial borders of the mastectomy defect, forming a muscular pocket (Fig. 5). The inferior border is closed over suction drains with pre-placed interrupted sutures, after expander/implant placement. This prevents inadvertent puncture of the prosthesis when suturing. As an alternative to inserting the expander or prosthesis between LD and PM, PM can be incorporated into the anterior aspect of the muscle pocket, so that the expander or implant lies behind both PM and LD. To do this PM is detached from its origins from the lower part of the sternum, and the lower border of the muscle is sutured to the upper border of LD. The expander or prosthesis will now lie directly on the rib cage, deep to both muscles. This modification helps to avoid upper pole fullness, due to direct compression of the underlying prosthesis by PM, but contraction of PM can produce an ugly deformity over this most visible portion of the reconstructed breast.

> *The position of the expander or implant will decide the final shape and contour of the breast mound.*

8.3. Selection and placement of expander or implant

Preoperative measurement ensures the selection of an appropriate expander or prosthesis. These dimensions should be checked again peroperatively by measuring the base width of the new muscular pocket and cross-referencing with the manufacturers charts. Any retained air is aspirated from the expander, which is then immersed in povidone–iodine solution and partially inflated with 100–200 ml of normal saline. The surgeon re-gloves, and the expander or prosthesis is placed in the submuscular pocket. As there is little movement of textured expanders after their placement, correct positioning and orientation at this stage is vital (Fig. 6).

> *Careful measurement, selection, handling and positioning of expanders or prostheses is essential.*

The inferior margin of the pocket is closed and after creation of a subcutaneous tunnel for the injection port (Fig. 7) if an expander is being used, the skin island is sutured into the mastectomy defect. The volume of the tissue expander is adjusted to a size which matches the remaining breast as closely as possible (Fig. 8). Seroma aspiration and tissue expansion are performed in the outpatient department and may require several visits. Maximum on-table expansion can help to limit the need for postoperative expansion, while "quilting" of the donor cavity may help to reduce seroma formation [10].

A variety of different problems may be encountered during LD reconstruction. These can be

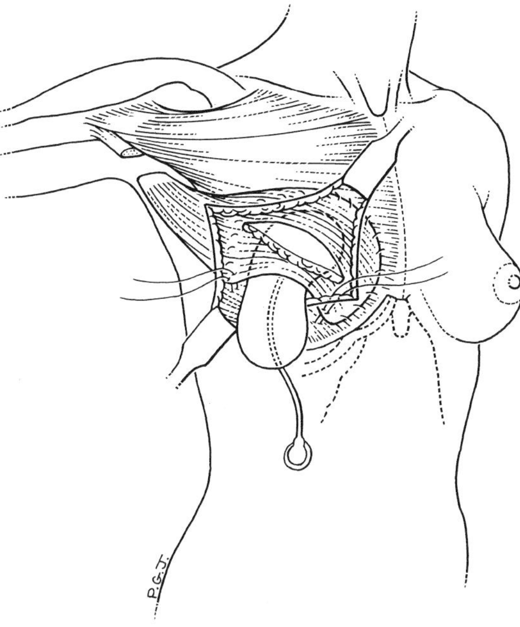

Fig. 6. Insertion and positioning of expander in intermuscular pocket (p14, under "Selection and placement of expander", line 18).

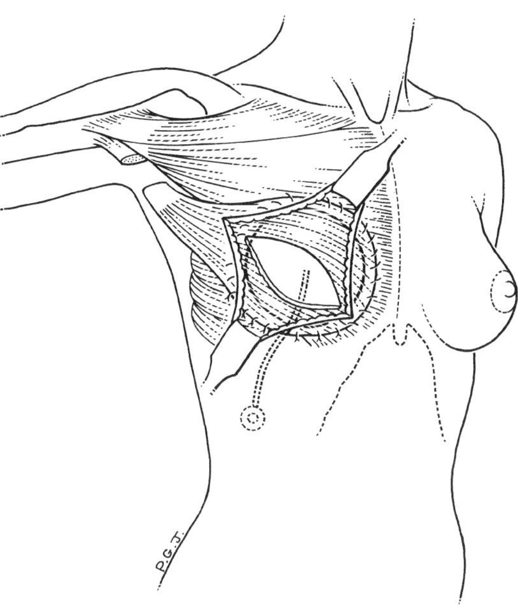

Fig. 7. Closure of muscular pocket and positioning of injection port (p15, under "expanders is essential", line 7).

avoided or solved in a number of ways, some of which have been summarised in Table 2.

9. Skin-sparing mastectomy

The combination of SSM with immediate LD reconstruction is an evolving new technique which adds a further dimension of sophistication to breast reconstruction. The increasing trend towards greater skin conservation has been underpinned by an understanding of the importance of preservation of as much of the breast envelope as possible. A total glandular resection and axillary dissection can be carried out through a small central aperture. This approach maximises skin conservation, minimises scar formation, and preserves the inframammary fold. The

Table 2. Problem solving in LD reconstruction

Problem	Solution
Synmastia	Avoid dissection over midline
Mastectomy flap necrosis	Gentle handling and sharp dissection
Malposition of expander	Careful preoperative mark-up and peroperative positioning
Difficult identification of pedicle	Dissect from cranial to caudal aspect axilla
Inadvertent elevation of SA muscle	Identify SA at tip of scapula
Malposition of skin paddle	Careful preoperative mark-up
Damage to pedicle during flap elevation	Identify pedicle and divide SA branches with patient supine before flap elevation
Inadequate muscle cover over expander	Careful preoperative mark-up and planning
Muscle fringe too short	De-epithelialise tip of donor skin paddle to create extra length
Badly orientated flap	Divide tendon, rotate and de-epithelialise if necessary
Wrongly-sized expander	Preoperative and peroperative measurement. Weigh breast. Use sizers and charts.

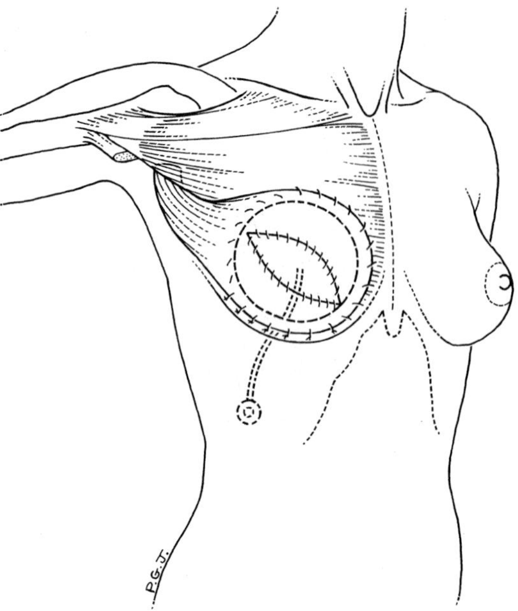

Fig. 8. Final closure and on-table expansion (p15, under "formation", line 15).

breast can then be reconstructed within its normal anatomical boundaries without increasing surgical complications [11] or compromising oncological safety [12].

The formation of a circular rather than an elliptical skin island greatly facilitates flap orientation and positioning. By retaining the ptotic shape of the skin envelope, an authentic reconstruction is more easily achieved. In practice, this results in a reduction of the number of contralateral procedures required to restore symmetry [1,6]. Moreover, the ugly "patch" effect of the more conventional elliptical LD skin island is avoided, as the circular disc of dorsal skin can be concealed by subsequent nipple reconstruction or by a silastic nipple prosthesis [13].

Although SSM carries a greater theoretical risk of incomplete mastectomy than non-SSM, rates of local recurrence do not appear to be influenced by the amount of skin removed when resecting T_1 and T_2 tumours [6,11,13–15]. Furthermore, identical amounts of residual glandular tissue remain after SSM and non-SMM [16]. Although a more detailed analysis of the medium and long-term results of this approach are eagerly awaited, early experience suggests an increasing future role for SSM combined with LD reconstruction.

SSM and immediate LD reconstruction preserves the breast shape and reduces scar formation without increasing complications or local recurrence rates.

10. Conclusion

The popularity of LD reconstruction in breast surgery is directly related to the usefulness of these myocutaneous flaps in a number of different clinical situations. Myocutaneous, myosubcutaneous and autogenous flaps can be used for a range of reconstructive procedures in the immediate and delayed setting. Their utility is related to their reliability and adaptability, and accounts for their expanding role in the surgical management of breast cancer.

Acknowledgements

The author thanks Mr Peter Jack, Medical Artist, for the illustrations, and the Winchester Cancer Research Trust (Registered Charity No. 1003252) for financial support.

References

1. Tansini I. Nuovo Processo per l'amputazione della mammella per cancre. La Reforma Medica 1896; 12: 3–12.
2. Muhlbauer W, Olbrisch R. The latissimus dorsi myocutaneous flap breast reconstruction. Chir Plast 1977; 4: 27–34.
3. Bostwick J, Carlson GW. Reconstruction of the breast. Surg Oncol Clin N Am 1997; 6: 71–89.
4. Slavin SA, Colen A. Sixty consecutive breast reconstructions with the inflatable expander: a critical appraisal. Plast Reconstr Surg 1990; 86: 910–9.
5. Knowlton EW, Gorey R, Taekman H. Total immediate breast reconstruction with "peg" latissimus dorsi flap. Contemp Surg 1992; 41: 15–19.

6. Slavin SA, Schnitt SJ, Duda RB et al. Skin-sparing mastectomy and immediate reconstruction: oncologic risks and aesthetic results in patients with early-stage breast cancer. Plast Reconstr Surg 1998; 102: 49–62.
7. Papp C, Zanon E, McCraw J. Breast volume replacement using the de-epithelialised latissimus dorsi myocutaneous flap. Eur J Plast Surg 1988; 11: 120–5.
8. Noguchi M, Taniya T, Miyasaki I, Saito Y. Immediate transposition of a latissimus dorsi muscle correcting a post-quadrantectomy breast deformity in Japanese patients. Int Surg 1990; 75: 166–70.
9. Raja MAK, Straker V, Rainsbury RM. Extending the role of breast conserving surgery by immediate volume replacement. Br J Surg 1997; 84: 101–5.
10. Titley OG, Spyrou GE, Fatah MFT. Preventing seroma in the latissimus dorsi donor site. Br J Plast Surg 1997; 50: 106–8.
11. Carlson GW, Bostwick J, Styblo TM et al. Skin-sparing mastectomy. Oncologic and reconstructive considerations. Ann Surg 1997; 225: 570–8.
12. Kroll SS, Schusterman MA, Tadjalli HE, Singletary SE, Ames FC. Risks of recurrence after treatment of early breast cancer with skin-sparing mastectomy. Ann Surg Oncol 1997; 4: 193–7.
13. Pyser PM, Abel JA, Straker VH, Hall VL, Rainsbury RM. Ultra-conservative skin-sparing "keyhole" mastectomy and immediate breast and areolar reconstruction. Ann R Coll Surg Eng 2000; 82: 227–235.
14. Sandelin K, Billgren AM, Wickman M. Management, morbidity and oncological aspects of 100 consecutive patients with immediate breast reconstruction. Am Surg Oncol 1998; 5: 159–65.
15. O'Brien W, Hasselgren P-O, Hummel RP. Comparison of post-operative wound complications and early cancer recurrence between patients undergoing mastectomy with or without immediate breast reconstruction. Am J Surg 1990; 125: 1303–8.
16. Barton FE, English JM, Kingsley WB, Fietz M. Glandular excision in total glandular mastectomy and modified radical mastectomy: a comparison. Plast Reconstr Surg 1991; 88: 389–94.

Breast Cancer: Diagnosis and Management
J.M. Dixon (Ed.)

CHAPTER 29

HRT and breast cancer

Klim McPherson

1. Introduction

Breast cancer is a hormonal disease with its aetiology involving manifestations of different determinants or consequences of the hormonal milieu. Early age at menarche and late age at first full term pregnancy both independently increase breast cancer risk later in life. Height, growth rate and aspects of diet, for instance alcohol consumption, also increase risk. Body mass index among post menopausal women and weight increase among pre menopausal women also increase the risk, reflecting a source of endogenous oestrogen in menopausal women and a less significant source in the premenopausal.

Crucially the incidence curve plotted against age, assumes a lower gradient at around the average age of menopause [1]. Incidence increases by about 8% per year of age before the menopause and by around 3% afterwards. On a log scale these graphs are linear with a reduction in rate of increase in incidence at around age 50. It is reasonable to assume that these changes have something to do with circulating hormone levels, and that the reduction that occurs at menopause results in a lower incidence than would have occurred had there been no reduction in hormonal levels. This implies that, among women of the same age, other risk factors being equal those who are post menopausal should have a lower risk than women who are still menstruating.

In such an analysis of the incidence of breast cancer it is easy to interpolate lines which, for example, begin the reduction in rate of incidence increase at age 45. Then the line simply rises in parallel with the observed line which reduced slope at age 50 and is lower by a constant amount. On a log scale this constant vertical distance represents a constant relative risk which in this case is equivalent to the relative risk of subsequent breast cancer among women with an early menopause (at age 45) compared with those whose menopause is at age 50. Thus the simple graph gives rise to the hypothesis that the ratio of incidence extrapolated from the higher observed line to that on the lower hypothetical line at any age represents the relative risk of breast cancer associated with early menopause compared with the average.

Breast cancer incidence increases as the age at menopause increases.

Indeed the same applies to a menopause occurring naturally later; for each year of delayed menopause so the subsequent risk of breast cancer increases by around 3%. Just as the extrapolated line beginning its reduced slope at age 53 say will be around 9% (1.03 cubed equals 1.093, i.e. 9.3%) higher than the observed line for women whose menopausal age is average.

2. Detecting any relationship of HRT with breast cancer

Clearly assessing risk is a matter for observational epidemiology, since randomizing women to take HRT and then comparing breast cancer incidence is not a practical option. However women take HRT largely for symptoms and the prevalence of use is very much determined by culture and the environment in which women find themselves. Moreover the nature and composition of preparations change — particularly with the addition of progestagen to mitigate the effect on the endometrium of unopposed oestrogen.

Women who take HRT might be at a different risk of breast cancer than those who do not. There is some evidence to suggest for example that women whose menopausal symptoms are less tolerable have lower circulating oestrogen levels than unsymptomatic women [2], and such women would be at lower intrinsic risk. On the other hand HRT users are likely to be of higher economic status and possibly to consume more alcohol, and together these factors give rise to a higher intrinsic risk [3]. Also taking HRT is associated with greater use of mammography and therefore higher detection rates, but the use of hormones is associated with lower specificity and sensitivity of mammography because of changes in density [4].

To complicate matters further the bulk of epidemiology, ie most of the studies which now exist, were conducted at a time when unopposed oestrogen was the dominant mode of replacement therapy. This means that most of the evidence on the effect of taking HRT comes from studies in which women took only oestrogen. Thus should the addition of progestagen affect the risk of breast cancer, this will be difficult to detect, since data may be immature or insufficient. In particular, in this complicated relationship, might the addition of progestagen not change the immediate risk but prolong the period for which a change in risk attributable to hormone replacement lasts? Such questions are not currently answerable.

Finally there are several interesting characteristics of possible risk which it might be sensible to distinguish, to help women make decisions. For example does HRT only increase risk while being taken and if not for how long does the change in risk last. Also are there subgroups of women for whom the risk of HRT on breast cancer is importantly different. Possibly more importantly, if there is an increase in risk of breast cancer, does that translate into a commensurate increased risk in mortality from breast cancer?

Assessing the impact of HRT on breast cancer incidence and mortality is not easy.

3. The estimated risk

Results of the effect on breast cancer risk are taken largely from the collaborative reanalysis of data from 51 studies conducted world wide among 52,705 cases and 108,411 women without breast cancer [5]. In these analyses close stratification and adjustment were made for study, age, parity and age at first birth. Some analyses also stratified for menopausal status and for body mass index. Most studies were carried out in North America or Europe, although studies from 21 countries were included in the combined analysis.

The main results of this collaboration can be summarised by the observation that the risk appears to be increased among women who are recent (within 5 years) or current users of HRT and that this increase is related to duration of use. For women who ceased HRT use more than five years age the risk is not increased even for long durations of use. The estimated relative risks are shown in Table 1.

These results suggest that the use of HRT does increase the risk of breast cancer, but only in the short to medium term suggesting a promotional affect. Indeed the average rate of increase in risk is estimated as 1.023 (standard error 0.006) per year, giving rise to cumulative relative risks of 1.023, 1.046, 1.071, 1.095, 1.12 etc for the 1st, 2nd, 3rd, 4th and 5th years of use. There is a cumulative

Table 1. Relative risk of breast cancer by use of HRT, adjusting for confounders

HRT use	Cases	Controls	Relative risk	95% confidence limits
Never use	12457	23568	1.00 (reference)	0.96–1.04
Last use < 5 years before diagnosis				
Duration of use				
< 1 year	368	860	0.99	0.82–1.16
1–4 years	891	2037	1.08	0.96–1.20
5–9 years	588	1279	1.31	1.16–1.46
10–14 years	304	633	1.24	1.03–1.45
≥ 15 years	294	514	1.56	1.31–1.81
Last use 5+ years before diagnosis				
Duration of use				
< 1 year	437	890	1.12	0.97–1.27
1–4 years	566	1256	1.12	0.99–1.25
5–9 years	151	374	0.90	0.67–1.13
≥ 10 years	93	233	0.95	0.67–1.23

increase at an annual rate of 2.3%. This excess risk is no different from the estimated risk of delayed menopause among women in these studies who have never use HRT, of 1.028 (standard error 0.003) per year (i.e. 2.8% per year). There could be no clearer demonstration that replacing endogenous hormones has the same effect on breast cancer risk as endogenous levels would have had. This latter estimate of the protective effect of early menopause in turn is not affected by whether the menopause is surgical or natural. However, these affects are somewhat modified by the age of diagnosis, that is each year of delayed menopause (past age 50 for example) exacts a 4.0% annual increase for breast cancer risk at age 50–59, 2.5% at age 60–69 and 1.3% at age 70–79 (suggesting that the lines in Fig. 1 are not quite parallel). It seems clear from Table 1 that similar results for HRT use might emerge from more information on past use. Five years use at the latter rate of increase would only yield a relative risk of 1.06 — well inside the confidence limits of the current estimate.

For every year of HRT use the relative risk of breast cancer increases by 1.023 which is approximately the same as the risk of a year later in menopausal age (1.028).

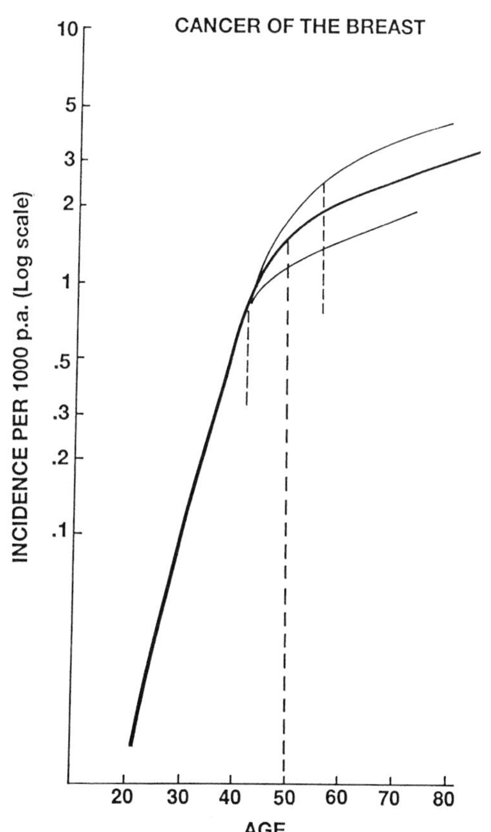

Fig. 1. Detecting any relationship to HRT with breast cancer.

In population terms these results indicate that for 1000 women who take hormone replacement therapy for ten years there will be 6 excess cases of breast cancer and for 15 years HRT use there will be 12 excess cases. In absolute terms among such a cohort some 64 women anyway, and around 70 women who have used HRT for ten years, will be diagnosed with breast cancer by age 70. This will give rise to more breast cancer than a natural delay in menopause might since a ten year delay is less common and does not guarantee less severe menopausal symptoms, for which HRT would be indicated.

While these estimates of effect appear consistent and are clearly the most reliable available, they must nonetheless be treated as preliminary. This is because today most women with a uterus will be taking opposed therapy and these data are based largely on experience gained from the use of unopposed oestrogen. In fact around 20% of the women in the category of use less than five years before diagnosis were using opposed therapy while less than 8% of the remainder were. Clearly this does not adequately represent current HRT use. The evidence as it stands would suggest that the addition of progestagen certainly does not decrease the risk of breast cancer [6].

The effects of HRT on breast cancer risk rely heavily on early studies where the majority of women were using unopposed oestrogen replacement therapy. This does not represent current HRT use.

When a systematic examination of potential modifiers of the above effect was undertaken the only significant finding was an apparent reduction in effect among women with a high body mass index (bmi). Thus the relative risk of five years or more of use completed less than five years before diagnosis was estimated as 1.73 for bmi<22.5, 1.29 for bmi between 22.5–24.9 and 1.02 for bmi>25.0. These differences were significant at 0.0001. Other potential effects modifiers, for instance a family history of breast cancer, were not apparent.

In terms of survival advantage, many would like to believe that notwithstanding an increase in incidence the mortality rate will be unchanged, and there is some evidence for this [7]. However there are serious problems of selection and bias (surveillance bias for example) in the reliable assessment of this question. For example it is too easy to observe from the few cohort studies, no significant increase in observed mortality together with a significant increases in incidence and to therefore conclude that this implies a more benign disease. Clearly however, since breast cancer is relatively slow growing, mortality effects are much more difficult to detect. This is another case of no evidence for an effect being confused with evidence for its absence [8]. While the collaborative study finds some evidence for a lower rate of the risk of disease having spread beyond the breast in HRT users the conclusion was nonetheless that the effect of HRT on mortality from breast was unknown. Where adjustment for stage at diagnosis is attempted the apparent survival advantage disappears [9]. In the Nurses Health Study [6] the relative risk of mortality is significantly increased at 1.45 for five years use or more.

Few studies of mortality from breast cancer and HRT use have long term follow up data. Long term (>10 years) use may be associated with a significant increase in breast cancer deaths.

References

1. Key TJ and Pike M. The role of estrogens and progestogens in the epidemiology of and prevention of breast cancer. Eur J Cancer Clin Oncol 1998; 24: 29–35.
2. Longcope C, Crawford S and McKinlay S. Endogenous estrogens: Relationship between estrone, estadiol, non-protein bound estradiol and hot flashes and lipids. Menopause 1996; 3: 77–80.
3. Isaacs A, Britton A and McPherson K. Why do women doctors in the UK take hormone replacement therapy? J Epidemiol Commun Health 1997; 51: 373–377.

4. Laya M, Larson E, Taplin S et al. Effect of estrogen replacement therapy on the specificity and sensitivity of screening mammography. J Natl Cancer Inst 1996; 88: 643–649.
5. Collaborative Group, Breast cancer and hormone replacement therapy: collaborative reanalysis of data from 51 epidemiological studies of 52705 women with breast cancer and 108411 without breast cancer. Lancet 1997; 350: 1047–1059.
6. Colditz GA, Hankinson SE, Hunter DJ et al. The use of estrogen and progestins and the risk of breast cancer in postmenopausal women. NEJM 1995; 332: 1589–1593.
7. Berkvist L, Adami HO, Persson I et al. Prognosis after breast cancer diagnosis in women exposed to estrogen and estrogen- progestin replacement therapy. Am J Epidemiol 1989; 139: 221–228.
8. McPherson K. Type 3 errors, pill scares, and the epidemiology of oral contraception and health. J Epidemiol Commun Hlth 1999; 5: 258–260.
9. Stickland D, Gambrell R, Butzin C et al. The relationship between breast cancer survival and prior menopausal estrogen use. Obstet Gynecol 1992; 80: 221.

Breast Cancer: Diagnosis and Management
J.M. Dixon (Ed.)

CHAPTER 30

Axillary surgery in breast cancer: an overview

Andrew J. Spillane and Nigel P.M. Sacks

1. Introduction

Axillary surgery has an established role in staging and therapy for early breast cancer (EBC) [1,2]. Despite this, the appropriate surgical management of the axillary lymph nodes (ALN) in EBC is a controversial subject amongst breast specialists [3–8] and patients alike. The nature of this controversy largely relates to:

(1) the best method for surgically staging the clinically negative axilla;
(2) when axillary surgery can be safely avoided in the clinically negative axilla;
(3) the current place of sentinel node biopsy;
(4) whether more extensive axillary treatment has a survival advantage in node positive breast cancer.

EBC can be defined as the presence of a mobile tumour within the breast with or without associated mobile enlarged ALN [9] and represents the vast majority ($\geq$ 90%) of patients who present with breast cancer. This chapter principally relates to those with EBC and a clinically negative axilla as it is generally agreed that the appropriate treatment of the clinically and/or cytologically involved ALNs is a well performed level II/III axillary dissection which both accurately stages and treats the axilla with minimal risk of local recurrence [10,11]. Women with a clinically negative axilla now represent an increasing proportion of the breast cancer caseload. This is occurring because the proven benefit of mammographic screening programmes [11–13] is now widely accepted and the population is more aware of breast cancer resulting in more frequent earlier stage diagnoses [5,14–18]. Until recently the frequency of histologically positive ALN in EBC has been of the order of 40–50% [19–23]. However with the increasing percentage of small invasive (T1a and b) tumours and a higher proportion of noninvasive breast cancer the marginal utility of axillary dissection may be reducing. To add to this there is some evidence that screen detected tumours, for any given size, may be associated with fewer ALN metastases than those detected in non-screened populations [24,25]. Much of the momentum to obviate the need for axillary dissection derives from reports in the literature of a low incidence of ALN positivity in these patients however these low rates have not been confirmed by all authors as shown in Table 1. Furthermore most women with EBC are offered some form of chemoendocrine adjuvant therapy based on factors independent of ALN status as data from the Early Breast Cancer Trialists' Collaborative Group (EBCTCG) demonstrate equivalent proportional benefit from adjuvant therapy independent of ALN status and age [33–35]. These data are controversial and are not as clear cut when one looks only at the unconfounded data. One

Table 1. Frequency of lymph node positivity in T1 breast cancer

Author	Comments	% Node positive			Ref.
T1 tumours:		T1a	T1b	All T1	
Carter et al.				21%	[26]
McGee et al.		12%			[27]
Dees et al.		8%	10%		[28]
Cox et al.	Sentinel nodes			16%	[29]
Silverman et al.		3%	17%		[6]
Silverman et al.	Screen detected	4%	6%		[6]
Tabar et al.	Screen detected			5%	[12]
Walls et al.	Screen detected			3%	[30]
DCIS	DCIS			DCIS	
Silverman et al.				0.6%	[31]
Cox et al.	Sentinel node			4.6%	[29]
Wong et al.				0/33	[32]

could argue there is no role for surgically staging the axilla if the result is not going to change a patient's management or if it offers a very limited therapeutic benefit to that patient. Alternatively by staging the axilla by pre-operative imaging or per-operatively with lesser procedures, most notably sentinel node biopsy (SNB) in recent years, are other potential approaches.

When ALN are heavily involved, or a patient is at high risk of loco-regional recurrence, radiotherapy to the chest wall and regional nodes following mastectomy and (limited) axillary dissection in pre-menopausal women has been shown by two groups to confer a survival advantage which is independent of the added benefit from systemic adjuvant therapy [36,37]. This recent evidence has challenged the current model of the biology of breast cancer spread and suggests that ALN involvement is not just a marker of systemic disease but if inadequately treated can affect overall survival. Whether or not an alteration in practice will follow as a result of these important studies remains to be seen.

- *With the increasing percentage of small invasive and in-situ carcinomas the marginal utility of axillary surgery in these women is reducing.*

- *Many women with EBC are offered adjuvant chemo-endocrine therapy independent of ALN status.*
- *There are widely varying reports about the incidence of positive lymph nodes in small invasive tumours.*
- *Radiotherapy following (limited) axillary dissection probably has a survival advantage in pre-menopausal high risk women.*

2. Axillary staging

2.1. The significance of axillary staging

Pathological data on tumour size, grade, oestrogen receptor level and ALN status taken in the context of the patient's age and menopausal status have formed the basis of clinical decision making in recent years. The ALN status has provided the single most reliable information on long-term recurrence and survival [26,38–42]. It is well established that the incidence of ALN metastases is directly related to the size of the primary tumour [6,26,38,43,44] or more specifically to the size of the invasive component [45]. To a lesser extent it is also related to the presence of lymphovascular invasion [41,46,47] and the grade of the primary tumour [41,48]. Prognosis is also directly related to the absolute number of involved ALN as well as the anatomical level of involvement [38–41].

The reported number of ALN metastases in a specimen is dependent to some extent on the technique of nodal examination [5]. Taking multiple sections and utilisation of immunohistochemical staining increases the incidence of positive nodes detected by pathological assessment of the axilla. However most of these occult new positive nodes contain micrometastatic disease only [41,49,50] representing a focus of 0.25 mm diameter or less in over 50% [41]. The biological clinical significance of occult ALN metastases detected by non-standard techniques is still debated with more information from long-term follow up needed [25,41,42,50,51]. The Ludwig Trial suggested that occult metastases detected by finer slicing of ALN and standard H and E staining imply a worse prognosis [41] but occult metastases detected by more sensitive tests have not been proven to be associated with a worse prognosis [42]. This is particularly important now with the increasing utilisation of SNB and multiple sectioning of ALN resulting in occult metastatic disease being reported more often. The reason for this is the pathologist can now focus in detail on a small number of lymph nodes rather than having to assess the entire axilla [51]. Reverse transcriptase–polymerase chain reaction technology has been shown to be even more sensitive than immunohistochemistry in detecting otherwise occult metastases but the significance of this is unknown [52,53] and it may be that these techniques will lead to a stage shift bias — the so called Will Rogers Phenomenon [54].

- *Prognosis for individual patients is directly related to the total number and anatomical level of nodes involved.*
- *The incidence of ALN metastases is dependent on the pathological technique of nodal examination.*
- *The clinical significance of occult metastatic disease is controversial. The debate will intensify as SNB is more widely utilised and techniques with increased sensitivity for detection of otherwise occult metastases are widely introduced.*

2.2. The arguments for and against axillary dissection

Axillary dissection involves clearance of all lymph node bearing tissue from the axilla to at least the medial border of pectoralis minor muscle. It remains the standard in breast cancer management perhaps with the exception of certain good prognosis groups such as patients with small, low grade tumours, especially those who are not eligible for adjuvant chemotherapy [28,55]. In Table 2 the arguments for and counter-arguments against axillary dissection for staging in EBC are enumerated.

Up to 50% of patients with ALN metastases at level I also have involved nodes at level II or III [20,38]. Proponents for level II/III axillary dissection in the clinically negative axilla argue that if a full axillary dissection is not performed higher level nodes and occasionally skip metastases can be missed [2]. Veronesi et al. reported skip metastases in only 1.3% of cases [21] but other authors have reported an incidence between 6% and 28% [23,71].

- *Currently axillary dissection is the 'gold standard' for staging in EBC management.*
- *In T1a and b invasive tumours the incidence of positive ALN is reported up to 21%. Therefore the majority of these women have no benefit from axillary surgery.*
- *Subsequent to the EBCTCG overviews many women are advised or elect to receive adjuvant therapy even if they are node negative.*
- *Neoadjuvant chemotherapy makes an alteration of management based on the information gained from staging axillary dissection less likely.*

Table 2. Assessment of arguments and counter-arguments for staging EBC by axillary dissection

Advant ages of axillary dissection for staging	Negatives against need for axillary dissection in staging
Axillary status is the best prognostic indicator in EBC [1,26,38–43,55]	Axillary status does not alter treatment in a large percentage of cases with EBC and a clinically negative axilla.
The reported percentage of lymph node involvement in small tumours varies considerably but up to 36% for small invasive tumours [56]	Higher prevalence of small invasive/non-invasive tumours results in more negative axillary dissections but the same attendant morbidity.
The number of ALN involved [28], or even positive SNB [57], alters the nature of adjuvant chemotherapy.	Most women get adjuvant chemotherapy independent of axillary node status [33–35].
High numbers of involved ALN is usually the entry criteria for enrollment in high dose chemotherapy (HDCT) trials [8].	HDCT has no proven survival advantage [58–60].
Identification of high numbers of involved ALN results in advising locoregional RT with its improved local control and possible survival advantage [36,37,61].	In the trials of SNB in EBC the sentinel node is the only one involved in 38–67% of cases [62,63].
Full axillary dissection makes extranodal extension more likely to be detected. Hence the patient may benefit from RT for local control [64,65].	Not proven [66].
Axillary lymph nodes status is still a major prognostic indicator following neoadjuvant chemotherapy [67].	Neoadjuvant chemotherapy makes an alteration in treatment less likely after axillary dissection [8,68–70], and may downstage axillary node status [8].
Information from axillary dissection is useful for audit and comparison of clinical trials of treatments and outcomes.	This may not benefit individual patients.

2.3. Overview of alternative axillary staging methods

Clinical assessment of the axillary status is notoriously unreliable with high false positive and false negative rates of approximately 30% [20,72,73].

Triple node biopsy involves sampling of an internal mammary, axillary and apical lymph node. It is utilised by several groups and shown to give very reliable prognostic information in EBC [74,75] but recurrence rates in the axilla of up to 21% have been reported [76].

Axillary sampling is often an ill-defined procedure ranging from blind biopsy in the vicinity of the axillary tail to a formal level I dissection. Kjaergaard et al. reported that in 40% of their cases sampled material contained insufficient or no nodal material [77]. Other data have demonstrated that the procedure can be reliably predictive of the ALN status [78–80]. Even after an adequately performed axillary sampling the problem remains how to treat the remaining ALNs in patients with positive sampling. This has been exemplified by a rate of arm swelling in excess of 30% when radiotherapy was added to axillary node sampling, resulting in some to recommend completion axillary dissection as the preferred option [79]. More recent data (see chapter by U Chetty) from a randomised trial of axillary sampling and post-operative radiotherapy compared with level III axillary dissection showed identical rates of axillary recurrence with more arm swelling following axillary clearance but some restriction in shoulder movement after radiotherapy.

Sentinel node biopsy identifies the first draining lymph node(s) after tracking blue dye or radiolabelled colloid, or both, injected around the primary tumour site. It has been shown by numerous investigators in non-randomised case series to be a reasonably reliable predictor of axillary status [29,51,63,64,81,82]. The sentinel node is the only lymph node involved in between 38–67% of cases [63,64], but as explained above, SNB results in upstaging of the axilla by finding otherwise occult metastases in a significant proportion of cases [29,51]. A potential advantage over axillary dissection is the identification and assessment of isolated non-axillary sentinel nodes which occur in about 8% of cases [81]. If the sentinel node is fully replaced by tumour it will not retain radiolabelled colloid. This may explain in part the reported false negative rate of up to 12% [43]. Difficulties in sentinel node identification may also arise when the sentinel node is not in the axilla or if the primary tumour is very medial or lateral in the breast making differentiation of the primary site hot spot difficult to separate from the sentinel node [81]. The high false negative rate of up to 12% is not acceptable unless the real risk of axillary node involvement is very low for an individual patient, or the consequences of a false negative result do not significantly affect the individual patient's management [43]. There needs to be further investigation of the technique including timing and dose of radiolabel injection; the ideal particle size; the significance of micrometastatic ALN disease; and long term follow up of local tumour control and patient survival when staged by this technique compared with traditional axillary management [10].

Other modalities of preoperative imaging such as high resolution duplex and colour flow doppler ultrasound [83–85], MRI [86], PET [87,88] and sestamibi nuclear scanning [89,90] have not been shown to reliably predict the ALN status.

- *Adequate axillary sampling and probably sentinel node biopsy can also reliably stage the axilla. Triple node biopsy gives reliable prognostic information but neither stages nor treats the axilla.*
- *Randomised controlled trials are required to establish the place of SNB.*

2.4. Other prognostic indices

Numerous attempts to negate the value of axillary staging by providing equally reliable prognostic information by other methods have been made. The systemic concept of breast cancer spread conceptually weakens the idea that axillary status should remain the most reliable predictor of systemic disease. Ravdin et al. attempted to develop a prognostic index based on the United States National Breast Cancer Tissue Resource Data for nearly 12,000 women. The authors were unable to reach 95% confidence limits for predicting ALN status using tumour size, patient age, S phase fraction and progesterone receptor level which was the most sensitive combination of factors identified from their analysis [91]. Other factors assessed individually without great success include S phase fraction [91], DNA ploidy [92,93], integrin expression [94], serum CA 15-3 concentrations [95], urokinase plasminogen activator concentration [96], MUC 1 epithelial mucin expression level [97], CD44 level [98], Cathepsin D levels [99], cell cycle inhibitor p27 level [100] and c-erb B2 (or HER-2/neu) oncogene overexpression [101,102].

More significantly the expression of high levels of c-erb B2 has recently been shown to be an independent predictor of worse prognosis and associated with poor response to chemotherapy. The receptor is being targeted for monoclonal antibody therapeutic intervention with early non-randomised trial reports of survival benefit [101–103].

- *As breast cancer is often a systemic disease from an early stage the concept that ALN status should remain the most reliable prognostic indicator is weakened.*
- *No tumour markers or combinations of tumour/patient factors have been identified which give equal prognostic information to ALN status.*

Table 3. Assessment of the axillary staging/treatment modalities and morbidity associated with their use in EBC

Modality (reference)	Staging	Local ax. rec. rate	Morbidity	Survival benefit
Axillary dissection	Gold standard if adequately performed $\geq$ 10 nodes	In EBC 1% or less [2,21,106]	WC 8% [2]; AS 8–16% [2,106]; CP 50% [107]; LSM 2% [69]	Possible small % benefit over no treatment [19], or inadequate treatment [108]
Axillary sampling	In expert hands reliable but 2nd operation if node positive	Up to 21% [77]	WC, AS, CP, LSM lower than axillary dissection [78–80]	Nil
Sentinel node biopsy	Probably good – no randomised controlled trials [29,51,63,81,82]	Unknown. False negative rate up to 12% [81]	Unknown – less than AD	Upstages axilla – may be advantageous if alters adjuvant therapy [29,58]
Radiotherapy	None – clinical/radiological	EBC 2–3% [19]. Clinically involved nodes 10% [109–111]	WC nil. AS/CP/LSM same axillary dissection [7,57,66,110–115]. BP 1.3% < 50 Gy; 5.5% > 50 Gy [117]; RIS-21/10^5 pt yrs [118,119]	Increased non-breast cancer deaths [120,121]). No overall survival difference compared to axillary dissection [120]
Ax dissection + RT	Same as axillary dissection	Low	WC $\geq$ AD; AS 40–56% [105,122,123]; CP $\geq$ AD; LSM > AD	Significant survival benefit after inadequate AD + RT vs inadequate AD [17,18]
No treatment	Nil	19–20% [19,124]	Nil	Nil

WC = wound complications, AS = arm swelling, CP = chronic pain, LSM = limitations shoulder movement, BP = brachial plexopathy, RIC = radiation induced sarcoma, AD = axillary dissection, RT = radiotherapy.

3. Therapy: comparison of axillary surgery vs radiotherapy vs no axillary treatment

The only randomised controlled trial comparing axillary dissection to axillary radiotherapy and no axillary treatment was the NSABP B04 Trial which demonstrated no significant overall survival difference between the three groups. The axillary relapse rate was 19% when the axilla was not treated. This rate of relapse when no treatment was given is much less than the 40% ALN positivity rate at histological assessment in the axillary dissection group [19]. This discrepancy is partly explained by many of the non-axillary dissection group effectively having an axillary sampling as part of the 'simple' mastectomy performed with up to a third of this group having a lower axillary dissection [7,104]. In comparing axillary surgery to radiotherapy and no axillary treatment Table 3 assesses the therapeutic effectiveness of each option for local control, the incidence of morbidity and long term survival implications. One important aspect of effective axillary treatment is the avoidance of the rare but impossible to treat scenario of uncontrolled axillary recurrence, the management of which is made more complicated by previous inadequate surgery or suboptimal radiotherapy.

After review of several trials, some of which utilised orthovoltage techniques that are now considered to be outdated, adjuvant radiotherapy was reported to be associated with a small increase in the rate of death from causes other than breast cancer [120,121]. This excess of non-breast cancer deaths was mostly related to internal mammary fields involving heart and lung exposure. Unfortunately the best data on this issue would have come from the NSABP B04 Trial but this has not been published. The 1995 EBCTCG demonstrated no overall survival difference between radiotherapy versus axillary dissection to the axilla [120]. It is obvious from other studies that the incidence of local recurrence following radiotherapy or surgery depends on the adequacy of the treatment. For example, in NSABP B-04 Trial data failure rates were 21%, 12% and 0% respectively when 0, 1–5 or 6 or more negative lymph nodes were found in axillary specimens [124].

There is evidence that ineffective axillary treatment may result in a survival disadvantage [3,7,107,108,125]. The corollary of this issue has been re-examined after recent publications suggesting that radiotherapy after mastectomy may have a survival advantage in high risk groups of premenopausal women [36,37] but also in pre and post-menopausal women who had greater than 10 positive lymph nodes [62]. These data raises questions about the biology of breast cancer spread and suggest that ALN status is more than just a marker of systemic disease. This concept is supported by a recently published study by Sosa et al. who found patients who were otherwise well matched, but who had a limited axillary dissection with < 10 ALN removed had a significantly worse survival than patients undergoing more extensive axillary surgery with > 10 ALN removed (75.7% vs 86.2%, $p < 0.01$) [107].

- *If untreated, axillary disease declares itself in around 20% of patients with EBC.*
- *Axillary dissection and radiotherapy are roughly equivalent in terms of local control, morbidity and effect on long term survival.*
- *More extensive axillary surgery or radiotherapy added to surgery may have a survival advantage for patients with positive ALN.*

4. Current recommendations

The surgical management of the axilla has to be determined on a case by case basis taking into account the patient's wishes. The decision will depend on patient and tumour characteristics, the technologies and local expertise of the institution, and whether the patient has consented to be enrolled in a properly designed prospective randomised controlled trial.

4.1. Early breast cancer with a clinically negative axilla

Fig. 1 proposes a schema for management of these patients. There is a need to justify not performing a recognised effective method of axillary staging on a case by case basis because axillary status remains the most reliable prognostic indicator for planning a patient's management. If the woman is at low risk of axillary metastases and axillary staging is highly unlikely to alter management then breast conservation surgery with radiotherapy to the breast and axilla is an alternative but will be overtreatment of the axilla in the majority of these women [116]. If mastectomy is being performed then it is sensible to perform a level II/III axillary dissection at that time.

4.2. Early breast cancer with clinically involved axilla

Despite what is reported as acceptable levels of local recurrence in the clinically involved axilla treated with radiotherapy (less than 10%), few would argue that full axillary dissection is the appropriate treatment in patients with a clinically positive axilla. Full axillary dissection is clearance of all the lymphatic bearing tissue that occupies the axilla below the lower margin of the axillary vein (unless gross disease is obvious above it) from the lower border of the latissimus dorsi posteriorly to the apex of the axilla (Halsted's ligament). Preservation of the thoracodorsal and long thoracic nerves is a minimum and some ad-

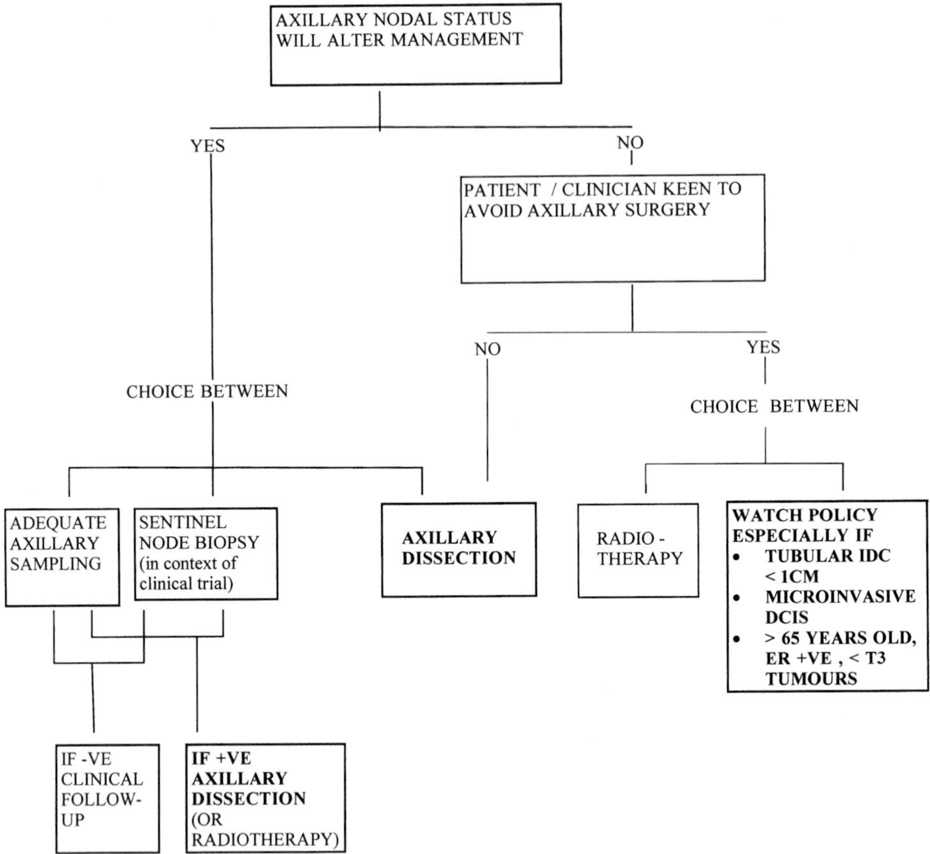

Fig. 1. Proposed management algorithm plan for axillary surgery in EBC with a clinically/cytologically negative axilla.

vocate the sparing of the intercostobrachial nerve although this is not conclusively of benefit. As most radiotherapy fields to the supraclavicular fossa extend to the coracoid process many would argue that level III dissection is not necessary unless there are obviously involved nodes in the third level. The role of adjuvant radiotherapy to the axilla when axillary dissection demonstrates a high number of nodes (> 4 usually) and/or extranodal spread should be made on a case by case basis after multidisciplinary discussion. There is no conclusive randomised controlled trial evidence of a survival advantage for radiotherapy in these women as debate surrounds both the extent of axillary surgery and the type of chemotherapy regimens used in trials to date which may lessen the impact of these studies [36,37].

4.3. Advanced breast cancer

The place of axillary surgery in advanced breast cancer is discussed in a separate chapter. The role of axillary surgery in this group is as part of a planned multimodality attempt to gain optimal local tumour control and to give the prognostic information of the number of nodes involved following systemic therapy [125,126].

References

1. Fisher ER. Prognostic and therapeutic significance of pathological features of breast cancer. NCI Monogr 1986; 1: 29–34.
2. Ball ABS, Waters R, Fish S, Thomas JM. Radical axillary dissection in the staging and treatment of

breast cancer. Ann R Coll Surg Engl 1992; 74: 126–129.
3. Fentiman IS, Mansel RE. The Axilla: not a no-go zone. Lancet 1991; 337: 221–223.
4. O'Dwyer PJ. Axillary dissection in primary breast cancer. Br Med J 1991; 302: 360–361.
5. Cady B, Stone MD, Schuler JG, Thakur R, Wanner MA, Lavin PT. The new era in breast cancer. Invasion, size and nodal involvement dramatically decreasing as a result of mammographic screening. Arch Surg 1996; 131: 301–308.
6. Silverstein MJ, Gierson ED, Waisman JR, Senofsky GM, Colburn WJ, Gamagam P. Axillary lymph node dissection for T1a breast carcinoma: is it indicated? Cancer 1994; 73: 664–667.
7. Harris JR, Osteen RT. Patients with early breast cancer benefit from axillary treatment. Breast Cancer Res Treat 1985; 5: 17–21.
8. Haffty BG, Ward B, Pathare P et al. Reappraisal of the role of axillary lymph node dissection in the conservative treatment of breast cancer. J Clin Oncol 1997; 15(2): 691–700.
9. Sacks NPM, Baum M. Primary management of carcinoma of the breast. Lancet 1993; 342(8884): 1402–1408.
10. Veronesi U. The sentinel node and breast cancer. Br J Surg 1999; 86(1): 1–2.
11. Tabar L, Fagerberg GJG, Gad A, et al. Reduction in mortality from breast cancer after mass screening with mammography. Lancet 1985; 1: 829–832.
12. Tabar L, Fagerberg G, Duffy SW et al. Update of the Swedish Two County Program of Mammographic Screening for Breast Cancer. Rad Clin N Am 1992; 30: 187–210.
13. Duffy SW, Tabar L, Fagerberg G et al. Breast screening, prognostic factors and survival – results from the Swedish Two County Study. Br J Ca 1991; 64: 1133–1138.
14. Solin LJ, Fowble BL, Schultz DJ et al. The impact of mammography on the patterns of patients referred for definitive breast irradiation. Cancer 1990; 65: 1085–1088.
15. Shapiro S. Determining the efficacy of breast cancer screening. Cancer 1990; 63: 1873–1880.
16. Cody HS. The impact of mammography in 1096 consecutive patients with breast cancer, 1979–1993: equal value for patients younger and older than age 50 years. Cancer 1995; 76(9): 1579–1584.
17. Schwartz GF, Carter DL, Conant EF et al. Mammographically detected breast cancer. Cancer 1994; 73: 1660–1665.
18. Cady B. Approach to mammographically discovered small breast cancer. Cancer 1996; 2: 56–58.
19. Fisher B, Redmond C, Fisher E et al. Ten year results of a randomized clinical trial comparing radical mastectomy and total mastectomy with or without radiation. N Engl J Med 1985; 312: 674–681.
20. Danforth DN, Findlay PA, McDonald HD et al. Complete axillary lymph node dissection for stage I–II carcinoma of the breast. J Clin Oncol 1986; 4: 655–662.
21. Veronesi U, Luini A, Galimberti V et al. Extent of metastatic axillary involvement in 1446 cases of breast cancer. Eur J Surg Oncol 1990; 16: 127–133.
22. Henderson IC. The treatment of metastatic breast cancer with adjuvant systemic therapy. Ann Oncol 1990; 1: 9–11.
23. Boova RS, Bonanni R, Rosato FE. Patterns of axillary nodal involvement in breast cancer. Ann Surg 1982; 196: 642–644.
24. Meterissian S, Fornage BD, Singletary SE. Clinically occult breast carcinoma: diagnostic approaches and role of axillary dissection. Ann Surg Oncol 1995; 2: 314–318.
25. Dowlatshahi K, Snider HC, Kim R. Axillary node status in nonpalpable breast cancer. Ann Surg Oncol 1995; 2: 424–428.
26. Carter CL, Allen C, Hensen DE. Relation of tumor size, lymph node status and survival in 24,740 breast cancer cases. Cancer 1989; 63(1): 181–187.
27. McGee JM, Youmans R, Clingan R, Malnar K, Bellefeuille C, Berry C. The value of axillary dissection in T1a breast cancer. Am J Surg 1996; 172(5): 501–504.
28. Dees EC, Shulman LM, Souba WW, Smith BL. Does information from axillary dissection change treatment in clinically node-negative patients with breast cancer? An algorithm for assessment of impact of axillary dissection. Ann Surg 1997; 226: 279–286.
29. Cox CE, Pendas S, Cox JM et al. Guidelines for sentinel node biopsy and lymphatic mapping of patients with breast cancer. Ann Surg 1998; 227(5): 645–653.
30. Walls J, Boggis CR, Wilson M, et al. Treatment of the axilla in patients with screen-detected breast cancer. Br J Surg 1993; 80(4): 436–438.
31. Silverstein MJ, Waisman JR, Gamagami P, et al. Intraductal carcinoma of the breast (208 cases). Clinical factors influencing treatment choice. Cancer 1990; 66: 102–108.
32. Wong J, Kopald K, Morton D. The impact of microinvasion on axillary node metastases and survival in patients with intraductal breast carcinoma. Arch Surg 1990; 125: 1298–1301.
33. Early Breast Cancer Trialists' Collaborative Group. Polychemotherapy for early breast cancer: an overview of the randomised trials. Lancet 1998; 352: 930–942.
34. Early Breast Cancer Trialists' Collaborative Group. Systemic treatment of early breast cancer by hormonal, cytotoxic, or immune therapy. 133 randomised trials involving 31,000 recurrences and

24,000 deaths among 75,000 women. Lancet 1992; 339: 1–15, 71–85.

35. Early Breast Cancer Trialists' Collaborative Group. Tamoxifen for early breast cancer: an overview of the randomised trials. Lancet 1998; 351: 1451–1467.
36. Overgaard M, Hansen PS, Overgaard J, et al. Postoperative radiotherapy in high-risk premenopausal women with breast cancer who receive adjuvant chemotherapy: Danish Breast Cancer Cooperative Group 82b Trial. N Engl J Med 1997; 337: 949–955.
37. Ragaz J, Jackson SM, Le N Pl, et al. Adjuvant radiotherapy and chemotherapy in node-positive premenopausal women with breast cancer. N Engl J Med 1997; 337: 956–962.
38. Veronesi U, Rilke F, Luini A et al. Distribution of axillary node metastases by level of invasion. An analysis of 539 cases. Cancer 1987; 59(4): 682–687.
39. Fisher B, Bauer M, Wickerham DL, Redmonds CK, Fisher ER. Relation of the number of positive axillary nodes to the prognosis of patients with primary breast cancer. Cancer 1983; 52: 1551–1557.
40. Henderson IC, Canellos GP. Cancer of the breast. N Engl J Med 1980; 302: 17–30.
41. International (Ludwig) Breast Cancer Study Group. Prognostic importance of occult axillary lymph node micrometastases from breast cancers. Lancet 1990; 335: 1565–1568.
42. McGuckin MA, Cummings MC, Walsh MD, Hohn BG, Bennett IC, Wright RG. Occult axillary node metastases in breast cancer: their detection and prognostic significance. Br J Cancer 1996; 73: 88–95.
43. McMasters KM, Giuliano AE, Ross MI, et al. Sentinel-lymph-node biopsy for breast cancer – not yet the standard of care. N Engl J Med 1998; 339(14): 990–995.
44. Ciatto S, Pacini P, Rosselli Del Turco M, et al. Patterns of axillary metastases in breast cancer. Radiother Oncol 1986; 5: 91–94.
45. Fisher B, Slack NH, Bross IDJ et al. Cancer and the breast; size of neoplasm and prognosis. Cancer 1964; 24: 1071–1080.
46. Seidman JD, Schnaper LA, Aisner SC. Relationship of the size of the invasive component of the primary breast carcinoma to axillary lymph node metastasis. Cancer 1995; 75(1): 65–71.
47. Weigand RA, Isenberg WM, Russo J, Brennan MJ, Rich MA. Blood vessel invasion and axillary lymph node involvement as prognostic indicators for human breast cancer. Cancer 1982; 50: 962–969.
48. Chadha M, Chabon AD, Friedmann P, Vikram B. Predictors of axillary lymph node metastases in patients with T1 breast cancer: a multivariate analysis. Cancer 1994; 73: 350–353.
49. Halverson KJ, Taylor ME, Perez CA, et al. Management of the axilla in patients with breast cancers one centimeter or smaller. Am J Clin Oncol 1994; 17: 461–466.
50. Nasser IA, Lee AKC, Bosari S, Saganich R, Heatley G, Silverman M. Occult axillary lymph node metastases in 'node-negative' breast carcinoma. Hum Pathol 1993; 24: 950–957.
51. Guiliano AE, Dale PS, Roderick R, Morton DL, Evans SW, Krasne DL. Improved axillary staging of breast cancer with sentinel lymphadenectomy. Ann Surg 1995; 222: 394–401.
52. Lockett MA, Metcalf JS, Baron PL, et al. Efficacy of reverse transcriptase-polymerase chain reaction screening for micrometastatic disease in axillary lymph nodes of breast cancer patients. Am Surg 1998; 64(6): 539–543.
53. Noguchi S, Aihara T, Nakamori S, et al. The detection of breast carcinoma micrometastases in axillary lymph nodes by means of reverse transcriptase–polymerase chain reaction. Cancer 1994; 74(5): 1595–1600.
54. Feinstein AR, Sosin DM, Wells CK. The Will Rogers Phenomenon. Stage migration and new diagnostic techniques as a source of misleading statistics for survival in cancer. N Engl J Med 1985; 312(25): 1604–1608.
55. Harris J, Morrow M, Norton L. Ch.36. Section 2. Malignant tumours of the breast. In Cancer: Principles and Practice of Oncology, 5th Edition, VT Devita Jr, Hellman S, Rosenburg SA. pp. 1557–1616.
56. Dewar JA, Sarrazin D, Benhamou E, et al. Management of the axilla in conservatively treated breast cancer: 592 patients treated at Institut Gustave-Roussy. Int J Radiat Oncol Biol Phys 1987; 13(4): 475–481.
57. Ollila DW, Brennan MB, Giuliano AE. Therapeutic effect of sentinel lymphadenectomy in T1 breast cancer. Arch Surg 1998; 133(6): 647–651.
58. Rodenhuis S, Richel DJ, van der Wall E et al. Randomised trial of high-dose chemotherapy and haemopoietic progenitor-cell support in operable breast cancer with extensive axillary lymph-node involvement. Lancet 1998; 352: 515–521.
59. Hortobagyi GN, Bazdar AU, Chaplin R et al. Lack of efficacy of adjuvant high-dose (HD) tandem combination chemotherapy (CT) for high-risk primary breast cancer (HRPBC): a randomised trial. Proc ASCO 1998; 17: abstr 417.
60. Peters WP, Berry D, Vredenburgh JJ et al. Five-year follow-up of high dose combination alkylating agents with autologous bone marrow transplantation as consolidation after standard dose cyclophosphamide, doxorubicin and fluorouracil for primary breast cancer involving >10 axillary lymph nodes. Proc ASCO 1995; 14: abstr 317.
61. Diab SG, Hilsenbeck SG, Moor C, et al. Radiation therapy and survival in breast cancer with 10 or more

positive axillary lymph nodes treated with mastectomy. J Clin Oncol 1998; 16: 1655–1660.

62. Veronesi U, Paganelli G, Galimberti V et al. Sentinel-node biopsy to avoid axillary dissection in breast cancer with clinically negative lymph-nodes. Lancet 1997; 349: 1864–1867.
63. Albertini JJ, Lyman GH, Cox C, et al. Lymphatic mapping and sentinel node biopsy in the patient with breast cancer. JAMA 1996; 276(22): 1818–1822.
64. Fisher BJ, Perera FE, Cooke AL, et al. Extracapsular axillary node extension in patients receiving adjuvant systemic therapy: an indication for radiotherapy? Int J Radiat Oncol Biol Phys 1997; 38(3): 551–559.
65. Leonard C, Corkill M, Tompkin J, et al. Are axillary recurrence and overall survival affected by axillary extranodal tumor extension in breast cancer? Implications for radiation therapy. J Clin Oncol 1995; 13(1): 47–53.
66. Recht A, Houlihan MJ. Axillary lymph nodes and breast cancer. A review. Cancer 1995; 76: 1491–1512.
67. Valagussa P, Zambetti M, Bonadonna G, Zucali R, Mezzanotte G, Veronesi U. Prognostic factors in locally advanced noninflammatory breast cancer. Long-term results following primary chemotherapy. Breast Cancer Res Treat 1990; 15(3): 137–147.
68. Fisher B, Mamounas EP. Preoperative chemotherapy: A model for studying the biology and therapy of primary breast cancer. J Clin Oncol 1995; 13: 537–540.
69. Powles TJ, Hickish TF, Makris A et al. Randomized trial of chemoendocrine therapy started before or after surgery for treatment of primary breast cancer. J Clin Oncol 1995; 13(3): 547–552.
70. Smith IE, Walsh G, Jones A et al. High complete remission rates with primary neoadjuvant infusional chemotherapy for large early breast cancer. J Clin Oncol 1995; 13(2): 424–429.
71. Smith JA, Gamez Aranjo JJ, Gallager HS, White EC, McBride CM. Carcinoma of the breast. Analysis of total lymph node involvement versus level of metastases. Cancer 1977; 39: 527–532.
72. Butcher H. Radical mastectomy for mammary carcinoma. Ann Surg 1969; 170: 883–884.
73. Haagensen CD. Diseases of the Breast (rev. 2nd Edn). Philadelphia, WB Saunders, 1971, pp. 384–390.
74. Du Toit RS, Locker AP, Ellis IO, Elston CW, Blamey RW. Evaluation of the prognostic value of triple node biopsy in early breast cancer. Br J Surg 1990; 77: 163–167.
75. Sauerbrei W, Hubner K, Schmoor C, Schumacher M. Validation of existing and development of new prognostic classification schemes in node negative breast cancer. German Breast Cancer Study Group. Breast Cancer Res Treat 1997; 42(2): 149–163.
76. Todd JH, Dowle C, Williams MR et al. Confirmation of a prognostic index in primary breast cancer. Br J Cancer 1987; 56: 489–492.
77. Kjaergaard J, Blickert-Toft M, Anderson JA, Rank R, Pedersen BV. (Danish Breast Cancer Cooperative Group). Probability of false negative nodal staging in conjunction with partial axillary dissection in breast cancer. Br J Surg 1985; 72(5): 365–367.
78. Stewart HJ, Everington D, Forrest APM. The Cardiff local therapy trial – results at 20 years. The Breast 1994; 3: 40–45.
79. Forrest APM, Everington D, McDonald CC, Steele RJ, Chetty U, Stewart HJ. The Edinburgh randomised trial of axillary sampling or clearance after mastectomy. Br J Surg 1995; 82: 1504–1508.
80. Steele RJC, Forrest APM, Gibson T et al. The efficacy of lower axillary sampling in obtaining lymph node status in breast cancer; a controlled randomised trial. Br J Surg 1985; 72: 368–369.
81. Krag D, Weaver D, Ashikaga T et al. The sentinel node in breast cancer – a multicenter validation study. N Engl J Med 1998; 339(14): 941–946.
82. Krag DN, Weaver DL, Alex JC et al. Surgical resection and radiolocalization of the sentinel lymph node in breast cancer using gamma probe. Surg Oncol 1993; 2: 335–340.
83. Bonnema J, van Geel AN, Ooijen B et al. Ultrasound-guided aspiration biopsy for detection of nonpalpable axillary node metastases in breast cancer patients: new diagnostic method. World J Surg 1997; 21(3): 270–274.
84. Yang WT, Ahuja A, Tang A, Suen M, King W, Metreweli C. High resolution sonographic detection of axillary lymph node metastases in breast cancer. J Ultrasound Med 1996; 15(3): 241–246.
85. Verbanck J, Vandewiele I, De Winter H, Tytgat J, Van Aelst F, Tanghe W. Value of axillary ultrasonography and sonographically guided puncture of axillary nodes: a prospective study in 144 consecutive patients. J Clin Ultrasound 1997; 25(2): 53–56.
86. Mussurakis S, Buckley DL, Horsman A. Prediction of axillary lymph node status in invasive breast cancer with dynamic contrast-enhanced MR staging. Radiology 1997; 203(2): 317–321.
87. Avril N, Dose J, Janicke F, et al. Assessment of axillary lymph node involvement in breast cancer patients with positron emission tomography using radiolabeled 2-(fluorine-18)-fluoro-2-deoxy-glucose. J Natl Cancer Inst 1996; 88(17): 1204–1209.
88. Smith IC, Ogston KN, Whitford P, et al. Staging of the axilla in breast cancer: accurate in vivo assessment using positron emission tomography with 2-(fluorine-18)-fluoro-2-deoxy-D-glucose. Ann Surg 1998; 228(2); 220–227.
89. Khalkhali I. New horizons in breast imaging: A complementary role of technetium 99m sestamibi for the

diagnosis and staging of breast carcinoma. Breast J 1996; 2: 23–25.
90. Taillefer R, Robidoux A, Lambert R, Turpin S, Laperriere J. Technetium-99m-sestamibi prone scintimammography to detect primary breast cancer and axillary lymph node involvement. J Nucl Med 1995; 36(10): 1758–1765.
91. Ravdin PM, De Laurentiis M, Vendely T, Clark GM. Prediction of axillary lymph node status in breast cancer patients by use of prognostic indicators. J Natl Cancer Inst 1994; 86(23): 1771–1775.
92. Zanon C, Durando A, Geuna M, et al. Flow cytometry in breast cancer: prognostic and surgical indications of the sparing of axillary lymph node dissection. Am J Clin Oncol 1998; 21(4): 392–397.
93. Noguchi M, Thomas M, Kitagawa H, et al. DNA ploidy and helix pomatia lectin binding as predictors of regional lymph node metastases and prognostic factors in breast cancer. Breast Cancer Res Treat 1993; 26(1): 67–75.
94. Gui GP, Wells CA, Browne PD, et al. Integrin expression in primary breast cancer and its relation to axillary nodal status. Surgery 1995; 117(1): 102–108.
95. Shering SG, Sherry F, McDermott EW, OHiggins NJ, Duffy MJ. Preoperative CA 15-3 concentrations predict outcome of patients with breast cancer. Cancer 1998; 83(12): 2521–2527.
96. Duffy MJ, Duggan C, Mulcahy HE, McDermott EW, OHiggins NJ. Urokinase plasminogen activator: a prognostic marker in breast cancer including patients with axillary node-negative disease. Clin Chem 1998; 44(6 Pt 1): 1177–1183.
97. McGuckin MA, Walsh MD, Hohn BG, Ward BG, Wright RG. Prognostic significance of MUC1 epithelial mucin expression in breast cancer. Hum Pathol 1995; 26(4): 432–439.
98. Jansen RH, Joosten Achjanie SR, Arends JW, et al. CD44v6 is not a prognostic factor in primary breast cancer. Ann Oncol 1998; 9(1): 109–111.
99. Foekens JA, Look MP, Bolt de Vries J, et al. Cathepsin D in primary breast cancer: prognostic evaluation involving 2810 patients. Br J Cancer 1999; 79(2): 300–307.
100. Tan P, Cady B, Wanner M, et al. The cell cycle inhibitor p27 is an independent prognostic marker in small (T1a,b) invasive breast cancer. Cancer Res 1997; 57(7): 1259–1263.
101. Ross JS, Fletcher JA. The HER-2/ neu oncogene in breast cancer: prognostic factor, predictive factor and target for therapy. Stem Cells 1998; 16(6): 413–428.
102. Pegram MD, Lipton A, Hayes DF, et al. Phase II study of receptor-enhanced chemosensitivity using recombinant humanized anti-p185HER2/neu monoclonal antibody plus cisplatin in patients with HER2/neu-overexpressing metastatic breast cancer refractory to chemotherapy treatment. J Clin Oncol 1998; 16(8): 2659–2671.
103. Slamon D, Leyland-Jones B, Shak S, et al. Addition of HerceptinTM (humanized Anti-HER2 antibody) to first line chemotherapy for HER2 overexpressing metastatic breast cancer (HER2+ / MBC) markedly increases anticancer activity: a randomized multinational controlled phase III trial. Proc ASCO 1998; abstract: 377.
104. Fisher B, Montague E. Comparison of radical mastectomy with alternative treatments for primary breast cancer. Cancer 1977; 39: 2829–2839.
105. Graverson HP, Blichert Toff M, Anderson JA et al. Breast cancer, risk of axillary recurrence in node negative patients following partial dissection of the axilla. Eur J Surg Oncol 1988; 14: 407–412.
106. Kissen MW, Querci della Rovere G, Easton D, Westbury G. Risk of lymphoedema following the treatment of breast cancer. Br J Surg 1986; 73: 580–584.
107. Tasmuth T, Blomqvist C, Kalso E. Chronic post-treatment symptoms in patients with breast cancer operated in different surgical units. Eur J Surg Oncol 1999; 25: 38–43.
108. Sosa JA, Diener West M, Gusev Y et al. Association between extent of axillary lymph node dissection and survival in patients with stage I breast cancer. Ann Surg Oncol 1998; 5(2): 140–149.
109. Bataini JP, Picco C, Martin M, Calle R. Relation between time-dose and local control of operable breast cancer treated by tumorectomy and radiotherapy or by radical radiotherapy alone. Cancer 1978; 42: 2059–2065.
110. Fletcher GH. Local results of irradiation in the primary management of localised breast cancer. Cancer 1972; 29: 545–551.
111. Amalric R, Santamaria F, Robert F, et al. Radiation therapy with or without primary limited surgery for operable breast cancer. Cancer 1982; 49: 30–34.
112. Mazeron JJ, Otmezguine Y, Huart J, Pierquin B. Conservative treatment of breast cancer: results of management of axillary lymph node area in 3353 patients (letter). Lancet 1985; 1: 1387.
113. Haffty BG, McKhann C, Beinfield M, et al. Breast conservation therapy without axillary dissection. A rational treatment strategy in selected patients. Arch Surg 1993; 128: 1315–1319.
114. Recht A, Pierce SM, Abner A et al. Regional nodal failure after conservative surgery and radiotherapy for early-stage breast carcinoma. J Clin Oncol 1991; 9: 988–991.
115. Cabanes PA, Salmon RJ, Vilcoq et al. Value of axillary dissection in addition to lumpectomy and radiotherapy in early breast cancer. Lancet 1992; 339: 1245–1248.
116. Wazer DE, Erban JK, Robert NJ et al. Breast conservation in elderly women for clinically negative lymph

nodes without axillary dissection. Cancer 1994; 74: 878–883.

117. Pierce SM, Recht A, Lingos T, et al. Long-term radiation complications following conservative surgery (CS) and radiation therapy (RT) in patients with early stage breast cancer. Int J Radiat Oncol Biol Phys 1992; 23: 915–923.

118. Kurtz JM, Amalric R, Brandone H, Ayme Y, Spitalier JM. Contralateral breast cancer and other second malignancies in patients treated by breast-conserving therapy with radiation. Int J Radiat Oncol Biol Phys 1988; 15(2): 277–284.

119. Taghiam A, Florent de Vathair P, Terrier P, et al. Long term risk of sarcoma following radiation treatment for breast cancer. Int J Radiat Oncol Biol Phys 1991; 21: 361–367.

120. Anonymous. Effects of radiotherapy and surgery in early breast cancer. An overview of the randomised trials. Early Breast Cancer Trialists' Collaborative Group. N Engl J Med 1995; 333(22): 1444–1455.

121. Cuzick J, Stewart H, Rutqvist L, et al. Cause-specific mortality in long-term survivors of breast cancer who participated in trials of radiotherapy. J Clin Oncol 1994; 12: 447–453.

122. Larson D, Weinstein M, Goldberg I, et al. Edema of the arm as a function of the extent of axillary surgery in patients with stage I–II carcinoma of the breast treated with primary radiotherapy. Int J Radiat Oncol Biol Phys 1986; 12: 1575–1582.

123. Delouche G, Bachelot F, Premont M, Kurtz J. Conservation treatment of early breast cancer: long term results and complications. Int J Radiat Oncol Biol Phys 1987; 13: 29–34.

124. Fisher B, Wolmark N, Bauer M, Redmond C, Gebhardt M. The accuracy of clinical nodal staging and of limited axillary dissection as a determinant of histologic nodal status in carcinoma of the breast. Surg Gynecol Obstet 1981; 152: 765–772.

125. Stotter A, Atkinson EN, Fairston B. Survival following locoregional recurrence after breast conservation therapy for cancer. Ann Surg 1990; 221(2): 166–172.

126. McCready DR, Hortobagyi GN, Kau SW, Smith TL, Buzdar AU, Balch CM. The prognostic significance of lymph node metastases after preoperative chemotherapy for locally advanced breast cancer. Arch Surg 1989; 124: 21–25.

Breast Cancer: Diagnosis and Management
J.M. Dixon (Ed.)

CHAPTER 31

Sentinel node biopsy

V. Galimberti, R. Gennari and F. Zerwes

1. Introduction

Following some years of controversy, and a number of important clinical trials, it is now accepted that breast conservation is the optimal approach for small-sized breast tumours [1–4]. Unfortunately things are not so straightforward when considering axillary dissection. Controversy has raged about axillary dissection for many years. Many surgeons today question the need for axillary dissection [5–7], while others, convinced by the findings of large-scale studies, continue to insist that axillary dissection is an integral part of the management of breast cancer; affirming that complete axillary dissection is important not only for staging, but also as a treatment [8–10].

Axillary lymph nodes are the most frequent site of metastases from breast cancer. Previous studies have shown that metastatic spread to the axilla proceeds in an orderly and progressive fashion from the first to the second level and then to the third level, with skip metastases occurring in only 2–6% of cases [11].

Skip metastases — involvement of level II or level III nodes in the absence of level I involvement is rare.

The number and level of axillary involvement is of independent prognostic value [12] and complete axillary dissection is a definitive treatment for the axilla, and is associated with a risk of local failure that is close to zero. However for patients who have non-involved nodes, the dissection is useless as a treatment and undesirable from the patient's point of view; it involves loss of immunocompetent tissue and there are potential immediate or late sequelae, including lymphoedema, paraesthesia, seroma, pain, infection and limitation of arm movement [13,14]. These considerations are becoming more important with the changing presentation of breast cancer. As breast malignancies are diagnosed earlier, the average size of lesions is smaller, and the probability of axillary involvement decreases [15–17]. Risk of axillary metastases is directly related to the size of the primary lesion. When the primary is less than 1 cm in diameter, the risk of axillary metastasis is about 10%; whereas in tumours larger than 5 cm in diameter, the risk increases to greater than 70% [18].

Considerations such as these have re-ignited the controversy over axillary dissection in breast cancer and point to the need for a non-invasive, or minimally invasive method to reliably predict the status of the axilla preoperatively. However, the currently available non-surgical methods for evaluating the axilla are inadequate. Neither ultrasonography (including colour Doppler) [19–21], nor lymphangiography, nor lymphoscintigraphy are able to determine the presence or extent of axillary lymph node involvement [22–24], while positron emission tomography (PET) [25–27] and magnetic resonance imaging (MRI) [28] are still experimental modalities being evaluated to assess the presence of micrometastases in axillary lymph nodes.

2. The sentinel node concept

The concept is that cancer cells from the primary tumour are carried in the lymph channels to the first lymph node to receive drainage from the cancer (Fig. 1). They are held in this node for some time but may migrate elsewhere later.

This concept is not new. Oliver Cope referred to the 'Delphian node' in 1963 as the node which could reveal the nature of a pathological process involving a nearby organ [29]. In 1977 Cabanes described a specific lymph node centre which he called the sentinel lymph node, in the context of penile cancer [30]. This node was identified by lymphangiograms and located anatomically around the superficial epigastric vein; it was almost always the first site of metastases and was frequently the only involved node. However, the validity of the sentinel node concept was first clearly demonstrated by Morton more than ten years ago. He and his colleagues injected blue dye close to the site of cutaneous melanoma and dissected along the blue lymphatic ducts to reach the first (blue) node [31]. Various dyes (patent blue and isosulfan blue) have been used in an attempt to optimise both the kinetics of transport in lymph channels and the uptake by the first lymph node (sentinel node).

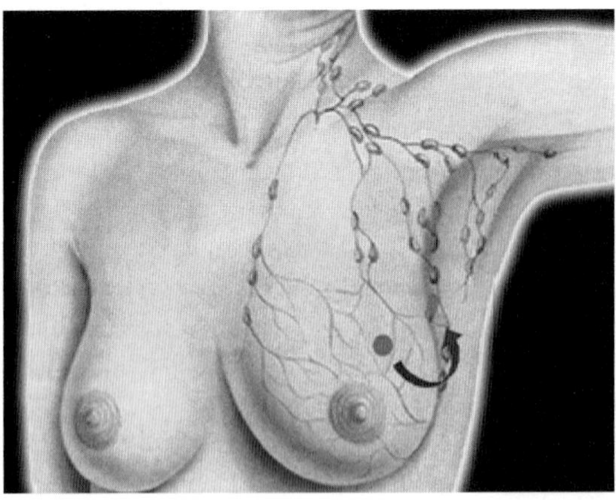

Fig. 1.

The sentinel node is the first lymph node to receive lymph from the area of the breast containing a cancer.

3. Methods for localising the sentinel node in breast cancer

The blue dye method is also used in breast cancer, alone or in association with other techniques [32] to identify the first node to receive lymph from the area containing the tumour. Our group and others have carried out extensive studies with microcolloid particles labelled with radioactive technetium [33–36]. Use of radioactive material allows identification of the sentinel lymph node by means of lymphoscintigraphy and, importantly, allows use of a gamma probe during surgery to locate precisely the sentinel node and guide its removal through a small incision. Following injection of colloid into the parenchyma or subdermis close to the primary tumour, the marker migrates to the sentinel node. Rates of identification of the sentinel node range from 94% to 98%, with false negative rates of 2.3% and 4.7% respectively [33,37]. Using the blue dye alone involves dissection along the blue-labelled lymphatic channels until the blue node (or nodes) are located; published rates of sentinel node identification using this technique are in the range 65% to 93%, with false negative rates from 0 to 12% [38,39].

The sentinel node can be identified using a blue dye, a radiolabelled colloid or a combination of the two.

Various types of colloid, of varying size ranges, have been used in the radioactive tracer method, including antimony sulphide average size < 50 nm, human serum albumin (HSA) < 80 nm and HSA 200–1000 nm. Studies are still underway to identify the most appropriate colloid particle for use in clinical practice. The characteristics required are mobility within lymphatic channels, and stable retention by the sentinel node, with little or no subsequent migration to other nodes in the lymphatic chain. Variations in these characteristics permit different centres to vary the time between particle injection, visualisation of the sentinel node by lymphoscintigraphy, and surgical removal of the sentinel node, according to their needs.

Our experience [40] is that large size HSA particles move relatively quickly within the lymph channels to reveal the lymphatic tree by lymphoscintigraphy in about 20 minutes, while they are retained fairly efficiently by the first node so that generally only one sentinel node is identified (Fig. 2). This is important for intraoperative frozen section analysis, which is time consuming and if several nodes are consistently revealed intraoperative analysis time is prolonged.

The colloid is injected into parenchyma around the breast mass with a long 25 gauge needle if the tumour is deep, otherwise it is injected subdermally above the lesion if the cancer is superficial. Following injection, the site is massaged for a few minutes to facilitate lymph flow. The total injection volume should not be more than 0.5 ml as larger volumes can impede flow.

Typically after just 20 minutes the lymphatic path to the sentinel node is visible on lymphoscintigraphic scans (as well as the injection site). Fig. 3 shows that the tracer has moved in two directions: towards the axilla and towards the internal mammary chain. This is a relatively rare occurrence. As soon as the sentinel node is identified, its position is marked on the overlying skin.

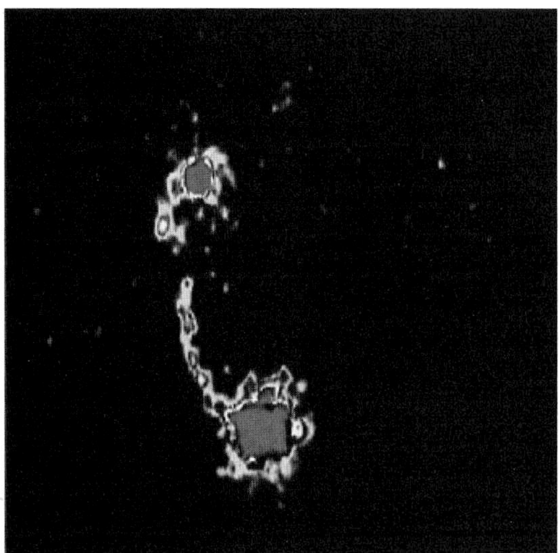

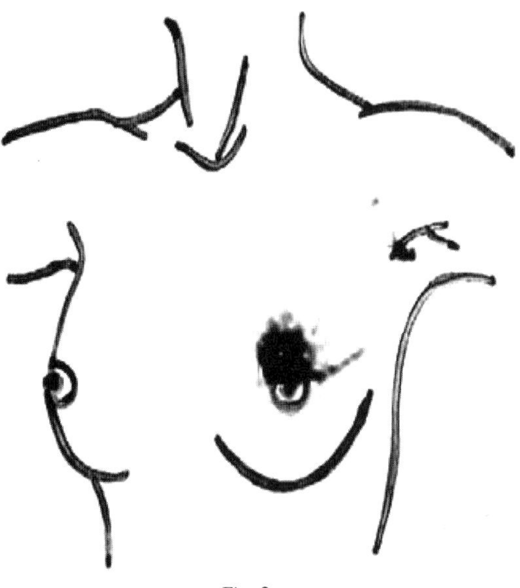

Fig. 2.

4. Surgery

Surgery is usually performed the next day. After removal of the primary tumour, sentinel node biopsy begins, using the previously made skin marker as a guide. The gamma probe in a sterile sleeve is used to locate the sentinel node precisely (the skin marker may move relative to the underlying tissue), and a 2–3 cm skin incision is made over the hot spot (Fig. 4). If the lesion is in the upper-outer quadrant, we use the probe to search for the sentinel node through the primary incision. Using the sounds emitted by the probe as a guide,

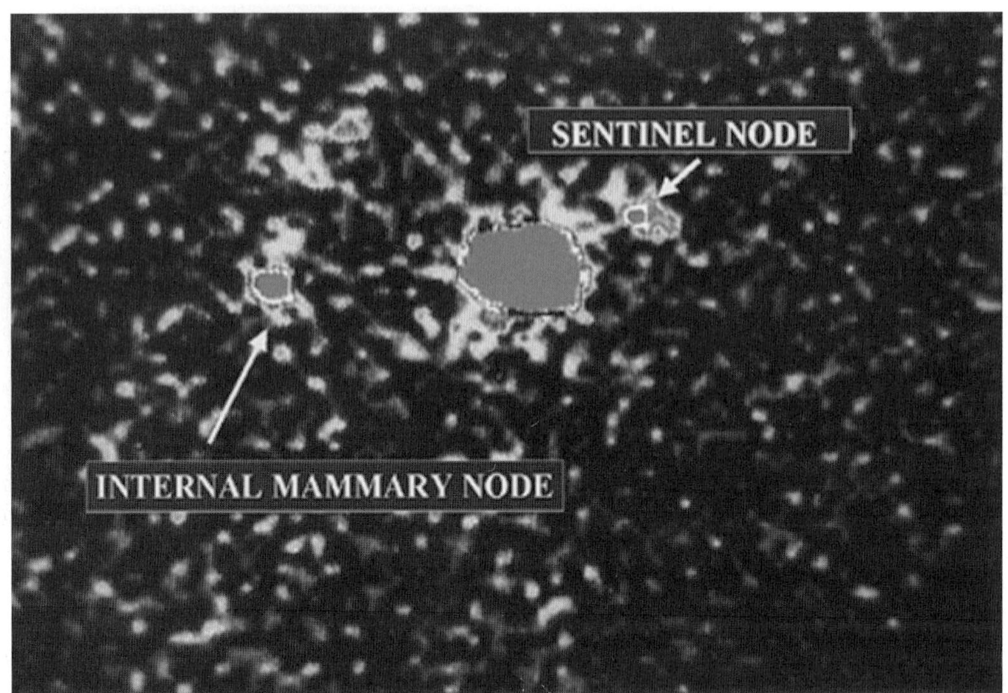

Fig. 3.

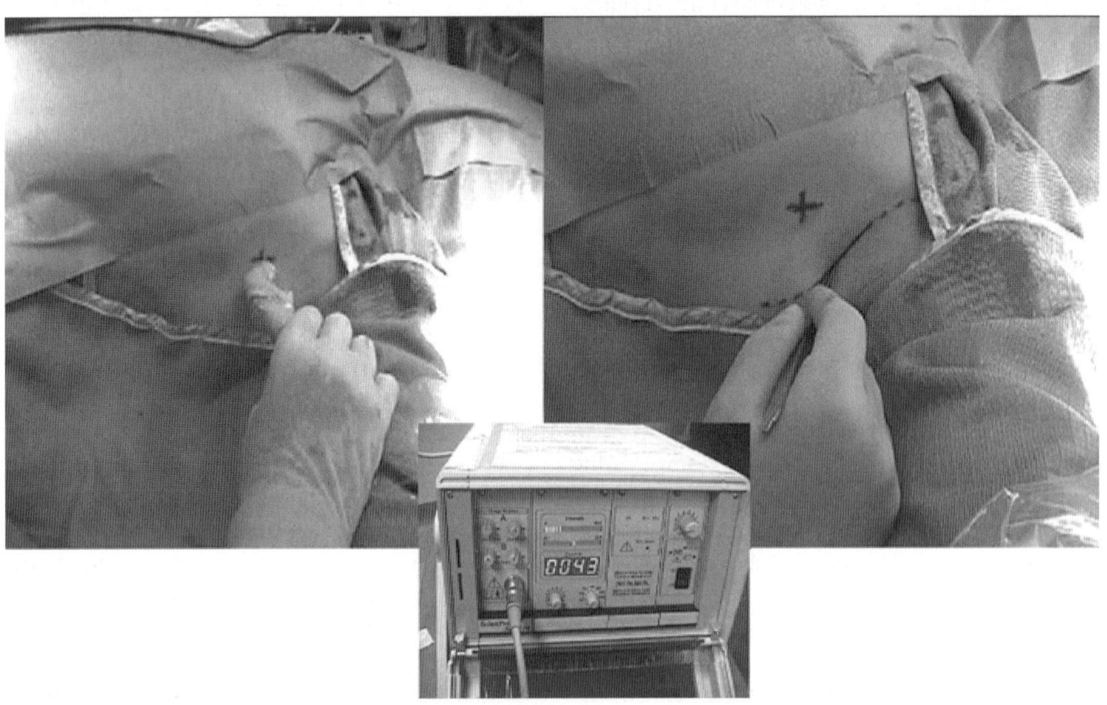

Fig. 4.

the sentinel node is isolated, removed and tagged separately and sent for frozen section analysis. After the sentinel node has been removed the operating field is checked for residual radioactivity: any remaining hot spots are removed and the node with greatest radioactivity is identified.

If the blue dye method is used, the time between injection and the axillary incision is critical: if performed too early no nodes are revealed, and if performed too late a large number of nodes have taken up the blue dye. Furthermore, with this method one has to dissect along the blue lymphatic which runs from the lesion until a blue node is found. This involves considerable surgical skill and a period of training before full competence is reached. By contrast, use of the gamma probe to identify and remove radioactive nodes, requires no additional training and no more than routine surgical skill.

However use of radioactive tracer does require the backup of a Nuclear Medicine Department. Both the blue dye and tracer methods seem to be equally accurate in identifying the sentinel node.

5. Pathological examination

If the sentinel method is to be used to select patients for complete axillary dissection the pathological examination of the sentinel node should be exhaustive and reliable, and should be performed intraoperatively. In our initial experience of 192 cases in which sentinel nodes were examined by conventional frozen section, we found 26 false negatives which had involvement on paraffin section histology, giving a concordance of 86.5%. This is too low to use the method to decide whether or not to perform axillary dissection.

Examination of the sentinel nodes by standard frozen section techniques is insufficiently sensitive for routine use.

We therefore devised a new method of intraoperative frozen section examination. This involves bisecting the node along its major axis. Both halves are embedded and frozen in liquid nitrogen–isopentane. Fifteen pairs of 4 μm sections are taken every 50 μm from each half node (total 60 sections). If material remains further pairs of sections are taken every 100 μm until all the node has been examined. One section of each pair is stained with hematoxylin and eosin. If these are negative or doubtful the other section of the pair is immunostained for cytokeratin. Our studies with this method have shown that the main factor which increases reliability of cancer cell detection has been increasing the number of sections examined, not the immunohistochemical staining [41]. From the surgical point of view the disadvantage is that it requires about 40 minutes, so that the surgeons can complete the breast surgery or breast reconstruction while waiting for the histological result.

6. Results obtained at the European Institute of Oncology

We now have sentinel node data on 376 patients [42]. Initially we performed a pilot study to determine the feasibility of isolating the sentinel node surgically with the aid of the gamma probe, and investigated how often the sentinel was metastatic in comparison to involvement of other axillary nodes. We enrolled patients scheduled to receive breast surgery combined with complete axillary dissection but with impalpable axillary nodes. The sentinel node was found and removed in all but five patients, where lymphoscintigraphy revealed no movement of radioactivity and it was impossible to identify any sentinel node using the gamma probe. A sentinel node was therefore identified in 98.7%.

The sentinel node was metastatic in 168 of the 371 patients. In 191 cases all axillary nodes were negative, while in 12 patients the sentinel node was free of disease but other nodes were positive for micrometastases, giving a concordance of 96.8% (Table 1). In 3 of these 12 patients the primary tumour was multifocal and in the other 9 patients there was peritumoural vascular invasion

Table 1.

PREDICTIVE VALUE OF SENTINEL NODE

Sentinel Node	Axillary nodes	N°
Positive	Positive	168
Negative	Negative	191
Negative	Positive	12
Total		371
Concordance	359/371 (96.8%)	

and/or the tumour location was in an inner quadrant. Following these findings we no longer use the sentinel node method in patients with multifocal tumours because they appear to be associated with a high rate of axillary involvement when the sentinel node is negative. From a biological point of view a multifocal tumour is likely to have more than one lymphatic pathway to the axilla so that a single sentinel node is less likely to predict the real state of the axilla in such patients.

Results with sentinel node assessment show that it is frequently the only axillary node involved and have confirmed that in the majority of patients it accurately reflects the status of all axillary nodes.

We have recently also started removing sentinel nodes from the internal mammary chain. Lymphoscintigraphy occasionally reveals that lymph flow from a tumour area is to the internal mammary chain. This occurs more often if the tumour is located in an inner quadrant. To remove a sentinel node in this chain the longitudinal fibres of the pectoralis major are separated to expose the rib cage. A section of intercostal muscle is removed above the hot spot and the sentinel node is located and removed without difficulty with the aid of the probe, taking care not to damage the underlying pleura.

Sentinel nodes can be in the internal mammary chain but are most commonly located in the lower axilla.

Our overall results indicate that the sentinel node can accurately predict the status of the axilla, so it would seem that when the sentinel node is negative axillary dissection can be avoided. Furthermore, in approximately 40% of cases with axillary involvement, the sentinel node is the only metastatic node, and this demonstrates the validity of the sentinel concept.

Following our initial findings we started a randomised trial in March 1998. For patients with pathological tumour size up to 2 cm, treatment consists of a Veronesi quadrantectomy plus radiotherapy. In the operating room patients are randomised to receive either immediate axillary dissection or sentinel node biopsy (Table 2). Patients with negative sentinel node biopsy receive quadrantectomy only, those with a positive sentinel node biopsy undergo axillary dissection. In all cases adjuvant treatment is decided on the basis of biological factors determined on the primary tumour and on nodal status. In all cases, even those randomised to receive total axillary dissection, lymphoscintigraphy is performed, and the sentinel node is identified and examined in exactly the same way as the sentinel node in the other arm of the trial so that the staging in both arms is identical.

Table 2.

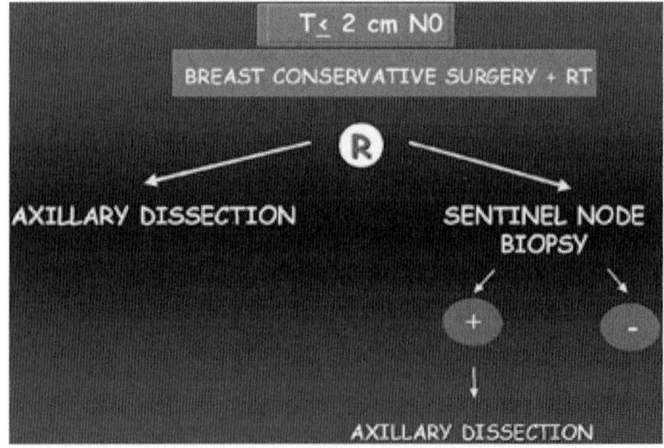

The objectives of the trial are (i) to compare the number of axillary relapses in the two study arms, and (ii) to assess overall survival and disease-free survival in both arms. We hope this study will validate sentinel node biopsy as a method of predicting the overall state of the axilla, so that if this node is negative the axilla can be safely left alone.

References

1. Veronesi U, Salvadori B, Luini A et al. Breast conservation is a safe method in patients with small cancer of the breast. Long-term results of three randomized trials on 1,973 patients. Eur J Cancer, 1995; 31(10): 1574–1579.
2. Fisher B, Redmond C, Poisson R et al. Eight years results of NSABP randomized clinical trial comparing total mastectomy and lumpectomy with or without radiation in the treatment of breast cancer. N Engl J Med, 1989; 320(13): 822–828.
3. Fisher B. Lumpectomy (segmental mastectomy) and axillary dissection. In Bland KI, Copeland EM (eds). The Breast, Saunders, Philadelphia, 1991; pp. 643–652.
4. Arriagada R, Le MG, Rochard F, Contesso G. Conservative treatment versus mastectomy in early breast cancer: patterns of failure with 15 years of follow-up data. Institute Gustave-Roussy Breast Cancer Group. J Clin Oncol 1996; 14(5): 1558–1564.
5. Fisher B, Redmond C, Fisher ER et al. Ten-years results of a randomized trial comparing radical mastectomy with or without radiation. N Engl J Med 1985, 14; 312(11): 674–681.
6. Cady B. The needs to reexamine axillary lymph node dissection in invasive breast cancer. Cancer 1994, 1; 73(3): 505–508.
7. Haffty BG, Ward B, Pathare P, Salem R et al. Reappraisal of the role of axillary lymph node dissection in the conservative treatment of breast cancer. J Clin Oncol, 1997; 15(2): 691–700.
8. Cabanes PA, Salomon RJ, Vilcoq JR, Durand JC et al. Value of axillary dissection in addition to lumpectomy and radiotherapy in early breast cancer. The Breast Carcinoma Collaborative Group of the Institut Curie. Lancet 1992, 23; 339(8804): 1245–1248.
9. Harris JR, Osteen RT. Breast Cancer Res Treat 1985; 5(1): 17–21.
10. Recht A. Nodule treatment for patients with early stage breast cancer: guilty or innocent? Radiother Oncol 1992; 25(2): 79–82.
11. Veronesi U, Rilke F, Luini A et al. Distribution of axillary node metastases by level of invasion: an analysis of 539 cases. Cancer 1986; 59: 682–687.
12. Veronesi U, Luini A, Galimberti V et al. Extent of metastatic axillary involvement in 1444 cases of breast cancer. Eur J Surg Oncol 1990; 16: 127–133.
13. Larson D, Weinstein M, Goldberg I et al. Edema of the arm as a function of the extent of axillary surgery in patients with stage I–II carcinoma of the breast treated with primary radiotherapy. Int J Rad Onc Biol Phys 1986; 12: 1575–1582.
14. Warmuth MA, Boven G, Prosnitz LR et al. Complications of axillary lymph node dissection for carcinoma of the breast: a report based on a patient survey. Cancer 1998, 1; 83(7): 1362–1368.
15. Tubiana M, Holland R, Kopans DB et al. Commission of the European Communities 'Europe Against Cancer' Programme. European School of Oncology Advisory Report. Management of non-palpable and small lesions found in mass breast screening. Eur J Cancer 1994; 30: 538–547.
16. Tabar L, Fageberg C, Duffy SW, Day NE, Gad A, Grontoft O. Update of Swedish two-country program of mammographic screening for breast cancer. Radiol Clin Nort Am 1992; 30: 187–210.
17. Baxter N, McCready D, Chapman JA et al. Clinical behavior of untreated axillary nodes after local treatment for primary breast cancer. Ann Oncol 1996; 3(3): 235–240.
18. Graversen HP, Toft MB, Andersen JA et al. Breast cancer: risk of axillary recurrence in node-negative patients following partial dissection of the axilla. Eur J Surg Onc 1998; 14: 497–412.
19. Ilkhanipour ZS, Harris KM, Staigler MJ, Ganott MA. Characteristics of axillary adenopathy as a predictor of malignancy at mammography and sonography [abstract]. Radiology 1993; 189(P): 244.
20. Allan SM, Kedar RP; Cosgrove DO, Sacks NPM. Axillary staging in breast cancer by colour Doppler ultrasound [abstract]. Br J Radiol 1993; 66(Suppl): 15.
21. Chang D, Chagla L, Lea R, Cade D. Can colour Doppler ultrasonography accurately assess axillary node status in breast cancer patients? Br J Surg 1994; 81(Suppl): 19.
22. Black RB, Taylor TV, Merrick MV, Forrest APM. Prediction of axillary metastases in breast cancer by lymphoscintigraphy. Lancet 1980; 2: 15–17.
23. Hill NS, Ege GN, Greyson ND, Mahoney LJ, Jirish DW. Predicting nodal metastases in breast cancer by lymphoscintigraphy. Can J Surg 1983; 26: 507–509.
24. Hughes K, Nabi H, Barron B et al. Radioimmunodetection (RAID) of operable breast cancer with 99mTc-labeled anti-CEA Fab fragment [abstract]. Proc Am Soc Clin Oncol 1995; 14: 101.
25. Hoh CK, Lee MH, Rege S, Glaspy J, Bassett LW, Hawkins RA. Whole-body PET with FDG: a potential complementary imaging technique to mammogra-

phy for detection of primary, recurrent, and metastatic breast cancer [abstract]. Radiology 1993; 189(P): 148.

26. Adler LP, Crowe JP, Al-Kaisi NK, Sunshine JL. Evaluation of breast masses and axillary lymph nodes with (F-18) 2-deoxy-2-fluoro-D-glucose PET. Radiology 1993; 187: 743–750.
27. Niewg OE, Kim EE, Wong W-H et al. Positron emission tomography with fluorine-18-deoxyglucose in the detection and staging of breast cancer. Cancer 1993; 71: 3920–3925.
28. Allan SM, McVicar D, Sacks NPM. Prospects for axillary staging in breast cancer by magnetic resonance imaging [abstract]. Br J Radiol 1993; 66 (Suppl): 15–16.
29. Cope O. Surgery of the Thyroid and its Diseases. JH Means, LJ DeGroot, JB Stamburry, Eds. McGraw-Hill, New York 1962; pp. 561–598.
30. Cabanas RM. An approach for the treatment of penile carcinoma. Cancer 1977; 39: 456–466.
31. Morton DL, Wen D-R, Wong JH et al. Technical details of intraoperative lymphatic mapping for early stagy melanoma. Arch Surg 1992; 127: 392–399.
32. Giuliano AE, Dale PS, Turner RR, Morton DL, Evans SW, Krasne DL. Improved axillary staging of breast cancer with sentinel lymphadenectomy. Ann Surg 1995; 222(3): 394–399.
33. Veronesi U, Paganelli G, Galimberti V et al. Sentinel node biopsy to avoid axillary dissection in breast cancer with clinically negative lymph nodes. The Lancet 1997; 349: 1864–1867.
34. Albertini JJ, Lyman GH, Cox C et al. Lymphatic mapping and sentinel node biopsy in the patient with breast cancer. JAMA 1996; 276: 1818–1822.
35. van der Veen H, Hoekstra OS, Paul MA, Cuesta MA, Meijr S. Gamma-probe-guided sentinel node biopsy to select patients with melanoma for lymphadenectomy. Br J Surg 1994; 81(12): 1769–1770.
36. Krag DN, Weaver DL, Alex JC, Fairbank JT. Surgical resection and radiolocalization of the sentinel node in breast cancer using a gamma probe. Surg Oncol 1993; 2: 335–339.
37. Pijpers R, Meijer S, Hockstra OS et al. Impact of lymphoscintigraphy on sentinel node identification with technetium 99m-colloidal albumin in breast cancer. J Nucl Med 1997; 38: 366–368.
38. Giuliano AE, Kirgan DM, Guenther JM, Morton DI. Lymphatic mapping and sentinel lymphadenectomy for breast cancer. Ann Surg 1994; 220: 391–398.
39. Giuliano AE, Jpnes RC, Brennan M, Statman R. Sentinale lymphadenectomy in breast cancer. J Clin Oncol 1997; 2345–2350.
40. De Cicco C, Cremonesi M, Luini A et al. Lymphoscintigraphy and radioguided biopsy of the sentinel axillary node in breast cancer. J Nucl Med 1998; 39(12): 2080–2084.
41. Viale G, Orvieto E, Bosari S. et al. Intraoperative examination of axillary sentinel nodes in breast cancer patients. Cancer (in press).
42. Veronesi U, Paganelli G, Viale G et al. Sentinel lymph node biopsy and axillary dissection in breast cancer: results in a large series. J Natl Cancer Inst 1999; 91(4): 368–373.

Breast Cancer: Diagnosis and Management
J.M. Dixon (Ed.)

CHAPTER 32

Axillary node sampling

U. Chetty

1. Introduction

In patients with invasive carcinoma of the breast the status of the axillary lymph nodes draining the tumour is an important factor predicting prognosis [1] and in planning both the locoregional and systemic therapy of the patient.

Many studies have been performed to find a pre-operative method of determining axillary lymph node status. Although some have shown promise there is no practical and reliable method available at present [2–4]. We therefore still require to examine the nodes histologically. Removing all the nodes (level III clearance) for examination is the gold standard. However, in those patients who are subsequently shown to be node negative, this is an unnecessary radical procedure. Several methods of axillary sampling have been tried. Cant and Forrest [5] initially reporting finding 'a constant' lymph node in the parenchymatous axillary tail, which if biopsied would stage the axilla. However, further studies from the same group [6] found no lymph nodes at this site in a third of cases and in those where a pectoral node was found, this did not reliably stage the axilla. They found that apparent node negative patients had a higher axillary node recurrence if no further treatment was given to the axilla. The technique of removing a single pectoral node was shown to be unsatisfactory. More extensive sampling was tried by several groups including a triple node sampling [7] and in Edinburgh, a four node sampling procedure. Targeted sentinel node biopsy using a combination of a blue dye and radiolabelled colloid or albumin has been shown to be promising and is discussed in detail in another chapter.

2. The four node sample technique

The aim of this procedure is to obtain at least four lymph nodes from the lower axillary fat. When performed at mastectomy the axillary tail is dissected off the serratus anterior muscle lying between the latissimus dorsi muscle posteriorly and the pectoral major muscle anteriorally. By palpating the axillary tail and lower axillary fat, four lymph nodes require to be identified and biopsied. If necessary the dissection is extended up to the intercostobrachial nerve which is preserved.

In patients being treated by a wide excision of the tumour (breast conservation) node sampling is performed through a separate transverse incision in the lower axilla, just below the hair bearing skin. The incision is deepened only through the subcutaneous fat being careful not to divide the axillary tail. The axillary tail is mobilised off the serratus anterior muscle between pectoralis major and latissimus dorsi. With fingers behind and in front of the axillary tail, starting inferiorally

Table 1.

Operation	No.	Mean no. of nodes	No. pts with involved nodes
Mx + ANS	203	4	88
Mx + ANC	203	20	80

Table 2.

Operation	No.	Mean no. nodes	No. pts with involved nodes
WLE + ANS	234	5	66
WLE + ANC	232	15	78

by palpation and inspection, at least four lymph nodes require to be identified and excised. It is the surgeon's responsibility to identify the nodes. Sending samples of fatty tissue and hoping lymph nodes are in it, has been shown to be inadequate [8,9].

3. Results

The efficacy of this technique was first assessed in patients being treated by a mastectomy [10]. 417 patients with operable breast cancer were randomised either to a node sample or a level III clearance. The rate of node positivity was the same in the two groups (Table 1).

The four node sample procedure was also evaluated in patients treated by breast conservation. 466 patients were randomised in the study of similar design to that above. This showed no statistical difference in survival or local recurrence (Table 2).

These two randomised studies demonstrate the efficacy of the axillary node sampling technique in determining the node status of the axilla.

Four node axillary sampling has been shown in prospective randomised studies to be an accurate method of assessing the presence or absence of involved axillary nodes.

Table 3.

Operation	Haematoma	Infection	Seroma	Hospital stay
Sample	3%	3%	0	2.25 days
Clearance	3%	9%	21%	7.5 days

4. Complications

We assessed the hospital in-patient stay and post-operative complications in 100 consecutive patients treated by breast conservation who were randomised either to a node sample or clearance. This showed that the node sample group had a shorter hospital stay and a lower incidence of wound infection and seroma infection (Table 3).

Patients in this randomised study were assessed pre-operatively and at 6, 12, 24 and 36 months after surgery for complications related to their range of movement, muscle power of the shoulder and swelling of the arm [11]. Some patients in the axillary node sample group were treated by radiotherapy to the axilla and assessment of morbidity was divided into three groups (node sample, no radiotherapy; node sample with radiotherapy; axillary node clearance with no radiotherapy). Patients who had a node sample without radiotherapy were found to have returned to pre-operative levels after six months with no detectable morbidity. Patients who had an axillary clearance were found to have an increased swelling of the arm and some restriction of abduction present three years after surgery. Patients who had a node sample and radiotherapy to the axilla had significant reduction in rotational movements of the shoulder.

Axillary sampling produces less short term and long term morbidity in node negative patients than axillary clearance. Axillary sampling followed in node positive patients by axillary radiotherapy is associated with significant reduction in rotational movements of the shoulder.

5. Conclusion

The four node sample technique has been shown in two randomised studies to stage reliably the axilla. However, others have reported difficulties using this technique [8,12]. The technique is operator dependent and relies largely on the surgeon to identify the nodes in a systematic way.

References

1. Carter CL, Allen C, Henson DE. Relation to tumour size, lymph node status and survival in 24,740 breast cancer cases. Cancer 1989; 63: 181–187.
2. Thompson CH, Stacker SA, Salehi N et al. Immunoscintigraphy for the detection of lymph node metastases from breast cancer. Lancet 1984; ii: 1245–1247.
3. Goldenberg DM, Wegner W. Studies of breast cancer imaging with radiolabelled antibodies to carcinoembryonic antigen. Immunomedics Breast Cancer Study Group. Acta Med Austr 1997; 24: 55–58.
4. Tjandra JJ, Russell IS, Collins JP et al. Immunolymphoscintigraphy for the detection of lymph node metastases from breast cancer. Cancer Res 1989; 49: 1600–1608.
5. Cant ELM, Shivas AA, Forrest APM. Lymph-node biopsy during simple mastectomy. Lancet 1975; i: 995–997.
6. Forrest APM, Roberts MM, Cant E. Simple mastectomy and pectoral node biopsy. Br J Surg 1976; 63: 569–575.
7. Du Toit RS, Coder AP, Ellis IO, Elston CW, Blamey RW. Evaluation of the prognostic value of triple node biopsy in early breast cancer. Br J Surg 1990; 77: 163–167.
8. Davies GC, Miller RR, Hayword JL. Assessment of axillary lymph node status. Ann Surg 1980; 192: 148–151.
9. Axelsson CK, Mouridsen HT, Zederler K. Axillary dissection of level I and II lymph node is important in breast cancer classification. Eur J Cancer 1992; 28a: 1415–1418.
10. Forrest APM, Everington D, McDonald CC, Steele RJC, Chetty U, Stewart HJ. The Edinburgh randomized trial of axillary sampling or clearance after mastectomy. Br J Surg 1995; 82: 1504–1508.
11. Chetty U, Jack W, Prescott RJ, Tyler C, Rodger A. Management of the axilla in patients with operable breast cancer treated by breast conservation: a randomized trial. Br J Surg 1999; in press.
12. Kissin MW, Price AB, Thompson EM, Scavin G, Kark AE. The inadequacy of axillary sampling in breast cancer. Lancet 1982; i: 1210–1212.

Breast Cancer: Diagnosis and Management
J.M. Dixon (Ed.)

CHAPTER 33

Axillary lymph node dissection: level I and level II

Patrick Ivan Borgen

1. Introduction

The status of the axillary lymph nodes is the most important prognostic indicator in the management of breast cancer [1,2]. Debate exists concerning the magnitude of the therapeutic benefit of removing axillary lymph nodes, despite substantial and credible evidence that axillary metastases can metastasise [3–6]. Chemotherapy is relatively unreliable in sterilising axillary disease, and although radiotherapy is effective, the axilla is infrequently radiated [7]. Given these diagnostic and therapeutic implications, it therefore remains critically important that a surgeon is skilled in the performance of a meticulous level I and level II lymph node dissection (removal of all nodes at levels I and II). In this chapter, the indications for a level I and level II node dissection will be considered and the technique of performing these procedures discussed.

2. Indications

Indications for a level I and level II lymph node dissection are summarised in Table 1. The most common indication for this type of axillary dissection is a positive sentinel lymph node in an axilla in which the other nodes are not suspicious for metastatic disease. Other indications for this operation are a breast cancer greater than one centimetre in diameter, or the presence of lymphovascular invasion and either a failed sentinel lymph node mapping procedure or patient preference for a standard axillary dissection procedure. This operation is also appropriate if, during a standard node dissection, a palpable node is encountered in level I that is positive on frozen section, but the remainder of the axilla appears to be clear. We convert the operation to a level III node dissection in the following situations: if multiple nodes are involved, if the patient has a stage III breast cancer, if there is a positive lymph node at level II, if there is a positive interpectoral (Rotter's) node, or if the patient has multiple positive level I nodes. Level III axillary node dissection is covered elsewhere in this book.

> *A level I and level II dissection is indicated where low level I nodes are positive but the remainder of the axilla is considered unlikely to be involved.*

3. Technique

Historically, axillary node dissections have been performed under general endotracheal anaesthesia. Patients typically spend one night in the hospital and are discharged the next morning. Patients are taught to care for their drain and

Table 1. Indications for level I and level II axillary node dissection

1.	Positive sentinel lymph node in level I (remaining lymph nodes are not clinically suspicious)
2.	Failed sentinel lymph node mapping in a patient with a tumour greater than one centimetre or if tumour has lymphovascular invasion
3.	Encountering positive lymph nodes during a routine axillary dissection in which the high level I and/or level II lymph nodes appear to be clear clinically
4.	Grossly palpable level II nodes encountered during a level I dissection
5.	Patient with invasive ductal or lobular carcinoma of the breast who refuses sentinel node mapping and opts for more conventional approach
6.	Suspicious level II nodes on preoperative CT scan (standard extent of disease work-up)
7.	Positive level I nodes

record its output and are discharged with the drain in place. The drain is removed when total drainage over a 24-hour period is less than 30 ml. The recent development of sentinel lymph node mapping (discussed elsewhere in this book), during which the sentinel lymph node is removed under local anaesthesia with the patient sedated has led to increased interest in performing a level I and level II node dissection under local anaesthesia. This is possible and is not difficult in a thin patient; however, it is to be discouraged in the obese patient. There are two reasons for this recommendation. First, airway management is much more critical in the obese patient and it is safer to perform this operation with the airway fully controlled. Secondly, the extent of tissue loss and the amount of dissection required may, even with sedation, exceed dose limitations of the local anaesthetic employed.

4. Operative technique

A curvilinear incision at the inferior-most border of the hair-bearing area of the axilla gives excellent access and ensures a good cosmetic scar. Alternative incisions include an 'S'-shaped incision beginning high in the axilla near the edge of the pectoralis major, curving down along the hair-bearing area of the axilla, and then turning inferiorly and following the anterior border of the latissimus dorsi muscle. The former incision is used over 90% of the time in our institution. The latter incision is much more popular when a microvascular anastomosis to a free flap is contemplated and wide exposure of the thoracodorsal neurovascular bundle is required. Using the 'U' shaped incision, we use six Adair clamps, two on the superior flap, two on the inferior flap, and one in each corner. The skin of the subcutaneous tissues are placed under tension laterally, and the flaps down to the superficial fascia are created with electrocautery.

Either a 'U' shaped incision around the hair bearing skin of the axilla or a lazy-'S'-shaped incision between the pectoralis major and latissimus dorsi provides adequate access for a level I and II dissection and leaves a good cosmetic scar.

We raise the inferior flap first and carry this down to the interdigitation of the serratus anterior and latissimus dorsi muscles. It is very common to encounter the inferior extension of the focal epigastric branch of the axillary vein, and it is worthwhile identifying this and controlling it prior to dividing it with the electrocautery. Using the same technique, flaps are created laterally to the interior border of the latissimus dorsi muscle and medially to the lateral border of the pectoralis major. After identifying the pectoralis major, the pectoralis minor is identified and the interpectoral space is entered and explored, first with digital palpation and inspected visually. The superior flap is created last and carried down onto the axillary vein. A number of techniques can be used to identify the vein. We discourage the time-honoured recommendation of identifying the latissimus dorsi and following it superiorly to the so called white tendon. A known anatomic variation called Langer's arch exists in which a slip of latissimus dorsi courses anterior to the axillary vein instead of along the usual course posterior to the vein. This can lead the surgeon across the top of the vein and into the neurovascular bundle to the arm, where great harm can occur. We prefer to identify the vein just under the pectoralis minor, just superior to the 'Y'-shaped vessels of the medial pectoral neurovascular bundle. Having identified the vein it is exposed along its entire anterolateral surface. This can often be done with dissection along the top of the vein, as virtually no large vessels ever come off in this direction. At this point the anatomic boundaries are well delineated. The axillary vein lies superiorly, and beyond it lie the axillary artery and the brachial plexus. Laterally, the length of the latissimus dorsi is exposed down to its interdigitation with the serratus anterior. Medially, we see the chest wall and the pectoralis major and minor.

After the interpectoral space has been cleared and the trapezoidal boundaries of the axilla have been identified, blunt dissection is employed to mobilise the pectoralis minor off the axillary vein and its accompanying tissue. A small window can be created medially near the origin of the pectoralis minor, and at this point, the muscle can be either divided or encircled with a Penrose drain or a rigid retractor to facilitate access to level II. In obese patients where there is limited assistance, the pectoralis minor can be divided just below its origin on the coracoid process of the scapula to facilitate access. The division of this muscle results in minimal disability, as it is primarily an accessory muscle of respiration. Even athletic patients who have undergone division of this muscle report no weakness or physical limitation because of the division of the muscle.

At this point, it is possible to visualise the top of level II of the axilla (the medialmost border of the pectoralis minor). Level III nodes are always palpated and, if not suspicious, dissection does not go into level III. Carefully dissect along the axillary vein using blunt dissection where possible, and then either clip or tie perforating veins entering the axillary vein. Axillary contents at their apex are marked with the appropriate level II metallic tag to alert the pathologist of the location of the uppermost limits of the dissection. As the axillary contents are swept laterally, one encounters the highest intercostobrachial cutaneous nerve. If one wishes to preserve this nerve, and if it has not been divided in a creation of a lateral flap, it can be preserved by carefully dissecting it from the surrounding axillary tissue. This can be accomplished without fear of leaving lymph nodes behind. Several studies have suggested, however, that the tension on the nerve required to remove the axillary lymph nodes results in a nerve that is not completely functional.

The highest intercostobrachial nerve can usually be preserved without compromising the axillary dissection. Division of the nerve or too much tension on a preserved nerve usually results in an area of anaesthesia at the top of the arm.

In a patient with multiple level I lymph nodes from whome a full axillary dissection is contemplated the highest intercostobrachial cutaneous nerve is usually divided. The resulting disability from this is an anaesthetic area on the arm. Clipping the nerve can result in a painful neuroma and is to be discouraged.

In looking for the long thoracic nerve (of Bell), which lies along the chest wall, it is worth noting that it has a constant anatomic relationship to the highest intercostobrachial cutaneous nerve. The long thoracic nerve always lies posterior to the intercostal nerve, so it is not necessary to look for this nerve until the intercostobrachial nerve has been identified. Once this has been done, blunt dissection along the chest wall helps to identify the long thoracic nerve, and the enveloping fascia that often accompanies it. The enveloping fascia is first incised, and then the nerve is swept from the axillary contents by blunt dissection along the length of the chest wall, both superiorly and inferiorly, until it is completely out of harm's way against the chest wall. Division of the long thoracic nerve results in a winged scapula because of loss of tone of the serratus anterior, which arises from the medial aspect of the scapula anteriorly. The clinical manifestations of this are difficulty in abducting the arm beyond 90 degrees at the shoulder joint. This is a very rare nerve injury, occurring in less than 1% of carefully performed axillary node dissections.

Next, move laterally along the axillary vein, dividing perforating vessels. The thoracoepigastric vein, which comes off the axillary vein, is a good landmark to the thoracodorsal neurovascular bundle, which usually lies just deep to this vein. The thoracoepigastric vein is sacrificed and is divided between 3-0 vicryl ties or ligaclips. Blunt dissection will usually reveal the thoracodorsal nerve, which then leads to the identification of the thoracodorsal artery and vein.

A small pocket just posterior and inferior to the axillary vein is created between the long thoracic nerve and the thoracodorsal neurovascular bundle. The tissue is clamped with a Kocher clamp and divided. It is tied with a 2-0 vicryl suture. At this point the axillary contents between the nerves can be swept bluntly using a swab on one's index finger. If the thoracodorsal neurovascular bundle is clinically involved by malignant nodes, it should be sacrificed. Otherwise, it is preserved in its entirety. The most important step at this point is to ensure that the axillary contents of the breast tissue are in the axilla along the chest wall, and thus outside of your incision as you skeletonise the thoracodorsal neurovascular bundle. This greatly facilitates identification of perforating vessels coming in and out of the bundle and speeds the dissection process. The accessory artery and vein that course from the rib cage across the axilla to anastomose with the thoracodorsal neurovascular bundle remain untouched as we complete this process.

The long thoracic nerve and the thoracodorsal vessels are preserved routinely during axillary dissection.

There are virtually never any lymph nodes posterior to the thoracodorsal neurovascular bundle structure, and dividing it is unnecessary in the majority of cases. Level I is then marked with the appropriate level metallic tag, and the specimen is sent for routine pathologic sectioning. We drain the axilla with a standard seven or ten millimetre Jackson Pratt drain, which can be brought out just above or just below the incision. The drain is secured to the skin with a proline or nylon suture. The wound is copiously irrigated. We check for bleeders and for residual lymphatic tissue, and when we are satisfied, the wound is closed in two layers using a 3-0 absorbable suture on the deep tissues and a running 4-0 absorbable suture subcuticularly on the skin.

Typical estimated blood loss would be less than 20 ml for this procedure, and the need for blood transfusion would be extremely rare. The patient typically spends one night in the hospital and goes home with her drain in place the next morning. The Jackson Pratt drain is removed when the recorded volume over any 24-hour period falls below 30 cc. This typically requires five to ten days. The patients are encouraged to begin a gentle range of motion exercises on the second or third postoperative day. The more vigorous the exercises are, however, the larger the volume of fluid produced and the longer the drain will remain in place.

5. Conclusion

It is a common misconception that once breast cancer reaches the axillary lymph nodes, the disease is uniformly fatal [8–11]. The strongest evidence against this assumption lies in the fact that for over the first three quarters of this century, surgery was capable of bringing about a cure in 30–50% of patients, the majority of whom had disease in their axillary lymph nodes. In Frank

Adair's landmark 30-year follow-up of 1200 patients in whom he performed radical mastectomies followed by no further treatment, there were 30-year survivors in every single subset of patients with positive nodes except in the group that had a primary tumour greater than five cm with multiple involved level III axillary nodes. In every other subset, surgery alone was capable of achieving a 30-year cure [12].

It has long been recognised that axillary recurrence is associated with a very poor prognosis. While some would argue that this is evidence that axillary nodes are a marker for systemic disease, it can also be argued that axillary metastases can metastasise, and that these nodes, containing recurrent or persistent diseases, are a source rather than a marker of systemic dissemination. Given these considerations, axillary node dissection remains an important component of the overall treatment strategy for invasive breast cancer [13,14].

References

1. Fisher B. The evolution of paradigms for the management of breast cancer: A personal perspective. Cancer Res, 1992; 52: 2371–2383.
2. Fisher ER. The impact of pathology on the biologic, diagnostic, prognostic, and therapeutic considerations in breast cancer. Surg Clin North Am 1984; 64: 1073–1093.
3. Fisher B, Redmond C, Fisher ER, et al. Ten-year results of a randomized clinical trial comparing radical mastectomy and total mastectomy with or without radiation. N Engl J Med 1985; 312: 674–681.
4. Lythgoe JP, Palmer MK. Manchester regional breast study: 5 and 10 year results. Br J Surg 1982; 69: 693–696.
5. Graversen HP, Blichert-Toft M, Anderson JA, et al. Breast cancer: Risk of axillary recurrence in node-negative patients following partial dissection of the axilla. Eur J Surg Oncol 1988; 14: 407–412.
6. Harris JR, Osteen RT. Patients with early breast cancer benefit from effective axillary treatment. Breast Cancer Res Treat 1985; 5: 17–21.
7. Goldhirsch A, Wood WC, Senn HJ, et al. Meeting highlights: International consensus panel on the treatment of primary breast cancer. J Natl Cancer Inst 1995; 87: 1441–1445.
8. Cancer Research Campaign Working Party. Cancer research campaign (King's/Cambridge) trial for early breast cancer. Lancet July 1980; 12: 55–60.
9. Forrest APM, Roberts MM, Preece P, et al. The Cardiff-St. Mary's trial. Br J Surg 1975; 61: 766–769.
10. Stewart HJ. South-east Scottish trial of local therapy in node negative breast cancer. Breast 1994; 3: 31–39.
11. White RE, Vezeridis MP, Konstadoulakis M, et al. Therapeutic options and results for the management of minimally invasive breast cancer: Influence of axillary dissection for the treatment of T1a and T1b lesions. J Am Coll Surg 1996; 183: 575–582.
12. Adair F, Berg J, Joubert L, et al. Long term follow-up of breast cancer patients: The 30 year report. Cancer 1974; 33: 1145–1150.
13. Hellman S. Dogma and inquisition in medicine. Cancer 1993; 71: 2430–2433.
14. Hellman S. Natural history of small breast cancer. J Clin Oncol 1994; 12: 2229–2234.

Breast Cancer: Diagnosis and Management
J.M. Dixon (Ed.)

CHAPTER 34

Level III axillary dissection in breast cancer

Wolfgang Gatzemeier and Virgilio Sacchini

1. Introduction

Level III refers to the apex of the axilla which is the topmost region of the axillary lymph node chain. A separate dissection of this area is rarely performed whereas a biopsy of the apex as a staging procedure to select patients for further surgical treatment depending on the node status has been described by van Tienhoven [1] et al. In most cases surgical treatment of level III is part of a complete axillary dissection when breast conserving therapy, a modified radical or a radical mastectomy is performed. Within a wafer-thin fascia in continuity with the lower levels of the axilla the area of the third level comprises a variable amount of lymph nodes and lymphatic structures. Anatomically the 3rd level is bordered medially by Halsted's ligament, laterally by the medial edge of the pectoralis minor muscle, superiorly by the anterior aspect of the axillary vein and posteriorly/ inferiorly by the anterior chest wall (see Fig. 1).

Complete axillary dissection involves removing all nodes at level I, II and III.

The Halstedian concept of radical surgery to cure breast cancer — which dominated surgical thinking for nearly one century — failed due to the clinical observation, that most women with axillary metastases treated only by surgery died of breast cancer. Axillary surgery is therefore regarded by many as a staging procedure but it is important for the maintenance of local control even though it does not appear to affect survival. Recent reports suggesting that untreated metastases in the axilla can serve as the source of new metastases and result in decreased survival have led to a resurgence of interest in the potential therapeutic role of more aggressive local treatment i.e. axillary dissection including level III. Retrospective long-term studies of patients with small breast cancers with metastases involving 1 to 3 axillary nodes have demonstrated prolonged survival in two thirds of these patients following loco-regional treatment alone [2].

The risk of metastatic lymph nodes in higher levels increases markedly when lower levels are involved. When level I lymph nodes are positive, the level II nodes are involved in 41% and the level III nodes in 21% [3]. Whenever level II lymph nodes are positive, metastases of the lymph nodes belonging to level III have been reported in 30–40% [3–5]. In patients with 1–3 positive level I lymph nodes involvement of level III is seen in up to nine percent. This increases to 47% when 4 or more lymph nodes are involved by metastases [6]. A higher incidence of level-III metastases is found when nodes of the lower levels are grossly involved when compared to those with only microscopic invasion (41% versus 15%) [7]. Tumour size also influences the probability of metastases to level III.

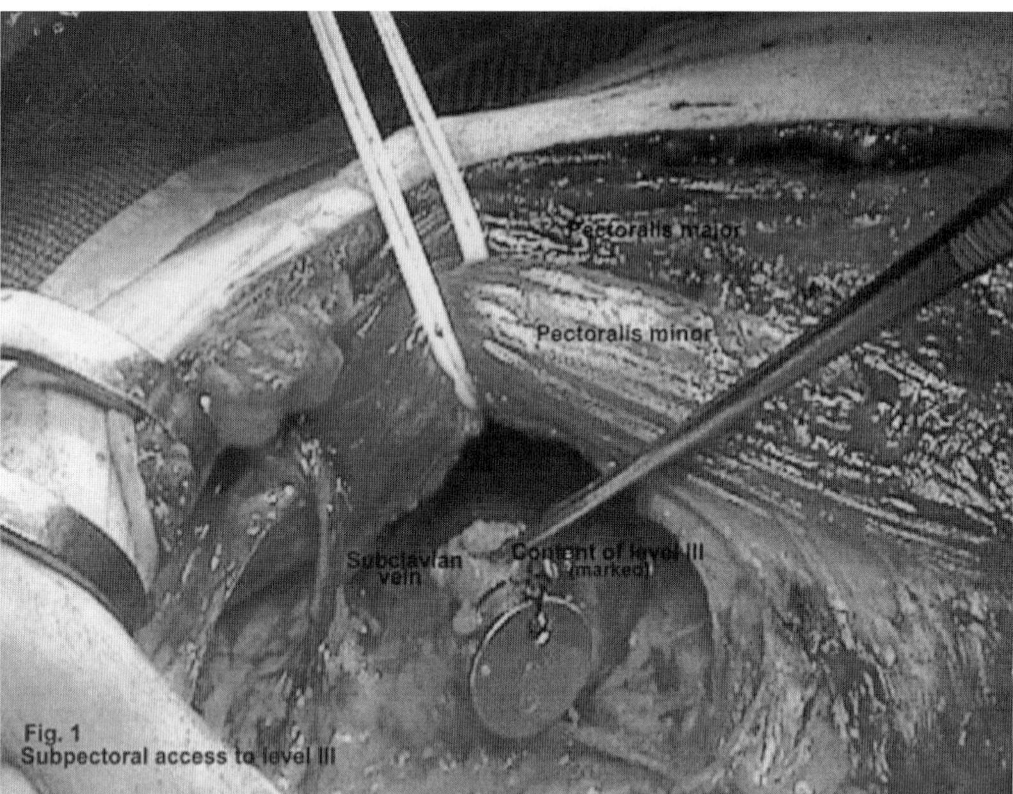

Fig. 1. Subpectoral access to level III.

In 14% a level III involvement is found in tumours smaller than 2 cm, compared to 36% in tumours of 2–3.9 cm in size [8]. Non-involved lymph nodes at level I and/or II but with 'skip' metastases to the third level are seen in between 0.4 [9] to 10% [10] of women. What remains to be clearly defined is the group of patients who obtain benefit from more aggressive surgical therapy to the axilla, i.e. from a level-III dissection.

> *When level II nodes are involved, 30–40% of women will have involved nodes at level III.*

1.1. Indications for level-III dissection

- Patients with clinically involved lymph nodes in the lower levels of the axilla (therapeutic/curative aspect).
- Patients with more advanced breast cancer and extensive but resectable nodal axillary involvement (maintenance of loco-regional control/prevention of axillary plexus damage).

1.2. Contraindications for level-III dissection

- Patients with minimal invasive breast cancer without clinically suspicious axillary nodes may not be candidates for a level III axillary dissection. In these cases, use of a sampling procedure such as a sentinel node biopsy technique should be considered [11,12].

2. Surgical procedure

Surgical access to level III of the axilla is the same as for the dissection of level I and II. The incision can be placed either in a transverse or longitudinal direction. In case of breast preserving treatment a separate transverse S-shaped incision at the lower end of the hair bearing area of the axillary skin or a longitudinal incision at the reverse side of the pectoral fold is feasible. Both incisions provide adequate exposure and excellent cosmesis after wound healing. We prefer the transverse access. When performing a mastectomy or a quadrantectomy in one of the lateral quadrants an axillary dissection can be performed in continuity. As a further alternative a transpectoral approach may be used (see technical remarks).

If the pectoralis minor muscle is to be preserved, the lateral borders of the pectoralis major and minor muscles and the medial pectoral nerve are preserved [14]. In this way it is possible in nearly every case to dissect the apex without division or removal of the pectoralis minor. Using a large retractor both pectoral muscles are retracted medially to allow exposure of the third level. After incision of the surrounding fascia anteriorly along the axillary vein to its junction with the chest wall, to a level just lateral to Halsted's ligament, careful traction in an inferior-lateral direction makes the dissection of the specimen from the surrounding structures possible. Small branches from the axillary vein and lymphatic vessels are cauterised whereas larger blood vessels should be clamped and ligated or clipped.

The content of level III can be removed in continuity with the specimen of levels I and II. For the purpose of the histological examination there are advantages in marking each level separately with metallic tags. If division of the tendon with or without removal of the pectoralis minor muscle is indicated or unavoidable, dissection ends as soon as the border of the pectoralis major is visualised. The pectoralis minor will remain in continuity with the breast and the axillary tissue. The lateral pectoral nerve, innervating the major pectoral muscle should be preserved. We prefer to leave the pectoralis minor in situ which results in a lower rate of subsequent problems (see below). After meticulous haemostasis a suction drainage is placed in the axillary cavity.

2.1. Technical remarks

Draping of the arm in a movable position may ease the access to the upper part of the axilla.

2.2. Removal of the pectoralis minor muscle

If bulky nodes are present or the patient is obese, division of the pectoralis minor tendon (with or without removal of the muscle) will ensure an adequate exposure of level III.

2.3. Transpectoral approach

Access to level III is possible using a transpectoral approach. After having dissected the lateral borders of the pectoralis major and minor muscles, they are separated from each other by blunt dissection. While retracting the pectoralis minor in a lateral direction, with a vessel loop, a direct approach to the axillary level III is possible through an infraclavicular window created by a blunt horizontal separation of the pectoralis major muscle bundles. To improve the exposure, the upper bundles of the muscle are retracted in a cranio-medial direction, the lower fibres are pulled in a caudo-lateral direction (see Fig. 2). During this manoeuvre attention should be paid to the coraco-acromial nerve and vessels, crossing the pectoralis muscle at this level.

Level III dissection can usually be performed without dividing the pectoralis minor muscle.

3. Complications

3.1. Brachial plexopathy

There are no data on brachial plexopathy after surgical treatment alone. After combined surgical/radiotherapeutical treatment in breast preserving therapy the reported incidence is 1% up to 5.9% and relates to fraction size and field overlap [13].

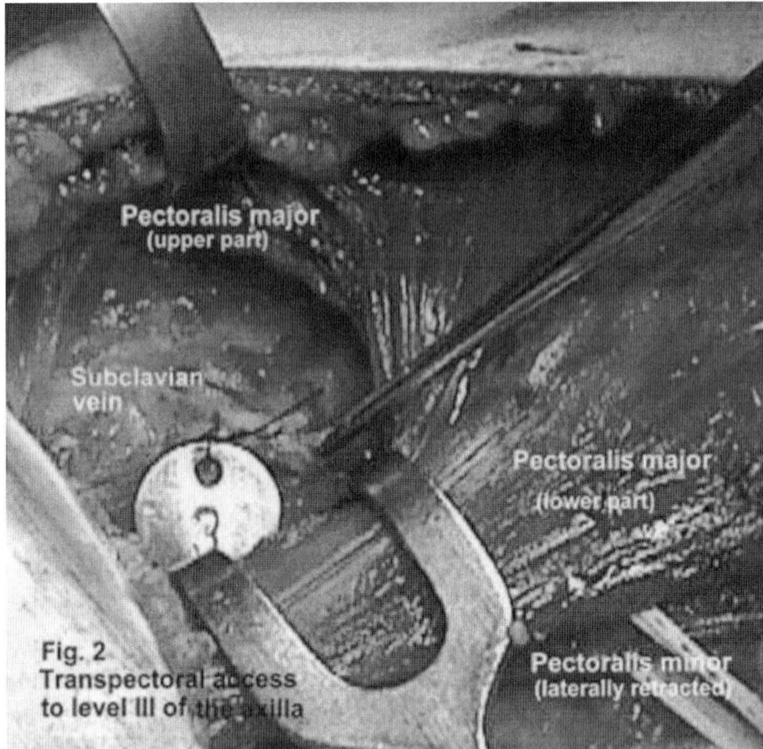

Fig. 2. Transpectoral access to level III of the axilla.

3.2. Lymphoedema

In a cumulative report the development of ipsilateral arm lymphoedema after complete axillary dissection varies between 7 and 16%. There is insufficient data to assess whether a complete axillary dissection leads to a higher incidence of lymphoedema than a level I and II dissection.

3.3. Complications related to the removal of pectoralis minor muscle

During the immediate postoperative period complications (shoulder pain, functional impairment, quantity or duration of serum drainage from the axilla) appear in the same percentage, with or without preservation of the pectoralis minor muscle. After longer follow up (more than 6 months) patients with removal of the muscle show a higher incidence of partial atrophy and fibrosis of the pectoralis major muscle, 54% versus 6% [14].

> *Lymphoedema affects between 7 and 16% of women following a level I, II and III axillary dissection.*

3.4. Incidence of axillary failure

The incidence of axillary failure after complete axillary dissection ranges from 0–3%.

4. Quality of life

Assessment of morbidity and the impact on quality of life when comparing a complete axillary dissection with a level I–II dissection have shown no relevant differences.

References

1. van Tienhoven G, Borger JH, Passchier DH et al. The prognostic significance of axillary apex biopsy in clinically operable breast cancer. Eur J Cancer. 1995; 31A (12): 1965–1968.
2. Quiet CA, Ferguson DJ, Weichselbaum RR et al. Natural history of node-positive cancer. The curability of small cancers with limited number of positive nodes. J Clin Oncol 1996; 14: 3105–3111.
3. Boova RS, Bonanni R, Rosato FE. Patterns of axillary nodal involvement in breast cancer: predictability of level one dissection. Ann Surg 1982; 196: 642–644.
4. Chevinsky AH, Ferrara J, James AG et al. Prospective evaluation of clinical and pathological detection of axillary metastases in patients with carcinoma of the breast. Surgery 1990; 108: 612–618.
5. Muller A, Mattfeld T, Engel K et al. Untersuchungen zur Radikalität der axillären Lymphonodektomie. Geburtsh Frauenheilk 1990; 50: 524–527.
6. Gaglia P, Bussone R, Caldarola B et al. The correlation between the spread of metastases by level in the axillary nodes and disease- free survival in breast cancer: a multivariate analysis. Eur J Cancer 1987; 23: 849–854.
7. Senofsky GM, Moffat FL, Davis K et al. Total axillary lymphadenectomy in the management of breast cancer. Arch Surg 1991; 126: 1336–1342.
8. Berg JW. The significance of axillary node levels in the study of breast cancer. Cancer 1955; 8: 776–778.
9. Veronesi U, Rilke F, Luini A et al Distribution of axillary node metastases by level of invasion. Cancer 1987; 59: 682.
10. Smith J, Gamex AJJ, Gallager H et al. Carcinoma of the breast: analysis of total lymph node involvement versus level of metastasis. Cancer 1977; 39: 527.
11. Veronesi U, Paganelli G, Galimberti V et al. Sentinel-node biopsy to avoid axillary dissection in breast cancer with clinical negative lymph-nodes. Lancet 1997; 349: 1864–1867.
12. Veronesi U, Paganelli G, Viale G, et al. Sentinel lymph node biopsy and axillary dissection in breast cancer: results in a large series. J Natl Cancer Inst 1999; 91(4): 368–373.
13. Powell S, Cooke J, Parsons C. Radiation-induced brachial plexus injury: follow up of two different fractionation schedules. Radiother Oncol 1990; 18: 213.
14. Merson M, Pirovano C, Balzarini A et al. The preservation of minor pectoralis muscle in axillary dissection for breast cancer: functional and cosmetic evaluation. Eur J Surg Oncol 1992; 18(3): 215–218.

Breast Cancer: Diagnosis and Management
J.M. Dixon (Ed.)

CHAPTER 35

The role of radiotherapy in the management of the axilla

A. Rodger

1. Introduction

Radiotherapy alone is as effective as surgical clearance alone in the prevention of axillary recurrences [1]. Surgical dissection of at least levels I and II of the anatomical axilla, however, gives in addition both qualitative and quantitative data on any histological involvement of the axilla. Qualitative information whether the axilla is involved or not gives only limited prognostic information. Quantitative information — i.e. the numbers of nodes that are involved — derived from a level I and level II or level I, II and III dissection gives additional prognostic information and is important in determining the nature and intensity of systemic adjuvant therapy. In general, therefore, the advantage of level I, II (and, if necessary III) dissection over axillary radiotherapy alone is that it provides full information on node status. Surgery rather than radiotherapy may, therefore, be preferred if such information is essential.

When less than a level I and II dissection is performed e.g. a formal sample with a minimum of 4 nodes [2] or level I dissection, qualitative information is not compromised but quantitative assessment of axillary involvement may be. There may, therefore, be an indication after such lesser surgical procedures for post operative axillary irradiation when lymph nodes are histologically involved.

There are also occasions when patients may require but refuse axillary surgery or where surgery is contraindicated. In these situations radiotherapy is a suitable alternative. More recently 3 trials have suggested that in high risk breast cancer post mastectomy radiotherapy that includes peripheral lymphatics may improve survival over chemotherapy [3–5].

2. Radiotherapy as sole axillary management

The Early Breast Cancer Triallists' Collaborative Group [1] has shown from their overview and meta-analysis of breast cancer trials that axillary irradiation alone has similar rates of axillary control to axillary clearance (at least levels I and II dissection). This applies whether local surgery was mastectomy or breast conserving surgery.

Because axillary radiotherapy without surgery does not provide the additional prognostic and management information that dissection provides, there are few circumstances where radiotherapy alone is recommended. These are when informed patients refuse surgery or where surgery is contraindicated for medical reasons. It is deemed preferable that palpable disease is excised, but there is no evidence to support this.

> *Radiotherapy alone to the axilla is equivalent in terms of axillary recurrence to at least level I and II axillary dissection.*

3. Radiotherapy after axillary surgery

Most women with invasive breast cancer will be advised to have and will undergo some degree of axillary surgery.

3.1. After axillary dissection (at least levels I and II)

The addition of axillary radiotherapy to at least a level I and II axillary dissection confers no additional benefit to surgery alone in terms of survival or axillary recurrence.

It will, however, increase local morbidity, particularly the risk of arm lymphoedema. The risk of arm lymphoedema after dissection alone is 6–18% but with additional radiotherapy will rise to 12–60% with most series reporting a rate of at least 30% [6].

> *Radiotherapy after extensive axillary surgery is associated with a rate of lymphoedema of at least 30%.*

Axillary radiotherapy after axillary dissection is considered when operative data or histopathological assessment of the axillary operative specimen suggest that dissection is incomplete. When a surgeon reports that he has left behind macroscopic disease or cut through tumour, axillary radiotherapy should be considered and discussed. It is important that there is close collaboration between breast surgeon and the radiation oncologist.

Of more debate is the importance of histopathological evidence of extracapsular extension (ECE) of malignant cells into axillary fat. While ECE has been shown to be a significant prognostic factor on univariate analysis for poorer overall survival, disease-free survival and locoregional recurrence, it was not independent of other adverse prognostic factors [7]. There is, however, no evidence that in general the presence of any degree of ECE indicates a need for axillary radiotherapy after surgery. There is also considerable debate about the relevance of the quantitative level of axillary involvement — i.e. the number of involved nodes — and the risk of axillary recurrence after dissection. In part the confusion is caused by series that do not separate local from regional recurrence. In NSABP trial BO6 [8] 90% of patients had less than 4 nodes involved and after axillary dissection alone only a 1–3% axillary recurrence. Other data from retrospective studies [9] give axillary recurrences rates for surgery alone at 2–6% for similar levels of axillary involvement. When more nodes are involved locoregional recurrence rates rise [9], with one study from the Royal Marsden Hospital describing axillary recurrence for patients with 4 or more positive nodes without radiotherapy at 6% and 0% with it. These studies, however, are nonrandomised and presumably subject to selection.

> *Radiotherapy to the axilla after at least a level I and II surgical dissection is NOT indicated unless*
> - *there is operative or histopathological evidence of macroscopic residual disease.*
> - *Extracapsular extension or heavy nodal involvement alone are not sufficient indication for post operative axillary radiotherapy.*

Whether lymph node irradiation given to poor prognosis ‘high risk’ patients improves survival over that obtained with systemic adjuvant therapy alone (after mastectomy) has been the subject of debate following recent publication of three trials. Two were in premenopausal patients who received CMF [3,4] and one in menopausal patients who received tamoxifen [5]. All patients underwent some degree of axillary dissection and radiotherapy to the mastectomy flaps, internal mammary chain, supraclavicular fossa and axilla. Locoregional recurrences were reduced and survival improved by the addition of radiotherapy. The trials have been criticised for the form of CMF used or duration of tamoxifen and the relatively low number of resected nodes.

In high risk patients radiotherapy to mastectomy flaps and IMC and supraclavicular fossa and axilla after modified radical mastectomy may improve survival over CMF (premenopausal patients) or tamoxifen for 1 year (postmenopausal patients).

3.2. After axillary sample or level I dissection

When a formal sample [2] or level I dissection is performed, and at least 4 nodes are obtained, if they are negative, radiotherapy is not indicated [10].

However, if these sampling procedures reveal involved lymph nodes, postoperative axillary radiotherapy is required. This will result in similar survival and axillary recurrences as full dissection (level I, II, III) [10].

After axillary sampling/level I dissection of at least 4 nodes, radiotherapy is indicated if nodes are involved. In this circumstance survival and axillary control are identical to full dissection.

4. Morbidity of axillary radiotherapy

The morbidity which is attributed to axillary radiotherapy is in part related to the extent of surgery. Comparisons of different approaches to axillary management are shown in Table 1.

Axillary radiotherapy can cause restriction in shoulder movement even if the shoulder joint is not irradiated; less lymphoedema if it is the sole treatment than a complete level I, II, II clearance alone; and rarely brachial plexopathy.

Table 1. Comparison of morbidity for different options for assessing and treating the axilla

Management option	Complications possible
Watch policy (e.g. clinically negative axilla)	None immediate Psychological morbidity of axillary relapse
Axillary sampling alone (e.g. node negative sample)	• Very low risk of arm oedema [10] • Minimal likelihood of neurological change
Axillary radiation after formal axillary sampling procedure (e.g. node positive sample)	• Arm oedema 6–32% [6] • Reduction in shoulder movement in some after XRT
Axillary radiation alone	• Arm oedema approx. 8% [6] • Pneumonitis 0.7–7% if given with breast or chest wall irradiation • Reduction in shoulder movement in some [10]
Axillary clearance (Levels I, II or levels I, II and III)	• Arm oedema 6–18% > than sampling + XRT but < clearance + XRT [6] • Reduction in shoulder movement in some [10] • Early pain • Numbness • Seroma/lymphocoele
Axillary radiation after a level I and II or I, II and III axillary clearance	• Arm oedema in 12–60%: most studies suggest at least 30% [6] • Reduction in shoulder movement in some • Early pain • Numbness • Seroma/lymphocoele

5. Radiotherapy details

The axilla is seldom irradiated alone. It is generally included in treatment fields which also encompass the supraclavicular fossa (and possibly the upper 2–3 internal mammary node levels). Axillary/supraclavicular fields are also frequently applied in conjunction with adjacent fields to mastectomy flaps or the breast. Care must be taken not to permit overlaps at junctions between chest wall/breast fields and the superior axillary/supraclavicular fields. To prevent any overlap patients should not be turned prone for posterior fields. The axillary nodes lie along the upper lateral rib cage. They lie at several centimetres depth. Single anterior fields are generally insufficient to deliver sufficient dose at depth. While such an anterior field is useful for supraclavicular and internal mammary node treatment, an adequate dose to the deeper axillary nodes may be ensured by applying a simulator planned small posterior field generally extending inferiorly from the level of the clavicle obliquely across the relevant superolateral rib cage. This should include up to 2 cm lung for adequate coverage of all nodes.

Doses of 45–50 Gray in 20–25 fractions, applied to all fields treated daily are required.

Radiotherapy fields should be simulated. Precautions to prevent field junction overlap are essential to reduce the risk of fibrosis or brachial plexus damage.

References

1. Early Breast Cancer Triallists' Collaborative Group. Effects of radiotherapy and surgery in early breast cancer. An overview of the randomised trials. New England Journal of Medicine, 1995; 333: 1444–1455.
2. Steele RJC, Forrest APM, Gibson T et al. The efficacy of lower axillary sampling in obtaining lymph node status in breast cancer: a controlled randomised trial. British Journal of Surgery, 1985; 72: 368–369.
3. Ragaz J, Stewart M, Jackson NL et al. Adjuvant radiotherapy and chemotherapy in node positive premenopausal women with breast cancer. New England Journal of Medicine, 1997; 337: 956–962.
4. Overgaard M, Hansen PS, Overgaard J et al. Postoperative radiotherapy in high risk premenopausal women with breast cancer who receive adjuvant chemotherapy. New England Journal of Medicine, 1997; 337: 949–955.
5. Overgaard M, Hansen PS, Overgaard J et al. Randomised trial evaluating postoperative radiotherapy in high risk postmenopausal breast cancer patients given adjuvant tamoxifen. Results from DBCG 82C trial. Radiotherapy and Oncology, 1998: 48 (suppl. 1): 586 (abstract).
6. Browning C, Thomas and Associates, Redman S, Pillar C et al. Lymphoedema: prevalence, risk factors and management: a review of research. NHMRC National Breast Cancer Centre, Sydney, 1998.
7. Fisher BJ, Perera FE, Cooke AL et al. Extracapsular axillary node extension in patients receiving adjuvant systemic therapy: an indication for radiotherapy. International Journal of Radiation Oncology, Biology and Physics. 1997; 38: 551–559.
8. Fisher B, Anderson S, Redmond C et al. Reanalysis and results after 12 years of follow up in a randomised clinical trial comparing total mastectomy with lumpectomy with or without irradiation in the treatment of breast cancer. New England Journal of Medicine, 1995; 333: 1456–1461.
9. Fowble B, Gray R, Gilchrist K et al. Identification of subgroups of patients with breast cancer and histologically positive axillary nodes receiving adjuvant chemotherapy who may benefit from postoperative radiotherapy. Journal of Clinical Oncology, 1988; 6: 1107–1117.
10. Chetty U, Jack W, Prescott R, Tyler C et al. Management of the axilla in patients with operable breast cancer being treated by breast conservation: a randomised trial. *B. J. Surgery* 2000; 87: 163–169.

Breast Cancer: Diagnosis and Management
J.M. Dixon (Ed.)

CHAPTER 36

Biological and biochemical factors in the prognosis of breast cancer

Massimo Gion and Giampietro Gasparini

1. Introduction

1.1. Breast cancer as a paradigm for the use of tissue biomarkers

Breast cancer is the first human malignancy in which a biological treatment, ablative endocrine therapy, has been successfully used [1]. This has led to intensive investigation, focused both on biological mechanisms underlying endocrine regulation of cell growth, and on optimising choices for more selective and effective endocrine manipulation. Nowadays endocrine options are a realistic effective alternative to cytotoxic chemotherapy in many women [2]. The identification of oestrogen (ER) and progesterone receptor (PgR) and the standardisation of methodology provides clinicians with specific and valid predictive factors for the selection of patients for endocrine therapy [3]. Over the last decade, knowledge and understanding of the molecular mechanisms controlling normal and cancer cell growth has increased sharply, leading to the identification of an ever increasing number of biomarkers which have been correlated with prognosis or used as predictors of response to specific treatments. Table 1 presents a partial list of the biomarkers associated with different cellular mechanisms whose clinical use has been investigated.

Table 1. Partial list of tissue biomarkers studied in breast cancer as prognostic or predictive factors

Cellular mechanism	Biomarker
Cell proliferation	^{3}H-thymidine labelling index BrdU labelling index cytometric S-phase Ki67, PCNA, AgNORs
Oncogenes/ oncosuppressor genes	c-erbB2, p53, EGFr, TGFβ, TGFα
Apoptosis	bcl-2, bax
Angiogenesis	VEGF, βFGF, metalloproteases, panendothelial markers and microvessels count
Proteases inhibitors/ proteases balance	cathepsin D, uPA, PAI- 1, tPA
Endocrine control	ER, PgR, pS2

1.2. What is the role of tissue biomarkers?

The interest in tissue biomarkers relates to prediction of response to specific treatments and prognosis (Table 2). Two factors have contributed to an increased interest in the potential role of tissue biomarkers in the assessment of the risk of relapse: first, the confirmation of the effectiveness of adjuvant treatments in both node-negative and node-positive patients, provided by the recent meta-analysis [4] and secondly the increasing

Table 2. Tissue biomarkers, in breast cancer: clinical applications

Patient groups	Outcome	Alternative choices
Node negative	prognosis	adjuvant therapies yes/no
Node positive	prognosis	aggressiveness of adjuvant therapies
Node negative and node positive	prediction of response to cytotoxic agent	adjuvant chemotherapy yes/no different chemotherapy regimens
Node negative and node positive	prediction of response to hormonal agent	adjuvant hormone-therapy yes/no different endocrine approaches
Node negative and node positive	prediction of response to biological therapies	humanised monoclonal antibodies against oncogene products yes/no anti-angiogenetic agents others

number of patients with early breast cancer whose axillary lymph nodes are free of disease [5]. In these patients, prognostic factors other than axillary lymph node status are important to help decide whether specific adjuvant therapies should be prescribed [6].

In the last few years, it has become common to treat almost all node-negative patients with systemic therapy and a consensus on this strategy has been achieved [7]. The prognostic role of tissue biomarkers is less critical in these patients but their role in deciding which node-negative patients should be given adjuvant treatment is increasing [8]. The expression of the c-erbB2 oncogene is an example of one such biomarker which has been evaluated. Several investigators have assessed the role of c-erbB2 as a predictor of response to cytotoxic chemotherapy. Results from two large, randomised, multicentric trials have been recently published. The Cancer and Leukemia Group B (CALGB) found that patients with c-erbB2 positive tumours benefited from dose intensive CAF (cyclophosphamide, doxorubicin, and 5-fluorouracil) [9]. These findings, although promising, did not reach statistical significance and need further confirmation. The National Surgical Adjuvant Breast and Bowel Project (NASBP) retrospectively examined the predictive value of c-erbB2 for doxorubicin-containing regimens. The results suggested that doxorubicin did not affect the clinical outcome of c-erbB2 negative cases. However, administration of doxorubicin was critical in patients with c-erbB2 positive tumours. Patients treated with doxorubicin-containing chemotherapy, had a clinical outcome similar to that found in patients who were c-erbB2 negative, while prognosis was less favourable in this group if doxorubicin was not administered [10]. Even though confirmatory studies are needed before clinical implementation, c-erbB2 seems a candidate biomarker to help with choosing an individually tailored chemotherapy regimen. Furthermore, c-erbB2 expression is also valuable when considering treatment with humanised anti-neu monoclonal antibodies (Herceptin) [11].

Tissue biomarkers will almost certainly have a role in the selection of patients eligible for anti-angiogenic therapy [12]. Concentrations of vascular endothelial growth factor (VEGF) significantly correlate with clinical outcome in both node-negative and node-positive breast cancer patients [13,14]. Independent studies have found that the use of panendothelial markers (such as factor VIII-RA, anti-CD31 or anti-CD34 antibodies) to assess microvessel density by immunohistochemistry provides important prognostic information.

Patients treated with the same adjuvant treatment but who have highly vascularised primary tumours have an increased risk of recurrence and death compared with those having tumours with low vascularity [15,16]. Because angiogenic activity is under control of pro- and anti-angiogenic factors, it is presumed that determination of angiogenic balance might more precisely predict biological aggressiveness of an individual tumour and help identify patients for therapy with specific anti-angiogenic agents. At least 25 inhibitors of angiogenesis having diverse mechanisms of action are under clinical evaluation [17]. The only way to rationalise the use of a specific anti-angiogenic compounds is to characterise the angiogenic steps which need to be inhibited in vivo to produce reductions in tumour size. For example, the clinical development of humanised anti-VEGF monoclonal antibody should include evaluation of certain surrogate markers such as VEGF levels in the cytosol and/or serum, VEGF-receptors in the tumour, tissue hypoxia etc. to provide a surrogate marker to help monitor patients following such a therapeutic approach [17].

Tissue biomarkers are being used increasingly in both prognosis and prediction of response to different treatments.

1.3. The need for standardisation

Despite the bulk of knowledge on the biology of breast cancer, the routine use of tissue biomarkers is limited and remains controversial. Loprinzi et al. carried out a survey among clinical oncologists in the USA and showed that ER, PgR and S-phase are in frequent use, while new biomarkers (i.e., cathepsin D, EGFR, erbB2 and p53 are only anecdotically determined [18]. In addition, in simulated clinical scenarios, the assessment of the risk of relapse in node negative patients based on traditional biomarkers is variable and differs among centres. Moreover, the availability of new biomarkers seems to have increased the variability of the decision process [18]. An Italian survey has confirmed the significant variability in clinical decisions driven by tissue biomarkers [19]. An additional issue emerged from the Italian survey was the use of a wide variety of methodologies to determine the same tissue biomarker which inevitably affects the comparability of results between laboratories.

Some additional problems emphasise the need for standardisation. First, tissue samples are progressively decreasing in size, due to the early diagnosis of breast cancer [5], and this may lead to subjective and arbitrary choices on which biomarkers should be measured. Secondly, the increasing reduction of resources means that the cost effectiveness of any biomarker should be assessed.

The American Society of Clinical Oncology (ASCO) has prepared and distributed clinical practice guidelines for the use of tumour markers in breast and colorectal cancer [20]. The ASCO recommendations, which are restrictive (Table 3), indicate that ER and PgR are the main tests which should be used for routine purposes for the prediction of hormone responsiveness but they are not recommended for the assessment of prognosis. The ASCO panel classified available studies according to the level of evidence, using a modification of the scale developed by the Canadian Task Force on the Periodic Health Examination, which scores evidences from Level I (highest) to Level V (lowest) [21]. The ASCO evaluation highlighted that the majority of studies on tumour biomarkers are small in size and retrospective and so they fall in the lowest evidence levels (IV and V), which prompts the need for guidelines for proper study design.

Improvement of the quality of study design will increase the strength of evidence available on the use of biomarkers in breast cancer.

Tissue biomarkers may be measured either by immunohistochemistry or biochemistry. Both approaches have advantages and drawbacks. Taking ER as an example immunohistochemistry provides determination on a qualitatively representative sample of tumour and shows the distri-

Table 3. ASCO Guidelines

- Oestrogen and progesterone receptors are relatively weak predictors of long-term relapse and breast cancer related mortality rates, and are not recommended to be used alone to assign a patient to prognostic groupings.
- Present data are insufficient to recommend routinely obtaining DNA flow cytometry-derived estimates of DNA content or S phase.
- DNA flow cytometry-derived ploidy is not recommended to be used to assign a patient to prognostic groupings. There is insufficient evidence to recommend the use of S-phase determination for assigning patients to prognostic groupings.
- Present data are insufficient to recommend the use of DNA flow-cytometry-derived ploidy (DNA index) or flow cytometric measures of proliferation (% S phase and related analysis) for selection of the type of adjuvant therapy to be given.
- Present data are insufficient to recommend the use of DNA flow cytometry-derived information to select among different treatment options for metastatic disease.
- Present data are insufficient to recommend the use of c-erbB2 (HER-2/neu) gene amplification or overexpression for management of patients.
- Present data are insufficient to recommend use of p53 measurements for management of patients.
- Present data insufficient to recommend use of cathepsin D measurements for management of patients.

(American Society of Clinical Oncology. J Clin Oncol, 1996; 14: 2843–2877).

Table 4. Tentative weight of tissue samples examined for biomarkers

Immunohistochemical methods			
Slice diameter (mm)	Slice weight[a] (mg)	Weight of examined tissue (mg) (no. of evaluated slices)	
		2	5
2	0.013	0.026	0.065
5	0.078	0.186	0.39
10	0.314	0.628	1.57
20	1.26	2.52	6.3
Biochemical methods			
Amount of tissue required for receptor assay: - minimum: 20 mg - standard: 100–200 mg			

[a] Approximately calculated assuming: slice thickness, 4 micron; tissue weight, 1 g/cm^3.

bution of the antigen in different tissue compartments. Results may be expressed either as a positive/negative or as both semi-quantitative or quantitative assessment [22]. Immunohistochemistry provides a genuinely qualitative approach since the amount of examined tissue is very small (Table 4). In contrast, biochemical methods provide biomarker determination in a quantitatively representative sample of tumour. Table 4 reports the difference in the amount of tissue actually examined by the two approaches. The cellular source of protein detected biochemically is not identifiable. Although generally providing a good correlation [23], the two methods should not be considered interchangeable [24]. Accordingly, the ASCO guidelines clearly state that the interchangeability of immunohistochemistry and biochemical assays has not yet been proven [20].

As regards biochemical methods, differences in values of any given biomarker can be due to a variety of factors. Major causes of variability relate both to assay techniques and to the reagents used. This issue is clearly demonstrated by comparing the radioligand binding assay and the enzyme immunoassay for ER determination. The two assays are based on totally different recognition of the receptor (binding with a radiolabelled ligand and recognition of the receptor protein by monoclonal antibodies, respectively). Results of the two methods showed a good correlation [25], but they are not superimposable [26] as they measure different functional forms of the same receptor [27].

The uPA/PAI-1 system provides another example of variability of results related to assay components. Different assays may provide different results in the same tissue sample, as demonstrated by a European multicentre study [28].

Both EGFR and p53 have been thoroughly investigated, although their prognostic and predictive values have not been as yet prospectively established. When reviewing these markers [29,30], a wide variety of laboratory methods have been used and this has almost certainly contributed to conflicting results in the literature.

Cathepsin D results were comparable in patients from different Institutions when Cathepsin D assays were performed in one laboratory [31]. However, results from different Institutions show a significant variability when samples were handled and assays were performed independently in each laboratory despite using the same assay [32]. It must be recognised that there is a degree of individuality in the way each laboratory performs assay protocols [33].

> *Centralisation of tissue biomarker assays in a few, highly specialised laboratories, accredited for specific assays and carefully monitored, is needed to ensure comparability of results.*

1.4. Quality assurance programmes

Quality control programmes are mandatory for tissue biomarkers. At present, a routine quality assurance programme exists only for ER and PgR, when measured by biochemical assays [34]. A great deal of work is in progress to set up quality control programmes for immunohistochemistry and for other markers measured biochemically. However, so far, they still lack routine-suited quality control programmes [35]. Effective quality assurance programmes have also been recently set up for certain proliferation indices [36].

> *There is variability in biomarker determination among different Institutions and a lack of consensus on the gold standard assay method or procedure.*
> *Quality assurance programmes are only available for a few biological markers.*

1.5. Implementing the clinical use of biomarkers other than ER and PgR

Cellular proliferation is a well known marker of prognosis and prediction of effectiveness of therapy in breast cancer. Historically, mitosis counting was used to assess tumour cell growth rate. Now, a number of other methods using different variables related to cellular proliferation are used: histochemical detection of proteins expressed only in cycling cells (Ki67, MIB1), silver staining of the nucleolar organising regions (AgNORs), uptake of labelled DNA precursors (tritiated thymidine and bromodeoxyuridine) and flow cytometry to assess the S-phase of the cell cycle [37]. Several studies have found a significant association between different cellular proliferation markers and clinical outcome in breast cancer [38,39]. In addition, some of these parameters have also been monitored by quality assurance programmes [36] and have been evaluated in prospective clinical settings [40]. Cellular proliferation indices are currently used in clinical decision making in several Institutions worldwide.

Several relevant studies on different biomarkers have been published since the latest updating of the ASCO guidelines [41]. Foekens et al. have confirmed the prognostic role of the serine protease Cathepsin D in a large, although retrospective, series. In 2810 cases, high Cathepsin D values were associated with a significantly shorter relapse-free survival in both node-negative and node-positive, as well as in pre- and in post-menopausal patients [42]. De Witte et al. have added further evidence on the prognostic role of uPA and PAI-1 in a series of 437 node-positive and 446 node-negative patients. Their data confirm previous findings which show a strong relationship between this protease-antiprotease system and clinical outcome in women with breast cancer [43]. The predictive role of c-erbB2 has been highlighted by several recent investigations [9–11].

2. Complexity of the biological mechanisms underlying biomarkers

The determination of tissue biomarkers, although analytically complex, provides biologically coarse information. ER was identified in the early '60s on the basis of the specific binding of radiolabelled oestradiol. Thereafter the radioligand binding assay was extensively used as the standard method for ER determination. In the late '80s ER specific monoclonal antibodies were produced, allowing both enzyme immunoassay and immunohistochemistry determination. Many studies demonstrated a clear association between tumour ER concentrations and hormone responsiveness of breast cancer. However, discrepant cases were noted, i.e. hormone unresponsive ER+ cases and, to a much lesser extent, hormone responsive ER- tumours. The reason for this is probably related to the complexity of the ER machinery. ER is a eteroholigomeric protein and the assembly of monomeric units and its quaternare structure is modified by activation [44]. The activation process modifies the epitopes exposition and their ultimate detectability by monoclonal antibodies [44]. The ER molecule contains at least seven functional domains [45]. Of these, two are hormone-independent activation domains that modulate the degree of hormone responsiveness [45]. In addition, the transcriptional activity of ER is modulated by several nuclear proteins, six acting as ER co-activators and two as ER co-repressors [46–48]. These molecules play a pivotal role in modulating anti-oestrogen activity. For example, ER positive tumours may have a hormone-resistant phenotype if they are deficient in co-activators [48]. Several variants of ER mRNA have been described [49,50]. Variants missing the hormone binding domain usually have hormone resistance and poor prognosis. Other variants with deletion of exon 7 and exon 5 in the hormone binding domain have been reported to be hormone resistant. It must be emphasised that these variants usually coexist with wild-type ER in the same tissue sample, making the interpretation of the ER assay uncertain [50].

In addition, beside the ERα gene discovered and sequenced several years ago [51], a second gene termed ERβ, has been recently identified. The tissue distribution of the two ERs is different, suggesting that ERα and ERβ may mediate different functions [3]. The two ER species show a high degree of homology of DNA-binding and hormone-binding domains. However, some differences have been found in translational domains, which may be related to a different response to anti-oestrogens. ERβ mRNA has also been isolated from human breast cancer tissues. Both ERα and ERβ are measured by the radioligand binding assay in an indistinguishable manner, making the interpretation of ER results 'biologically imprecise' [3].

The situation is similar, if not more complicated, when exploring other tissue biomarkers. The angiogenic cascade is a typical example, because it includes many molecular mechanisms in a complex network in which the assay of a limited array of biomarkers provides only a partial informative view [52,53]. The gap between the complexity of biological machinery and the information provided by certain tissue biomarkers is great and justifies the relatively high uncertainty of results of any association between these specific tissue biomarkers assays and clinical outcome.

> *The identification of key biomarkers in a pathway and choice of a comprehensive panel of biomarkers for that given biological pathway is a promising area of investigation.*

3. To explore the complexity of biological machinery

Prognostic and predictive factors may be dichotomised according to cut-off points or, alternatively, examined as continuous variables. Cut-off based criteria have been widely adopted for several biomarkers. They are easy to use since they give a clear-cut presentation of laboratory results and are commonly used to express results of routine immunohistochemistry. Indeed, they allow for an easy comparison between different studies and there are well accepted interpretation criteria for many clinical chemistry tests.

> *The use of a cut-off point may lead to erroneous information where continuous and/or non-linear, and/or non-monotonous associations between a biomarker and clinical outcome are present.*

The drawbacks for using cut-offs are the following: (i) no method for obtaining a reliable cut-off point has been established. Commonly used criteria have drawbacks and weaknesses that have been recently reviewed [54]; (ii) biological variables should not necessarily be expected to behave in a dichotomous manner. A relationship between prognosis and continuous variations of tissue biomarker concentrations has been demonstrated for ER [55] PgR [55], VEGF [13,14], c-erbB-2 [56,57], pS2 and cathepsin D [58,59]; (iii) the use of a cut-off point may lead to erroneous information in the case of non-monotonous associations between biomarkers and clinical parameters. Hupperets et al. reported that very high ER levels are associated with a worse prognosis [55]; the inclusion of patients with very high ER values as positive with reference to a cut-off point may cause an underestimate of the favourable prognostic value of intermediate receptor levels. A similar behaviour has been described by Gasparini et al. for VEGF in node-negative patients [13]. Increasing VEGF concentrations were associated with a poorer prognosis. However, in cases with very high VEGF values, prognosis tended to improve. Dittadi et al. first showed an association between very low c-erbB-2 and poor prognosis in breast cancer [56]. These findings were later confirmed by others [57]. Growing evidence suggests that the use of a dichotomous cut-off point could force together cases in which biomarkers provide opposite information and lead to a misleading assessment of prognosis or prediction of response to therapy.

The problem is further complicated by possible interactions between different biomarkers and has been highlighted in postmenopausal women with node-positive breast cancer. In these patients, the predictive value of high levels of cathepsin D for tamoxifen response varies in pS2 poor or in pS2 rich tumours [58,59]. The use of more complex and innovative statistical approaches seems a promising approach to explore the biological complexity of biomarkers [60].

4. Future directions

The more promising prognostic or predictive variables in node-negative and node- positive breast cancer have been recently highlighted in a special issue of Breast Cancer Research and Treatment [61]. These include markers of tumour cell proliferation (mainly S-phase fraction by cytometry and thymidine labelling index); growth factors such as c-erbB-2 and epidermal growth factor receptor, p53 protein, the uPA/PAI-1 system and surrogate markers of angiogenesis [62–70]. The development of more precise prognostic and predictive indexes is advocated instead of continuous research of single markers [71].

Recent guidelines and recommendations by Altman and Lyman [72] and Hayes et al. [73], represent a robust basis for an international consensus to standardise the statistical approach and to evaluate the clinical impact of a prognostic/predictive variable.

Acknowledgements

The studies of Dr Gasparini have been supported by grants from the Associazione Italiana per la Ricerca sul Cancro (AIRC), Milan, Italy. The studies of Dr Gion have been supported by the Regione Veneto and by the Associazione per l'Applicazione delle Biotecnologie in Oncologia (grupppo ABO), Venice, Italy. We thank Mrs Antonia Falzea for typing the manuscript.

References

1. Beatson GT. On the treatment of inoperable cases of carcinoma of the mamma: suggestions for a new method of treatment with illustrative cases. Lancet, 1896; ii: 104–107.
2. Osborne CK, Clark GM, Ravdin PM. Adjuvant systemic therapy of primary breast cancer. In: Harris JR, Lippman ME, Hellman S (eds) Diseases of the Breast. Lippincott–Raven Publishers. Philadelphia PA, 1996, 546–576.
3. Osborne CK. Steroid hormone receptors in breast cancer management. Breast Cancer Res Treat 1998, 51: 227–238.
4. EBCTC Group. Tamoxifen for early breast cancer: an overview of the randomised trials. Lancet 1998; 351: 1451–1467.
5. Tubiana M, Koscielny S. Natural history of human breast cancer: recent data and clinical implications. Breast Cancer Res Treat 1991, 18: 125–140.
6. Silvestrini R, Daidone MG, Luisi A et al. Biologic and clinico pathologic factors as indicators of specific relapse types in node-negative breast cancer. J Clin Oncol 1995; 13: 697–704.
7. Goldhirsch A, Glick JH, Gelber Rd et al.: Meeting Highlights: International consensus panel on the treatment of primary breast cancer. J Natl Cancer Inst 1998; 90: 1601.
8. Henderson IC, Patek AJ. The relationship between prognostic and predictive factors in the management of breast cancer. Breast Cancer Res Treat 1998; 52: 261–288.
9. Thor Ad, Berry DA, Budman DR et al. ErbB-2, p53, and the efficacy of adjuvant therapy in lymph node-positive breast cancer. J Natl Cancer Inst 1998; 90: 1346–1360.
10. Paik S, Bryant J, Park C et al. ErbB-2 and response to doxorubicin in patients with axillary lymph node-positive, hormone receptor-negative breast cancer. J Natl Cancer Inst 1998; 90: 1361–1370.
11. Pengram MD, Lipton A, Hayes DF et al. Phase II of receptor-enhanced chemosensitivity using recombinant humanized anti-p185HER2/neu monoclonal antibody plus cisplatin in patients with HER2/neu-overexpresing metastatic breast cancer refractory to chemotherapy treatment. J Clin Oncol 1998; 16: 2659–2671.
12. Gasparini G, Harris AL. Clinical importance of the determination of tumor angiogenesis in breast carcinoma: much more than a new prognostic tool. J Clin Oncol 1995; 13: 765–782.
13. Gasparini G, Toi M, Gion M et al. Prognostic significance of vascular endothelial growth factor protein in node-negative breast carcinoma. J Natl Cancer Inst 1997; 89: 139–147.
14. Gasparini G, Toi M, Miceli R et al. Clinical relevance of vascular endothelial growth factor and thymidine phosphorylase in patients with node-positive breast cancer treated with either adjuvant chemoterapy or hormone therapy. Cancer J Sci Am 1999; 5: 101–111.
15. Gasparini G. Barbareschi M, Boracchi P et al. Tumor angiogenesis predicts clinical outcome of node-positive breast cancer patients treated with adjuvant hormone therapy or chemotherapy. The Cancer Journal from Scientific American, 1, 131–141, 1995, Scientific American Inc, New York.
16. Gasparini G, Fox SB, Verderio P et al. Determination of angiogenesis adds information to estrogen receptor status in predicting the efficacy of adjuvant tamoxifen in node-positive breast cancer patients. Clinical Cancer Research — An official Journal of the American Association for Cancer Research, 2; 1191–1198, 1996. Cadmus Journal Services, Charlotte, U.S.A.
17. Gasparini G. The rationale and future potential of angiogenesis inhibitors in neoplasia. Drugs, 58: 17–38, 1999.
18. Loprinzi Cl, Ravdin PM, De Laurentiis M et al. Do American oncologist know how to use prognostic variables for patients with newly diagnosed primary breast cancer? J Clin Oncol 1994; 12: 1422–1426.
19. Gion M, Barioli P, Ponti A et al. How tumor markers are used in the routine follow-up of breast and col-

orectal cancer. A survey of 29 Italian Hospital. Int J Biol Markers 1998; 13: 124–138.

20. American Society of Clinical Oncology. Clinical practice guidelines for the use of tumor markers in breast and colorectal cancer. J Clin Oncol 1996; 14: 2843–2877.
21. Canadian Task Force on the periodic Health Examination. The periodic health examination. Can Med Assoc J 1979; 12: 1193–1254.
22. van Diest P, van Dam P, Henzen–Logmans SC et al. A scoring system for immunohistochemical staining: consensus report of the task force for basic research of the EORTC–GCCG. J Clin Pathol 1997; 20: 801–804.
23. de Mascarel I, Soubeyran G, MacGrogan J et al. Immunohistochemical analysis of estrogen receptors in 938 breast carcinomas: concordance with biochemical assay and prognostic significance. Appl Immunohistochem 1995; 3: 222–231.
24. Stierer M, Rosen H, Weber R et al. Comparison of immunohistochemical and biochemical measurement of steroid receptors in primary breast cancer: evaluation of discordant findings. Breast Cancer Res Treat 1998; 50: 125–134.
25. Blankenstein MA. Comparison of ligand binding assay an enzyme immunoassay of estrogen receptor in human breast cancer cytosols. Experience of the EORTC Receptor Group. Breast Cancer Res Treat 1990; 17: 91–98.
26. Gion M, Dittadi R, Leon AE et al. Comparison between single saturating dose ligand binding assay and enzyme immunoassay for low-salt extractable oestrogen and progesterone receptor in breast cancer: a multicentre study. Eur J Cancer 1991; 27: 996–1002.
27. Dittadi R, Meo S, Amoroso B et al. Detection of different estrogen receptor forms in breast cancer cytosol by enzyme immunoassay. Cancer Res 1997; 57: 1066–1072.
28. Sweep CGJ, Geurts–Moespot J, Grebenschikov N et al. External quality assessment of trans-European multicentre antigen determinations (enzyme-linked immunosorbent assay) of urokinase-type plasminogen activator (uPA) and its type 1 inhibitor (PAI-1) in human breast cancer tissue extracts. Brit J Cancer 1998; 78: 1434–1441.
29. Klijn JGM, Berns PMJJ, Schmitz PIM et al. The clinical significance of epidermal growth factor receptor (EGFr) in human breast cancer: a review on 5232 patients. Endocrine Review 1992; 13: 3–17.
30. Barbareschi M. Prognostic value of the immunohistochemical expression of p53 in breast carcinomas — A review of the literature involving over 9,000 patients. Appl Immunohistochem 1996; 4: 106–116.
31. Gion M, Mione R, Dittadi R et al. Relationship between cathepsin D and other pathological and biological parameters in 1752 patients with primary breast cancer. Eur J Cancer 1995; 31A: 671–677.
32. Pelizzola D, Gion M, Paradiso A et al. Cathepsin D versus other prognostic factors in breast cancer. Results and controversies of a multicenter study on 2575 cases. Int J Biol Markers 1996; 11: 139–147.
33. Thorpe SM, Poulsen HS, Pedersen KO et al. Impact of standardization of estrogen receptor assays of breast cancer biopsies in Denmark. Eur J Cancer and Clin Oncol 1988; 24: 1263–1269.
34. Romain S, Spyratos F, Goussard J et al. Improvement of quality control for steroid receptor measurements: analysis of distributions in more than 40000 primary breast cancers. Breast Cancer Res Treat 1996, 41: 131–139.
35. Barnes, DM, Millis RR, Beex LVAM et al. Increased use of immunohistochemistry for oestrogen receptor measurement in mammary carcinoma: the need for quality assurance. Eur J Cancer 1998; 34: 1677–1682.
36. Silvestrini R. Quality control for the evaluation of the S-phase fraction by flow-cytometry: a multicentric study. The SICCAB Group for Quality Control of Cell Kinetic determination. Cytometry 1994b; 18: 11–16.
37. Elias JM. Cell proliferation indexes: a biomarker in solid tumors. Biotech Histochem 1996; 72: 78–85.
38. Silvestrini R, Daidone MG, Luisi A et al. Cell proliferation in 3,800 node-negative breast cancers: consistency over time of biological and clinical information provided by 3H-thymidine labelling index. Int J Cancer 1997; 74: 122–127.
39. Gasparini G., Boracchi P., Verderio P. and Bevilacqua P. Cell kinetics in human breast cancer: Comparison of the prognostic value between the cytofluorimetric S-phase fraction and that of the antibodies to Ki-67 and PCNA antigens detected by immunocytochemistry. International Journal of Cancer. Official Journal of the Union Internationale Contre le Cancer (U.I.C.C.), 57, 822–829, 1994. J. Wiley and Sons Publisher, New York, U.S.A.
40. Amadori D, Volpi A, Maltoni R et al. Cell proliferation as a predictor of response to chemotherapy in metastatic breast cancer: a prospective study. Breast Cancer Res Treat 1997; 43: 7–14.
41. American Society of Clinical Oncology. 1997 update of recommendations for the use of tumor markers in breast and colorectal cancer. J Clin Oncol 1998; 16: 793–795.
42. Foekens JA, Look MP, Bolt de Vries J et al. Cathepsin D in primary breast cancer: prognostic evaluation involving 2810 patients. Br J Cancer 1999; 79: 300–307.
43. de Witte JH, Sweep CGJ, Klijn JGM et al. Prognostic impact of urokinase-type plasminogen activator (uPA) and its inhibitor (PAI-1) in cytosol and pellet extracts derived from 892 breast cancer patients. Br J Cancer 1999; 79: 1190–1198.
44. Giambiagi N, Pasqualini JR. Interaction of three monoclonal antibodies with the nonactivated and activated

forms of the estrogen receptor. Endocrinology 1991; 126: 1403–1409.

45. Osborne CK, Elledge RM, Fuqua SAW. Estrogen receptors in breast cancer therapy. Sci Med 1996; 3: 32–41.
46. Horovitz KB, Jakson TA, Bain DL et al. Nuclear receptor coactivators and corepressors. Mol Endocrinol 1996; 10: 1167–1177.
47. Li H, Leo C, Schroen DJ, Chen JD. Characterization of receptor interaction and transcriptional repression by the corepressor SMRT. Mol Endocrinol 1997; 11: 2025–2037.
48. Jakson WA, Richer RK, Bain DL et al. The partial agonist activity of antagonist-occupied steroid receptors is controlled by a novel hinge domain-binding coactivator L7/SPA and the corepressor N-CoR or SMRT. Mol Endocrinol 1997; 11: 693–705.
49. Clarke CL, Balleine RL, Auchus RJ et al. Estrogen and progesterone receptor variants in human breast cancer. Curr Opin Endocrinol Diabetes 1995; 2: 398–403.
50. Fuqua SAW, Wiltschke C, Castles C et al. A role for estrogen receptor variants in endocrine resistance. Endocr-Relat Cancer 1995; 2: 19–25.
51. Mosselman S, Polman J, Dijkema R. ER beta: dentification and characterization of a novel human estrogen receptor. FEBS Lett 1996; 392: 49–53.
52. Senger DR. Molecular Framework for angiogenesis. A complex web of interactions between extravasated plasma proteins and endothelial cell proteins induced by angiogenic cytokines. Am J Pathol 1996; 149: 1–7.
53. Bussolino F, Albini A, Camussi G et al. Role of soluble mediators in angiogenesis. Eur J Cancer 1996; 14: 2401–2412.
54. Altman DG, De Stavola BL, Love SB et al.: Review of survival analyses published in cancer journals. Br J Cancer 1995; 72: 551–518.
55. Hupperets PS, Volovics L, Schouten LJ et al. The prognostic significance of steroid receptor activity in tumor tissue of patients with primary breast cancer. Am J Clin Oncol 1997; 20: 546–551.
56. Dittadi R, Brazzale A, Pappagallo G et al. ErbB2 assay in breast cancer: possibly improved clinical information using a quantitative method. Anticancer Res 1997; 17: 1245–1248.
57. Koscielny S, Terrier P, Spielmann M et al. Prognostic importance of low c-erbB2 expression in breast tumors. J Natl Cancer Inst 1998; 90: 712.
58. Corradini D, Biganzoli E, Boracchi P et al. Effect of steroid receptors, pS2 and cathepsin D on the outcome elderly beast cancer patients: an exploratory investigation. Int J Cancer 1998; 79: 305–311.
59. Dittadi R, Biganzoli E, Boracchi P et al. Impact of steroid receptors, pS2 and cathepsin D on the outcome of N^+ postmenopausal breast cancer patients treated with tamoxifen. Int J Biol Markers 1998; 13: 30–41.
60. Biganzoli E, Boracchi P, Daidone MG, Gion M, Marubini E: Flexible modelling in survival analysis. Structuring biological complexity from the information provided by tumor markers. Int J Biol Markers 1998; 13: 107–123.
61. Gasparini G. Prognostic variables in node-negative and node-positive breast cancer. Special Issue Part I and II, Breast Cancer Res Treat 1998; 51 (n. 3) and 52 (n. 1–3).
62. Bryant J., Fisher B., Gunduz N., et al. S-phase fraction combined with other patient and tumour characteristic for the prognosis of node-negative, estrogen-receptor-positive breast cancer. Breast Cancer Res Treat 1998; 51: 239–253.
63. Wenger C.R., Clark G.M. S-phase fraction and breast cancer — a decade of experience. Breast Cancer Res Treat 1998; 51: 255–265.
64. Amadori D., Silvestrini R. Prognostic and predictive value of thymidine labelling index in breast cancer. Breast Cancer Res Treat 1998; 51: 267–281.
65. De Placido S., Carlomagno C., De Laurentiis M. et al. c-erbB2 expression predicts tamoxifen efficacy in breast cancer patients. Breast Cancer Res Treat 1998; 52: 55–64.
66. Pegram M.D., Pauletti G., Slamon D.J. HER-2/neu as a predictive marker of response to breast cancer therapy. Breast Cancer Res Treat 1998; 52: 65–77.
67. Elledge R.M., Allred D.C. Prognostic and predictive value of p53 and p21 in breast cancer. Breast Cancer Res Treat 1998; 52: 79–98.
68. Stephens R.W., Brunner N., Janicke F. et al. The urokinase plasminogen activator system as a target for prognostic studies. Breast Cancer Res Treat 1998; 52: 99–111.
69. Heimann R., Ferguson D., Gray S. et al. Assessment of intratumoral vascularization (angiogenesis) in breast cancer prognosis. Breast Cancer Res Treat 1998; 52: 147–188.
70. Locopo N., Fanelli M., Gasparini G. Clinical significance of angiogenic factors in breast cancer. Breast Cancer Res Treat 1998; 52: 189–173.
71. Gasparini G. Prognostic variables in node-negative and node-positive breast cancer — editorial. Breast Cancer Res Treat 1998; 52: 321–331.
72. Altman D.G., Lyman G.H. Methodological challenges in the evaluation of prognostic factors in breast cancer. Breast Cancer Res Treat 1998; 52: 289–303.
73. Hayes D.F., Trock B., Harris A.L. Assessing the clinical impact of prognostic factors: When is "statistically significant" clinically useful? Breast Cancer Res Treat 1998; 52: 305–319.

Breast Cancer: Diagnosis and Management
J.M. Dixon (Ed.)

CHAPTER 37

Primary systemic chemotherapy in early breast cancer

Ian E. Smith

1. Introduction

Primary systemic therapy before surgery in early breast cancer (sometimes also referred to as pre-operative or neoadjuvant chemotherapy) is a new concept with important implications for future management. Currently, the technique is used mainly in patients with large breast cancers who have a relatively poor prognosis [1], and who would therefore be candidates for adjuvant chemotherapy.

The most immediate advantage of this approach is that the primary tumour be downstaged with the opportunity for conservative surgery rather than mastectomy. A second theoretical advantage lies in the potential for survival improvement, based on experimental data that pre-operative chemotherapy might inhibit surgically stimulated growth factors that might also promote residual tumour growth [2]. Third, and potentially the most important advantage, is that the tumour itself can be used as an in vivo measure of response to treatment, in contrast to adjuvant therapy where treatment is given "blind" with no way of assessing individual clinical benefit. Conventional adjuvant trials of new drug therapy furthermore take many years to mature with disease-free survival as the key endpoint. If short-term response to pre-operative chemotherapy can be shown to be an effective surrogate marker for long term outcome, then this would have important implications both for individualising therapy and for the more rapid evaluation of new treatments (Table 1).

There are theoretical advantages for giving systemic therapy as the initial treatment even in operable breast cancer.

2. Does pre-operative chemotherapy reduce the need for mastectomy?

There is no doubt that preoperative chemotherapy is very active in early breast cancer. Overall objective response rates are generally higher than in metastatic disease, ranging from 70% to more than 90% [3–11] (Table 2). Complete clinical remissions are less frequent and generally occur only in a minority of patients, but have been reported in up to 66% of patients using an infusional chemotherapy schedule [8]. A key finding in all studies is that tumour progression during primary chemotherapy is rare, generally occurring in less than 5% of patients; early arguments that this approach might jeopardise subsequent operability have therefore proved invalid.

Results from non-randomised studies suggest that the high response rate is associated with a reduced need for mastectomy. In our own ex-

Table 1. Theoretical advantages and disadvantages of primary chemotherapy

Advantages
- Downstaging to avoid mastectomy
- Improved survival?
- Tumour as an in vivo measure of treatment response

Disadvantages
- Loss of traditional prognostic criteria including axillary node status (but recent overview data suggest axillary nodes no longer critical in deciding adjuvant therapy)
- Potential over-treatment of women with non-invasive breast cancer diagnosed on FNA alone but core needle biopsy would distinguish

Table 2. Pre-operative chemotherapy response rates

Reference	Tumour size	Schedule	Patients	Response
Jacquillat Cancer 1990	Operable	Vinblastine, Thiotepa, 5FU, Methotrexate	250	71%
Bonadonna JCO 1998	≥3 cm	CMF Doxorubicin	536	76%
Smith JCO 1995 [a]	3–12 cm	ECF	123	96%
Cameron Br J Cancer 1997	>4 cm	CHOP	94	70%
Fisher JCO 1998 [b]	Operable	Adriamycin Cyclophosphamide	749 (1523)	80%
Scholl Eur J Cancer 1994 [b]	3–7 cm	Adriamycin, 5FU, Cyclophosphamide	200 (390)	65%
Powles JCO 1995 [b]	Operable	Mitozantrone, Methotrexate	105 (309)	85%
Semiglazov Ann Oncol 1994 [b]	>2 cm	Thiotepa, Methotrexate, 5FU	134 (271)	57%
Mauriac Ann Oncol 1991 [b]	>3 cm	Epirubicin, Vincristine, Mitomycin C, Thiotepa, Vindesine	138 (272)	81%

[a] Updated results.
[b] Randomised (Total number randomised in trial).

perience at the Royal Marsden using infusional ECis F (Table 3) the main entry criterion was the need for mastectomy. Following infusional chemotherapy, only 8% of patients in a pilot study required mastectomy as first-line surgical treatment following chemotherapy [8]. A group from Milan likewise selected patients on the need for mastectomy and found that only 15% of patients subsequently required this treatment following adriamcyin/CMF chemotherapy [5]. In their experience the likelihood of conservative surgery was inversely related to the size of the original tumour; patients whose presenting tumours were <4 cm in maximum diameter had a >90% chance

Table 3. Frequently used pre-operative chemotherapy schedules

AC	
Adriamycin	60 mg/m^2 iv bolus day 1, repeating 3 weekly
Cyclophosphamide	600 mg/m^2 iv bolus day 1, repeating 3 weekly
Treatment continuing 3-weekly for 6 courses	
Infusional ECis F	
Epirubicin	60 mg/m^2 iv q. 21 days
Cisplatin	60 mg/m^2 iv q. 21 days
5FU	200 mg/m^2 iv by continuous infusion via Hickman line
Treatment continuing 3-weekly for 8 courses (phase II trial) and subsequently 6 courses (randomised phase III trial)	

of conservative surgery compared with around 60–70% in patients with tumours >5 cm.

Results from randomised trials confirm that the need for mastectomy can be reduced with primary chemotherapy, but the extent of benefit is considerably less than in non-randomised studies. In the NSABP B-18 trial lumpectomy was achieved in 67% of patients in the group treated with pre-operative chemotherapy compared with 60% in the immediate surgery group ($p = 0.002$). The difference was particularly evident in the group with tumours >5.1 cm (22% v. 8%). In a Royal Marsden Hospital trial using mitozantrone, methotrexate and tamoxifen mastectomy was reduced from 22% in the adjuvant group to 10% in the pre-operative group ($p < 0.003$) [12]. Likewise, a French randomised study of pre-operative CAF chemotherapy showed a reduced tendency for patients treated with pre-operative chemotherapy to undergo mastectomy (23% v. 36% in the adjuvant arm, $p < 0.003$) [10].

Preoperative systemic chemotherapy given to patients with large operable breast cancers reduces the need for mastectomy.

Local recurrence rates are an important issue in the context of avoiding mastectomy. Currently, three randomised trials have compared these in patients treated with chemotherapy pre-operatively versus post-operatively and none have shown any significant difference between the two treatments in the rate of local disease recurrence [7,10,12].

3. Does primary chemotherapy influence survival?

Initial results from two randomised French trials of primary chemotherapy suggested a small survival benefit [4,10]. In contrast, the largest and most important trial in this field, the NSABP B-18 trial, has so far shown no survival difference between primary and post-operative chemotherapy with overall survival rates of 80% in both arms at 5 years of follow-up [7]. Likewise the smaller Royal Marsden trial has also failed shown any survival difference related to the timing of chemotherapy [12]. Current results do suggest however that there is no survival disadvantage of primary chemotherapy, even if the weight of evidence does not so far indicate a survival benefit.

Randomised studies have not shown any survival advantage for preoperative compared with postoperative systemic chemotherapy.

4. The tumour as an in vivo measure of treatment response

Potentially, this could be the major long term benefit of primary chemotherapy, allowing for individualised treatment for each patient and permitting more rapid assessments of new therapies in the overall management of early breast cancer. This can be assessed at three levels; clinical, pathological and biological.

Clinical tumour response is an important predictor of outcome for primary chemotherapy and several groups have shown that responders have improved disease free survival and overall survival compared with non-responders [5,6,13]. In some [7] but not all [13] studies, complete clinical responders have likewise been shown to carry an additional predictive survival benefit over partial responders.

In contrast to complete clinical response, complete pathological remission (pCR) after surgery is emerging as a clear-cut predictor for survival. In the NSABP B-18 trial the 5 year disease-free survival for patients achieving pCR was 85% compared with an estimated 70% for those achieving a clinical but not pathological response and 58% for those not responding clinically [7]. Likewise the Edinburgh group, in a much smaller series of patients, reported an 88% 8 year survival for patients achieving pCR to chemotherapy compared with 60% for those achieving a clinical response and 35% for non-responders [6].

The practical limitation to pCR as a predictive end-point for survival is that generally less than 20% of patients achieve this. Furthermore, these data are only available at the time of surgery after medical treatment has been completed and do not allow the opportunity to make early adjustments in therapy.

Tumour response to primary chemotherapy is an important predictive factor.

5. Biological predictive factors

Primary chemotherapy offers important possibilities for the study of biological mechanisms underlying chemo-resistance and response. In addition, early changes in biological markers during therapy might predict for long-term outcome, and offer advantages over the clinical and pathological markers described above. Indeed anatomically breast cancer is the ideal clinical model for such studies because of the ease of access to serial fine needle aspirates and biopsies.

At the Royal Marsden we have compared apoptotic index (A1) before and 24 hours after infusional ECis F chemotherapy. Ten patients (59%) showed >50% increase in AI 24 hours following chemotherapy, 5 showed <50% change (considered no significant change) and 2 showed a decrease by >50%. Nine of 13 clinical responders (69%) showed a >50% increase in AI compared with only 1 of 4 clinical non-responders to chemotherapy (25%) [14]. If the trend found in this study is confirmed in a larger ongoing study then it might be possible to predict a patient's subsequent clinical outcome shortly after starting treatment, and modify therapy appropriately. In a similar study, serial sampling has shown that late decreases in proliferation indices following chemo-endocrine therapy help to predict for complete clinical response [15]. With the speed of current developments in molecular biology and biotechnology, it seems likely that biological predictive markers for pre-operative therapy will emerge to allow individual adjustment of treatment and to enable more rapid assessment of new drugs in the management of early breast cancer.

6. Conclusions

Primary chemotherapy is active in early breast cancer and current evidence suggests that some but not all patients with large breast primaries can avoid mastectomies with this approach. Longer term follow up is required, however, to establish whether this approach is associated with high local recurrence rates.

At present there appears to be neither a survival advantage nor a disadvantage in pre-operative medical treatments. This justifies further study with the aim of defining clinical, pathological and biological surrogate markers predicting for long term outcome. If these can be established, then treatment for the individual patient can be individualised with potential survival advantage over adjuvant therapy which must inevitably be given "blind". In addition surrogate markers could prove valuable in assessing the role for new therapies in early breast cancer; this could allow progress to be made much more rapidly than is possible with current adjuvant trials.

References

1. Haagensen DC, Bodian C: A personal experience with Halsted's radical mastectomy. Ann Surg 1984: 143–150, 1984.
2. Fisher B, Gunduz N, Coyle J, et al: Presence of a growth-stimulating factor in serum following primary tumour removal in mice. Cancer Res 49: 1996–2001, 1989.
3. Jacquillat C, Weil M, Baillet F, et al: Results of neoadjuvant chemotherapy and radiation therapy in the breast-conserving treatment of 250 patients with all stages of infiltrative breast cancer. Cancer 66: 119–127, 1990.
4. Mauriac L, Durand M, Avril A, et al: Effects of primary chemotherapy in conservative treatment of breast cancer patients with operable tumors larger than 3 cm. Results of a randomized trial in a single centre. Ann Oncol 2: 347–354, 1991.
5. Bonadonna G, Valagussa P, Brambilla C, et al: Primary chemotherapy in operable breast cancer: eight-year experience at the Milan Cancer Institute. J Clin Oncol 16 (1): 93–100, 1998.
6. Cameron DA, Anderson EDC, Levack P, et al: Primary systemic therapy for operable breast cancer in 10-year survival data after chemotherapy and hormone therapy. Br J Cancer 76: 1099–1105, 1997.
7. Fisher B, Bryant J, Wolmark N, et al: Effect of preoperative chemotherapy on the outcome of women with operable breast cancer. J Clin Oncol 16: 2672–2685, 1998.
8. Smith IE, Walsh G, Jones A, et al: High complete remission rates with primary neoadjuvant infusional chemotherapy for large early breast cancer. J Clin Oncol 13: 424–429, 1995.
9. Powles TJ, Hickish TF, Makris A, et al: Randomised trial of chemoendocrine therapy started before or after surgery for treatment of primary breast cancer. J Clin Oncol 13: 547–552, 1995.
10. Scholl SM, Fourquet A, Asselain JY, et al: Neoadjuvant versus adjuvant chemotherapy in premenopausal patients with tumours considered too large for breast conserving surgery: Preliminary results of a randomised trial: S6. Eur J Cancer 30A: 645–652, 1994.
11. Semiglazov VF, Topuzov EE, Bavli JL et al: Primary (neoadjuvant) chemotherapy and radiotherapy compared with radiotherapy alone in stage IIb–IIIa breast cancer. Ann Oncol 5: 591–595, 1994.
12. Makris A, Powles TJ, Ashley SE, et al: A reduction in the requirements for mastectomy in a randomized trial of neoadjuvant chemoendocrine therapy in primary breast cancer. Ann Oncol 9: 1179–1184, 1998.
13. Ellis P, Smith I, Ashley S, et al: Clinical prognostic and predictive factors for primary chemotherapy in operable breast cancer. J Clin Oncol 16: 107–114, 1998.
14. Ellis PA, Smith IE, McCarthy K, et al: Preoperative chemotherapy induces apoptosis in early breast cancer. Lancet 349–849, 1997.
15. Chang J, Powles TJ, Allred DC, et al: Predictive molecular markers for clinical outcome following primary chemotherapy for operable breast cancer. Proc Am Soc Clin Oncol 17: 384, 1998.

Breast Cancer: Diagnosis and Management
J.M. Dixon (Ed.)

CHAPTER 38

Neoadjuvant endocrine therapy

J.M. Dixon

1. Introduction

In patients with large operable or locally advanced breast cancer successful neoadjuvant therapy has the potential advantage of down staging the primary tumour and permitting a more conservative approach with less extensive surgery [1]. Studies to date have concentrated principally on neoadjuvant chemotherapy and only a few studies have evaluated neoadjuvant endocrine therapy in hormone sensitive, large operable or locally advanced breast cancers [2–4]. Those studies that have been performed in this group of patients have shown substantial reductions in tumour volume over a 12 week period with agents such as tamoxifen, aminoglutethimide, 4-hydroxandrostenedione and more recently letrozole and anastrozole.

Primary endocrine therapy has potential theoretical and practical advantages over chemotherapy. Inhibition of oestrogen stimulated enzyme release (plasminogen activator and collagenases) may reduce tumour cell shedding. In addition, there is strong evidence that oestrogen withdrawal not only reduces growth factor synthesis but also disrupts the function of a number of other growth factors [5,6] and hormone receptors and/or their second messenger signalling pathways [7–9]. Although there are only limited data from randomised trials of preoperative endocrine therapy, there a number of small phase II studies [10–24].

Primary (neoadjuvant endocrine therapy given to women with large operable or locally advanced oestrogen receptor positive tumours can produce substantial reductions in tumour volume.

2. Randomised trials

The randomised trials of primary endocrine therapy have all been in elderly patients [6–8,25]. In two trials, tamoxifen therapy was compared with immediate surgery and no tamoxifen and in the other two trials tamoxifen alone was compared with surgery and tamoxifen [6,7]. Not surprisingly the time to local relapse was significantly shorter in the tamoxifen alone arm but what was surprising was the number of patients with distant relapse was less in three out of four trials in patients who had no immediate surgery. A more recent combined analysis [26] did show a significant reduction in deaths from breast cancer in patients having immediate surgery. None of these trials set out to answer the question whether endocrine therapy followed by surgery results in a better or worse survival than surgery followed by endocrine therapy.

3. Problems with assessment of response

A problem with endocrine studies has been evaluating response. In general, clinical response has been described using UICC criteria, attempts have been made to assess response using mammography or ultrasound [27]. The problem with UICC criteria is that it demands that any reduction in the product of the two tumour diameters to be present for at least one month. Such a method of assessing response is inappropriate for treatment periods which are often only three months long. For this reason, studies have looked at different methods of assessing response, either by measuring multiple diameters or assessing volume using mammography or ultrasound [27]. In series published to date, complete response rates have varied between 8 and 58%, partial response rates from 15 to 75% with stable disease being reported in 7 to 50% of patients. Progressive disease has been noted in between 0 and 23% of patients [10–19] [20–24]. The median duration of response to tamoxifen in the studies where this has been reported has been approximately two years [8,27–29]. The durations of response in each category has been variable but often prolonged and may relate to how rigorously response was assessed.

Assessing response to primary systemic therapy by changes in tumour volume is a more accurate way of assessing response than using standard UICC criteria.

4. Selection of patients

In most studies, oestrogen receptor status was not measured and thus an unknown proportion of patients with ER-negative tumours were included. Data from the world overview has demonstrated that patients who are ER-negative get little beneficial effect from endocrine therapy. In those series that have selected patients on the basis of ER-positivity, complete and partial response rates have been much higher and when combined have ranged from 72 to 92% [2,11,30–32]. These data emphasise the need to select patients with ER-positive tumours when using primary endocrine therapy [33].

A small study of 12 patients treated with neoadjuvant exemestane has produced similar results to those obtained with letrozole and anastrozole. A randomised study of tamoxifen versus letrozole has now been completed and preliminary data presented at meetings but not yet published had demonstrated that letrozole produces a significantly higher response rate and significantly more patients in the letrozole group underwent conserving surgery.

5. The use of breast conservation after neoadjuvant endocrine therapy

The majority of preoperative endocrine trials have been performed in the elderly and have not been designed to assess whether breast conservation is possible after a period of primary endocrine therapy. Although in some studies it has been reported that endocrine therapy takes many months to produce a clinically evident response, other studies have shown impressive reductions in tumour size within a three month period of neoadjuvant endocrine therapy [2,11,26,30]. In studies of neoadjuvant chemotherapy it appears that breast conserving surgery is associated with satisfactory local control rates following a period of tumour shrinkage with chemotherapy. In one series of 226 patients with breast cancer with tumours larger than 3 cm in greatest dimension, 90% had a reduction in tumour size sufficient to justify breast conservation. 203 patients subsequently underwent breast conservation and in this series there were only 12 local recurrences (5.9%) compared with 5 local recurrences in 23 patients who were not suitable for breast conservation and were treated by mastectomy (21.7%). The median follow up in this study was 6 months [34].

Table 1. Median percentage in tumour volume as assessed by ultrasound

Drug	No	No >50% reduction	No <50% reduction <25% increase	No >25% increase
Tamoxifen	65	30	34	1
Letrozole	24	21	2	1
Anastrozole	23	18	5	0

There are few data on the use of breast conserving surgery following neoadjuvant endocrine therapy: data do show that breast conserving treatment following neoadjuvant chemotherapy produces acceptable local disease control.

One potential problem with using tamoxifen as neoadjuvant therapy is that it takes up to five weeks to attain steady state levels in plasma. In contrast, the newer aromatase inhibitors, letrozole and anastrozole, build up rapidly in plasma and reach effective concentrations within a few days of starting treatment. In one study, 65 patients were treated as part of a standard protocol with three months of tamoxifen, 24 patients were treated with letrozole and 24 patients with anastrozole. In this study patients were monitored at monthly intervals and outcomes were expressed as a percentage change in tumour volume over the three month period as assessed by clinical, ultrasound and mammographic assessments. The numbers of patients who had reductions in tumour volume of more than 50% as assessed by ultrasound are shown in Table 1. Only 2 patients progressed during treatment, one of the 65 patients treated with tamoxifen and one of the 24 patients treated with letrozole. 35 of the 65 patients treated by tamoxifen (46%), 21 out of 24 women treated with letrozole (88%) and 18 out of 23 treated with anastrozole (78%) had a reduction in tumour volume of greater than 50% as assessed by ultrasound. 41 of 65 women were considered to require mastectomy prior to any treatment in the tamoxifen group. At the end of treatment, 21 of these 42 actually underwent breast conservation. In the letrozole group, 15 out of 24 would have required a mastectomy and all patients underwent breast conservation after three months of treatment. Similar results were obtained with anastrozole, 15 patients being considered to require mastectomy at the outset with only 2 patients undergoing mastectomy at the end of the three month treatment period. Follow up data on these patients is short but at a median follow up of four years in the letrozole group two patients have developed local recurrence. Neither of these two patients had radiotherapy following their wide excision. In the anastrozole group all patients received post-operative radiotherapy after breast conserving surgery and after a median of 2 years there have been no local recurrences.

Most studies of neoadjuvant endocrine therapy have been with tamoxifen but there is evidence that aromatase inhibitors may be more effective in postmenopausal women because of the speed at which effective blood levels are achieved.

6. Conclusion

Neoadjuvant therapy is effective. Toxicity in studies to date has been low and the number of patients who have ceased treatment because of side effects is very small. Reductions in tumour volume seen with neoadjuvant endocrine therapy are not dissimilar to those reported with neoadjuvant chemotherapy. From a surgical aspect, the ability to perform less mutilating surgery is an advantage of this approach. The little data available to date suggest that breast conserving surgery followed by radiotherapy produces adequate local control of disease. Further studies of neoadjuvant endocrine therapy are ongoing and the results of these studies are awaited with interest.

References

1. Miller WR, Anderson TJ, Hawkins RA, Keen J, Dixon JM. Neoadjuvant endocrine treatment: the Edinburgh experience. In: Howell A, Dowsett M, editors. ESO Scientific Updates, volume 4. Primary Medical Therapy for Breast Cancer. Amsterdam, Elsevier Science BV, 1–11, 1999.
2. Anderson EDC, Forrest APM, Levack PA, Chetty U, Hawkins RA. Response to endocrine manipulation and oestrogen receptor concentration in large operable primary breast cancer. Br J Cancer 1989; 60: 223–226.
3. Leal da Silva JM, Cardosa F, Oliveira F, Cunha H, Pinton Ferreira E. Neoadjuvant hormonal therapy in locally advanced breast cancer. Eur J Cancer 1998; 34 (suppl 5): S15 Abs 52.
4. Valero V, Hoff PM, Singletary SE, Buzdar AU, Theriault RL, Strom E, Booser DJ, Asmar L, Frye D, McNeese MD, Hortobagyi GN. Combined modality treatment of locally advanced breast cancer (LABC) in elderly patients (PTS) using tamoxifen (TAM) as primary therapy. Proc Am Soc Clin Oncol 1989; 17: 105a, Abs 403.
5. Gaskell DJ, Hawkins RA, de Carteret S, Chetty U, Sangster K, Forrest APM. Indications for primary tamoxifen therapy in elderly women with breast cancer. Br J Surg 1992; 79: 1317–1320.
6. Mustacchi G, Milani S, Pluchinotta A, De Matteis A, Rubagott A, Perrota A. Tamoxifen or surgery plus tamoxifen as primary treatment for elderly patients with operable breast cancer. The GRETA trial. Anticancer Res 1994; 14: 2197–2200.
7. Gazet JC, Ford HT, Coombes RC, Bland JM, Sutcliffe R, Quilliam J, Lowndes S. Prospective randomized trial of tamoxifen vs surgery in elderly patients with breast cancer. Eur J Surg Oncol 1994; 20: 207–214.
8. Van Dalsen AD, De Vries J. Treatment of breast cancer in elderly patients. J Surg Oncol 1995; 60: 80–82.
9. Bergman L, van Dongen JA, van Ooijen B, van Leeuwen FE. Should tamoxifen be a primary treatment choice for elderly patients with locoregional disease. Breast Cancer Res and Treat 1995; 34: 77–83.
10. Ciatto S. Tamoxifen as primary treatment of breast cancer in elderly patients. Neoplasma 1996; 43–45.
11. Dixon JM, Love CDB, Tucker S, Bellamy C, Cameron DA, Miller WR, Leonard RCF. Letrozole as primary medical therapy for locally advanced and large operable breast cancer. Breast Cancer Res and Treat 1997; 46 (suppl): 54.
12. Clemons M, Leahy M, Valle J, Jayson G, Ransopn M, Howell A. Review of recent trails of chemotherapy for advanced breast cancer: studies excluding taxanes. Eur J Cancer 1997; 13: 2171–2182.
13. Fisher B, Mamounas EP. Preoperative chemotherapy: a model for studying the biology and therapy of primary breast cancer. J Clin Oncol 1995; 13: 537–540.
14. Gunduz N, Fisher S, Saffer EA. Effect of surgical removal on the growth and kinetics of residual tumour. Cancer Res 1979; 39: 3861–3865.
15. Fisher B, Gunduz N, Coyle J, Rudock C, Saffer E. Presence of a growth-stimulating factor in serum following primary tumor removal in mice. Cancer Res 1989; 49: 1996–2001.
16. Fisher B, Saffer E, Rudock C, Coyle J, Gunduz N. Effect of local or systemic treatment prior to primary tumour removal on the production and response to a serum growth-stimulating factor in mice. Cancer Res 1989; 49: 2001–2004.
17. Goldie JH, Coldman AJ. A mathematical mode for relating the drug sensitivity of tumors to their spontaneous mutation rate. Cancer Treat Rep 1979; 63: 1727–1733.
18. Skipper HE. Kinetics of mammary tumour cell growth and implication for therapy. Cancer 1971; 28: 1479–1499.
19. Gregory H, Thomas CE, Willshire IR, Young JA, Anderson H, Baildam A, Howell A. Epidermal and transforming growth factor alpha in patients with breast tumours. Br J Cancer 1989; 59: 605–609.
20. Noguchi S, Motomura K, Inaji H, Imaoka S, Koyama H. Down-regulation of transforming growth factor alpha by tamoxifen in human breast cancer. Cancer 1993; 72: 131–136.
21. Vignon F, Bouton MM, Rochefort H. Antiestrogens inhibit the mitogenic effect of growth factor on breast cancer cells in the total absence of estrogen. Biochem Biophys Res Commun 1987; 146: 1502–1508.
22. Ignar-Trowbridge DM, Nelson KG, Bidwell MC, Curtis SW, Washburn TF, McLachlan JA, Korach KS. Coupling of dual signalling pathways: epidermal growth factor action involves the estrogen receptor. Proc Natl Acad Sci USA 1992; 89: 4685–4662.
23. Katzenellengoven BS, Montano MM, Ekena K, Herman ME, McInerney EM. Antiestrogen: mechanism of action and resistance in breast cancer. Breast Cancer Res Treat 1997; 44: 23–48.
24. Early Breast Cancer Trialists' Collaborative Group. Tamoxifen for early breast cancer: an overview of the randomised trials. Lancet 1998; 35: 1451–1467.
25. Bates T, Riley DL, Houghton J, Fallowfield L, Baum M. Breast cancer in elderly women: a Cancer Research Campaign trial comparing treatment with tamoxifen and optimal surgery with tamoxifen alone. Br J Surg 1991; 78: 591–594.
26. Kenny FS, Robertson JFR, Ellis IO, Elston CW, Blamey RW. Primary tamoxifen versus mastectomy

and adjuvant tamoxifen in fit elderly patients with operable breast cancer of high ER content. Breast 1999; 8: 216.

27. Forouhi P, Walsh JS, Anderson TJ, Chetty U. Ultrasound as a method of measuring breast tumour size and monitoring response to primary systemic therapy. Br J Surg 1994; 81: 223–225.
28. Preece PE, Wood RAB, Mackie CR, Cuschieri A. Tamoxifen as initial sole treatment of localised breast cancer in elderly women: a pilot study. BMJ 1982; 284: 869–970.
29. Bradbeer JW, Kyndon J. Primary treatment of breast cancer in elderly women with tamoxifen. Clin Oncol 1983; 9: 31–34.
30. Keen JC, Dixon JM, Miller EP. Cameron DA, Chetty U, Hanby A, Bellamy C, Miller WR. The expression of Ki-s1 and BCL-2 and the response to primary tamoxifen therapy in elderly patients with breast cancer. Breast Cancer Res Treat 1997; 44(2): 123–133.
31. Allan SG, Rodger A, Smyth JF, Leonard RCF, Chetty U, Forest APM. Tamoxifen as primary treatment of breast cancer in elderly or frail patients: A practical management. BMJ 1985; 29: 358.
32. Low SC, Dixon AR, Bell J, Ellis IO, Elston CW, Robertson JFR, Blamey RW. Tumour oestrogen receptor content allows selection of elderly patients with breast cancer for conservative tamoxifen treatment. Br J Surg 1992; 79: 1314–1316.
33. McCarty KS Jr, Miller LS, Cox EB, Konrath J, McCarty KS Sr. Estrogen receptor analyses: correlation of biochemical and immunohistochemical methods using monoclonal antireceptor antibodies. Arch Pathol Lab Med 1985; 109: 716–721.
34. Veronesi U, Bonadonna G, Zurrida S, Galimberti V, Greco M, Brambilla C, Luini A, Andreola S, Rilke F, Rasaelli R, Merson M, Sacchini V, Agresti R. Conservation surgery after primary chemotherapy in large carcinomas of the breast. Ann Surg 1995; 222: 612–618.

Breast Cancer: Diagnosis and Management
J.M. Dixon (Ed.)

CHAPTER 39

Adjuvant chemotherapy for early breast cancer

R.C.F. Leonard and F.E. Nussey

1. Introduction

Adjuvant chemotherapy is given to patients with early breast cancer to eradicate putative micrometastatic of disease which would otherwise result in incurable metastatic disease despite successful local disease control provided by surgery and/or radiotherapy. Systematic overviews of randomised trials for more than a decade and a half have shown that some months of polychemotherapy improves the survival of women presenting with apparently localised breast cancer. Uncertainties remain however as to which women derive most benefit, which regimen should be targeted at which patients, how intensive chemotherapy needs to be and finally how this should be combined with endocrine therapy for patients who have potentially hormone sensitive cancers.

After some 25 years of clinical trials, certain conclusions can be drawn concerning the value of adjuvant chemotherapy for operable breast cancer. The evidence from meta-analysis of randomised clinical trials confirms that poly-chemotherapy given for several months to patients with or without pathological nodal involvement whether pre or post menopausal substantially reduces the risk of recurrence and improves the survival for as long as 10 to 15 years after diagnosis. The broad effect of this chemotherapy is to reduce the recurrence rates by about 25 to 35% and the mortality rate between 25 and 30%.

Recent overview data published in the Lancet [1] confirms that polychemotherapy based on CMF (Cyclophosphamide, Methotrexate, 5 Fluorouracil) produces consistent benefit in terms of reduction of risk of relapse and improvement in mortality across all age groups regardless of ER status or the simultaneous use of endocrine therapy. These data are based on the effect of the CMF regimen, a treatment that in advanced disease only shows modest anti-cancer activity compared with many other polychemotherapies particularly those based on anthracyclines. There is growing evidence for benefit from the use of anthracyclines, both in advanced disease and in the adjuvant setting. New agents are showing even further protective effects notably the recent CALGB Trial in 1998 [2] which shows the additional benefit of adding paclitaxel following an adriamycin/cyclophosphamide regimen.

2. Overview data

In 1998 the Early Breast Cancer Trialists Collaborative Group [1] published the results of an overview of randomised trials of chemotherapy. By definition the trials had to have 5 years of maturity being commenced before 1990 with a comparison differing only in respect of the chemotherapy regimens being compared. This analysis of 18,000 women in 47 trials of prolonged polychemotherapy compared against noth-

Table 1. Proportional risk reductions with polychemotherapy subdivided by age at randomisation (A) and proportional risk reductions in mortality with polychemotherapy during first five years of follow up (years 0–4) and later years (≥5) subdivided by age at randomisation and nodal status (B)

Age at randomisation	% Proportional risk reductions		
	Recurrence (SD)	Mortality (SD)	
(A)			
< 40	37 (7)	27 (8)	
40–49	34 (5)	27 (5)	
50–59	22 (4)	14 (4)	
60–69	18 (4)	8 (4)	
(B)			
	Nodal status	% Proportional risk reduction in mortality	
		0–4 years (SD)	≥5 years (SD)
< 50	−ve	18 (11)	23 (14)
< 50	+ve	24 (7)	39 (8)
50–69	−ve	23 (10)	17 (12)
50–69	+ve	10 (4)	9 (5)

ing included 6,000 patients in 11 trials of long versus short duration polychemo-therapy and 6,000 in 11 trials of anthracycline containing regimens compared against the CMF (cyclophosphamide, methotrexate and 5 fluorouracil) regimen. Results substantially define the benefit of chemotherapy for women under the age of 70 and the results show that for women under the age of 50 at randomisation the reduction in recurrence achieved by chemotherapy was approximately 35%; this reduction is significantly lower for those between the ages of 50 and 69 at around 20%. The mortality reductions for the under 50s were 27% and over 50s 11%. Reductions in recurrence are seen mainly in the first 5 years whereas improvements in survival continue for the first 10 years. The proportional benefit is similar for both node negative and node positive disease. For women under the age of 50 this impact of chemotherapy changes the 10 year survival from about 71% for node negative disease to 78% and for node positive disease from 42% to 53%. For women aged between 50 and 60 at randomisation the absolute benefits change from 67% to 69% i.e. an absolute gain of just 2% for node negative disease and for node positive disease an absolute gain of 3% from 46% to 49% (Table 1A,B).

The age specific benefits of chemotherapy are largely regardless of menopausal status at presentation, the oestrogen receptor status of the primary tumour and whether or not adjuvant tamoxifen had been given. Further conclusions of the overview are that contralateral breast cancer is also influenced by polychemotherapy reducing the occurrence by about a fifth and there is no excess death attributed to the side effects of chemotherapy. There was no benefit to prolonging chemotherapy by more than about 6 months. One new finding which emerged compared to the previous analysis that is when anthracycline containing regimens are compared against the CMF regimen there is an improvement in recurrence and mortality from using anthracyclines.

Polychemotherapy for operable breast cancer reduces relapse and death rates by nearly a third and mortality by a quarter, the effect lasting for more than a decade after diagnosis.

2.1. Interpretation of the overview

The importance of the overview data cannot be overstated. Patients whose data were analysed in this overview had source records reviewed and information on axillary nodal status obtained by pathological review for 98% of patients. One common misunderstanding of the way these data are presented is interpreting the absolute as opposed to the proportional risk reduction for death or recurrence. In the methodology for the trials reported it is stated that the ratio of the absolute to the proportional mortality reduction during the first 10 years is about two fifths for the higher risk (node positive) patients and one fifth for the lower risk (node negative) patients. Thus a 25% reduction in the death rate corresponds to an absolute benefit of 10% for the high risk patients and 5% for the lower risk node negative patients.

3. Importance of age

There is a clear trend for greater risk reductions in younger compared to older patients. Roughly speaking the benefit for those under the age of 40 is twice as large as the relative benefit for those aged between 60 and 69, a 37% risk reduction for recurrence versus an 18% risk reduction respectively for the two age groups. A similar trend is noted for the impact on mortality. Women who are still free of recurrence 5 years after randomisation appear to have a better prognosis beyond 5 years than those who did not have chemotherapy. Although significant in women under the age of 50 this did not reach significance in the over the 50s. In neither age group was there any evidence of loss of these early benefits with longer follow up. Conversely for mortality the gains seen in the first 5 years appear to continue to accrue with time. The absolute gain for node negative disease compared to node positive disease in younger patients is less but there is little difference in gain between node negative and node positive disease in the older age group. For women aged between 50 and 69 the women with node negative disease who appear to gain more in reduction in mortality than those with node positive disease.

Menopausal status did not seem to interact strongly with the chemotherapy effect once age had been taken into account. There were less than 10% of women under the age of 50 who were post menopausal and less than 10% over the age of 50 who were premenopausal so data in these subgroups of patients are somewhat unreliable. Oestrogen receptor status was important only in the post menopausal group where patients who had ER poor disease had nearly twice as much benefit with a risk reduction at 30% when compared to those with ER positive disease where the risk reduction was only 18%.

The effect of chemotherapy is most powerful in the under-50 age group.
Anthracyclines provide some further benefit but in the overview analysis the effect is small.

4. Chemoendocrine therapy

The findings of the meta-analysis were that whether or not tamoxifen is used, polychemotherapy provides an additional benefit in delaying recurrence and death. Excluding patients who had ER poor tumours from the analysis did not materially affect the findings. The Early Breast Cancer Trialists Collaborative Group published an overview of the randomised trials of tamoxifen for early breast cancer in 1998. This showed that the addition of tamoxifen to chemotherapy produced further benefits. Chemotherapy plus about 5 years of tamoxifen was substantially better than the same chemotherapy alone. There is however some concern that tamoxifen, as it slows the division of cancer cells, might make concurrent chemo or radiotherapy less effective. To answer this question will require trials of concurrent versus consecutive chemoendocrine therapy which are not yet available [30].

5. Chemotherapy variants

There is little evidence of benefit for prolonging chemotherapy beyond 6 months. However in the 11 trials which compared CMF against anthracycline containing regimens, a further 12% gain in proportional reduction of recurrence was seen for anthracyclines. These trials are less mature than many of the other trials but the modest gain from anthracyclines in terms of mortality suggest a benefit. They varied from showing an insignificant benefit up to about 5.5% absolute improvement in survival compared to non anthracycline chemotherapy at 5 years.

There is little benefit for prolonging chemotherapy in most patients beyond six months.

The benefits of polychemotherapy confirmed in the overview analysis answers some basic questions but raises many others. The increasing confidence in the validity of the observations concerning benefit help to define more clearly what threshold should be adopted in selecting systemic therapy which is inevitably toxic, time consuming, expensive and not without acute risk. In 1998 the Journal of the National Cancer Institute published a consensus from St Gallen Meeting of the same year, one of whose aims was to redefine thresholds for systemic therapy [3]. At the St Gallen conference, women with a less than 10% chance of relapse at 10 years were considered low risk and therefore not routinely candidates for systemic chemotherapy. This policy recognises the avoidance of relapse as the goal of treatment. The trend of course is to apply systemic therapy to an increasingly good prognostic group. At the very beginning adjuvant therapy was offered only to patients with lymph node positive disease who had a survival at 10 years between 30 and 50%. Ten years ago there was increasing recognition of the need to look at the possibility of adjuvant therapy in women with lymph node negative disease, a group with an approximate 70% overall survival at 10 years. In 1995, the International Consensus Panel recommended chemotherapy for patients with more than 10% mortality at 10 years. This has now been converted to a recommendation for the use of chemotherapy for patients with a 10% risk of relapse as opposed to 10% mortality. The philosophy behind re-examining the thresholds for benefit has emerged from the observation that even disease perceived to have low risk of mortality is in reality associated with a significant disease-specific morbidity. Thus the National Surgical Adjuvant Breast and Bowel Project (NSABP) examined the disease free survival of lymph node negative patients who have received no adjuvant systemic therapy according to tumour size. In the ER negative trial (B13) [4] the 5 year disease free survival for untreated patients with less than 1 cm sized tumours was only 77%. In the ER positive trial (B14) [5] the 5 year disease free survival for the same sized tumours was 82%. Others have also examined the survival of lymph node negative T1 breast cancers treated by mastectomy, and after 10 years women with tumours less than 1 cm had a mortality of 7% and a relapse-free survival of 91%. At 20 years these figures had become 10% and 88% respectively. For larger tumours up to 2 cm, at 10 years the mortality was 18% and the disease free survival 78% and at 20 years survival was 76% and disease free survival 74%. Interestingly the pattern of relapse for the smallest tumours showed a proportionally higher risk of late relapse when compared to larger tumours. This means that in good and intermediate risk, lymph node negative breast cancer the 20 year survival statistics are very important. An important survey by Ravdin and colleagues [6] of breast cancer patients concerning their knowledge and expectations of adjuvant chemotherapy suggest that the recipients of treatment would judge an improvement of relapse rates as low as 1% to be an acceptable outcome for toxic treatment (Table 2 and Table 3).

Node negative breast cancer has an approximate 10 year survival of 70%.
Node positive breast cancer has an approximate 10 year survival of 30–50%.
Tumour size and oestrogen receptor status are also prognostic factors.
For tumours of < 1 cm diameter, node status is the critical determinant of outcome.

Table 2. Definitions of risk groups and associated risk of relapse

Risk group	Age	Survival without relapse at 5 years
Node −ve patients		
Low risk	> 35 tumour ≤ 1 cm in diameter	> 90%
Intermediate risk	≤ 35 tumour ≤ 1 cm in diameter	75–80%
	> 35 tumours > 1 cm grade I or II	
High risk	≤ 35 tumour > 1 cm grade I or II	50–60%
	Any tumour > 1 cm grade III	
Node +ve patients		
Low + intermediate	> 35 1–3 positive nodes	40–50%
High risk	≤ 35 1–3 positive nodes	20–30%
	> 35 4–9 positive nodes	
Very high risk	≤ 35 4 + nodes involved	10–15%
	> 35 10 + nodes involved	

Table 3. Adjuvant treatment for patients with breast cancer

	ER	Premenopausal	Postmenopausal
Node −ve patients			
Low risk	+ve	Tam or nil	Tam or nil
	−ve	Nil	Nil
Intermediate risk	+ve	Tam	Tam
	−ve	Chemotherapy	Chemotherapy
High risk	+ve	Chemo + Tam	Tam +/− Chemo
	−ve	Chemo	Chemo
Node +ve patients			
Low + intermediate risk	+ve	Chemo + Tam +/− LHRH	Chemo +Tam
	−ve	Chemo	Chemo
High + very high risk	+ve	More intensive chemo + Tam + LHRH	More intensive chemo + Tam if fit

The trend has been to extend the use of systemic therapy to a wide range of patients. These long term data for patients with low risk disease are extremely important in that all units are now seeing patients with earlier stage disease due to the impact of Screening Programmes. The question of selection becomes more important, the hope being to identify the sub set of patients with disease which really has poor risk in the long term as opposed to that which can be safely watched and not treated with adjuvant therapy. Various clinical factors are recognised, can be reproducibly measured and are powerful; namely hormonal status of the tumour, pathological grade and age, as well as node status. With the advent of new therapies such as the antibody transtuzumab ('Herceptin') bio markers which predict response as well as prognosis are being sought and maybe of great importance [8,28].

6. Intensive adjuvant chemotherapy for breast cancer

6.1. Selection of adjuvant therapy

In making decisions about selecting adjuvant chemotherapy, clinical as well as biological factors have to be taken into account. The most important relates to the selection of patients. Treatment that can be offered to a 40 year old is not necessarily appropriate for a 69 year old although they might have the same biological risk

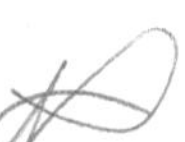

factors. The patient's age therefore and general fitness have a major impact on the decision making. Furthermore, no two patients have the same needs and whereas one patient may be prepared to accept a high incidence of side effects for a small statistical gain, another patient may make an informed decision not to have treatment.

The search for biological factors that predict chemotherapy benefit continues. ER/PgR remains the only useful predictive factor for adjuvant therapy, its major benefit being the ability to select patients who will not benefit from adjuvant hormone therapy as revealed by the recent EBCTG overview [7]. CerbB2 (HER2) might be the chemotherapy equivalent and is under investigation. In a well publicised study by Muss et al. in 1994 [8], there appeared to be an interaction between HER2 over-expression and a benefit from intensified anthracycline chemotherapy in the adjuvant setting. Although further studies have claimed to substantiate this effect, this is not borne out by a close examination of these reports [28].

The most powerful biological predictor of outcome is the pathological involvement of the axillary lymph nodes at the time of primary surgery [9]. In the absence of any other factors, patients with uninvolved lymph nodes at the time of surgery have a better than 70% chance of disease free survival at 10 years. In contrast, patients with more than 20 lymph nodes involved have a less than 10% chance of being disease free at 10 years. All other levels of nodal involvement from 1–20 show a gradation in survival according to node number involved (Table 2). The Nottingham Prognostic Index also suggests that tumour grade and tumour size may add further prognostic information in addition to nodal involvement. This has been verified by independent studies (see chapter by Pinder).

> *The index is less useful for small [e.g. screen-detected tumours] < 1 cm [10].*

6.2. Selection of appropriate adjuvant chemotherapy

The overview data show that although the relative benefit of chemotherapy is constant the absolute benefit is necessarily less for the patients with a good prognosis than for those with a poor prognosis. Furthermore the benefit seen in the under 50s is much stronger than the benefit seen in the over 50s. There is therefore uncertainty as to whether cytotoxic chemotherapy is justified in older patients with good risk disease whereas there is no doubt that in younger patients with poor risk disease the benefit is worthwhile. Complete protection is not however provided by CMF based polychemotherapy and for poor risk patients delaying the onset of an inevitable recurrence has to be regarded as an inadequate outcome. The 1998 overview statistics [1] confirmed what individual trials have directly indicated that appropriately used anthracyclines significantly improve the relapse and survival outcomes for patients in the adjuvant setting when compared to standard CMF treatment. In the overview data, the relative benefits of anthracyclines over CMF are modest with a 12% reduction in the rate of relapse and 11% relative improvement in survival at 5 years. This translates to only 2–3% gain in absolute benefit for the risk groups examined. Although a statistically powerful effect, the clinical benefit is very modest. Two individual trials have indicated that these small benefits from anthracyclines may be related to the quality of the chemotherapy. The International Collaborative Cancer Group (ICCG) trial reported by Coombes in 1996 [11] looked at 2 forms of CMF chemotherapy against 2 matched forms of FEC chemotherapy (5 fluorouracil, epirubicin and cyclophosphamide). It is only the relatively intensive form of FEC (5 fluorouracil and cyclophosphamide on day 1 and 8 at 600 mg/m^2 each and epirubicin 50 mg/m^2 on day 1 out of a 28 day cycle) which when compared against the more intensive form of CMF showed a clear benefit at 5 year with an improved survival at 5 years of 73.8% for CMF to 86.6% for FEC. A similar dose intense programme by Levine et al in Canada [12] also showed substantial benefits for CEF (cyclophosphamide 75 mf/m^2 d1–14, epirubicin 60 mg/m^2 d1 and d8, 5 fluorouracil 500 mg/m^2 d1 and d8) compared with CMF.

The most impressive results from anthracycline therapy come from Buzzoni and colleagues updated by Bonadonna in 1995 [13]. In this trial the sequencing of chemotherapy was examined by comparing alternating CMF and doxorubicin over 12 cycles and against a sequential regimen comprising 4 cycles of doxorubicin initially followed by 8 cycles of CMF. The total dose intensity and dose rate were identical in both arms. The outcomes however were very different with a disease free survival for the alternating regimen at 10 years of 28% compared to 42% for the sequential therapy; the overall survivals were 44% and 58% respectively. Furthermore the shape of the survival curve for the sequential regimen indicates that there may be long term cured patients as opposed to simply delaying relapse. The price in terms of cardiotoxicity was not heavy with 4 cases [< 2%] of clinical heart failure, 2 fatal. Other studies have confirmed the activity of the Bonadonna regimen but have only short follow up. Our own experience in Edinburgh [14] of 75 patients with a 3 year follow up has confirmed 95% overall survival for patients with 4–9 nodes involved and 70% for patients with more than 10 nodes affected. The disease free survivals for both groups are 62% and 60% respectively. Toxicity from this therapy has proved to be predictable and to date there have been no cardiac or treatment related deaths. Other studies [15] published in the last 12 months have confirmed that provided that the cumulative dose of epirubicin or doxorubicin is kept within the guidelines, the risk of congestive heart failure is very low at less than 4%. One issue of concern in relation to dose intensity of anthracyclines is the risk of acute myeloblastic leukaemia which is thought to be related to the topoisumimane II inhibition effect of anthracylcines. The acute leukaemia is (characteristic of 11 q23 translocation pattern) seen at a frequency of up to 5–7% in the very dose intense anthracycline programmes published by Berg [16] and to a lesser extent by Levine [12]. This is compared to a CMF-associated leukaemia risk of 0.23% over a 15 year period [17] with reports from the ICCG and NSABP B15 [18] groups of less than 1%. The overall risk of leukaemia in association with standard doses of anthracyclines is around 1.4%. Providing the use of anthracyclines is not at excessive dose rates, but at the levels suggested by Coombes [11] and Levine [12], the beneficial effects of anthracycline combination therapy seems to outweigh the late risks and may substantially reduce the risk of relapse of breast cancer. Anthracycline regimens remain the most potent anticancer treatments for breast disease in the neoadjuvant setting.

Adequate dose intensity and scheduling appear necessary for best effect of anthracyclines.
There is a small risk of leukaemia from the highest achievable intensity with anthracyclines.
The evidence for HER2 — anthracycline interaction is weak.

7. cerbB2/HER2 and immunotherapy

The presence of HER2 gene amplification and/or associated oncoprotein over-expression in the cell membrane is associated with a worse outcome regardless of adjuvant treatment. This pattern of expression is seen in about 30% of breast cancers. Whereas the interaction of this protein expression with anthracycline dose remains controversial it becomes clear that patients with this biological feature with advanced breast cancer obtain a real benefit from the use of a humanised antibody to HER2 which has been in clinical trials for the last 5 years. ‘Herceptin’ (trastuzumab) is a humanised IgG3 anti-cerbB2 antibody which was demonstrated to have good single agent activity in chemotherapy failed patients with a 15% overall objective response rate according to studies by Slamon et al. [19]. The antibody on its own produces very few side effects apart from some protein associated chills and fevers. In the last 12 months 2 reports on a trial combining 'Herceptin' with chemotherapy have shown a higher response rate of around 60% compared to 47% for the chemotherapy alone (doxorubicin, cyclophosphamide) and a recent update by Norton [20] has confirmed that this translates to a 20% improvement in the median survival of patients of about 25 months compared to about 20 months on the chemotherapy alone. This benefit was seen both for adding the antibody to adriamycin and cyclophosphamide and also to Taxol for those patients who had prior anthracycline exposure. The one problem at the moment seems to be an enhanced risk of cardiotoxic complications for those patients on simultaneous anthracyclines and 'Herceptin'. Trials looking at the impact of 'Herceptin' in the adjuvant setting are about to start.

'Herceptin' is an effective immunotherapeutic agent in selected [HER2+] advanced disease. There is no information on its effect in adjuvant setting. Caution is advised and cardiac effects have been reported when it is used in combination with anthracyclines.

8. Bisphosphonates

Intravenous bisphosphonates have shown unequivocal benefit for patients with symptomatic metastases in the bones both in combination with endocrine therapy and with cytotoxic chemotherapy. Their place in the adjuvant therapy setting is less clear. There was a very strikingly positive report by Diel and colleagues in 1998 [21] indicating that clodronate by mouth, reduced not only the incidence of bone metastases but also visceral metastases with associated benefits on survival regardless of the other adjuvant therapy employed. However, a similar study by Saarto and colleagues [22] has shown exactly the opposite effect. Trials looking at intravenous as well as oral therapy with bisphosphonates in the high risk adjuvant setting need to start soon to address this potentially important further modification of standard protocols.

Bisphosphonates, especially intravenously, are effective for bone palliation in advanced disease. Their effect in adjuvant setting remains uncertain.

9. High dose chemotherapy

Apart from two inadequately powered trials reported in 1998, there were no large scale randomised control studies on high dose chemotherapy in the adjuvant setting until this year. These data have been long awaited, particularly in view of the very encouraging reports from Duke University [25] and from Milan when high dose chemotherapy in the adjuvant setting was compared against historical control data. At the ASCO meetings in 1999 three randomised controlled trials were reported in the adjuvant setting. Bergh [23] reported a Swedish study of 525 patients with node positive disease who were randomly assigned to 5 fluorouracil, epirubicin and cyclophosphamide (FEC) chemotherapy ×3 followed by high dose chemotherapy (cyclophosphamide, thiotepa and carboplatinum) compared against a 'tailored' FEC arm of 9 cycles where the dose was increased to tolerance levels supported by GCSF on an individual patient basis. The median term results show a clear advantage for the tailored FEC combination compared against high dose chemotherapy with 50 relapses and 40 deaths against 78 relapses and 40 deaths for the high dose chemotherapy. There were 2 deaths due to high dose chemotherapy in one arm against 8 deaths from acute myeloid leukaemia (AML) or myelodysplastic syndrome (MDS) when using the intensified FEC regimen (see previous). The Bergh trial is interesting. The results of the tailored arm FEC are impressive although this would not be regarded as standard therapy. Further analysis is unlikely to show benefit for the high dose chemotherapy but the incidence of AML/MDS in the tailored therapy arm raise major concerns about this sort of intensity of anthracycline therapy as a standard treatment.

The Cancer and Acute Leukaemia Group B (CALGB) trial reported by Peters [24] was basically the randomised version of the Duke University study which had shown promise when compared against the historical controls. 783 patients with more than 10 involved nodes were randomly assigned to cyclophosphamide, adriamycin and 5 fluorouracil (CAF) plus high dose cyclophosphamide, carmustine (BCNU) and platinum (CBP) compared against the same induction followed by standard doses of CBP. The disease free survival at 3 years was 68% against 64% (not significant) but there were 29 deaths in the high dose arm (7.4%). This trial was analysed earlier than planned and the next analysis will not be for another 2 years. It is also noted that the high dose results are similar to those seen with the high dose treatment at 3 years in the pilot study (72% DFS). What has changed is the DFS in the control group. The level of mortality is totally unacceptable given that results elsewhere show a 0–2% treatment complication rate but there is a hint of a late benefit although not significant for the high dose arm. It is unlikely that this trial will show a substantial benefit for high dose chemotherapy partly due to the high mortality of the treatment.

The third trial to be reported was that of Bezwoda [26], showing benefit for the high dose therapy. On the basis of these seemingly important positive findings it was decided to perform an international confirmatory study, but before this an on site review of records was sought. The essential findings were that the trial was seriously flawed and the results have been discounted [32]. At the AsCO meeting in 2000, preliminary results were presented from the NWAST group (Netherlands Working Party on Autotransplantation in Solid Tumours) trial. A total of 885 patients have been randomised into this phase III study comparing 5 courses of standard adjuvant chemotherapy against 4 courses of the same chemotherapy and a 5th course of high dose chemotherapy plus a peripheral blood progenitor cell transplant. All patients have now completed adjuvant chemotherapy and early analysis of the data shows a benefit in the high dose arm. Obviously this data is not yet mature, and full results are awaited [33].

There are several major European trials continuing which have not yet reported on high dose chemotherapy which include the Anglo–Celtic 1 trial which compares the Bonadonna sequential adriamycin and CMF regimen as the standard treatment against 4 cycles of doxorubicin followed by cyclophosphamide/thiotepa. This has just closed having recruited 600 patients. A similarly powered Dutch study is due to report on 850 patients and there are 3 other German studies and one other British study (recruiting 300 patients) all with basically similar lines of induction plus high dose compared against an alkylating combination as the standard arm.

The general view of high dose chemotherapy at the moment is that the trials are still immature and several have not even had their first analysis. A major (30%) benefit from high dose chemotherapy compared against standard dose therapy is highly unlikely and trials need to be meta-analysed to show a clinically significant but smaller benefit. One problem with all this sort of argument about high dose chemotherapy is that the standard treatment has probably changed over the years and nowadays a trial would probably have to include taxoids with anthracyclines as standard treatment in a comparative study.

High dose chemotherapy has not been proved to provide major benefit in the initial reports of adjuvant trials. Further trials and probably meta-analysis are awaited.

10. Primary systemic therapy

There are several theoretical advantages to primary systemic therapy as opposed to post operative chemotherapy. One is the early action of cytotoxic drugs against micrometastatic disease, secondly the chance of assessing response effectiveness of the chosen treatment and thirdly the down staging of the primary tumour avoiding mastectomy or converting inoperable to operable disease and improving local control. In endocrine therapy there is also interest in studying the impact of tamoxifen or aromatase inhibitors on ER and BCL2 as mediators of endocrine therapy effects at the cellular level. In contrast, in the chemotherapy studies, intense interest has been expressed in the effect of cytotoxics on p53, HER2 and p-Glycoprotein (over expressed in some chemotherapy resistant cancers). In addition, by studying tumour biopsies during treatment, the pharmacodynamic effects of cytotoxics and endocrine agents can be assessed directly on human cancer tissue. Clinical and ultrasonic examination of tumour response patterns give the possibility of mathematical modelling of tumour response against outcome [27]. The most active regimens reported include anthracyclines with response rates of between 75 and 90%. However looking at randomised trials there is no evidence yet of a survival gain for patients treated this way compared against standard treatment. There is undoubtedly however a gain in terms of surgical benefit for many patients [29,31]. The interest in primary therapy remains intense because of the possibility of experimenting and finding early indicators of benefit or resistance. What is quite clear from these results is that patients who have had nodes involved at the end of primary therapy have a very poor prognosis and trials are underway to examine the potential benefit of high dose chemotherapy compared against standard treatment for this group of patients whose prognosis is dismal.

Despite theoretical benefits randomised trials have not shown primary systemic therapy to be superior to standard postoperative chemotherapy. It is however a productive area for research into the effects of treatments and may lead to more rapid assessment of benefit with new policies.

11. General conclusion

Anthracyclines at appropriate dose and schedule have now established a clear place in the treatment of poor risk disease in the adjuvant setting. Bone protecting compounds and immunotherapy approaches are also being examined in the adjuvant setting. There is no clear advantage for primary chemotherapy apart from down staging the primary tumour and providing a good research tool to investigate new treatment designs. The debate on high dose chemotherapy remains.

References

1. Early Breast Cancer Trialists Group. Polychemotherapy for early breast cancer — overview of the randomised trials. Lancet 1998; 352: 930–942.
2. Henderson IC, Berry D, Demetri G, Cirrincione C, Goldstein L, Martino S et al. Improved disease free and overall survival from the addition of sequential paclitaxel but not from the escalation of doxorubicin dose level in the adjuvant chemotherapy of patients with node positive primary breast cancer. Proc Am Soc Clin Oncol 1998; 17: 101.
3. Goldhirsch A, Glick J H, Gelbe R, Senn H J. Meeting highlights International Consensus Panel on the treatment of breast cancer. JNCI 1998; 19: 1601–1608.
4. Fisher B, Redmond C, Dimitrov N, Bowman D, Legant–Poisson S, Wickerham L et al. A randomised clinical trial evaluating sequential methotrexate and 5 flurouracvil in the treatment of patients with node negative breast cancer who have oestrogen receptor negative tumours. NEJM 1989; 320(8): 473–478.
5. Fisher B, Costantino J, Redmond C, Poisson R, Bowman D, Couture J, et al. A randomised controlled trial evaluating tamoxifen in the treatment of patients with node negative breast cancer who have oestrogen receptor positive tumours. NEJM 1989; 320(8): 479–484.
6. Ravdin P M, Siminoff I A, Harvey J A. Survey of breast cancer patients concerning their knowledge and expectations of adjuvant therapy. J Clin Oncol 1998; 16(2): 515–521.
7. Early Breast Cancer Trialists Group. Tamoxifen for early breast cancer: an overview of randomised trials. Lancet 1998; 351: 1451–1467.
8. Muss HB, Thor AD, Berry DA, Kute T, Liu ET, Koerner F et al. c-erbB-2 expression and response to adjuvant therapy in women with node-positive early breast cancer. N Engl J Med 1994; 330(18): 1260–1266.

9. ABC of Breast Diseases. Dixon JM, ed. BMJ Publishing Group 1995.
10. Kollias J, Murphy CA, Elston CW, Ellis IO, Robertson JFR, and Blamey RW. The Prognosis of Small Primary Breast Cancers. Eur J Cancer 1999; 35(6): 908–912.
11. Coombes RC, Bliss JM, Wils J, Morvan F, Espie M, Amadori D et al. Adjuvant cyclophosphamide, methotrexate and fluorouracil versus fluorouracil, epirubicin, cyclophosphamide chemotherapy in premenopausal women with axillary node positive operable breast cancer: results of a randomised trial. The International Collaborative Cancer Group. J Clin Oncol 1996; 14: 35–45.
12. Levine MM, Bramwell VH, Pritchard KI, Norris BD, Shepherd LE, Abu–Zahra H et al. Randomised trial of intensive cyclophosphamide, epirubicin and 5 fluorouracil chemotherapy compared with cyclophosphamide, methotrexate and fluorouracil in pre menopausal women with node positive breast cancer. J Clin Oncol 1998; 16(8): 2651–2658.
13. Bonadonna G, Zambetti M, Valagussa P. Sequential or alternating doxorubicin and CMF regimens in breast cancer with more than 3 positive nodes: 10 year results. JAMA 1995; 273(7): 542–547.
14. Anderson A, Cameron DA, Massie C, Dillon P, Leonard RCF. A single centre experience of adjuvant doxorubicin-CMF chemotherapy for multiple node positive breast cancer. Unpublished data.
15. Neilson D, Jensen JB, Dombernowsky P et al. Epirubicin cardiotoxicity: A study of 135 patients with advanced breast cancer. J Clin Oncol 1990; 8: 1806–1810.
16. Bergh J, Wiklund T, Erikstein B, Fornander T, Bengtsson N O, Malmstrom P et al. Dosage of adjuvant G-CSF (filgrastim)-supported FEC polychemotherapy based on equivalent haematological toxicity in high risk breast cancer patients. Scandinavian Breast Group SBG 9401. Ann Oncol 1998; 9(4): 403–411.
17. Valagussa P, Moliterni A, Tereziani M, Zambetti M, Bonadonna G. Second malignancies following CMF-based adjuvant chemotherapy in resectable breast cancer. Ann Oncol 1994; 5(9): 803–808.
18. Fisher B, Brown AM, Dimitrov NV, Poiisson R, Redmond C, Margolese RG, et al. Two months of doxorubicin-cyclophosphamide with and without interval reinduction therapy compared with 6 months of cyclophosphamide, methotrexate, and flurouracil in positive-node breast cancer patients with tamoxifen-nonresponsive tumors: results from the National Surgical Adjuvant Breast and Bowel Project B-15. J Clin Oncol 1990 Sep; 8(9): 1483–1496.
19. Cobleigh MA, Vogel CL, Tripathy D, Robert NJ, Scholl S, Frenbacher L et al. Efficacy and Safety of Herceptin (Humanized Anti-Her2 Antibody) As A single Agent in 222 Women with Her2 Overexpression Who Relapsed Following Chemotherapy for Metastatic Breast Cancer. Proceedings of American Society of Clinical Oncology 1998; #376: p97a.
20. Norton L, Slamon D, Leyland–Jones B, Wolter J, Fleming T, Eirmann W et al. Overall survival (OS) advantage to simultaneous chemotherapy plus humanised anti HER2 monoclonal antibody Herceptin in HER2 — overexpressing metastatic breast cancer. Proceedings of ASCO 1999(18); Abstract 483: p127a.
21. Diel IJ, Solomayer EF, Costa SD, Gollan C, Goerner R, Wallwiener D et al. Reduction in new metastases in breast cancer with adjuvant clodronate treatment. N Engl J Med 1998; 339(6): 357–363.
22. Saarto T, Blomquvist C, Virkkunen P, Elomaa I. No reduction of bone metastases with adjuvant clodronate in node positive breast cancer patients. Proceedings of ASCO 1999 (18); Abstract 489: 128a.
23. Scandanavian Breast Cancer Study Group. Results from a randomised adjuvant breast cancer study with high dose chemotherapy with CTCb supported by autologus bone marrow stem cells versus dose escalating and tailored effect therapy. Proceedings of ASCO 1999; 18: Abstract 3. p2a.
24. Peters W, Rosner G, Vredenburgh J, Shpall E, Crump M, Richardson P, et al. A prospective randomised comparison of 2 doses of combination alkylating agents (AA) as consolidation after CAF in high risk primary breast cancer involving 10 or more axillary lymph nodes: Preliminary results of CALGB9082/SWOG91104/NCICMA-13. Proceedings of ASCO 1999; (18): Abstract 2. p1a.
25. Peters W, Ross M, Vredenburgh J, Meisenberg B, Marks L, Winer E et al. High-dose chemotherapy and autologous bone marrow support as consolidation after standard dose adjuvant therapy for high risk primary breast cancer. J Clin Oncol 1993 11(6) 1132–1143.
26. Bezwoda WR. Randomised controlled trial of high dose chemotherapy (HD-CNVp) versus standard dose (CAF) chemotherapy for high risk, surgically treated, primary breast cancer. Proceedings of ASCO 1999; 18: abstract 4. p2a.
27. D Cameron et al. Mathematical model of response in primary chemotherapy for breast cancer. British Journal of Cancer. 1996. 73 1409–1416.
28. Cameron DA, Leonard RC. Re; erbB-2, p53, and efficacy of adjuvant therapy in lymph node-positive breast cancer. J Natl Cancer Inst 1999; 91(8): 728–729.
29. Fisher B, Bryant J, Wolmark N, Mamounas E, Brown A, Fisher ER et al. Effect of preoperative chemotherapy on the outcome of women with operable breast cancer. J Clin Oncol 1998; 16(8): 2672–2685.
30. Early Breast Cancer Trialists Collaborative Group. Tamoxifen for early breast cancer: an overview of the randomised trials. Lancet 1998; 351: 1451–1465.
31. Scholl S, Beuzeboc P, Harris AL, Pierga JY, Asselain B, Palangis T, et al. Is Primary Chemotherapy Useful for All patients with Primary Invasive Breast Cancer?

Recent Results in Cancer Research 1998; 152: 217–226.

32. Weiss RB, Rifkin RM, Stewart FM, Theriault RL, Williams LA, Herman AA, et al. High dose chemotherapy for high risk primary breast cancer: an on site review of the Bezwoda study. *Lancet* 2000; 355(18): 999–1003.

33. Rodenhuis S, Bontenbal M, Beex LVAM, van der Wall E, Richel DJ, Nooij MA, et al. Randomized phase III study of high dose chemotherapy with cyclophosphamide, thiotepa and carboplatim in operable breast cancer with 4 or more axilliary lymph nodes. *Proc. ASCO* 2000; 19: abstract 286.

Breast Cancer: Diagnosis and Management
J.M. Dixon (Ed.)

CHAPTER 40

Adjuvant endocrine therapy for early breast cancer

F. Nussey and R.C.F. Leonard

1. Introduction

It has been known for over 100 years that hormones have an important influence on the behaviour of breast carcinoma [1]. At first presentation breast carcinoma is considered in many women to be a systemic disease with micrometastases thought to be present at the time of diagnosis. Systemic treatment needs to be considered for these women and may involve the use of chemotherapy, endocrine therapy or both.

2. Selection of endocrine treatment

The decision to use endocrine therapy is based on a number of factors. The first being the oestrogen receptor (ER) status of the tumour. This helps to identify those patients who are most likely to benefit from the currently available forms of endocrine therapy. The choice of agent depends on the menopausal status of patient. The major site of oestrogen production changes from being primarily ovarian in pre-menopausal women to being produced peripherally from precursor androgens released by the adrenal glands, with subsequent conversion by the aromatase enzyme in fat and muscle in post-menopausal women [2]. Many women will not derive benefit from the adjuvant endocrine therapy they will receive but as yet it is impossible to determine those in whom either the disease is truly localised or those whose disease will be affected by the treatment [3].

3. Oestrogen receptor status

This should be assessed in every patient with breast carcinoma. It is usually assessed either by an ELISA based biochemical assay or by immunohistochemistry. The latter has superseded the former because of convenience and the ability to assay routinely processed paraffin embedded tissue. Unfortunately there is a lack of consistency between laboratories as to what constitutes ER positivity. The potential for significant error in evaluating ER, particularly during the era of biochemical assays, resulted in poor standardisation of quantitative data. Thus many women have been misclassified as being ER negative and have either not been offered potentially beneficial therapy or have been given tamoxifen despite being "ER negative".

> *About 60% of breast cancers express significant amounts of ER protein.*
> *Endocrine therapy is a valuable treatment for early and advanced breast cancers.*

4. Current practice for use of tamoxifen

Tamoxifen is the most widely prescribed anti cancer drug in clinical use and its widespread adoption is thought to be the major contributor to the fall in mortality from breast cancer in the UK [6]. Tamoxifen is thought to work by competing with oestradiol for the high affinity oestrogen receptor and binding to it. In this way it leaves the cell refractory to oestrogenic stimulation, and may result in the death of cells that are dependent on oestrogen for their survival [4].

Over the last 30 years there have been a multitude of studies reporting the effects of hormonal treatments in early breast carcinoma. The first adjuvant trial reported was in 1977. The NATO (Nolvadex Adjuvant Treatment Organisation) trial showed that tamoxifen given for 2 years after mastectomy reduced the risk of relapse and death [12,13]. In an attempt to clarify statistically variable data the Early Breast Cancer Trialists Collaborative Group was established in Oxford in the middle 1980s. They have produced several meta-analyses which have provided overview consensus data on which current practice is based. The most recent publication in 1998 reviewed world-wide data on over 30,000 patients who had received tamoxifen with early breast cancer who had a minimum of 10 years of follow up. This showed a beneficial effect from the use of tamoxifen in the adjuvant setting in both pre- and post-menopausal ER-positive women. It had been previously thought that pre-menopausal women derived less benefit. This review showed that for ER-positive women there were proportional reductions in the risk of recurrence at 1 year, 2 years and 5 years of 21%, 29%, and 47% respectively and that the proportional reductions in mortality were 12%, 17% and 26% at the same time intervals (Table 1). In the group who were ER positive or ER poor there was a proportional reduction in the risk of contralateral breast carcinoma of 13%, 26% and 47% at 1, 2 and 5 years respectively (Table 3). There was some data to suggest that a positive progesterone receptor might identify a tamoxifen responsive subset who were ER poor, but the number of patients was too small, and it was felt that further research was required into the benefits of tamoxifen in ER-negative patients. The authors advised caution in applying the results in those found to be ER negative (mainly for the reasons previously described) and suggested that if might be prudent to re-test these patients [5]. Similar benefits were found in node-negative and node-positive patients. The only subgroup who appeared to derive no benefit from adjuvant tamoxifen were the truly ER-negative women aged less than 50 years.

Table 1. Proportional risk reduction during the first 5 years for ER-positive and ER unknown patients, subdivided by tamoxifen duration

Duration of tamoxifen	Recurrence (SD)	Mortality from any cause (SD)
1 year	20% (3)	12% (3)
2 years	28% (2)	17% (6)
5 years	47% (3)	26% (4)

Adapted from Ref. [5].

Endocrine therapy has been used in randomised controlled trials for over 25 years. There is unequivocal evidence for a significant benefit for the use of tamoxifen in early breast cancer. At 10 years there is a reduction in risk of recurrence by 47% and of death by 28% in ER-positive patients.

5. Duration of tamoxifen therapy

Currently most patients are given 5 years of adjuvant tamoxifen. The overview data shows that 2 years of treatment is suboptimal, and the hope that a longer duration of tamoxifen therapy is beneficial is based on disease free and overall survival trends in the overview data supported by pre-clinical studies showing that it might be a cytostatic agent [3]. The true optimum duration however remains controversial. The NSABP-B14 trial reported that disease free survival was worse in patients treated for 10 years rather than those treated for 5 years [7], an ECOG trial showed the opposite [8], whereas a Scottish trial [9] showed no appreciable differences in recurrence between

5 years or more than 5 years of treatment. Several concerns have been raised about these trials; one of them closed early and the follow up was too short for any potential late benefits of tamoxifen to be identified. There is a benefit which continues after tamoxifen therapy is stopped, so delayed events may have important bearing on interpretation of these trials. The EBCTCG agree that it may take several more years to establish whether tamoxifen should be given for more than 5 years as there have not been enough deaths in the groups studied.

The precise duration of tamoxifen treatment is uncertain.
The minimum duration is 5 years.
Trials are underway to define the optimum duration of therapy.

Any potential benefits of longer treatment periods must be balanced against the risk of relapse of the original breast cancer and the increased incidence of "side effects", including endometrial cancer. Two large studies are in progress, which aim to answer the question of how long adjuvant tamoxifen should be given. One million patients now take adjuvant tamoxifen and many of these are discharged from hospital follow up whilst still on tamoxifen [6,10,11].

6. Safety issues with tamoxifen

The commonest side effects reported with Tamoxifen are hot flushes, vaginal discharge, irregular menses and endometrial changes. Tumour flare, visual disturbances, leucopenia, ovarian cysts in pre-menopausal women and liver enzyme abnormalities have been reported but are not common [11]. Many of these are minor and not harmful. There are some "side effects" of concern.

6.1. Endometrial cancer risk

It is known that unopposed oestrogen promotes the development of endometrial cancer. Approximately 250 cases have been reported world wide in women on adjuvant tamoxifen trials [2]. In the untreated control groups there were 80 cases. This is an important issue when giving adjuvant tamoxifen because we are treating some women who will not derive any benefit and are at risk of side effects. The EBCTCG addressed this issue recently [5]. In their meta-analysis the incidence of endometrial cancer was doubled with one or two years of adjuvant tamoxifen, and increased by a factor of four with five years of therapy. The increased risk of endometrial cancer at five years is approximately one case annually per 1000 women on tamoxifen (Table 2). The absolute reduction in the risk of contralateral breast cancer was however twice as great as the absolute increase in endometrial cancer. Other groups have looked at endometrial cancer risk [17]. In a series of 825 patients screened annually by cervical cytology and endometrial aspiration/curettage, tamoxifen did not appear to be associated with an increased risk of endometrial cancer when compared to the general population [14]. Others feel the increase is in part due to greater surveillance reflecting heightened awareness and increased use of screening procedures in this population [11,15]. This is corroborated by the fact that these cancers, once detected, have the same characteristics in terms of stage, grade, histology and outcome as endometrial cancers detected in the general population [15,16]. Nevertheless, the American College of Obstetricians and Gynaecologists has issued

Table 2. Endometrial cancer risk in women taking tamoxifen, irrespective of ER status (10-year risk per 1,000)

Tamoxifen duration	Endometrial cancer incidence	Control incidence	Endometrial cancer mortality	Control mortality
1 year	5	2	2	1
2 years	4	2	1	0
5 years	11	3	2	0
Total	6	2	1.7	0.4

Adapted from Ref. [5].

guidelines on the management of patients on tamoxifen [16].

There is a small increased risk of endometrial carcinoma with tamoxifen, but this risk is it is outweighed by the beneficial effects.

One Swedish study showed an elevated risk of gastrointestinal cancers (particularly colorectal and stomach) in association with tamoxifen, but a large retrospective analysis of 101,390 patients [17] did not support this or any increase in the incidence of liver cancer which was of concern because tamoxifen is recognised to be a carcinogen in rats.

6.2. Ocular toxicity

Rarely macular oedema and reversible retinal lesions are seen with tamoxifen, and there is some experimental evidence to suggest that it may promote cataract formation [10].

6.3. Interaction with radiotherapy

A non-hormonal effect of tamoxifen is the induction of TGF beta secretion. TGF beta has been implicated in the pathogenesis of radiation induced fibrosis. A recent study [18] used optical density changes on pre- and post-treatment chest X-rays to monitor the development of lung fibrosis. In the series of 196 patients there was a significant association ($p = 0.01$) between tamoxifen and the incidence of lung fibrosis. A further increased risk was found for patients who received tamoxifen simultaneously with radiotherapy ($p = 0.007$). This has implications for breast cancer patients, many of whom now receive adjuvant radiotherapy following breast conservation surgery in addition to adjuvant tamoxifen.

6.4. Cardiovascular risk

Tamoxifen has beneficial effects on serum lipids which in Swedish and Scottish studies have translated to a reduction in the risk of fatal myocardial infarction [19]. Some of the newer anti oestrogens also appear to confer similar benefit.

6.5. Prevention of post-menopausal bone loss

This has been well established and there is some evidence of a reduction in fracture rate [10].

6.6. Reduction in risk of contralateral breast cancer

In the EBCTCG meta-analysis [5] the proportional risk reduction for development of a contralateral breast cancer in patients who are ER positive of ER poor at 1, 2 and 5 years is 13%, 26%, and 47% respectively (Table 3). It is on the basis of these figures that the use of tamoxifen as a preventative agent for women at high risk of breast cancer is now being investigated.

Ancillary Benefits of Tamoxifen.
Reduced risk of myocardial infarction.
Reduction in fracture rate.
Reduction in the risk of contralateral breast cancer.

6.7. Prediction of response to tamoxifen

Women who get no benefit from tamoxifen are exposed to the potential side effects. The ability to predict who might respond to tamoxifen would allow us to decrease this unnecessary exposure. One study [20] has shown that adjuvant tamoxifen

Table 3. Contralateral breast cancer risk, irrespective of ER status (10-year risk per 1,000)

Scheduled tamoxifen duration	Contralateral breast cancer incidence	Control
1 year	23	26
2 years	21	28
5 years	26	47
Total	23	32

Adapted from Ref. [5].

significantly prolonged survival (disease free and overall survival) in patients who were cerbB2 negative, whereas it had no effect on those who were cerbB2 positive. cerbB2 is a transmembrane oncoprotein which is overexpressed in about 30% of breast cancer and associated with a poor prognosis and may be a signal of resistance to tamoxifen.

> *CerbB2 is a transmembrane protein which is over expressed in 30% of breast cancer and associated with a poor prognosis.*
> *Patients who are cerB2 positive may have less benefit form tamoxifen.*

A humanised monoclonal antibody which targets cerbB2 has been trialled successfully in metastatic breast cancer, and it may eventually be given in an attempt to overcome resistance conferred by the presence of cerbB2 overexpression in the adjuvant setting.

6.8. Uses in other groups

A large number of women who develop breast carcinoma are elderly. Tamoxifen seems to be an adequate option in those patients who are ER positive irrespective of node status [21]. Controlled trials are needed to look at disease free survival, overall survival and perhaps most importantly in this group of patients toxicity. There are a small number of men who suffer form breast carcinoma. Unfortunately no large randomised controlled trials are available, but several small randomised studies suggest that adjuvant tamoxifen increases survival in this group [3].

6.9. Variations in the use of tamoxifen

A postal survey undertaken in 1997, was published in the Lancet last year [22], of people who attended meetings and were involved in clinical trials (the so called "opinion leaders"). They were asked about their use of Tamoxifen. 3000 were approached and 1053 replied. Of those who replied 99% who treated patients with breast carcinoma said they would generally use tamoxifen in older, node-positive women, but only 54% would do so in younger node-positive women (78% and 33% respectively for node-negative women). 75% said that they would treat for 5 years and 12% reported themselves as prescribing a longer duration of therapy. These variations in practice in a group of "opinion leaders" are disturbing, and it would be interesting to repeat this survey following the 1998 publication of the world-wide meta-analysis [5].

7. Medical and surgical oophorectomy

The role of ovarian ablation in the management of pre-menopausal women (the group who have primarily ovarian production of oestrogen) with early breast cancer has been well established. A 1995 EBCTCG meta analysis looked at adjuvant oophorectomy trials in early breast cancer [23], and found that adjuvant oophorectomy reduced the relative risk of death by 12% for an absolute decrease in death of 6.3 per 100 women ($p = 0.001$).

LHRH analogues are established in the treatment of relapsed disease in both pre- and post-menopausal women. They act on the hypothalamo-pituitary axis to cause ovarian suppression by gonadotrophin receptor down regulation in the pituitary resulting in profound suppression of LH which in turn leads to a decline in levels of oestradiol to post-menopausal levels within 21 days. One of the major advantages is this effect is reversible, so allowing future child bearing (although the extent of reversibility might depend upon age at which they were first introduced). Drug company data is convincing that menopause is not permanently brought forward by goserelin. Another advantage is the lack of stimulatory effect on the endometrium or ovaries. Having no pro-oestrogenic properties these agents avoid the risk of endometrial cancer which has been reported with tamoxifen [24]. One particular example is goserelin, which is given by a depot sub-cutaneous injection every four weeks. As promoters of early menopause there are however some concerns about their effect on lipids and bone mineral density.

Oophorectomy cuts the relative risk of death by 12% in the adjuvant setting.
LHRH analogues have a similar but reversible effect, allowing the maintenance of fertility.

8. The potential role of aromatase inhibitors

Aromatase inhibitors cause selective and potent inhibition of the aromatase enzyme with a subsequent profound suppression of oestrogen levels in women who have no ovarian function. Oestrogen levels fall towards the lower limits of detection of current assays, and third generation aromatase inhibitors, such as anastrozole and letrozole, are substantially more potent than aminoglutethemide in inhibiting aromatase activity in vitro. Their side effects include nausea, enhanced menopausal flushing and sweating. There is theoretically a potential detrimental effect on lipids and bone mineral density due to heavily suppressed oestrogen levels and lack of oestrogen agonist properties. Concerns about this are currently being addressed in ongoing trials. The acceptability of adjuvant therapy depends on its lack of adverse effects. Their role as second line hormonal therapy in the management of relapsed disease has been well established and they have largely replaced progestins in these patients. Experimental evidence exists that giving them in combination with tamoxifen might be superior to tamoxifen alone. However, there is some evidence for a negative pharmacological interaction between aromatase inhibitors and tamoxifen. The combined use of aminoglutethemide and tamoxifen has been found to increase the clearance rate of tamoxifen twofold, such that circulating levels of tamoxifen when combined with aminoglutethemide are only 50% of those with monotherapy [29]. This may explain the disappointing results of combination therapy in the advanced disease setting, but the relevance to the adjuvant setting is unclear. In an experimental tumour model letrozole (a third generation aromatase inhibitor) was found to be significantly more effective than antioestrogens in suppressing tumour growth, but when an aromatase inhibitor was combined with tamoxifen then tumour growth was only suppressed to about the same extent as that of aromatase inhibitor alone [31]. Two large multi-centre trials are currently in progress to further evaluate the role of this class of drugs in the adjuvant setting. Large trials of aromatase inhibitors alone vs tamoxifen alone vs the two combined are underway [10,25,26].

The triazole aromatase inhibitors encourage the over production of aromatase but the importance of this in the generation of aromatase inhibitor resistance is not known. The steroidal suicide inhibitor of aromatase, exemestane does not induce aromatase, but it has been less well studied although trials are ongoing.

Aromatase inhibitors may have a role in the adjuvant setting.
Trials are underway to address this question.

9. Other newer agents

New anti-oestrogens are being developed. Faslodex is a steroidal antioestrogen currently in trials which has no oestrogenic activity and therefore a potential advantage of lack of effect on the endometrium, however it does lack the beneficial effects in terms of lipids and bone mineral density which tamoxifen does have [2]. A Lavender extract (perillyl alcohol) is also under investigation. It is known to block cell division, induce apoptosis and in some cases induce cell differentiation. When fed to rats it prevented tumours from developing and caused complete regression of advanced mammary tumours. A Phase 1 study is in progress, with the eventual aim being that it may be an alternative to tamoxifen in adjuvant therapy of early breast cancer [28].

References

1. G.T. Beatson et al. On the treatment of inoperable cases of carcinoma of the mamma. Suggestion for a new method of treatment with illustrative cases. Lancet 1896. 104–107.
2. A.U. Buzdar, G. Hortobagyi. Update of endocrine therapy for breast carcinoma. Clin. Cancer Res. 1998; 4: 527–534.
3. C.K. Osbourne. Tamoxifen in the treatment of breast carcinoma. N.E.J.M. 1998. 339; 22: 1609–1617.
4. I.F. Tannock and R. Hill. Hormones and Cancer. In: The Basic Science of Oncology. 2nd edition 1992. McGraw-Hill.
5. The Early Breast Cancer Triallists Collaborative Group. Tamoxifen for Early Breast Cancer. An overview of the randomised Trials. Lancet 1998; 351: 1451–1465.
6. D. Rea, C. Poole, R. Gray. Adjuvant tamoxifen: How long before we know how long? BMJ 1998; 316: 1518–1519.
7. B. Fisher, J. Dingham, J. Bryant, A. Decillis, D. Wickeham, N. Wolmark et al. Five versus more than Five years of Tamoxifen therapy for Breast Cancer patients with negative lymph nodes and ER positive tumours. J. Natl. Cancer Inst. 1996; 88: 1529–1542.
8. D. Tormey, R. Gray, H. Falkson for E.C.O.G. Postcemotherapy adjuvant tamoxifen beyond 5 years in patients with lymph node positive breast cancer. J. Natl. Cancer Inst. 1996; 88: 1828–1833.
9. H.J. Stewart, A.P. Forrest, D. Everington, C.C. McDonald, J. Dewar, R. Hawkins. Randomised comparison of 5 years of adjuvant tamoxifen with continuous therapy for operable breast cancer. The Scottish Cancer Trials Breast Group. Br. J. Cancer 1996; 74: 297–299.
10. G.Y. Locker. Hormonal therapy of breast cancer. Cancer Treat. Rev. 1998; 24: 221–246.
11. M. Baum. Tamoxifen in the treatment of choice. Why look for alternatives. Br. J. Cancer 1998; 78(4s): 1–4.
12. T.J. Powles. Adjuvant therapy for early breast cancer: a time to refine. J. Natl. Cancer Inst. 1997; 89(22): 1652–1654.
13. Controlled Trial of Tamoxifen as Adjuvant Agent in Management of Early Breast Cancer. Interim analysis at 4 years of Nolvadex adjuvant trial organisation. Lancet 1983; 1: 257–261.
14. K. Katase, Y. Sugiyama, K. Hasumi, M. Yoshimoto, F. Kasumi. The incidence subsequent endometrial cancer with tamoxifen use in patients with primary breast carcinoma. Cancer; 82(9); 1698–1703.
15. J. Zeigler. Endometrial cancers from tamoxifen use are not more aggressive. J. Natl. Cancer Inst. 1998; 88(16): 1100–1102.
16. V.J. Assikis, P. Neven, V.C. Jordan, I. Vergote. A realistic clinical perspective of tamoxifen and endometrial carcinogenesis. Eur. J. Cancer 1996; 32A(19): 1464–1476.
17. R.E. Curtis, J.D. Boile Jr., D.A. Shriner, B.F. Harkey, J.F. Fraumeni Jr. Second cancers after adjuvant tamoxifen for breast cancer. J. Natl. Cancer Inst. 1996; 88(12): 832–834.
18. S.M. Bertzen, J.Z. Skocylas, M. Overgaard, J. Overgaard. Radiotherapy related lung fibrosis enhanced by tamoxifen. J. Natl. Cancer Inst. 1996; 88(13): 918–920.
19. T. Saarto, C. Blomguvist, C. Ehnholm, M.R. Taskinen, I. Elomaa. Anti-atherogenic effect of adjuvant anti-oestrogens. J. Clin. Oncol. 1996; 14(2): 429–433.
20. C. Carlomagno, F. Pennone, C. Gallo, M. De Laurentis, R. Lauria, A. Morabito et al. CerbB2 Overexpression decreases the benefit of adjuvant tamoxifen in early stage breast carcinoma without lymph node metastasis. J. Clin. Oncol. 1996; 14(10): 2702–2708.
21. P. Manchei, V. Bianco, E. Pignatelli, S. Chiodini, D. Santini, E. Carico et al. Adjuvant treatment for breast cancer in the elderly. Anticancer Res. 1996; 16: 911–914.
22. C. Davies, P. McGale, R. Peto. Variation in the use of adjuvant tamoxifen. Lancet 1998; 351: 1189–1196.
23. Early Breast Cancer Triallists Collaborative Group. Ovarian ablation in early breast cancer. Overview of randomised trials. Lancet 1996; 348: 1189–1196.
24. W. Jonat. LHRH analogues in the rational for adjuvant use in premenopausal women with early breast cancer. Br. J. Cancer 1998; 78(4s): 5–8.
25. R.W. Blamey. The role of selective nonsteroidal aromatase inhibitors in future treatment strategies. Oncology 1997; 54(2s): 27–31.
26. P.E. Lonning. Aromatase inhibitors and their future role in post-menopausal women with early breast cancer. Br. J. Cancer 1998; 78(4s): 12–15.
27. A. Howell, S. Downey, E. Anderson. New endocrine therapies for breast cancer. Eur. J. Cancer 1996; 32A(4): 576–588.
28. J. Zeigler. Raloxifene, retinoids and lavender; 'metoo' tamoxifen alternatives under study. J. Natl. Cancer Inst. 1996; 88(16); 1100–1102.
29. E.A. Lien, G. Anker, P.E. Lonning, E. Solheim, P.M. Ueland. Decreased serum concentrations of tamoxifen and its metabolites induced by aminoglutethemide. Cancer Res. 1990; 50: 5851–5857.
30. Endocrine Related Cancer. Published in Journal of Endocrinology 1997 Vol. 4 (3). Editor V.H.T. James.
31. A. Brodie, O. Lu, Y. Liu, B. Long. Aromatase inhibitors and the antitumour effects in model systems. Endocrine Related Cancer 1999; 6: 205–210.
32. W. Miller. Aromatase inhibitors. Endocrine Related Cancer 1996; 3: 65–79.

Breast Cancer: Diagnosis and Management
J.M. Dixon (Ed.)

CHAPTER 41

Role of high-dose chemotherapy as an adjuvant in high-risk early breast cancer

John Crown

1. Introduction

Most breast cancer patients are diagnosed with stages I–II disease. While loco-regional therapy will cure many, approximately 50% of patients with node-positive, and approximately 30% with node-negative disease, will ultimately die from metastases, and thus must have had occult dissemination at presentation. Systemic "adjuvant" therapy is thus necessary to effect cure. Support for this approach came from the work of Skipper and Schabel [1], whose experiments, revealed that chemotherapy killed a constant proportion of cells, and that there was an inverse relationship between the size of a tumour and its curability by chemotherapy. Their model appeared to be particularly relevant to breast cancer, in that metastatic disease is partially chemo-sensitive, but is rarely cured [2]. Adjuvant chemotherapy regimens do produce a benefit in patients with earlier stage disease [3], but the magnitude is modest, and stages I–II breast cancer remain frequently fatal.

Norton and Simon proposed an explanation for this observation. They hypothesised that tumours grew, and regressed according to Gompertzian kinetics, i.e. the growth rate varied inversely with the size of the tumour, i.e., large tumours had lower growth fractions than did smaller ones, and hence were less sensitive to drugs. Thus cell kill is directly related to the size of the dose, and to the growth rate of the unperturbed tumour at that point in its growth curve [4]. They proposed that patients should first be treated with "induction" therapy to reduce their tumour burden, at which point eradication might be attempted with "intensified" therapy. Several randomised trials have tested this hypothesis [5,6], using generally modest intensification, with modest benefit.

2. Chemotherapy dose–response effect

Experimental models show that there is a relationship between dose and cell-kill [7,8]. The degree of dose-escalation which is required to eradicate cancers is in general of a log order of magnitude. Colony-stimulating factors (CSFs) facilitate relatively modest increases in dose and intensity [9]. Moderately dose intensified regimens (i.e. increases in dose which do not require autograft support) have not surprisingly, produced marginal and inconsistent results [10–17].

3. Haematopoietic support of high-dose chemotherapy

Very high-dose chemotherapy with haematopoietic autograft support has been reported to produce exceptionally high rates of complete response in patients with metastatic breast cancer, with some of these remissions remaining durable at five years [18]. Treatment-related death was a relatively frequent occurrence [19,20]. The use of haematopoietic colony-stimulating factors (CSFs) following marrow re-infusion resulted in a dramatic abbreviation of the period of neutropenia, and a consequent fall in mortality [21]. They also mobilize large numbers of haematopoietic progenitors (PBP) into the peripheral blood [22], from whence they can be harvested, and used as a substitute for autologous bone marrow (ABM). These PBP were demonstrated to be superior to growth factors alone, or to marrow in prospective random assignment trials [23,24].

As discussed below, single arm studies of high-dose chemotherapy produced promising, provocative results in early stage, high-risk breast cancer, and in patients with metastatic disease. The possibility of case-selection bias mandated that these results be confirmed in randomized trials [25]. Before analysing the randomised trials which have been reported, it is necessary to outline the various high-dose chemotherapy strategies which have been developed.

4. High-dose chemotherapy strategies

4.1. Primary high-dose chemotherapy

In this strategy, HDC is administered as one (or uncommonly, two or more), definitive cycles of "stand alone" treatment to patients with cancer. High rates of usually short-lived response were reported in several of these studies, especially in metastatic breast cancer [26]. Primary high-dose chemotherapy has had rather little investigation, due primarily to the fact that late-intensification rapidly became the dominant strategy for high-dose chemotherapy.

4.2. Late-intensification

This model, is an adaptation of the work of Norton and Simon. Obviously autografting allowed a substantial degree of dose-escalation, and during the 1980s, late intensification became the most widespread application of high-dose chemotherapy. In addition to the kinetic rationale, several other clinical arguments were advanced in support of using high-dose chemotherapy as a form of late-intensification. It was proposed that the cytoreduction which was achieved by conventional chemotherapy might increase the ability of the subsequent high-dose cycle to eradicate the cancer, by presenting it with a smaller tumour burden. Conventional chemotherapy might also improve the performance status of patients with advanced cancer prior to their being subjected to high-dose treatment. However, a historical comparison using identical HDC regimens either with or without conventional induction, did not suggest a major benefit for the induction component of a late-intensification regimen [27,28].

Peters and colleagues treated patients with breast cancer involving at least ten axillary lymph nodes with an aggressive doxorubicin-based adjuvant regimen followed by a single cycle of high-dose late-intensification chemotherapy supported by an autograft of bone marrow or peripheral blood, and reported a 70% rate of long-term remission [29].

There have now been seven randomised trials in which late-intensification, autograft-supported high-dose chemotherapy has been compared to non-high-dose approaches in the therapy of either high-risk early stage, or metastatic breast cancer. These will be discussed in detail later, all have been either negative, or ambiguous.

4.3. High-dose sequential

The high-dose sequential (HDS) approach devised by Gianni and colleagues in Milan enables very high-doses of drugs to be delivered in a fashion which does not pre-dispose to overlapping toxicity, and which also attempts to deal with the clonal heterogeneity predicted by Goldie and Coldman. In this approach, patients are treated with a number of different drugs and regimens given at, or close to, maximum dose. Gianni and colleagues studied HDS (see below) in patients with stage II breast cancer involving 10 or more axillary lymph nodes. In their study, 65% of patients remained free of relapse [30].

4.4. Multi-cycle high-dose chemotherapy (MCHDC)

The multi-cycle high-dose chemotherapy model has its origins both in a critical analysis of the general development of clinical chemotherapy theory and practice, and in an alternative interpretation of the Norton–Simon model [31].

Curative chemotherapy has generally involved the identification of highly active regimens, and then, the application of a sufficient number of cycles of those regimens to achieve tumour eradication. Thus, in the early MOPP program of chemotherapy for Hodgkin's disease, patients achieved remission after an average of three cycles of therapy. Another observation that emerged in early studies in Hodgkin's disease was that the initial use of non-curative therapy compromised the ability of subsequent potentially curative therapy to effect cure.

Investigators in New York demonstrated the feasibility of accelerated, progenitor-supported, multi-cycle high-dose chemotherapy in breast cancer. In one small study which employed four cycles of high-dose alkylating agents as a treatment for metastatic breast cancer, a high-rate of remission was achieved, but with a high rate of fatal pulmonary drug toxicity [32].

5. Randomised trials of high-dose chemotherapy in breast cancer

The results of five randomised trials of high-dose chemotherapy as a treatment for high-risk early stage breast cancer have been reported. Four have studied late-intensification [33–36]. In the Scandinavian study, patients received either standard FEC chemotherapy followed by a single high-dose cycle, or individually escalated doses of FEC. Patients on the "low-dose" arm received higher doses of anthracycline, cyclophosphamide and 5-fluorouracil than did patients on the "high-dose" arm [37]. The study was negative, but in fact compared two high-dose strategies.

Peters et al. randomised patients to receive either high-dose cisplatin, BCNU and cyclophosphamide with an autograft, or, lower doses of the same drugs with filgrastim support following induction therapy. At early follow-up, no advantage was seen for the high dose treatment. Patients on the high-dose arm of this study, however, had an unusually high, (8%) rate of treatment-related mortality. Two other very small studies in which late-intensification HDC was compared to conventionally dosed therapy were also negative.

The fifth trial, conducted by Bezwoda et al., compared primary multi-cycle (two cycles) of HDC to conventional FAC therapy. Conventional induction therapy was not used, and the first chemotherapy patients received was high-dose. Although this study was reported as showing an advantage for high dose [38] there are doubts about the scientific integrity of the data which mean that until confirmed, these results should be disregarded.

Four randomized trials comparing HDC to CDC have been carried out in patients with metastases. Three used the late intensification approach and were all either negative or ambiguous [38–40]. The sole study of primary multi-cycle HDC which showed a striking advantage for high-dose [41] comes again from the South African group whose data is now considered flawed.

> *Single cycle late-intensification cannot be regarded as an evidence based approach for patients with metastatic or multi-node-positive breast cancer. Multi-cycle high-dose chemotherapy needs further study.*

6. Research priorities and future directions

Two broad strategies need to be addressed in successor trials:

(1) Improving results of treatment. The impact

of new high-dose regimens, engineered autograft products [42,43], adjuvant immunotherapy [44], gene therapy [45], anti-angiogenics [46], allogenic transplantation [47], multiple high-dose cycles, and late-intensification versus HDS and primary high-dose chemotherapy strategies should all be studied.

(2) There have also been substantial advances in conventionally-dosed therapy in recent years. Thus control groups will also have to be optimised [48]

The current literature does not invalidate high-dose therapy, but rather suggests a possible route for future investigations.

References

1. Skipper HE, Schabel FM. Quantitative and cytokinetic studies in experimental tumor systems. In Holland J, Frei FE (eds.): Cancer Medicine. Philadelphia, Lea and Febiger, 1988, pp. 663–84.
2. Greenberg PAC Hortobagyi GN, Smith TL, et al. Long-term follow-up of patients with complete remission of patients with complete remission following combination chemotherapy for metastatic breast cancer. J Clin Oncol 14: 2197–2205, 1996.
3. Early Breast Cancer Trialist's Collaborative Group. Systemic treatment of early breast cancer by hormonal, cytotoxic or immune therapy: 133 randomized trials involving 31,000 recurrences and 24,000 deaths among 75,000 women. Lancet 1992; 339: 1–15.
4. Norton L, Simon R, Brereton HD, et al. Predicting the course of Gompertzian growth. Nature (Lond.) 1976; 264: 542–45.
5. Perloff M, Norton L, Korzun AH, et al. Post surgical adjuvant chemotherapy of stage II breast carcinoma with or without crossover to a non-cross-resistant regimen: a cancer and leukemia Group B study. J Clin Oncol 1996; 14: 1589–1598.
6. Cocconi G, Bisagni G, Bacchi M, Buzzi F, Canaletti R, Carpi A, Ceci G, Colozza A, De Lisi V, Lottici R, et al. A comparison of continuation versus late intensification followed by discontinuation of chemotherapy in advanced breast cancer. A prospective randomized trial of the Italian Oncology Group for Clinical Research (G.O.I.R.C.). Ann Oncol 1990; 1(1): 36–44.
7. Skipper HE, Schabel FM. Quantitative and cytokinetic studies in experimental tumor systems. In Holland J, Frei FE (eds.): Cancer Medicine. Philadelphia, Lea and Febiger, 1988, pp. 663–84.
8. Teicher BA, Holden SA, Cucchi CA, et al. Combination thiotepa and cyclophosphamide in vivo and in vitro. Cancer Res 1988; 48: 94–100.
9. O'Dwyer PJ, LaCreta FP, Schilder R, et al. Phase I trial of thiotepa in combination with recombinant human granulocyte-macrophage colony-stimulating factor. J. Clin Oncol 1992; 10: 1352–1358.
10. Bastholt L, Dalmark M, Gjedde S. Dose–response relationship of epirubicin in the treatment of postmenopausal patients with metastatic breast cancer: a randomized study of epirubicin at four different dose levels performed by the Danish Breast Cancer Cooperative Group. J Clin Oncol 1996; 14: 1146–1155.
11. Hortobagyi GN, Buzdar AU, Bodey GP, et al. High-dose induction chemotherapy of metastatic breast cancer in protected environment units: a prospective randomized study. J Clin Oncol 1987; 5: 178–184.
12. Ardizzoni A, Venturini M, Sertoli MR, et al. Granulocyte-macrophage colony-stimulating factor (GM-CSF) allows acceleration and dose-intensity increase of CEF chemotherapy: a randomized study in patients with advanced breast cancer. Br J Cancer 1994; 69: 385–391.
13. Henderson IC, Berry D, Demetri G, Cirrincione C, Goldstein L, Martino S, Ingle JN, Cooper MR, Canellos G, Borden E, Fleming G, Holland JF, Graziano S, Carpenter J, Muss H, Norton L. Improved disease-free survival and overall survival from the addition of sequential Paclitaxel but not from the escalation of doxorubicin dose in the adjuvant chemotherapy of patients with node-positive primary breast cancer. Proc Am Soc Clin Oncol 1998; 17: 101a.
14. Fisher B, Anderson S, Wickerham DL, et al. Increased intensification and total dose of cyclophosphamide in a doxorubicin-cyclophosphamide regimen for the treatment of primary breast cancer: Findings from National Surgical Adjuvant Breast and Bowel Project B-22. J Clin Oncol 1997; 15: 1858–1869.
15. Levine MN, Gent M, Hryniuk WM, Bramwell V, Abu-Zahra H, DePauw S, Arnold A, Findlay B, Levin L, Skillings J, et al. A randomized trial comparing 12 weeks versus 36 weeks of adjuvant chemotherapy in stage II breast cancer. J Clin Oncol 1990; 8(7): 1217–25.
16. Bonneterre J, Roché H, Bremond A, Kerbrat P, Namer M, Fumoleau P, Goudier M-J, Fargeot P, Bardonnet M, Marcillac I, Luporsi E. Results of a randomised trial of adjuvant chemotherapy with FEC 50 vs FEC 100 in high-risk node positive breast cancer patients. Proc Am Soc Clin Oncol 1998; 17: 124a.
17. Tannock IF, Boyd NF, Deborer G, et al. A randomized trial of two dose levels of CMF chemotherapy for patients with metastatic breast cancer. J Clin Oncol 1988; 6: 1377–87.

18. Peters WP, Shpall EJ, Jones RB, et al. High-dose combination alkylating agents with bone marrow support as initial treatment for metastatic breast cancer. J Clin Oncol 1988; 6: 1368–1376.
19. Eder JP, Antman K, Peters WP, et al. High-dose combination alkylating agent chemotherapy with autologous marrow support for metastatic breast cancer. J Clin Oncol 1986; 4: 1592–1597.
20. Lazarus H, Reed MD, Spitzer TR, et al. High-dose iv thiotepa and cryopreserved autologous bone marrow transplantation for therapy of refractory cancer. Cancer Treat Rep 1987; 71: 689–695.
21. Peters WP, Rosner G, Ross M et al. Comparative effects of granulocyte-macrophage colony-stimulating factor (GM-CSF) and granulocyte colony-stimulating factor (G-CSF) on priming peripheral blood progenitor cells for use with autologous bone marrow after high-dose chemotherapy. Blood 1993; 81: 1709–1719.
22. Socinski MA, Elias A, Schnipper L, Cannistra SA, Antman KH, Griffin JD. Granulocyte-macrophage colony-stimulating factor expands the circulating haemopoietic progenitor cell compartment in man. Lancet 1988; i 1194–1198.
23. Beyer J, Schwella N, Zingsem J, et al. Bone marrow versus peripheral blood stem cells as rescue after high-dose chemotherapy. Blood 1993; 82 (suppl 1): 454a.
24. Kritz A, Crown J, Motzer R. Beneficial impact of peripheral blood progenitor cells in patients with metastatic breast cancer treated with high-dose chemotherapy plus GM-CSF: a randomized trial. Cancer 1993; 71: 2515–2521.
25. Zia U Rahman, Debra K Frye, Aman U Buzdar. Impact of selection process on response rate and long-term survival of potential high-dose chemotherapy candidates treated with standard-dose doxorubicin-containing chemotherapy in patients with metastatic breast cancer. J Clin Oncol 15: 3171–3177.
26. Eder JP, Antman K, Peters WP, et al. High-dose combination alkylating agent chemotherapy with autologous marrow support for metastatic breast cancer. J Clin Oncol 1986; 4: 1592–1597.
27. Peters WP, Shpall EJ, Jones RB, et al. High-dose combination alkylating agents with bone marrow support as initial treatment for metastatic breast cancer. J Clin Oncol 1988; 6: 1368–1376.
28. Jones RB, Shpall EJ, Ross M, Bast R, Affronti M, Peters WP. AFM induction chemotherapy followed by intensive alkylating agent consolidation with autologous bone marrow support for advanced breast cancer. Current results. Proc Am Soc Clin Oncol 1990; 9: 9.
29. Peters WP, Ross M, Vredenburgh JJ, et al. High-dose chemotherapy and autologous bone marrow support as consolidation after standard-dose adjuvant therapy for high risk primary breast cancer. J Clin Oncol 1993; 11: 1132–1144.
30. Gianni AM, Siena S, Bregni M, et al. Growth factor supported high-dose sequential adjuvant chemotherapy in breast cancer with >10 positive nodes. Proc Am Soc Clin Oncol 1992; 11: 60.
31. Crown J, Norton L. Potential strategies for improving the results of high-dose chemotherapy in patients with metastatic breast cancer. Ann Oncol 1995; 6(suppl 4): s21–s26.
32. Crown J, Raptis G, Vahdat L, et al. Rapidly administration of sequential high-dose cyclophosphamide. melphalan, thiotepa supported by filgrastim and peripheral blood progenitors in patients with metastatic breast cancer: a novel and very active treatment strategy. Proc Am Soc Clin Oncol 1994; 13: 110 (abst).
33. Rodenhuis S, Richel DJ, van der Wall E, Schornagel JH, Baars JW, Koning CC, Peterse JL, Borger JH, Nooijen WJ, Bakx R, Dalesio O, Rutgers E. Randomised trial of high-dose chemotherapy and haemopoietic progenitor-cell support in operable breast cancer with extensive axillary lymph-node involvement. Lancet 1998; 352: 515–21.
34. The Scandinavian Breast Cancer Study Group 9401. Results from a randomized adjuvant breast cancer study with high-dose chemotherapy with CTC_b supported by autologous bone marrow stem cells versus dose escalated and tailored FEC therapy. Proc ASCO 1999; 2a.
35. Peters W, Rosner G, Vredenburgh J, Shpall E, Crump M, Richardson P, Marks L, Cirrincone C, Wood W, Henderson I, Hurd D, Norton L for CALGB, SWOG and NCIC. A prospective, randomized comparison of two doses of combination alkylating agents as consolidation after CAF in high-risk primary breast cancer involving ten or more axillary lymph nodes: Preliminary results of CALGB 9082/SWOG 9114/NCIC MA-13. Proc ASCO 1999; 18: 1a.
36. Hortobagyi GN, Buzdar AU, Champlin R. Lack of efficacy of adjuvant high-dose tandem combination chemotherapy for high-risk primary breast cancer a randomised trial. Proc Am Soc Clin Oncol 1998; 17: 123a, 1998.
37. Scandinavian Breast Cancer Study Group. Results from a randomized adjuvant breast cancer study with high dose chemotherapy with CTCb supported by autologous bone marrow stem cells versus dose escalated and tailored FEC therapy'. Proc Am Soc Clin Oncol 1999; 18: 2a.
38. Stadtmauer EA, O'Neill A, Goldstein LJ, Crilley P, Mangan KF, Ingle JN, Lazarus HM, Erban J, Sickles C, Glick JH. Phase III randomized trial of high-dose chemotherapy (HDC) and stem cell support (SCT) shows no difference in overall survival or severe toxicity compared to maintenance chemotherapy with cyclophosphomide, methotrexate and 5-fluorouracil (CMF) for women with metastatic breast cancer who

are responding to conventional induction chemotherapy: The Philadelphia Intergroup Study (PBT-01), Proc Am Soc Clin Oncol 1999; 18: 1a.

39. Lotz J-P, Cure H, Janvier M, Morvan F, Asselain B, Guillermot M, Laadem A, Maraninchi D, Gisselbrecht C, Roche H, and the PEGASE Group. High-dose chemotherapy (HD-CT) with hematopoietic stem cells transplantation (HSCT) for metastatic breast cancer: results of the French Protocol Pegase 04'. Proc Am Soc Clin Oncol 1999; 18: 43a.
40. Peters WP, Jones RB, Vredenburgh J et al. A large, prospective, randomized trial of high-dose combination alkylating agents (CBP) with autologous cellular support as consolidation for patients with metastatic breast cancer achieving complete remission after intensive doxorubicin-based induction therapy (AFM). Proc ASCO 1996; 15: 121.
41. Bezwoda WR, Seymour L, Dansey RD. High-dose chemotherapy with hematopoietic rescue as primary treatment for metastatic breast cancer: a randomised trial. J Clin Oncol 1995; 13: 2483–89.
42. Brugger W, Heimfeld S, Berenson RJ, Mertelsmann R, Kanz L. Reconstitution of hematopoiesis after high-dose chemotherapy by autologous progenitor cells generated ex vivo. N Engl J Med 1995; 333: 283–287.
43. Shpall EJ, Jones RB, Bearman SI et al. Transplantation of enriched CD34-positive autologous marrow into breast cancer patients following high-dose chemotherapy: influence of CD34-positive peripheral-blood progenitors and growth factors on engraftment. J Clin Oncol 1994; 12: 28–36.
44. Kennedy MJ, Vogelzang G, Beveridge R, et al. Phase I trial of intravenous cyclosporine to induce graft versus host disease in women undergoing autologous bone marrow transplantation for breast cancer. J Clin Oncol 1993; 11: 478–484.
45. Hesdorffer C, Ayello J, Ward M, Kaubisch A, Vahdat L, Balmaceda C, Garrett T, Fetell M, Reiss R, Bank A, Antman K. Phase I trial of retroviral-mediated transfer of the human MDR1 gene as marrow chemoprotection in patients undergoing high-dose chemotherapy and autologous stem-cell transplantation. J Clin Oncol 1998; 16: 165–172.
46. O'Reilly MS, Holmgren L, Chen C, Folkman J. Angiostatin induces and sustains dormancy of human primary tumors in mice. Nat Med 1996; 2(6): 689–92.
47. Ueno N, Rondón G, Mirza NQ. Allogeneic peripheral-blood progenitor-cell transplantation for poor-risk patients with metastatic breast cancer. J Clin Oncol 1998; 16: 2817–2824.
48. Chan S, Friedrichs K, Noel D, Pintér T, Van Belle S, Vorobiof D, et al. Prospective randomized trial of docetaxel versus doxorubicin in patients with metastatic breast cancer. J Clin Oncol 1999; 17: 2341–2354.

Breast Cancer: Diagnosis and Management
J.M. Dixon (Ed.)

CHAPTER 42

The management of the side-effects of adjuvant therapy including chemotherapy and endocrine effects

Anthony Maraveyas and Janine L. Mansi

1. Introduction

Adjuvant therapy is given to prolong the disease-free and overall survival of patients with operable breast cancer. Unfortunately the major treatment modalities involved in chemotherapy and endocrine therapy are associated with toxicities, which can cause significant morbidity, both short- and long-term, and mortality.

The giving of such agents and the range of agents available continues to increase as randomised trails confirm significant survival advantages (see Chapters 24, 25, 26). In conjunction with this the identification, prevention and management of potential and established toxicities has become an increasingly important feature.

Adjuvant therapy can cause significant short and long term morbidity and mortality.

2. Chemotherapy

The majority of patients with breast cancer will receive combination chemotherapy. The drugs used and most commonly encountered side-effects are summarised in Table 1.

Toxicity can be graded using a number of systems (Common Toxicity Criteria [CTC] or WHO) with a range of options from 0 to 4 (0 indicating no symptoms). Patients who experience grade 3 or 4 toxicities usually require a dose reduction of the responsible drug(s) with or without a delay in administration until recovery has occurred. Identification of patients at risk either before commencing adjuvant chemotherapy or during treatment is essential.

3. Specific toxicities of chemotherapy and their management

3.1. Short-term (acute toxicities)

3.1.1. Nausea and vomiting

One of the most important advances in our ability to give combination chemotherapy has been the effective use of antiemetics (e.g. incorporating dexamethasone), and the development of potent new agents such as the $5HT_3$ antagonists [1]. Nowadays this side-effect should be prevented in the majority of patients [2]. Nausea and vomiting may be acute (commencing within 24 h after treatment), delayed (occurring 24 h or more after chemotherapy), and anticipatory (conditioned reflex which reflects unsuccessful control of chemotherapy induced nausea and vomiting) [3].

There is a greater risk of vomiting with young age, female sex and previous adverse experience with chemotherapy. A history of regular alcohol

Table 1. Agents used in the adjuvant treatment of breast cancer and their side-effects

Drug	Potential side-effects
Cyclophosphamide	Myelosuppression, haemorrhagic cystitis, gastrointestinal (nausea/vomiting/anorexia), alopecia (50%), cardiac (high dose only), reproductive failure, SIADH
Methotrexate	Myelosuppression, gastrointestinal (nausea/vomiting/diarrhoea), hepatotoxicity (high dose only), rashes, skin pigmentation changes (hypo/hyper), renal, pneumonitis, conjunctivitis
Doxorubicin	Myelosuppression, alopecia (>90%), vesicant, cardiotoxicity (max 550 mg/m^2), gastrointestinal (nausea/vomiting/mucositis), urine discolouration, radiation recall effects (skin)
Epirubicin	Similar side-effects to doxorubicin although slightly less myelosuppression and cardiotoxicity (max dose 900 mg/m^2)
5FU	Myelosuppression, gastrointestinal (diarrhoea/nausea/anorexia/stomatitis), skin rash, conjunctivitis, neurological, palmar plantar erythema, hyperpigmentation of veins and nail beds, mild alopecia, neurological side-effects (rare)
Vinorelbine	Myelotoxicity, gastrointestinal (usually mild), peripheral neuropathy (30%), alopecia (25%), vesicant
Paclitaxel	Myelotoxicity, peripheral neuropathy, hypersensitivity (6% of infusions), cardiovascular, alopecia (100%), flu-like symptoms
Mitoxantrone	Myelosuppression, gastrointestinal (nausea/vomiting/mild stomatitis), alopecia (25%), cardiac (above 140–160 mg/m^2)
Docetaxel	Myelosuppression, hypersensitivity, cardiovascular (less than paclitaxel), alopecia (80%), rash, phlebitis, gastrointestinal (nausea/vomiting) mild
Tamoxifen	Endocrine (menopausal symptoms — menstrual irregularity — vaginal bleeding), weight gain, endometrial cancer (rare), rare myelosuppression, transaminitis, acute flare of breast cancer symptoms, bone pain, hypercalcaemia, elevated ALT, alk phos and bilirubin (uncommon), rare ophthalmological side-effects (retinitis, macular degeneration)
GnRH	Endocrine (menopausal symptoms), stops ovulation and menstruation

The treatment of breast cancer with these agents predisposes to a hypercoagulable state; therefore, patients are at increased risk of deep vein thromboses, arterial thrombo-embolism and pulmonary emboli.

intake reduces the level of nausea and vomiting [4].

Patients are treated based on the emetogenic potential of the regimen used. Most drugs used for the treatment of adjuvant breast cancer are of moderate (doxorubicin, epirubicin, cyclophosphamide) to low (methotrexate, 5-FU, mitoxantrone) emetogenic potential. Table 2 provides a guide to the use of antiemetics for such patients. Lorazepam can be given 24 h before the start of chemotherapy where anticipatory nausea is troublesome. Additional helpful agents include haloperidol and the cannabinoids. Furthermore, the recent development of novel antiemetics based on neurokinin-1 receptor antagonists may offer greater scope of nausea and vomiting control in refractory patients and delayed emesis [5].

Effective antiemetic combinations should significantly protect against chemotherapy induced nausea and vomiting.

3.1.2. Myelosuppression

Bone marrow suppression is commonly encountered with the majority of cytotoxic chemotherapeutic drugs given. Conventional chemotherapy combinations used for the adjuvant treatment of breast cancer have a relatively low risk of profound myelosuppression and associated morbidity.

Table 2. Combination antiemetic therapy for acute emesis for adjuvant/neo-adjuvant regimens* in breast cancer patients

Regimen	Start at level	Antiemetic policy (SGHMS)		Most emetogenic drug in regimen	Start at level
Adriamycin, cyclophosphamide	4	Level 1	Domperidone 20 mg tds 3–5 days (±	Carboplatin	3/4
CMF	2		Cyclizine 25–50 mg tds)	Cisplatin	4
ECF-epirubicin, cisplatin, 5-fluorouracil	4	Level 2	Dexamethasone 8 mg × 1	Cyclophosphamide	2
Epirubicin	3		+ Domperidone 20 mg tds 3–5 days		
Epirubicin, Cyclo	4	Level 3	Dexamethasone 8 mg × 1	Doxorubicin	2/3
Epirubicin, Taxol	4**		+ Dexamethasone 2 mg tds 3 days	5-FU/Capecitabine	1/2
			+ Domperidone 20 mg tds 5 days		
FEC — 5-fluorouracil, epirubicin, cyclophosphamide	4	Level 4	Dexamethasone 8 mg × 1	Mitoxantrone	1/2
			+ Ondansetron 8 mg × 1		
5-FU/Capecitabine	1		+ Dexamethasone 2 mg tds 3 days	Methotrexate	1/2
			+ Domperidone 20 mg tds 5 days		
5-FU/Folinic acid	2	Level 5	As Level 4	Methotrexate (high dose)	4
			+ Lorazepam 1 mg × 2	Mitomycin-C	2/3
			+ Dexamethasone 4 mg tds 3 days		
MMM — mitomycin C, methotrexate, mitoxantrone	2	Level 6	As Level 5	Paclitaxel	1/2
			+ Cyclizine 50 mg tds		
				Vinorelbine	1/2

** no additional dexamethasone if already on steroids as part of chemotherapy regimen

Notes: All acute failures (within 24 h of chemo) should have iv Ondansetron 8 mg + iv Dexamethasone 8 mg as rescue.
If a patient fails at one level they should receive premedication at the next level for their next course.
Oral antiemetic premedication should be given 1 hr before chemo for pharmacokinetic reasons when high-dose steroids are given as part of the regimen or for other reasons (cf. paclitaxel) additional dexamethasone is not required

* St George's Hospital Medical School — local policy

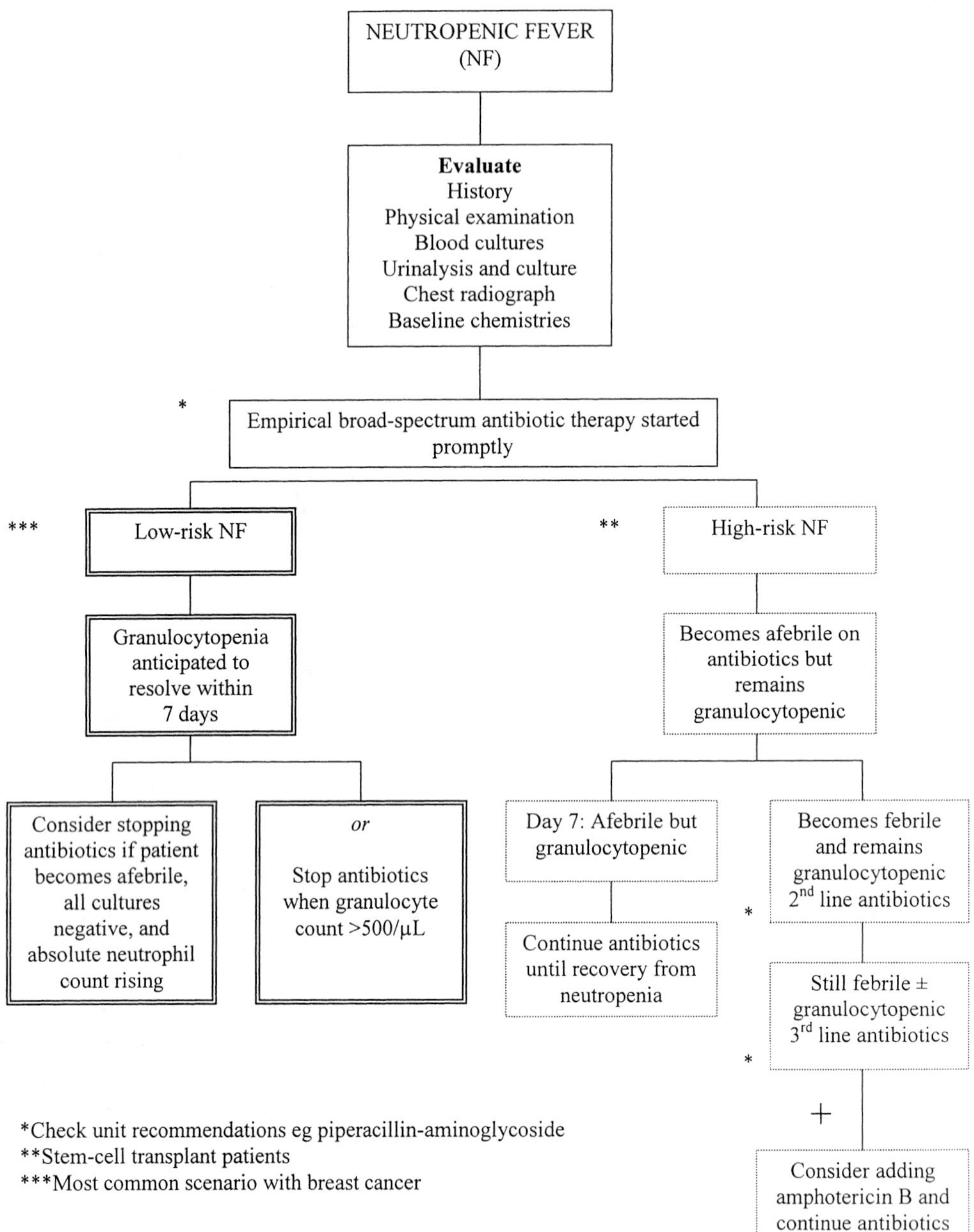

Fig. 1. Neutropenic sepsis management flow chart.

Neutropoenia is responsible for a significant proportion of life threatening events and should be anticipated. Patients should be warned to report symptoms of fevers, sweats or rigors particularly occurring at the time of the nadir (usually between day 7 to 14 of each treatment cycle). Aggressive treatment of sepsis with appropriate broad spectrum antibiotics as outlined in Fig. 1 should be initiated promptly. The use of growth factors (such as G-CSF) is still a matter of debate but there is no rationale for their use in established neutropoenic sepsis [6], although there is some evidence for reduction in the length and morbidity of the neutropoenic period. Growth factors also allow increase in dose intensity but as yet this approach has not been shown to translate into a survival benefit [7]. Many centres give prophylactic antibiotics, such as ciprofloxacin 250 mg bd or septrin 960 mg (2 tablets) bd on alternate days, for patients who are either considered to be at risk or where an episode of neutropoenic infection or sepsis has occurred.

Neutropoenic infection or sepsis is responsible for a significant proportion of life threatening events and should be anticipated and when suspected treated aggressively and promptly.

Thrombocytopoenia is not a common occurrence, but if symptomatic (e.g. petechiae, epistaxis), and/or platelet counts are rapidly decreasing (usually to less than $20 \times 10^9/l$) particularly in the presence of infection, patients can be supported with platelet transfusions. Anaemia is also uncommon occurring as a late event following a number of cycles of chemotherapy and can be corrected by blood transfusions or in exceptional circumstances erythropoietin can be prescribed [8].

3.1.3. Mucositis

Mucosa is characterised by rapid cell turnover following the cytotoxic insult. Early symptoms and signs of sore mouth and pale mucosa, are followed by erythema and sometimes ulceration. Abnormal bacterial, fungal (candidiasis) and viral (Herpes simplex) colonization is a risk especially if dentition is bad. Oral and dental hygiene is thus essential. Frequent mechanical cleansing of the mouth using normal saline is probably of equivalent value or even safer than mouthwashes containing local anaesthetic and anti-inflammatory properties [9–12]. Diet should exclude hot and spicy items. Nystatin can prevent oral candidiasis, but if severe, fluconazole may be required. If ulceration is the prominent manifestation sucralfate is helpful to relieve oral discomfort [12]. Future directions may include prevention of mucositis with local cryotherapy [13] and prostaglandin E_2 [14]. Promising results have recently been obtained with topical non-absorbable antibiotics [15] topical and systemic G-CSF [16] or GM-CSF [17,18] and TGFβ-3 [19]. Liposomal encapsulation of anthracyclines have also been shown to have a mucosa-sparing effect [20].

Mouth assessment and preventative dental and oral hygiene measures are necessary to reduce the incidence of mucositis. The treatment is supportive including frequent mechanical cleansing with mouth washes or N saline and avoidance of noxious substances/foods.

3.1.4. Alopecia

Alopecia is an especially distressing side-effect for this population of patients. Although it is not universally a major problem with CMF the greater reliance on anthracycline-based adjuvant regimens for high-risk patients, and the increasing probability of other drugs such as the taxanes becoming agents of choice for adjuvant treatment are set to change the situation. Hair loss from chemotherapy usually starts 2–3 weeks into treatment, reaching maximum loss within 2 months. Hair always regrows and this can start whilst the patient is still receiving treatment. Mechanical means such as scalp cooling have variable efficacy and are useful only for short duration infusions of anthracyclines. Supportive services such as wigs and counselling should be at hand and used early in the management. Recently an immunomodulating agent, AS101 has been shown to have protective effects both in animal (Ara-C treated rats) and in human hosts in small non-controlled trials [21,22]. A further area of research includes the prophylactic use of propylthiouracil which has shown hair-sparing effects in rats treated with cyclophosphamide [23].

Alopecia is set to increase in incidence. Currently supportive measures remain the best management.

3.1.5. Neurotoxicity

The incidence of dose-limiting neurotoxicity in patients treated with adjuvant chemotherapy (CMF) for breast cancer is low, and is not a problem with anthracyclines. This may change as the newer agents such as the taxanes becoming more widespread in use. This is a reversible side-effect although improvement may be slow and delayed and sometimes not complete. Dose-reduction should be undertaken if grade III toxicity ensues. Of note are the very promising results of glutathione prevention of neurotoxicity from at least two randomised trials [24,25].

3.1.6. Conjunctivitis

This may occur with methotrexate administration. Folinic acid rescue (15 mg 6 hourly for 6 doses) starting 24 h after administration of methotrexate usually prevents this side-effect, although some patients may require a prolonged course with or without folinic acid eye drops; commonly hypermellose eye-drops are used to maintain lubrication.

3.1.7. Diarrhoea

5-fluorouracil is the most commonly used drugs in breast cancer responsible for causing diarrhoea. Treatment is usually symptomatic with codeine phosphate or loperamide. If severe, admission may be required for rehydration. An underlying infective cause (including Clostridium Difficile) should be excluded.

3.1.8. Venous thrombosis and pulmonary emboli

There is a small but increased risk of thrombosis and pulmonary emboli with chemotherapy administration. A substantive diagnosis should be made and treatment started immediately with intravenous heparin or subcutaneous fragmin followed by oral anticoagulants for the duration of the chemotherapy.

4. Fatigue

Fatigue is one of the most frequent and distressing symptoms experienced by patients receiving adjuvant chemotherapy [26]. Interest in this hitherto poorly recognised symptom is increasing, and is consistent with a greater awareness of quality of life as an important measure of outcome. There have been a small number of studies which have also addressed the presence of fatigue after completion of chemotherapy [27–29]. Broeckel et al. have shown that levels of fatigue are 50% greater in women who have previously received adjuvant chemotherapy (an average of 471 days following completion) than those reported by women with no history of cancer [29], and that this may be exacerbated by menopausal symptoms. Correlation of severity of fatigue with age, time since treatment completed and additional treatment with radiotherapy or current use of tamoxifen has not been clearly defined. The challenge is to further identify the causes of fatigue and to develop interventions that are effective in preventing or reducing fatigue. Self-care strategies such as exercise [30], diversional therapies [31] and psychosocial interventions [29] to change maladaptive cognitive and behaviourial responses are currently the most helpful.

Fatigue is one of the most frequent and distressing symptoms associated with adjuvant chemotherapy. Strategies such as increased exercise, diversional therapies and psychosocial interventions are currently the most helpful methods of reducing fatigue.

5. Long-term toxicities

5.1. Cardiotoxicity

There is some evidence that anthracyclines in the adjuvant setting may impact positively on survival and thus their use is increasing. The main concern is that these agents are also cardiotoxic, usually causing heart failure, and that this side-effect may be a latent morbidity problem for many women who will become long-term survivors. This toxicity is thought to be mediated by the generation of free radicals possibly through an iron–anthracycline complexation [32]. The incidence of toxicity increases exponentially above 550 mg/m^2 of doxorubicin and 900 mg/m^2 of epirubicin [33]. Schedule of administration (bolus vs infusion), radiotherapy to the mediastinum, cardiac co-morbidity, age and concurrently administered cytotoxics may be other risk factors for this toxicity. Avoidance of this by strict adherence to the maximum cumulative dose, and monitoring patients with MUGA scans or echocardiography for assessment of the ejection fraction as a measure of cardiac function is currently the best management. Liposomally encapsulated anthracyclines may be less cardiotoxic [20] and dexrazoxane (ICRF-187, a novel bisdioxopiperazine free radical scavenger, which works through intracellular hydrolysis to form a bidentate chelator), has shown evidence of cardioprotection in initial randomised studies [34–36]. This is, however, at the expense of increased myelosuppression.

Cardiotoxicity can be avoided. Cardiac co-morbidity and other risk factors should be assessed rigorously. Patients at risk should be monitored with MUGA or echocardiography. The recommended total dose of any drug should not be exceeded.

5.2. Infertility

For pre-menopausal women receiving adjuvant chemotherapy the risk of long-term or permanent infertility increases with increasing age. For younger pre-menopausal women menstruation may be unaffected, altered in terms of the regular cycle or stop temporarily. All at risk women should be warned of these potential changes and advised regarding appropriate contraception during their chemotherapy. The symptoms of the menopause should also be explained.

Research into storage of fertilised eggs is in progress and can be discussed with the younger patients ie less then 35 years and in a stable relationship. However, this group of women are less likely to become infertile as a result of treatment and this should be stressed when discussing such options [37]. These new approaches are not yet widely available.

Premenopausal women should be warned that their menstrual cycles may be affected by chemotherapy and this could result in infertility. Conversely information should be given about the need for contraception during and after treatment.

5.3. Second malignancy

Although a recognised long-term toxicity for patients receiving chemotherapy for lymphomas this has not been a feature for those women receiving adjuvant breast cancer chemotherapy [38]. Caution, however, should be exercised regarding the follow-up of women who have received prolonged or high dose treatments where long-term information is not available. This also applies to the long-term effects of some of the newer agents being explored in an adjuvant setting such as the taxanes.

The development of second malignancies is uncommon in this group of patients but may be a problem in women receiving more intensive or prolonged chemotherapy regimens.

6. Endocrine treatment

6.1. Tamoxifen

Tamoxifen is the most commonly used hormonal manipulation in an adjuvant setting and has proven efficacy (Chapter 25). In general it is very well tolerated with the majority of women not experiencing major toxicities. The most commonly encountered are shown in Table 1. Women should be given information regarding the potential side-effects and in particular to report any post-menopausal bleeding in view of the low, but significant increased, risk of uterine malignancies in women on long-term tamoxifen [39].

The treatment of menopausal symptoms can be difficult and remains empirical. Agents such as clonidine, evening primrose oil, or vitamin E have been advocated to be helpful but there is no strong evidence from randomised trials that these are effective. At present detailed counselling should be provided [40]. A recent randomised trial looking at oral versus depot injection medroxyprogesterone showed suppression of menopausal symptoms in at least 80% of women receiving these treatments [41]. This is consistent with the studies which have shown megestrol acetate given in a dose of 20 mg twice per day is effective in controlling hot flushes in two thirds of women. The addition of hormone replacement therapy to tamoxifen is to be the subject of a multi-centre study; the results of this study could be extrapolated to ongoing studies evaluating the use of newer and purer antioestrogens.

Ovarian ablation in pre-menopausal women either surgically, with radiotherapy or with gonadotrophin-releasing hormone (GnRH) agonists are universally associated with menopausal symptoms. This is reversible only in women given GnRH analogues.

7. Conclusion

Our ability to control chemotherapy side-effects has led to improved dose intensity, more extensive use of effective drugs and better patient compliance. Although many pharmaceutical advances are emerging which promise an even better quality of life for patients during chemotherapy, management by experienced sympathetic and supportive staff, patient individualisation, clear instructions and counselling where appropriate, remain the cornerstones of symptom control.

References

1. Soukop M, McQuade B, Hunter E et al. Ondansetron compared with metoclopramide in the control of emesis and quality of life during repeated chemotherapy for breast cancer. Oncology 1992; 49: 295–304.
2. Fouser AA, Fellhauver M, Hoffman M et al. Guidelines for anti-emetic therapy: acute emesis. Eur J Cancer 1999; 35: 361–366.
3. Wilcox PM, Fetting JH, Nettesheim KM et al. Anticipatory vomiting in women receiving cyclophosphamide, methotrexate and 5-FU (CMF) adjuvant chemotherapy for breast carcinoma. Cancer Treat Rep 1982; 66: 1601–1604.
4. Sullivan JR, Leydon MJ, Bell R. Decreased cisplatin-induced nausea and vomiting with alcohol ingestion. N Eng J Med 1983; 309(13): 796.
5. Navari RM, Reinhardt RR, Gralla RJ et al. Reduction of cisplatin-induced emesis by a selective neurokinin-1-receptor antagonist. L-754,030 Antiemetic Trials Group. N Engl J Med 1999; 340(3): 190–5.
6. Ozer H, Miller LL, Schiffer CA et al. American Society of Clinical Oncology update of recommendations for the use of hematopoietic colony-stimulating factors: evidence-based, clinical practice guidelines. J Clin Oncol 1996; 14: 1957–1960.
7. Savarese DM, Hsieh C, Stewart FM. Clinical impact of chemotherapy dose escalation in patients with haematologic malignancies and solid tumors. J Clin Oncol 1997; 15: 981–2995.
8. Maraveyas A, Pettengell R. What is the role of erythropoietin in patients with solid tumours? Ann Oncol 1998; 9: 239–241.
9. Epstein JB, Vickars L, Spinelli J et al. Efficacy of chlorhexidine and nystatin rinses in prevention of oral complications in leukaemia and bone marrow transplantation. Oral Surg Oral Med Oral Pathol 1992; 73: 682–689.
10. Foote RL, Loprinzi CL, Frank AR et al. Randomised trial of a chlorhexidine mouthwash for the alleviation of radiation induced mucositis. J Clin Oncol 1994; 12: 2630–2633.
11. Feber RL. Management of mucositis in oral irradiation. Clin Oncol 1996; 8: 106–111.
12. Makkonen TA, Bostron P, Vilja P et al. Sucralfate mouth washing in the prevention of radiation induced mucositis: a placebo-controlled double blind randomised study. Int J Radiat Oncol Biol Phys 1994; 30: 177–182.
13. Mahood DJ, Dose AM, Loprinzi C et al. Inhibition of

fluorouracil-induced stomatitis by oral cryotherapy. J Clin Oncol 1991; 9: 449–452.

14. Kuhrer I, Kuzmits R, Linkesch W, Ludwig H. Topical PGE2 enhances healing of chemotherapy associated mucosal lesions. Lancet 1986; 1: 622.
15. Symonds RP, McIlroy P, Khorrami J et al. The reduction of radiation mucositis by selective decontamination antibiotic pastilles: a placebo controlled double blind trial. Br J Cancer 1996; 74: 312–317.
16. Johnston EM, Crawford J. Hematopoietic growth factors in the reduction of chemotherapeutic toxicity. Semin Oncol 1998; 25(5): 552–561.
17. Nicolatou O, Sotiropoulou–Lontou A, Skarlatos J et al. A pilot study of the effect of granulocyte-macrophage colony-stimulating factor on oral mucositis in head and neck cancer patients during X-radiation therapy: a preliminary report. Int J Radiat Oncol Biol Phys 1998; 42(3): 551–556.
18. Ibrahim EM, Al-Mulhim FA. Effect of granulocyte-macrophage colony-stimulating factor on chemotherapy-induced oral mucositis in non-neutropenic cancer patients. Med Oncol 1997; 14(1): 47–51.
19. Sonis ST, Van Vugt AG, Brien JP et al. Transforming growth factor-beta 3 mediated modulation of cell cycling and attenuation of 5-fluorouracil induced oral mucositis. Oral Oncol 1997; 33(1): 47–54.
20. Batist G, Rao SC, Ramakrishnan G et al. Phase III study of liposome-encapsulated doxorubicin (TLC-D-99) versus doxorubicin (Dox) in combination with cyclophosphamide in patients with metastatic breast cancer (MBC). ASCO Proceedings 1999; 18: 127a Abs 486.
21. Sredni B, Xu RH, Albeck M et al. The protective role of the immunomodulator AS101 against chemotherapy-induced alopecia studies on human and animal models. Int J Cancer 1996; 65(1): 97–103.e
22. Sredni B, Albeck M, Tichler T et al. Bone marrow-sparing and prevention of alopecia by AS101 in non-small cell lung cancer patients treated with carboplatin and etoposide. J Clin Oncol 1995; 13(9): 2342–2353.
23. Linscheer WG, Murthy VK, Alvarez-Moratilla S. Prevention of cyclophosphamide-induced baldness by propylthiouracil in a new rat model. Proceedings of ASCO 1999; 18: 453a Abs 1749.
24. Cascinu S, Cordella L, Del Ferro E et al. Neuroprotective effect of reduced glutathione on cisplatin based chemotherapy in advanced gastric cancer: a randomized double-blind placebo-controlled trial. J Clin Oncol 1995; 13: 26–32.
25. Smyth JF, Bowman A, Perren T et al. Glutathione reduces the toxicity and improves quality of life of women diagnosed with ovarian cancer treated with cisplatin: results of a double-blind, randomised trial. Ann Oncol 1997; 8: 569–573.
26. Greene D, Nail LM, Fieler VK et al. A comparison of patient-reported side effects among three chemotherapy regimens for breast cancer. Cancer Pract 1994; 2: 57–62.
27. Berglund G, Bolund C, Fornander T et al. Late effects of adjuvant chemotherapy and postoperative radiotherapy on quality of life among breast cancer patients. Eur J Cancer 1991; 27: 1075–1081.
28. Beisecker A, Cook MR, Ashworth J et al. Side effects of adjuvant chemotherapy: perceptions of node-negative breast cancer patients. Psychooncology 1997; 6: 85–93.
29. Broeckel JA, Jacobsen PB, Horton J et al. Characteristics and correlates of fatigue after adjuvant chemotherapy for breast cancer. J Clin Oncol 1998; 16: 1689–1696.
30. Berger AM. Patterns of fatigue and activity and rest during adjuvant breast cancer chemotherapy. Oncol Nurs Forum 1998; 25: 51–62.
31. Cimprick B. Developments of an intervention to restore attention in cancer patients. Cancer Nursing 1993; 16: 83–92.
32. Singal PW, Iliskovic N. Doxorubicin-induced cardiomyopathy. New Engl J Med 1998; 339: 900–905.
33. Ryberg M, Nielsen D, Skovsgaard T et al. Epirubicin cardiotoxicity: an analysis of 469 patients with metastatic breast cancer. J Clin Oncol 1998; 16: 3502–3508.
34. Swain SM, Whaley FS, Gerber MC et al. Cardioprotection with dexrazoxane for doxorubicin-containing therapy in advanced breast cancer. J Clin Oncol 1997; 15: 1318–1332.
35. Swain SM, Whaley FS, Gerber MC et al. Delayed administration of dexrazoxane (ADR-529, ICRF-187) provides cardioprotection for patients with advanced breast cancer treated with doxorubicin-containing therapy. J Clin Oncol 1997; 15: 1333–1340.
36. Venturini M, Micelotti A, Del Mastro L et al. Multicentre randomized controlled clinical trial to evaluate cardioprotection of dexrazoxane versus no cardioprotection in women receiving epirubicin chemotherapy for advanced breast cancer. J Clin Oncol 1996; 14(12): 3112–3120.
37. Dnistrian AM, Schwartz MK, Fracchia AA, Kaufman RJ, Hakes TB, Currie VE. Endocrine consequences of CMF adjuvant therapy in premenopausal and postmenopausal breast cancer patients. Cancer 1983; 51: 803–807.
38. Valagussa P, Moliterni A, Terenziani M, Zambetti M, Bonadonna G. Second malignancies following CMF-based adjuvant chemotherapy in resectable breast cancer. Ann Oncol 1994; 5: 803–808.
39. Van Leeuwen FE, Bernraadt J, Coebergh JW et al. Risk of endometrial cancer following breast cancer treatment with tamoxifen. Lancet 1994; 343: 448–452.

40. Zahasky KM, Loprinzi CL, Sloan J, Novotny PJ, Quella SK. Detailed prospective data regarding tamoxifen associated hot flashes. ASCO proceedings 1999; 18: 591, Abs 2283.
41. Bertelli G, Venturini M, Mastro LD et al. Depot intramuscular medroxyprogesterone acetate (MAP) vs oral megestrol acetate for the treatment of hot flashes in breast cancer survivors: results of GONO (Gruppo, Oncologico Nord Ovest) MIG-4 Phase III trial. ASCO Proceedings 1999; 18: 592a, Abs 2286.

Breast Cancer: Diagnosis and Management
J.M. Dixon (Ed.)

CHAPTER 43

Management of side effects associated with radiotherapy

Ian Kunkler

1. Introduction

The side effects of radiotherapy relate to the tissues which are included within the irradiated volume when the breast/chest wall and/or peripheral lymphatics are treated. These are the skin, soft tissues, ribs, lung, heart and brachial plexus. Side effects are usually classified into acute and late. These side effects are listed in Table 1. Acute side effects occur during radiotherapy or within a few weeks of its completion (e.g. skin reactions, oesophagitis and acute radiation pneumonitis). Late effects occur months or years after treatment (e.g. telangiectasia, soft tissue fibrosis and necrosis, rib fractures, lung fibrosis, myocardial ischaemia, lymphoedema, brachial plexopathy and radiation induced malignancy). Most of the side effects of radiotherapy are irreversible. For this reason prevention of toxicity is a key element of management. The usage of fractionated megavoltage radiotherapy (e.g. 45–50 Gy over 4–5 weeks) to respect normal tissue tolerance, good field matching between axillary and chest wall/breast fields to avoid overdosage from overlapping fields in the axilla (a potential cause of radiation induced brachial plexopathy) and minimising the volume of lung and heart irradiated are of paramount importance.

Table 1. Side effects of loco-regional irradiation for breast cancer

(a) Acute
Acute skin reaction
Cellulitis
Oesophagitis
Pneumonitis
(b) Late
Telangiectasia
Cellulitis
Soft tissue fibrosis
Soft tissue necrosis
Rib fractures
Lung fibrosis
Myocardial ischaemia
Brachial plexopathy
Second malignancy

> *Side effects of radiotherapy are irreversible. Careful attention to total dose and fractionation and techniques to minimise the volume of critical normal structures is of paramount importance.*

2. Management of acute skin reactions

The typical acute skin reaction which accompanies radical radiotherapy is mild in the majority of patients. More intense reactions are more common in women with larger breasts and a small number of individuals with increased intrinsic radiosensitivity. Dry desquamation may progress to painful patchy or confluent moist desquamation, particularly in the submammary fold. During the period of acute skin reaction, pressure on the irradiated area should be minimised by wearing loose fitting clothing. A variety of topical ointments (paraffin, almond, aqueous cream, herb oils or corticosteroids) have been used. However there is no convincing evidence of their benefits. Although most departments discourage washing or application of ointments during treatment, a randomised trial comparing washing versus not washing with soap [1] found that acute reactions were milder in patients who washed with soap.

Cellulitis of the breast characterised by erythema, warmth, oedema and tenderness of the breast may occur before, during or after radiotherapy in patients treated by breast conserving surgery. In contrast to a radiation reaction, it may extend outwith the irradiated area and has to be distinguished from the normal skin reaction to radical radiotherapy. The incidence is reported to be 1.25%–9% [2]. Skin erythema due to radiotherapy is unusual at a dose of 20 Gy or less [2]. The relative contribution of surgery and radiotherapy to this phenomenon is unclear. A bacteriological diagnosis should be sought, although this is rarely positive [3]. The commonest organisms are staph. aureus and group A and B haemolytic streptococci. Appropriate antibiotics should be used. Recurrence is common and symptoms tend to respond slowly to antibiotics [4].

Skin reactions to radiotherapy are common and include dry and moist desquamation. There is no convincing evidence that washing the treated area increases skin reaction.

3. Oesophagitis

Radiation induced oesophagitis is normally a transient side effect settling within 2–3 weeks of completion of radiotherapy. Symptomatic treatment with mucaine (which contains a local anaesthetic) 10 ml prn and before meals is recommended.

4. Late effects

4.1. Skin and soft tissue necrosis

With conventionally fractionated megavoltage radiotherapy to the breast/chest wall, necrosis of the skin and underlying soft tissues is extremely unusual. Problems currently seen are usually late complications occurring among women treated in the 1960s and 1970s with orthovoltage radiotherapy (where the full dose was delivered to the skin or when the dose per fraction of radiotherapy was higher and skin bolus was used to overcome the skin sparing effect of megavoltage irradiation). Occasionally small areas of necrosis may heal with conservative measures (standard wound care, simple debridement and antibiotics). Infection and chronic discharge is common at the site of necrosis and should be treated with appropriate antibiotics. For areas of necrosis failing to respond to conservative measures excision of the affected skin with a myocutaneous flap is the best option. There is some limited evidence for the efficacy of pentoxifylline, a methyl xanthine derivative used in the treatment of a variety of vasculo-occlusive disorders in chest wall necrosis [5]. It appears to work by improving blood flow within irradiated tissue by two mechanisms. The first is by increasing red cell deformability [6] and the second by stimulating prostacyclin release [7]. In a pilot study of pentoxifylline at a variety of sites of soft tissue radionecrosis Dion et al. described two cases of chest wall necrosis which healed within 4 and 7 weeks respectively. Pain which was a feature of the second case resolved within 3 weeks. However it is possible that this necrosis might have healed with conservative treatment. A multicentre randomised trial is required to confirm the efficacy of pentoxifylline. In the pilot study at a dose of 400 mg tds (the same as used for intermittent claudication) the only toxicity was gastrointestinal.

Late effects on skin and soft tissues are uncommon with conventional fractionated radiotherapy but are still seen in patients treated by earlier orthovoltage radiotherapy.

4.2. Cosmesis

Impaired cosmesis in women managed by breast conserving therapy is a consequence of both surgery, radiotherapy and chemotherapy [8]. Cosmesis is commonly impaired initially by breast oedema and subsequently by the skin changes of telangiectasia and fibrosis. Fibrosis results in retraction of the breast and distortion of its contour [9]. Bolus should be avoided except in T_4 tumours or where there is histological evidence of skin involvement following mastectomy to avoid the development of telangiectasia. Dose homogeneity is also thought to be important to minimising breast fibrosis.

4.3. Pneumonitis

Radiation pneumonitis is a clinical syndrome usually occurring 1–3 months following radiotherapy. Its incidence varies from 0 to 10% [10]. Pneumonopathy is perhaps a better term as McDonald et al. [11] point out since it is not an infective process. Cytokine release may be important in the generation of radiation fibrosis [12]. Typical symptoms are a nonproductive cough, associated with progressive or acute dyspnea. There are usually no abnormal respiratory signs. The use of internal mammary node photon fields increased the risk of pneumonitis in one series to 12.8% [13]. Investigations should include a chest radiograph which may show a diffuse infiltrate within the irradiated volume [14], CT scanning (Fig. 1), is a more sensitive method of detecting radiological changes, and is abnormal in more than 50% of patients [15] and pulmonary function tests. The latter usually show a restrictive pattern with impairment of gas transfer due to a change in the alveolar capillary barrier [11]. Lung fibrosis is identifiable at 20 weeks after radiotherapy and stabilises after approximately 34 weeks [16]. A central lung distance (the perpendicular distance from the posterior beam edge of the tangential fields to the inner aspect of the chest wall) in excess of 3 cm is associated with a high risk of pneumonitis and should be avoided [36].

Treatment is with steroids (Prednisolone 30–60 mg per day) tapered off according to clinical response. Antibiotics have been commonly added but there is no good evidence of their value. Drugs such as interferon [17] that antagonise or inhibit the action of growth factors which promote fibrosis have the potential to improve the symptoms of pneumonitis but studies have yet to establish their clinical value.

Radiation pneumonitis or pneumonopathy affects patients 1–3 months after radiotherapy and presents with an irritating nonproductive cough. Treatment is with oral prednisolone.

4.4. Cardiac effects

The role of loco-regional radiotherapy for breast cancer in the development of coronary artery disease is controversial. The study of Paszat et al. [18] from the Surveillance, Epidemiology and End Results database in the United States shows that adjuvant radiotherapy for left sided breast cancer is associated with a relative risk of 1.1 for fatal myocardial infarction. Gyenes et al. [19] have shown myocardial scintigraphic defects using ^{99m}Tc SestaMIBI suggesting hypoperfusion corresponding to the irradiated volume of the left ventricle after regional radiotherapy. However these changes did not correspond with any defect on ECG or of ventricular function. Radiotherapy planning should attempt to minimise the volume of the heart irradiated. In particular direct fields to cover the internal mammary chain should be treated predominantly with electrons rather than with photons to reduce the dose to the heart. However in many patients it is not possible using

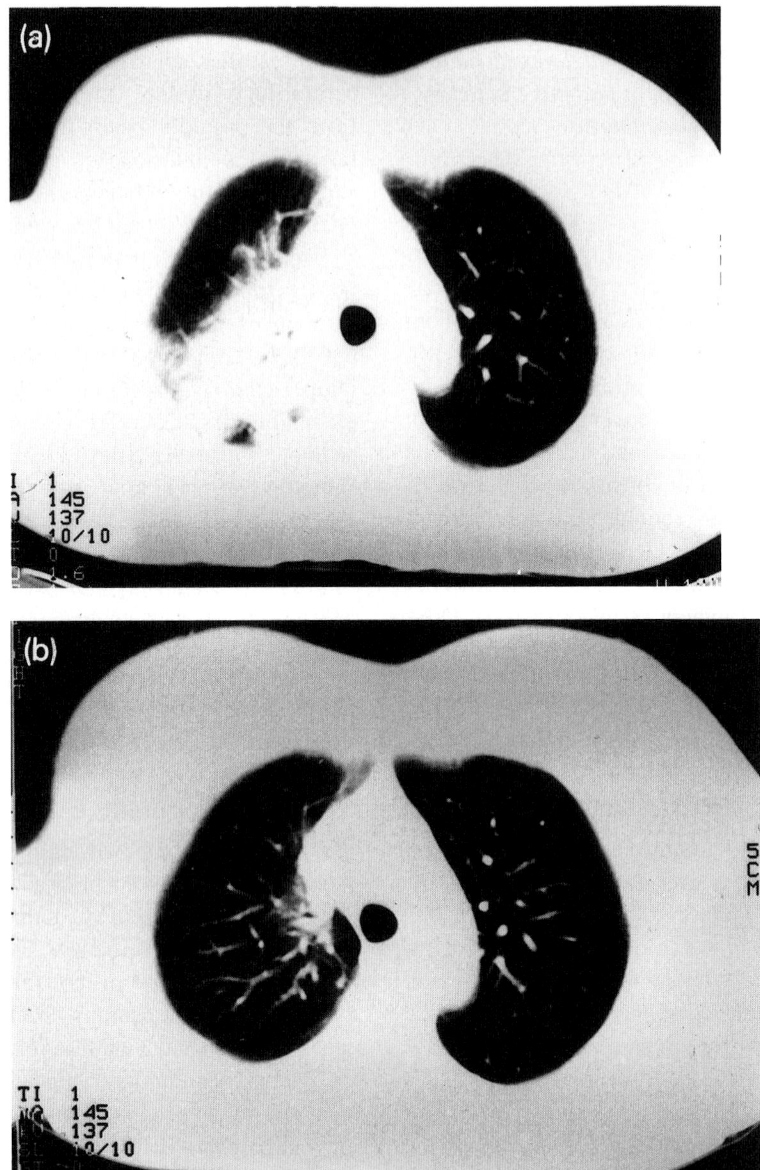

Fig. 1. Radiation pneumonitis. CT scan of the thorax of patient with exertional dyspnea (a) 4 weeks after completion of radical radiotherapy to the axilla and supraclavicular fossa showing opacification of right upper lobe and (b) 8 weeks later showing resolving radiological changes which corresponded to reduction in dyspnea.

tangential fields to avoid irradiating some part of the myocardium in order treat the breast/chest wall adequately.

The use of internal mammary chain irradiation with photons increases the dose to the heart and lung should be discouraged.

Table 2. Summary of management of lymphoedema

Good skin hygiene, prompt treatment of skin cuts and abrasions to reduce risk of cellulitis
(a) Moderate severity
Compression bandaging to reduce limb size
Elastic hosiery to maintain limb size
Manual lymphatic drainage
(b) Complicated cases
Phase 1:
2–3 weeks of daily skin care, multilayer bandaging, exercises and manual lymphatic drainage
Phase 2:
Maintenance skin care
Elastic hosiery
Simplified manual lymphatic drainage

4.5. Lymphoedema

Lymphoedema of the upper limb has been reported in 9.1% of patients whose axilla has been irradiated following an axillary sample and 8.3% in the absence of axillary surgery [20]. Radiotherapy causes obstruction of the axillary lymphatics and lymphatics do not regenerate following radiation damage. Cellulitis is a common complication of lymphoedema. Good skin care, hygiene and prompt cleaning of wounds and skin abrasion is important to reduce the risk of infection (Table 2). The main handicaps of lymphoedema are pain, heaviness of the arm, reduced arm mobility and function [21]. Secondary joint and musculoskeletal problems may result from the size and weight of the limb. Referral to a experienced physiotherapist for assessment at an early stage is important before chronic and irremediable lymphoedema becomes established. There is no curative treatment for lymphoedema. However, using a variety of physical therapies, it is possible to control symptoms. These therapies aim to keep the swelling under control and facilitate drainage through existing lymphatics and collateral routes. Elastic hosiery (e.g. a Jobst armlet) helps to maintain limb size by containment. Individualised fitting is essential for good compliance. At least 30 mm Hg pressure is needed. Compression bandaging is also of value. A strong nonelastic bandage is applied (Fig. 2). This exerts high pressure during muscular contraction and low pressure at rest [21]. Manual lymphatic drainage by gentle massage beginning proximal to the site of obstruction is used to stimulate lymph flow through residual normal lymphatic channels. For the more complicated cases intensive treatment over 2–3 weeks with a daily regime involving skin care, multilayer bandaging, exercises and manual lymphatic drainage is recommended [22]. Pneumatic compression may be helpful in conjunction with other physical therapies. It helps to promote the flow of lymph through tissue channels. However it does not stimulate lymph drainage. Consequently proteins are not removed from the interstitium and the osmotic imbalance remains. Once the machine is discontinued, the swelling will return. Long term use of pneumatic compression results in a fibrotic cuff at the shoulder which impedes lymphatic drainage. In the second phase of treatment (maintenance) daily skin care, wearing a compression garment, exercises and a simplified form of manual lymphatic drainage (simple lymphatic drainage exercises are taught). Milder cases may start directly on the maintenance regime.

> *Axillary radiotherapy can cause fibrosis of lymphatics resulting in lymphoedema. As fibrosis develops over a period of years the onset of lymphoedema can occur many years after radiotherapy.*

> *Manual lymphatic drainage, bandaging and support hosiery are the most useful treatments for lymphoedema.*

4.6. Rib fractures

Rib fractures occur in about 5% of patients treated with breast/chest wall radical radiotherapy [23]. Analgesia may be required in symptomatic cases.

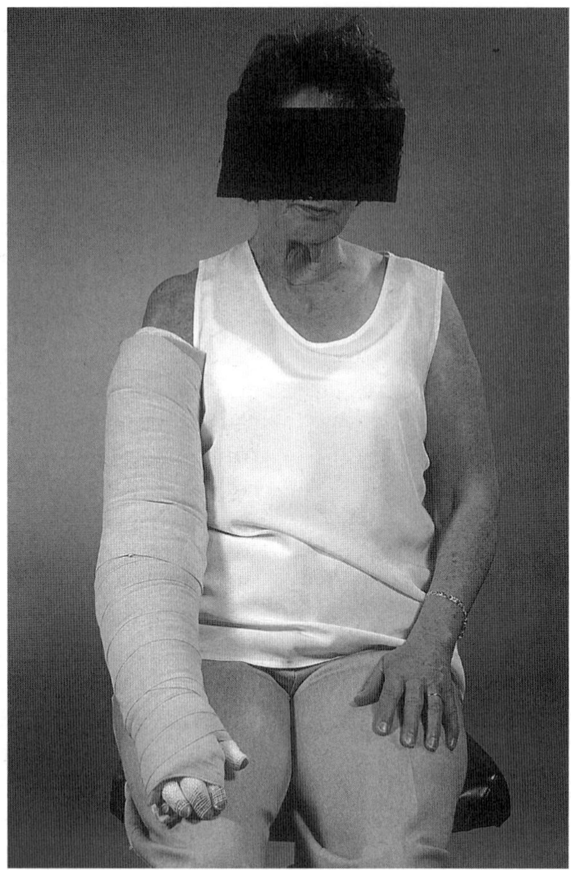

Fig. 2. Bandaging of lymphoedematous arm, a late complication of axillary irradiation.

4.7. Brachial plexopathy

Radiation induced brachial plexopathy should occur in less than 1% of patients treated with conventional fractionation regimes (e.g. 50 Gy in 2 Gy fractions over 5 weeks). Its incidence rises to approximately 5% at a total dose of 60 Gy to the brachial plexus. Typical features are persistent shoulder pain, tingling and numbness of the thumb and forefinger and wasting and weakness of the small muscles of the hand. Management should be multidisciplinary involving surgeons, oncologists, neurologists, palliative care physicians, anaesthetists, physiotherapists and occupational therapists. Investigations should include chest and cervical spine radiographs, CT/MRI scanning of the axilla with biopsy under CT control of suspicious areas and nerve conduction studies to identify the site of the block. Systematic management of pain is essential. Tricyclic antidepressants, anticonvulsants (carbamazepine, sodium valproate), topical non-steroidal anti-inflammatory drugs, transcutaneous electrical nerve stimulation (TENS), acupuncture, psychological support all play a role. Assessment by an occupational therapist for adaptations to the home and car may be required. Physiotherapists can advise on the use of pain relieving techniques such as heat, ice, TENS and use of massage, advise on positioning, splinting, skin care, supportive aids and graded exercises. First line therapy should be with TENS with or without a tricyclic antidepressant (amitryptaline, dothiepin or clomipramine). Temporary (e.g. regional guanethidine) or permanent dorsal root entry zone (DREZ) ablation nerve blocks may be appropriate for a small number of highly selected patients [24].

The role of surgery [25] in decompressing the brachial plexus and revascularising nerves is controversial and its value has yet to be established.

Brachial plexopathy is an uncommon complication of axillary radiotherapy; <1% when standard doses (<50 Gy) are used but it increases in frequency with increasing dose.

5. Treatment of late complications

Hyperbaric oxygen (HBO) has been shown to be beneficial in some cases of radiation induced tissue damage (e.g. osteoradionecrosis of the mandible [26]. Such irradiated tissues have been shown to have 20–30% of the capillary density of normal tissue [27]. During HBO treatment, a 7–10 fold increase in oxygen tension and a steep oxygen gradient can be achieved within the irradiated area. Angiogenesis appears to be stimulated by these steep gradients [28]. In animal models a prompt rise in lumenised capillaries ensues reaching 75–80% of normal tissue levels. There is very limited evidence of its value in radiation induced neurological damage. Some improvement in sensory symptoms was reported in 5 cases of radiation myelopathy but there was no improvement in motor function [29]. The value of HBO is being assessed in a randomised phase III study in patients with radiation induced brachial plexopathy [30].

The management of radiation induced brachial plexus plexopathy requires a multidisciplinary approach involving specialist surgeons, oncologists, palliative care physicians, anaesthetists, physiotherapists and occupational therapists.

5.1. Second malignancies

Sarcomas of bone in the shoulder girdle and ribs may arise as a rare late complication of loco-regional irradiation for breast cancer. Histologies include osteosarcomas, fibrosarcomas, malignant fibrous histiocytoma and chondrosarcoma. Most cases occur in the scapula followed by humerus and clavicle. Doherty et al. [31] reported a 0.26% incidence (2 cases) among 3199 cases of breast cancer treated by simple mastectomy and radiotherapy or primary radiotherapy from 1954 to 1964. Average latency was 10 years 9 months. Treatment following restaging to exclude metastases involves a forequarter amputation. Survival is poor among patients not receiving treatment for this complication (on average 8 months). Radiation induced soft tissue sarcomas also occur within the irradiated fields. These include angiosarcoma and leiomyosarcoma. Treatment is by radical excision where possible. Taghian et al. [32] reported a series of 11 cases of radiation induced bone and soft tissue sarcomas from 6919 patients treated by radiotherapy for breast cancer at Institut Gustave Roussy, Paris between 1954 and 1983. The relative risk of developing a sarcoma was 1.81 with a cumulative incidence of 0.2% at 10 years and 0.43% at 20 years and 0.78% at 30 years after radiotherapy. The latent period for developing a sarcoma was 10 years. Radiation induced sarcomas are aggressive with a high tendency for local recurrence and distant metastases. A few long-term survivors treated by forequarter amputation are described [33]. Oesophageal cancer has also been reported [34]. Neugut et al. [35] reported a threefold increase in lung cancer in both smoker and non-smokers treated more than 10 years previously by adjuvant loco-regional irradiation for breast cancer. Radical oesophagectomy or pneumonectomy should be considered where feasible. An increased incidence of breast cancer has also been reported in patients treated at a young age for lymphoma by mantle radiotherapy.

Radiation induced malignancies (usually soft tissue sarcomas) are uncommon (<0.5% at 20 yrs) and occur on average 10 years following radiotherapy.

References

1. Campbell IR, Illingworth MH. Can patients wash during radiotherapy to the breast or chest wall? A randomised controlled trial. Clin Oncol 1992; 4: 78–82.
2. Hughes LL, Styblo TM, Thoms WW et al. Cellulitis of the breast as complication of breast conserving surgery and irradiation. Am J Clin Oncol 1997; 20: 338–41.
3. Simon MS, Cody RL. Cellulitis after axillary lymph node dissection for carcinoma of the breast. Am J Med 1992; 93: 543–8.
4. Rescigno J, McCormick B, Brown AE and Myskowski PL. Breast cellulitis after conservative surgery and radiotherapy. Int J Radiat Oncol Biol Phys 1994; 29: 163–168.
5. Dion MW, Hussey DH, Doornbos JF, Vigliotti, Chen Wen B, Anderson B. Preliminary results of a pilot study of pentoxifylline in the treatment of late radiation soft tissue fibrosis. Int J Radiat Oncol Biol Phys 1990; 19: 401–407.
6. Ehrly AM. The effect of pentoxifylline on the flow properties of human blood. Curr Med Res Opin 1978; 5: 608–613.
7. Jarrett PE, Moreland M, Browse NL. The effect of oxypentifylline on the fibrinolytic activity and plasma fibrinogen levels. Curr Med Res Opin 1977; 4: 492–95.
8. Ray GR, Fish VJ, Marmor JB et al. Impact of adjuvant chemotherapy on cosmesis and complications in stage 1 and 11 carcinoma of the breast treated biopsy and radiation therapy. Int J Radiat Oncol Biol Phys 1984; 10: 837–41.
9. Kurtz JM. Impact of radiotherapy on breast cosmesis. Breast 1995; 4: 163–169.
10. Polansky SM, Ravin CE, Prosnitz LR. Pulmonary changes after primary radiation for early breast carcinoma. Am J Radiol 1980; 134: 101.
11. McDonald S, Rubin P, Phillips TL, Marks LB. Injury to the lung from cancer therapy: clinical syndromes, measurable endpoints, and potential scoring systems. Int J Radiat Oncol Biol Phys 1995; 31: 1187–1203.
12. Rubin P, Finkelstein, J, McDonald S, Horowitz S, Sinkin R. The identification of new early molecular mechanisms in the pathogenesis of radiation induced pulmonary fibrosis. Int J Radiat Oncol Biol Phys 1991; 21: (S1) 163.
13. Halverson KL, Taylor ME, Perez CA et al. Regional nodal management and patterns of failure following conservative surgery and radiation therapy for stage 1 and 11 breast cancer. Int J Radiat Oncol Biol Phys 1993; 26: 593–9.
14. Gross NJ. Pulmonary effects of radiation therapy. Ann Intern Med 1981; 159: 115–125.
15. Mah K, Van Dyk J, Keane T et al. Acute radiation-induced pulmonary damage: a clinical study on the response to fractionated radiation therapy. Int J Radiat Oncol Biol Phys 1987; 13: 179–188.
16. Herrmann T, Schorcht J, Molls M. Radiation pneumonopathy- experimental and clinical data. In: Dunst J, Sauer R (Eds), Late Sequelae in Oncology. Berlin: Springer, pp. 123–131, 1993.
17. McDonald S, Rubin P, Chang A et al. Pulmonary changes induced by combined mouse b-interferon and radiation in normal mice — toxic versus protective effects. Radiother Oncol 1993; 26: 212–8.
18. Paszat LF, Mackillop WJ, Groome PA, Boyd C, Schulze K, Holowaty E. Mortality from myocardial infarction after adjuvant radiotherapy for breast cancer in the Surveillance, Epidemiology and End-Results Cancer Registries. J Clin Oncol 1998; 2625–31.
19. Gyenes G, Fornander T, Carlens P, Glas U, Rutquist LE. Myocardial damage in breast cancer patients treated with adjuvant radiotherapy: a prospective study. Int J Radiat Oncol Biol Phys 1996; 4: 899–905.
20. Kissin MW, Querci della Rovere G, Easton D et al. Risk of lymphoedema following treatment of breast cancer. Br J Surg 1986; 73: 580–4.
21. Mortimer PS. Investigation and management of lymphoedema. Vasc Med 1990; 1: 1–20.
22. Todd JE. A study of lymphoedema patients over their first six months of treatment. Physiotherapy 1999; 85: 65–76.
23. Hellman S, Harris J, Cannellos GP, Fisher B. Cancer of the breast. In: DeVita VT, Hellman S, Rosenberg SA (Eds), Cancer Principles and Practice of Oncology. JP Lippincott, 1982, p. 941.
24. Maher Committee. Management of adverse effects following breast radiotherapy. London: Royal College of Radiologists, 1995.
25. Narakas AO. Operative treatment for radiation-induced and metastatic brachial plexopathy in 45 cases, 15 having an omentoplasty. Bull Hosp J Dis Orthop Inst 1984; 44: 354–75.
26. Mountsey RA, Brown DH, O'Dwyer TP et al. Role of hyperbaric oxygen in the management of mandibular osteoradionecrosis. Laryngoscope 1993; 103: 605–8.
27. Marx RE, Ehler WJ, Tayapongsak PT et al. Relationship of oxygen dose to angiogenesis induction in irradiated tissues. Am J Surg 1990; 16: 519–524.
28. Knighton DR, Hunt TK, Schenestuhl H et al. Oxygen tension regulates the expression of angiogenesis factor by macrophages. Science 1983; 221: 1283–89.
29. Hart GB, Minous EG. The treatment of radiation

necrosis with hyperbaric oxygen. Cancer 1976; 37: 2580–2585.
30. Yarnold J. Personal communication, 1999.
31. Doherty MA, Rodger A, Langlands AO. Sarcoma of bone following therapeutic irradiation for breast cancer. Int J Radiat Oncol Biol Phys 1986; 12: 103–6.
32. Taghian A, De Vathaire F, Terrier P et al. Long term risk of sarcoma following radiation treatment for breast cancer. Int J Radiat Oncol Biol Phys 21: 361–367.
33. Sim FH, Cupps RE, Dahlin DC, Ivins JC. Post-irradiation sarcoma of bone. J Bone Joint Surg 54-A: 1479–1489.
34. Ferguson DJ, Sutton HG, Dawson PJ. Late effects of adjuvant radiotherapy for breast cancer. Cancer 1984; 54: 2319.
35. Neugut AI, Robinson E, Lee WC, Murray T, Karwoski K, Kutcher G. Lung cancer after radiation therapy for breast cancer. Cancer 1994; 73: 1615.
36. Bartelink H, Garavaglia G, Johanson K-A et al. Quality assurance in conservative treatment of early breast cancer. Radiother Oncol 1991; 22: 323–6.

Breast Cancer: Diagnosis and Management
J.M. Dixon (Ed.)

CHAPTER 44

Follow-up of patients after treatment for breast cancer

Stefano Ciatto

1. Aims of follow-up

Performing regular follow-up examinations of breast cancer patients after primary treatment has been a common practice over the past few decades. Regular follow-up (FU) has a number of aims and goals including

- obtaining information on the natural history of the disease,
- improving prediction of prognostic factors by assessing detailed course of disease,
- reassuring the patient of the absence of detectable metastatic disease,
- monitoring disease status for clinical trials,
- allowing patients to discuss side effects of therapy and to prescribe treatments to combat these,
- providing psychological support and providing an opportunity for early recognition of psychological problems.

The major goal however is to detect early symptomatic local or distant recurrence and to attempt to improve prognosis through early treatment. If early detection of local or systemic disease has no significant impact on prognosis, then the regular FU examinations could be reduced at least outside clinical trials.

Early detection of local or distant recurrences when asymptomatic is possible with a variety of diagnostic tests, but as breast cancer recurs most frequently locally or in bone and lung (Table 1), FU of breast cancer patients has usually involved physical examination, mammography, chest X-ray and a skeletal survey. The latter, originally based on radiography of the skeleton, has been more recently replaced by bone scintigraphy, which is more sensitive than radiography [2]. Due to the increased risk of contralateral breast cancer, contralateral mammography is also commonly included in FU protocols.

Table 1. Relative frequency of first relapse by relapse site: consecutive series of 1120 breast cancer patients [1]

Relapse site	Cases	Relative frequency (%)
Isolated, loco-regional	349	31.2
Bone, isolated	299	26.7
Lung, isolated	171	15.3
Soft tissues, isolated	51	4.5
Liver, isolated	50	4.5
Brain, isolated	29	2.6
Multiple sites [a]	171	15.3
Total	1120	100.0

[a] Bone and/or lung mostly involved.

2. Evidence of follow-up efficacy

No direct scientific evidence of the efficacy of FU was available until a few years ago. FU was presumed to be effective as it achieves early detection of some recurrences which are usually less advanced than symptomatic recurrences, and it does allow earlier treatment, and it was assumed that this would be beneficial and would improve survival.

A number of studies have shown that the average interval from primary treatment to recurrence detected by FU is significantly shorter than for symptomatic recurrences, the average detection lead time ranging between 6 and 12 months [1,3]. Based on the view that early detection of metastases of a limited extent should have a better survival when compared to more diffuse symptomatic metastases, the benefits of early detection were taken for granted. The few retrospective studies which have reported a survival advantage in the group with asymptomatic metastases [1,5], did not take account of lead time bias. Slow-growing metastases have a longer preclinical detectable phase and are more likely detected by regular FU investigations whereas fast-growing metastases tend to present with symptoms between two consecutive FU visits (Fig. 1). Thus finding a better survival for asymptomatic metastases may be just a consequence of identifying less aggressive lesions, rather than an effect of early detection. When survival is measured from primary treatment the majority of retrospective studies show no survival difference between asymptomatic and symptomatic metastases, in spite of earlier diagnosis (Table 2).

Most of the evidence on the efficacy of regular follow up has shown no benefit for early detection of local and distant recurrence and early positive studies were retrospective and suffer from length time bias sampling and lead time bias. When survival is compared from the time of primary treatment retrospective studies show no improvement in survival for patients having regular investigations during follow up.

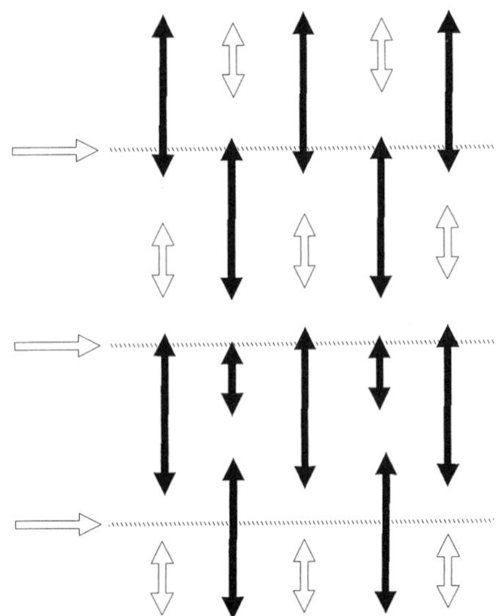

Fig. 1. Scheme illustrates length biased sampling. Metastases growing at different speeds are represented as short (fast growth) or long (slow growth) arrows. Arrow length indicates the length of the preclinical detectable phase. Periodic follow-up (horizontal arrows) has a higher chance to detect (black arrow) slow-growing metastases (large targets) whereas fast-growing metastases are more likely to surface as symptomatic (white arrows) in the interval between two consecutive follow-up controls.

3. Prospective trials of regular follow-up

The common practice in the 1980s was to perform regular FU examination and investigations despite no direct evidence of its efficacy and some indirect evidence from poorly constructed studies that it may not influence overall survival. Two controlled randomised studies were started in Italy in an attempt to provide reliable evidence of the efficacy of regular follow up assessments. The two studies had a similar design with subjects being randomly allocated either to intensive FU, undergoing tests aimed at early detection of distant metastases, or to minimal FU, where physical examination and mammography only were performed. One of the two studies [10] failed in its main objective in that metastatic disease was not detected at an earlier stage in the active FU arm, possibly because bone scintigraphy was repeated

Table 2. Estimates of the prognostic impact of follow-up based on a comparison of survival from primary treatment in cases with metastases detected as asymptomatic or symptomatic

Author	Relapse site	Survival (asymptomatic vs symptomatic)
Ciatto [4]	lung	median NS [a]
Ciatto [1]	bone	10-years +17% ($P < 0.05$)
	other sites	10-years NS
Buzdar [7]	all sites	median +12% ($P = 0.2$)
Broyn [6]	all sites	median NS
Hietanen [7]	lung	median NS
Zwaveling [8]	all sites	5-years NS
Rutgers [9]	all sites	5-years NS
Andreoli [3]	lung	10-years NS

[a] NS = statistically not significant difference.

with too infrequently, on an annual basis, an interval far exceeding the average detection lead time [1]. However, whatever the cause of the failure to diagnose asymptomatic metastatic disease the study failed to demonstrate any impact on survival and mortality of the more intensive follow up regimen.

The second study [11] in contrast, achieved a significant rate of early metastatic disease detection of bone and lung metastases (these two metastatic sites were investigated by bone scintigraphy and chest X-ray) and allowed earlier treatment of these women (Table 3). Despite apparent earlier detection and treatment of metastatic breast cancer, no difference in mortality was observed in the two study arms at five years (Table 3). No difference is also apparent on a preliminary evaluation of results at 10 years.

Table 3. Evidence of early diagnosis of asymptomatic metastases by an intensive follow-up programme and of the prognostic impact of intensive vs. minimal follow-up (data from the Florence randomised trial [11])

	Intensive	Minimal	Total
Distant metastases	164	125	289
bone, isolated	84	53	137
lung/pleura, isolated	28	18	46
other sites, isolated	22	21	43
multiple sites	30	33	63
Loco-regional recurrences	55	49	104
No recurrence reported	403	447	850
Total subjects in study	622	621	1243
Alive	503	498	1001
Dead	116	121	237
Unknown	3	2	5

> *Evidence from controlled randomised studies show that regular follow up investigations can result in early detection of asymptomatic metastases but these studies have failed to show any impact on prognosis of intensive follow up programmes.*

The only explanation of these results is that early detection and treatment of breast cancer metastases does not result in a significant improvement in survival and does not affect mortality. Of course, such findings are related to the diagnostic techniques utilised and the therapies available at the time these studies were performed. FU identifies recurrences which can be regarded as "early" with respect to their symptomatic onset but they are still too advanced to be managed with currently available therapeutic modalities. Hopefully, either diagnostic or therapeutic progress might change this scenario in the future, but presently there is no evidence to support regular FU by chest X-ray and bone scintigraphy in breast cancer patients. Intensive FU programmes have no significant impact on

Table 4. Evidence of early diagnosis and prognostic impact of regular FU for contralateral metachronous breast cancer (data from a retrospective study of cases detected as asymptomatic or symptomatic [13])

	Asymptomatic	Symptomatic
No. of cases	89	86
Disease-free interval from first primary (months)	68.9	96.8
Proportion of pTIS, pT1 (%)	55	37
Proportion of pN0 (%)	76	67
5 year survival (%) [a]	82	90
10 year survival (%) [a]	72	80

[a] Measured from the date of primary treatment of first cancer.

prognosis and its only effect is to make the patient aware of recurrent disease earlier and to expose them earlier to the side effects of treatment.

Existing scientific evidence does not support the use of regular investigations to detect asymptomatic metastases in breast cancer patients.

4. Regular assessment to detect local recurrences and contralateral breast cancer

FU protocols commonly include physical examination and mammography, aimed at early detection of local recurrences and contralateral breast cancer. Both conditions are known to be curable, the chance of cure being higher if disease is detected in a less advanced stage. From our experience the effects of early detection of breast or local recurrences on survival, as results from a retrospective study [12] may be limited. Similar results have been observed in a retrospective study of contralateral breast cancer [13]: FU allows detection at an earlier stage than symptomatic local recurrence but early treatment does not seem to increase survival, and patients seem to die "with" rather than of metachronous contralateral breast cancer (Table 4). As controlled studies are lacking, a definitive statement of the benefits of FU aimed at early detection of local recurrence and contralateral cancer is not possible. Periodic physical examination and mammography are generally regarded as "minimal" FU and are often motivated by the assumption that patients feel better if some sort of regular surveillance is available.

There is no scientific evidence that early detection of local recurrences or contralateral breast cancer is beneficial. Indirect evidence suggests that any benefit is limited.

References

1. Ciatto S, Rosselli Del Turco M, Pacini P et al. Early detection of breast cancer recurrences through periodic follow-up. Is it useless? Tumori 1985; 71: 325–329.
2. Freundlich IM, O'Mara R, Pitt MJ. Thermographic, radionuclide and radiographic detection of bone metastases. Radiology 1977; 122: 665–668.
3. Andreoli C, Buranelli F, Campa T et al. Chest X-ray survey in breast cancer follow-up — a contrary view. Tumori 1987; 73: 463–466.
4. Ciatto S, Herd-Smith A. The role of chest X-ray in the follow-up of primary breast cancer. Tumori 1983; 60: 161–163.
5. Buzdar A, Mahajan S, Hortobagyi C, Blumenschein G. Role of staging procedure for detection of recurrent disease in breast cancer patients and its impact on survival. In: Biomarkers, Diagnosis, Epidemiology, ASCO Reports 9, Abst-C, 1984.
6. Broyn T, Froyen J. Evaluation of routine follow-up after surgery for breast carcinoma. Acta Chir Scand 1982; 148: 401–404.
7. Hietanen P. Chest radiography in the follow-up of breast cancer. Acta Radiol (Oncol) 1986; 25: 15–18.
8. Zwaveling A, Albers GH, Felthuis W, Hermans J. An evaluation of routine follow-up for detection of breast cancer recurrences. J Surg Oncol 1987; 34: 194–197.
9. Rutgers EJ, van Slooten EA, Kluck HM. Follow-up

after treatment of primary breast cancer. Br J Surg 1989; 76: 187–190.

10. The GIVIO investigators. Impact of follow-up testing on survival and health related quality of life in breast cancer patients — A multicenter randomised trial. JAMA 1994; 271: 1587–1592.
11. Rosselli Del Turco M, Palli D, Cariddi A et al. Intensive diagnostic follow-up after treatment of primary breast cancer: A randomised trial. JAMA 1994; 271: 1593–1597.
12. Ciatto S, Rosselli Del Turco M, Pacini P et al. Early detection of local recurrences in the follow-up of primary breast cancer. Tumori 1984; 70: 179–183.
13. Ciatto S, Ambrogetti D, Bonardi R et al. Prognostic impact of early detection of contralateral primary breast cancer. Tumori 1990; 76: 370–373.

Breast Cancer: Diagnosis and Management
J.M. Dixon (Ed.)

CHAPTER 45

Treatment of breast recurrence after breast conservation

Elaine D.C. Anderson

1. Incidence

Breast conservation treatment, i.e. wide local excision of tumour and breast radiotherapy is now accepted treatment for early breast cancer. Randomised studies have shown survival rates comparable to those achieved after radical mastectomy but with possibly a slightly higher rate of local recurrence [1–3]. The exact incidence of intrabreast tumour recurrence (IBTR) after breast conserving surgery and radiotherapy is complicated by the tendency to report all local recurrences, including breast and axillary recurrences together. True breast recurrence increases with time since original treatment and has been reported in 5–10% of patients at 5 years and in 10–22% after 10 years [4–11].

Local recurrence following breast conserving therapy develops in 5–10% of women by 5 years.

2. Prognosis

Previous reports [8,10,12] have suggested that an isolated breast recurrence, in comparison to chest wall recurrence post mastectomy, is less likely to be associated with simultaneous distant metastases and is associated with a more favourable prognosis. The effect of breast relapse after conservative treatment on survival remains controversial. Some authors have reported no adverse effect on survival [13,14], but others have [15–17]. Fisher suggested that patients who developed IBTR had a 3.41 times greater risk of distant relapse [19] and suggested IBTR is a marker but not a cause of distant metastases. More recent reports have demonstrated that patients with IBTR have a second peak of distant metastases suggesting that IBTR can act as a source of systemic disease and influence subsequent mortality [17].

Local recurrence may be a marker for distant metastases.

3. Diagnosis

Between 25 and 35% [7,18–20] of breast recurrences are detected by mammography alone, the majority however are clinically apparent. The median interval to breast recurrence is variable. Some authors report a median interval of 34–37 months [20–22] while others report longer intervals of 53 months [6] and 44 months [7]. Interval to recurrence is related to location of recurrence with true or marginal recurrences occurring earlier than cancer elsewhere in the treated breast [18,20,23]. Recht [10] reported a median time to local failure of 38.5 months for true or marginal recurrences compared to 68.5 months for those elsewhere. The majority of recurrences occur in the vicinity of the original primary [4,5,7,8,10,20,24–26] with the incidence of disease elsewhere in the breast increasing as the time interval since surgery increases. Kurtz [27] observed that 32% of recurrences occurring after 5 years were elsewhere in the breast compared with 14% before 5 years. The majority of recurrences occurring after 10 years are at a different site and are almost certainly new primary tumours [8].

Approximately 80% of local recurrences in the conserved breast occur at the site of original breast cancer. The remainder are probably second primary tumours. As time since surgery increases, so the likelihood increases that a breast 'recurrence' will be distant from the original tumour site and a second primary.

As with all breast lesions confirmation of diagnosis is by triple assessment, i.e. clinical examination, imaging including ultrasound when appropriate and cytology or core biopsy. Open biopsy may be required if a diagnosis cannot be achieved by other means. Magnetic resonance imaging (MRI) is of value in differentiating scar from recurrent malignancy in patients where completion of radiotherapy is greater than one year from examination [28]. For the majority of patients developing breast recurrence, the histology is that of invasive cancer with approximately 10% having only DCIS [20].

90% of local recurrences following breast conserving therapy are invasive.

4. Staging

Approximately 10% of patients with breast recurrence following conservative surgery and radiation will have simultaneous or antecedent distant metastases [4,5,8,12,20,29] and prior to a therapeutic decision, the patient should be screened for the presence of occult metastatic disease. Patients confirmed to have concomitant systemic disease should receive treatment appropriate for the stage of their disease.

5. Treatment

The relative frequency of operable recurrence is between 90 and 94% [8,12,24,30–32]. Features which exclude operability are those of locally advanced disease, i.e. peau d'orange, skin nodules or skin fixation, signs of inflammation, chest wall fixation or the presence of fixed axillary or malignant supraclavicular lymph nodes. The management of locally advanced disease is covered in Ch. 50. The standard surgical procedure for operable intrabreast recurrence is salvage mastectomy [1–3]. Loco-regional control rates with salvage mastectomy were 88% with recurrences occurring within 5 years and 96% for those after 5 years in one study [31]. The 5-year actuarial survival following salvage mastectomy in another study was 84.5% with a disease free survival of 59% [20]. Kurtz [31] reported that although recurrences occurring after 5 years had no effect on long term prognosis, recurrences within the first 5 years was associated with a poorer survival.

Reconstruction following mastectomy for local recurrence either immediate or delayed does not appear to be associated with a significant increase in complications compared to primary mastectomy and reconstruction [2]. Patients undergoing subpectoral implant placement in this situation have been reported to have no increased incidence of dehiscence or capsular formation but these must be used with caution in patients following radiotherapy. Myocutaneous flap reconstruction may give better results in these women particularly if there is evidence of significant radiotherapy effect.

Although total mastectomy is considered the treatment of choice for local failure in the breast after breast conservation therapy, some IBTR are small and localised, and occasional patients desire breast preservation despite local failure. Salvadori [32] reported recently a group of 57 patients presenting with IBTR treated by re-excision of whom 84% had a solitary recurrent lesion and 60% had a tumour size of 1 cm or less. The risk of a second local recurrence following operation was higher following excision alone (19%) compared to a 4% recurrence rate following mastectomy. The risk of distant metastases was 74% after mastectomy compared to 20% after re-excision but this series was not randomised and the difference is likely to be a function of patient selection. A second group have reported a locoregional failure rate of 38% at 5 years after breast conserving salvage procedures in 50 selected intramammary recurrences following standard breast conserving treatment [33]. The 5-year local control was however better at 92% for recurrences occurring after 5 years compared with 49% for recurrence developing within 5 years; recurrence following re-excision was 7% for negative compared with 36% for positive or indeterminate margins. No other determinants for second local failures were identified. An important finding of this study was the poor prognosis of patients who developed a second failure in the breast. Median survival after second local failure in this study was 33 months. One-quarter of second local recurrences were inoperable, and in another 31% there was extensive recurrence detected in the mastectomy specimen. Ultimate local control can be achieved by tertiary treatment in only half of the 16 patients failing locally after conservative salvage surgery. The authors suggest that re-excision after IBTR may be appropriate in selected patients, i.e. small solitary recurrences in large breasts developing more than 5 years after primary therapy but clear margins are essential. Further confirmatory reports are necessary before re-excision becomes accepted as a definitive option. If re-excision is offered, the woman must be appropriately counselled as to the further risks of IBTR. The long-term effects on survival of re-excision when compared to mastectomy remain uncertain.

> *The treatment of choice for breast recurrence after breast conserving therapy is mastectomy.*

At the time of salvage breast surgery, axillary dissection in those who have not previously had a full level III clearance shows that approximately one third of patients have positive axillary nodes [7,8,12,21]. Fowble [20] reported a figure of 58%. In women who have had previous axillary radio-

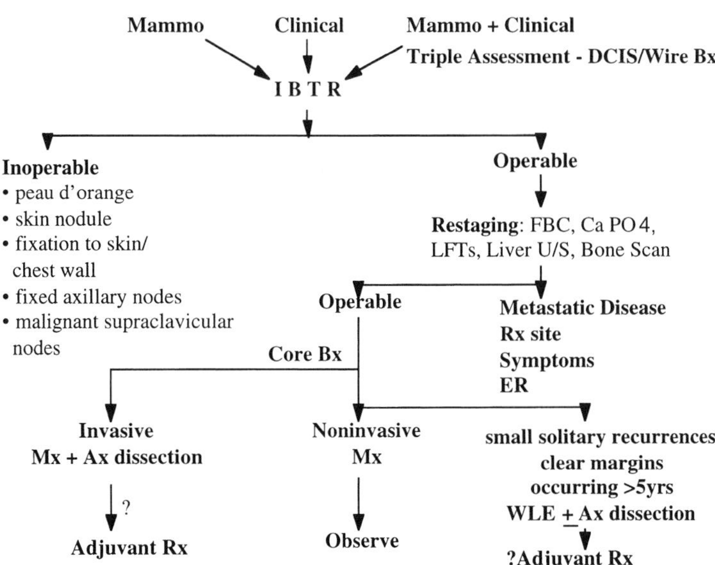

Fig. 1. Management of locoregional recurrence.

therapy a high incidence of arm lymphoedema may result (up to 30%) following completion axillary dissection and patients should be warned of this. Frozen section examination of axillary nodes to avoid unnecessary axillary dissection results in a 27% false negative rate and must be used with caution [34].

The presence of histologically positive nodes and their effect on survival remains controversial. Some authors report no effect [20,35] whereas others suggest a negative effect which in studies to date has failed to reach significance because of the small numbers [12,24].

6. Systemic therapy

The role of adjuvant systemic therapy at the time of local recurrence is not well studied. Fowble [20] reports a 5-year actuarial survival following recurrence of 76% for those who received chemotherapy because of positive axillary lymph nodes, extensive involvement of the breast, or dermal lymphatic, vascular or lymphatic invasion, compared to 89% who did not. The authors suggested that the difference reflected patient selection but a comparable group with poor prognostic signs who did not receive chemotherapy was not available for comparison. Adjuvant systemic therapy is not appropriate for those who develop purely non-invasive recurrence. Similarly patients whose interval to recurrence is greater than 5 years, whose initial tumour size was T1, or whose tumour recurrence is located in a separate quadrant of the breast and who do not have poor prognostic signs have a very good prognosis with a 5-year survival in excess of 90%. These patients do not appear to require adjuvant systemic therapy [20].

The role of systemic therapy following mastectomy for apparently localised breast recurrence is unclear.

The management of breast recurrence after breast conservation is summarised in Fig. 1.

References

1. Fisher B, Redmond C, Poisson R et al. Eight-year results of a randomised clinical trial comparing total mastectomy and lumpectomy with or without radiation in the treatment of breast cancer. N Eng J Med 1989; 320: 822–828.
2. Veronesi U, Banfi A, Del Vecchio M et al. Comparison of Halsted mastectomy with quadrantectomy, axillary dissection and radiotherapy in early breast cancer: long-term results. Eur J Cancer Clin Oncol 1986; 22: 1085–1089.
3. Sarrazin D, Le M, Rouesse J et al. Conservative treatment versus mastectomy in breast cancer tumours with macroscopic diameter of 20 millimeters or less. Cancer 1984; 53: 1209–1213.
4. Clark RM, Wilkinson RH, Mahoney LJ, Reid JG, MacDonald WD. Breast cancer: a 21-year experience with conservative surgery and radiation. Int J Radiat Oncol Biol Phys 1982; 8: 967–975.
5. Clark RM, Wilkinson RH, Miceli PN, MacDonald WSD. Breast cancer: experience with conservative therapy. Am J Clin Oncol 1987; 10: 461–468.
6. Fourquet A, Campana F, Zafrani B, Mosseri V, Vielh P, Durand JC, Vilcoq JR. Prognostic factors in the conservative management of early breast cancer: a 25-year follow-up at the Institut Curie. Int J Radiat Oncol Biol Phys 1989; 17: 719–725.
7. Hafty BG, Goldberg NB, Fischer D, McKhann C, Bienfield M, Weissberg JB, Carter D, Gerald W. Conservative surgery and radiotherapy therapy in breast carcinoma: local recurrence and prognostic implications. Int J Radiat Oncol Biol Phys 1989; 17: 727–732.
8. Kurtz JM, Amalric R, Brandone H, Ayme Y, Jacquemier J, Pietra JC, Hans D, Pollet JF, Bressac C, Spitalier J. Local recurrence after breast-conserving surgery and radiotherapy. Frequency, time course and prognosis. Cancer 1989; 63: 1912–1917.
9. Pierquin B. Conservative treatment for carcinoma of the breast: Experience of Creteil-ten-year results. In: Harris J, Hellman S, Silen W, eds. Conservative management of breast cancer. Philadelphia, PA, Lippincott, 1988, pp 11–14.
10. Recht A, Silen W, Schnitt SJ, Connolly JL, Gelman RS, Rose MA, Silver B, Harris JR. Time course of local recurrence following conservative surgery and radiotherapy for early stage breast cancer. Int J Radiat Oncol Biol Phys 1988; 15: 255–261.
11. Solin LJ, Fowble B, Martz K, Goodman RL. Definitive irradiation for early stage breast cancer: the University of Pennsylvania experience. Int J Radiat Oncol Biol Phys 1988; 14: 235–242.
12. Recht A, Schnitt SJ, Connolly JL, Rose MA, Silver B, Come S, Henderson IC, Slavin S, Harris JR. Prognosis following local or regional recurrence after conserva-

tive surgery and radiotherapy for early stage breast carcinoma. Int J Radiat Oncol Biol Phys 1989; 16: 3–9.

13. Amalric R, Santamari F, Robert F, Seigle J, Altschuler C, Kurtz JM, Spitalier JM, Brandone H, Ayme Y, Pollet JF, Burmeister R, Abed R. Radiation therapy with or without primary limited surgery for operable breast cancer: a 20-year experience at the Marseilles Cancer Institute. Cancer 1982; 49: 30–34.
14. Clarke RM, Wilkinson RH, Mahonety LJ, Reid JG, MacDonald WD. Breast cancer: a 21-year experience with conservative surgery and radiation. Int J Radiat Oncol Biol Phys 1982; 8: 967–975.
15. Fisher B, Anderson S, Fisher ER, Redmond C, Wickerham DL, Wolmark N, Mamounas EP, Deutsch M, Margolese R. Significance of ipsilateral breast tumour recurrence after lumpectomy. Lancet 1991; 338: 327–331.
16. Chauvet B, Reynaud-Bougnoux A, Calais G, Panel N, Lansac J, Bougnoux P, Le Flak O. Prognostic significance of breast relapse after conservative treatment in node-negative early breast cancer. Int J Radiat Oncol Biol Phys 1990; 19: 1125–1130.
17. Fortin A, Larochelle M, Laverdiere J, Lavertu S, Tremblay D. Local failure is responsible for the decrease in survival for patients with breast cancer treated with conservative surgery and postoperative radiotherapy. J Clin Oncol 1999; 17: 101–109.
18. Bartelink H, Border JH, van Dongen JA, Peterse JL. The impact of tumour size and histology on local control after breast conserving therapy. Radiother Oncol 1988; 11: 297–303.
19. Stomper PC, Recht A, Berenberg AL, Tochels MS, Harris JR. Mammographic detection of the recurrent cancer in the irradiated breast. AJR 1987; 148: 39–43.
20. Fowble B, Solin LJ, Schultz DJ, Rubenstein J, Goodman RL. Breast recurrence following conservative surgery and radiation: patterns of failure, prognosis and pathologic findings from mastectomy specimens with implications for treatment. Int J Radiat Oncol Biol Phys 1990; 19: 833–842.
21. Bluming AZ, Dosik G, Lowiz B, Newman S, Citronbaum R, Zeitz B et al. Treatment of primary breast cancer without mastectomy. The Los Angeles community experience and review of the literature. Ann Surg 1986; 204: 136–147.
22. Sarrazin D, Dewar JA, Arriagada R, Benhamou S, Benhamou E, Lasser PO, Fontaine F, Travagli JR, Spielmann M, le Chevalier T, Contesso G. Conservative management of breast cancer. Br J Surg 1986; 73: 604–606.
23. Veronesi U, Banfi A, Del Vecchio M, Saccozzi, Clemente C, Greco M, Luini A, Maruloini E, Micolina G, Rilke F, Sacchini V, Salvadori B, Zecch A, Zucali R, Comparison of Halsted mastectomy with quadrantectomy, axillary dissection and radiotherapy for early breast cancer: long-term results. Eur J Cancer Clin Oncol 1986; 22: 1085–1089.
24. Leung S, Otmezguine Y, Calitchi E, Mazeron JJ, Le Bourgeois JP, Pierquin B. Local regional recurrences following radical external beam irradiation and interstitial implantation for operable breast cancer — a 23 year experience. Radiother Oncol 1986; 5: 1–10.
25. Nobler MP, Venet L. Prognostic factors in patients undergoing curative irradiation for breast cancer. Int J Radiat Oncol Biol Phys 1985; 11: 1323–1331.
26. Schnitt SJ, Connolly JL, Recht A, Silver B, Harris JR. Breast relapse following primary radiation therapy for early breast cancer II. Detection, pathologic features and prognostic significance. Int J Radiat Oncol Biol Phys 1985; 11: 1277–1284.
27. Kurtz JM, Spitalier J, Amalric R, Brandone H, Ayme Y, Jacquemier J, Hans D, Bressac C. The prognostic significance of late local recurrence after breast conserving therapy. Int J Radiat Oncol Biol Phys 1990; 18: 87–93.
28. Mussurakis S, Buckley DL, Bowsley SJ, Carleton PJ, Fox JN, Turnbull LW, Horsam A. Dynamic contrast-enhanced magnetic resonance imaging of the breast combined with pharmokinetic analysis of gadolinium-DTPA uptake in the diagnosis of local recurrence of early stage breast carcinoma. Invest Radiol 1995; 30: 650–662.
29. Mate TP, Carter D, Fischer DB, Hartman PV, McKhann C, Merino M, Prosnitz LR, Weissberg JB. A clinical and histopathologic analysis of the results of conservation surgery and radiation therapy in stage I and II breast carcinoma. Cancer 1986; 58: 1995–2002.
30. Salvadori B. Local recurrences after breast-conserving treatment: an open problem. Semin Surg Oncol 1996; 12: 46–52.
31. Kurtz JM, Amalric R, Brandone H, Ayme Y, Jacquemier J, Pietra J-C, Hans D, Pollet J-F, Bressac C, Spitalier J-M. Local recurrence after breast-conserving surgery and radiotherapy. Cancer 1989; 63: 1912–1917.
32. Salvadori B, Marubini E, Mieli R, Conti AR, Cusumano F, Andreola S, Zucali R, Veronesi U. Reoperation for locally recurrence breast cancer in patients previously treated with conservative surgery. Br J Surg 1999; 86: 84–87.
33. Kurtz JM, Jacquemier J, Malaric R, Brandone H, Ayme Y, Hans D, Bressac C, Spitalier J-M. Is breast conservation after local recurrence feasible? Eur J Cancer 1991; 27: 240–244.
34. Dixon JM, Mamman U, Thomas J. Accuracy of intraoperative frozen-section analysis of axillary nodes. Br J Surg 1999; 86: 392–395.
35. Kurtz JM, Amalric R, Brandone H, Ayme Y, Spitalier JM. Results of salvage surgery for mammary recurrence following breast-conserving therapy. Ann Surg 1988; 207: 347–351.

Breast Cancer: Diagnosis and Management
J.M. Dixon (Ed.)

CHAPTER 46

Breast cancer in elderly patients

J.M. Dixon and M. Aapro

1. Introduction

Over one third of all breast cancers occur in women over 70. Although these elderly women have usually been excluded from breast cancer trials, women aged 70 have a life expectancy of 15.5 years. Several studies have indicated that breast cancer survival is poor for older women [1–3]. The overall 10 year survival for all patients with breast cancer in a Swedish study was 51% but only 44% of older women survived 10 years. Although some of this difference in breast cancer survival may be related to a difference in stage at diagnosis a major part of the difference was related to failure to treat older patients in a similar manner to their younger counterparts. Looking at stage specific survival data from the Surveillance, Epidemiology and End Results (SEER) Program only patients aged 85 years or older had a worse survival [4]. Both older and younger women with breast cancer which is localised to the breast or to the breast and axillary nodes fair equally well.

In general, older patients have biologically less aggressive cancers (Table 1) [5]. These women have cancers with lower breast cancer cell proliferation rates, they have a higher frequency of hormone receptor positivity and a lower rate of node positivity for tumours of the same size. From a biological viewpoint, these older patients should have cancers which if treated appropriately are associated with a better survival. Why is it then that mortality from breast cancer in older patients is no better and in many series worse than younger patients?

Table 1. Biology of breast cancer in the elderly (Clark J, Gerontology 1992; 47: 19–23)

In patients 65 or over ($n = 2919$)	Parameter	In younger patients ($n = 6309$)
84%/52%	ER+/PgR+	67%/45%
58%	NO	50%
33%/20%	>2/5 cm	44%/13%

2. Co-morbidity and patient evaluation

The number of co-existing illnesses increases with advancing age and these co-morbid conditions have an influence on how individual patients are treated. Although breast cancer increases in frequency with age, the percentage of women dying from breast cancer decreases with age; this is because patients who have breast cancer over the age of 65 are more likely to die of unrelated causes than younger women [6]. The correct assessment of a cancer patient is a key step in the treatment process. In older people, this assessment entails not only the patient's basic medical history and standard cancer staging, but also a comprehensive evaluation of all facets of the patient's health and environment as this may be important to consider when selecting most appropriate therapeutic approach for the patient. Patient fitness for elective surgery, radiation therapy and chemotherapy have to be considered using scientifically validated methods.

Both the Charlson and the CIRS-G scale are well defined and validated scales for measuring co-morbidity in older patients and have been shown to correlate with outcomes such as mortality, hospitalization duration, or disability in various populations outside geriatric oncology [7]. They represent two different approaches to co-morbidity. The Charlson scale focuses on a short list of selected diseases, and is aimed at simplicity. It is based on the one year mortality of patients admitted to a medical hospital service. The CIRS-G scale is aimed at giving a comprehensive assessment and allows rating of all diseases encountered. The CIRS-G has a structure analogous to the WHO or the NCI toxicity scales which are well known to medical and radiation oncologists. This scale classifies co-morbidities into 14 organ systems, and grades each condition from 0 (no problem) to 4 (severely incapacitating or life-threatening condition). Scores may be summarised in different ways, with comparable results and it encompasses both potentially lethal and non-lethal co-morbid conditions.

A multidimensional assessment is a key part of the approach to older cancer patients. Co-morbidity, functional loss, depression, cognitive impairment, nutritional status and insufficient social support have all been demonstrated to affect survival of elderly and/or cancer patients, with relative risks of death often in the 2 to 4 times range with values even higher in patients with co-morbidity [7].

More than one third of all breast cancer occur in women over the age of 70. The assessment of co-morbidity in elderly patients is an important part of managing their breast cancer.

3. Fitness for surgery

While operating upon the elderly, and even the very elderly, for orthopaedic or cardiovascular diseases is increasingly accepted, there have been a reluctance to recommend adequate intervention for breast cancer. Careful evaluation of renal and cardiovascular function is essential and may lead to an adaptation of drug dosages, specific types of anaesthesia and delivery of pre- and post-anaesthesia care [8]. While acute surgery remains a major cause of perioperative death in the elderly, elective operations are a well-controlled procedure with hazards similar to those of the younger patients [9]. Age appears to be an independent predictor for management. As women age, their preferences for treatment change and these need to be considered when planning treatment. Older women tolerate breast surgery well [10] but have operative mortality rates of between 1 and 2% [11,12]. The main factor influencing surgical morbidity and mortality is not age but the presence of co-existent disease. Standard treatments for breast cancer produce similar outcomes and studies to date have shown low rates of local recurrence in elderly patients after breast conserving surgery. In one study in women aged 70 or older who were given the choice of breast conservation or mastectomy, more women chose breast conserving surgery [13].

Elderly patients who are suitable for breast conservation should be given the choice of breast conserving treatment or mastectomy.

4. Radiation therapy

Older women tolerate breast radiation [14,15] as well as younger women and should be offered the option of breast preservation as body image and loss are important issues regardless of age. A possible problem for elderly patients treated with radiotherapy is the need to attend hospital five times a week and to adopt the supine position for prolonged periods. Patient transportation often depends on family or partner support, community support or the availability of public transportation.

5. Fitness for chemotherapy

Recent studies have shown that patients who are carefully screened for underlying disease have less functional loss than reported traditionally [16]. Changes in renal and hepatic function, as well as modifications of lean body mass and bone marrow reserves are important to consider when chemotherapy is contemplated. One should always calculate the actual creatinine clearance in a particular patient using for example the formula of Cockroft and Gault [17] which is more reliable in this population than an evaluation based on standard 24 hour urine collections. Hepatic function is modified in several respects by ageing with decreased blood flow, decreased albumin production and decreased cytochrome P450 function [18,19]. As elderly people often take several drugs concomitantly, this can lead to clinically significant changes in cytochrome P450 function and may affect the activity of the cytotoxic agents cyclophosphamide and ifosfamide.

As many cytotoxic agents (vinca alkaloids, epipodophyllotoxins, taxanes and platinum derivatives) are neurotoxic, it is important to understand that an elderly person may be considerably handicapped by loss of peripheral sensitivity, as well as by ototoxicity which can result in a clinically significant hearing loss [20].

6. Tamoxifen alone as primary treatment

Uncontrolled studies published in the early 1980s suggested that tamoxifen as the sole treatment was effective in elderly patients with breast cancer [21–24]. Following these studies it became standard practice to treat elderly patients with tamoxifen. Follow up in these studies was short and it became clear that tamoxifen alone does not provide adequate long-term local control of disease in two thirds of patients [25]. In these studies the response rate even in an unselected population was high with up to 73% responding sufficiently to continue treatment.

Studies comparing the efficacy of tamoxifen therapy with surgery with or without tamoxifen therapy have found similar survival rates but much higher local recurrence rates with tamoxifen alone (Table 2). Response rates to tamoxifen alone have varied from 28 to 67% compared with wide excision alone in older women which has produced local control rates ranging from 71 to 97% [26–29].

Two randomised trials have examined the effect of surgery in addition to tamoxifen [30,31]. In the Cancer Research Campaign trial surgery was

Table 2. Survival and local control rates after treatment with tamoxifen alone and surgery with or without tamoxifen

	n	Median follow-up	Overall survival (%)		Local recurrence (%)	
			Tam	Surg	Tam	Surg
Retrospective review						
Van Dalsen and deVries [30]	171	41 mo	68	72	27	6
Tamoxifen vs surgery without tamoxifen						
Nottingham group [31]	135	2 yr	85	74.6	44	24
St George's Hospital [32]	116	3 yr	78.3	80.3	25	37.5
St George's Hospital [33]	200	6 yr	66	72	56	44
Tamoxifen vs surgery and tamoxifen						
British Cancer Research Campaign [16]	381	34 mo	82.5	84.8	23	7.5
Group for Research on Endocrine Therapy in the Elderly [17]	473	36 mo	82.6	79.7	25.4	6.3

necessary in 35 patients treated with tamoxifen and 15 patients managed by tamoxifen combined with surgery requiring a second operation for recurrence, $p = 0.001$ [14]. In a multicentre trial by the group researching endocrine therapy in the elderly, there were significantly less recurrences in patients treated with both surgery and tamoxifen compared with those treated with tamoxifen alone [15]. One problem with these studies is that they have not selected patients for treatment on the basis of the oestrogen receptor concentration. Much higher response rates have been reported if patients who are only oestrogen receptor positive are treated by tamoxifen and in these patients a much higher rate of long-term local control has been reported by tamoxifen alone.

Tamoxifen alone is not satisfactory treatment. Older patients tolerate surgery and radiotherapy as well as younger patients but are at higher risk of surgical morbidity and mortality.

7. Neoadjuvant therapy in the elderly

Studies with tamoxifen and the new aromatase inhibitors letrozole and anastrozole have shown that in oestrogen receptor-positive patients, between 75 and 92% [30,31] get a response to neoadjuvant endocrine therapy. Following such treatment, breast cancers initially only suitable for mastectomy can be reduced in volume over a three month period to a size at which breast conservation is possible. Data suggest that patients who do not respond to endocrine treatments within the first three months are unlikely to gain any significant reduction in volume by continuing with treatment for a longer period before surgery [30].

Neoadjuvant endocrine therapy in appropriate selected patients can significantly reduce tumour size and allow breast conservation in patients who otherwise would require a mastectomy.

Table 3. Benefit of tamoxifen citrate adjuvant therapy in women 70 years and older

Approximate duration of tamoxifen use (yr)	Reduction in risk of relapse (%)	Reduction in risk of death (%)
1	22 (9)	8 (8)
2	42 (8)	36 (7)
5	54 (13)	34 (13)

Numbers in parentheses are standard deviations.
Adapted from Ref. [25].

8. Current consensus treatment

Elderly patients should be treated in a similar manner to younger patients unless there is significant co-morbidities which limit their overall likely survival. If they are suitable for breast conservation, they should be offered this. Unless there are specific contra-indications, patients should have radiotherapy to the breast following breast conserving surgery.

With regard to adjuvant therapy, the 1998 overview showed the benefits of adjuvant tamoxifen therapy in women aged 70 years or older (Table 3) [30]. The proportional reduction in breast cancer relapse and mortality appear similar for women with node-negative and node-positive disease. The benefits of tamoxifen are almost exclusively restricted to patients with oestrogen receptor-positive tumours.

In the adjuvant chemotherapy trials considered in the meta-analysis [32], only 600 women were included over 70 years or older and the sample size was insufficient to determine the benefits of chemotherapy in this age. However, the proportional benefits of chemotherapy in patients aged over 70 are unlikely to be significantly different from postmenopausal women from 50 to 60 years old and for these women the proportional risk reductions following chemotherapy were 20% (SD 3) for recurrence and 11% (SD 3) for overall mortality. This translates to a 2% absolute gain in 10 year survival for a woman with node-negative and a 3% net gain in 10 year survival for node-positive breast cancer.

Table 4. Recommendation for adjuvant therapy for women older than 70 years

Risk category	Definition	Treatment
Node −ve		
Minimal/low	<1 cm, ER and/or PR +ve, Grade I	No treatment or tamoxifen
Moderate	>1 cm and <2 cm, Grade I or II, ER and/or PR +ve	Tamoxifen + chemotherapy
High	>2 cm, ER and/or PR −ve or Grade I or III	Tamoxifen chemotherapy if ER/PR −ve
Node +ve		
ER +ve	Any	Tamoxifen
ER −ve	Any	Chemotherapy

ER, oestrogen receptor; PR, progesterone receptor, −ve, negative; +ve, positive.
Grades: 1, well differentiated; II, moderately differentiated; III, poorly differentiated.
Modified from Ref. [27].

The consensus view from the St Gallen meeting in 1998 for adjuvant therapy in women over 70 years of age is presented in Table 4 [27]. Adjuvant hormonal therapy with tamoxifen should be considered for all postmenopausal women with hormone receptor-positive tumours. Only older women who have a very low risk of distant metastases (<10%), have an oestrogen receptor zero tumour or severe co-morbid conditions should not be offered tamoxifen. Adjuvant systemic chemotherapy should be considered for elderly women whose risk of systemic relapse is high and/or the tumour is oestrogen receptor negative.

Patients with oestrogen receptor-positive tumours should receive adjuvant tamoxifen.

Chemotherapy in elderly patients should be restricted to those patients at high risk of local recurrence and/or those with oestrogen receptor negative tumours.

9. Treatment of metastatic disease

Endocrine therapy is the standard primary treatment for women with hormone receptor-positive metastatic disease. In elderly patients with hormone receptor-negative metastatic breast cancer whose disease is not rapidly progressive or life threatening then endocrine therapy again should be considered. The use of chemotherapy in elderly patients with metastatic breast cancer should be considered only for patients with symptomatic disease who have progression on endocrine therapy or are truly oestrogen receptor zero. The additive therapies of radiation therapy and bisphosphonates should be used in appropriate patients.

Acknowledgements

The authors thank Dr. Martine Extermann (Moffitt Cancer Center, Tampa, Florida, for her suggestions).

References

1. Adami HO, Malker B, Holmberg L, Persson I, Stone B. The relation between survival and age at diagnosis in breast cancer. New Engl J Med 1986; 315: 559.
2. Holli K, Osola J. Effect of age on the survival of breast cancer patients. Eur J Cancer 1997; 33: 425.
3. Host H, Lund E. Age as a prognostic factor in breast cancer. Cancer 1986; 57: 2217.
4. Yancick R, Ries LG, Yates JW. Breast cancer in age-

ing women. A population-based study of contrasts in stage, surgery and survival. Cancer 1989; 63: 976.

5. Clark GM. The biology of breast cancer in older women. J Gerontol 1992; 47: 19–23.
6. Fish EB, Chapman JA, Link MA. Competing causes of death for primary breast cancer. Ann Surg Oncol 1998; 5: 368.
7. Extermann M, Oversash J, Lyman GH, Parr J, Balducci L. Comorbidity and functional status are independent in older cancer patients. J Clin Oncol 1998; 16: 1582–7.
8. Yeager M, Glass D, Neff R, Brinck-Johnsen T. Epidural anaesthesia and analgesia in high-risk surgical patients. Anaesthesiology 1987; 66: 729–736.
9. Audisio RA, Cazzaniga M, Robertson C, Veronesi P, Andreoni B, Aapro MS. Elective surgery for colorectal cancer in the aged: a clinical-economical evaluation. Br J Cancer 1997; 76: 382–4.
10. Wazer DE, Erban JK, Robert NJ et al. Breast conservation in elderly women for clinically negative axillary lymph nodes without axillary dissection. Cancer 1994; 74: 878.
11. Amsterdam E, Birkenfield S, Gilad A, Krispin M. Surgery for carcinoma of the breast in women over 70 years of age. J Surg Oncol 1987; 35: 180.
12. Svastics E, Sulyok Z, Besznyak I. Treatment of breast cancer in women older than 70 years of age. J Surg Oncol 1989; 41: 19.
13. Sandison AJ, Gold DM, Wright P, Jones PA. Breast conservation or mastectomy: treatment choice of women aged 70 years and older. Br J Surg 1996; 83: 994.
14. Lindsey AM, Larson PJ, Dodd MJ, Brecht ML, Packer A. Comorbidity, nutritional intake, social support, weight and functional status over time on older cancer patients receiving radiotherapy. Cancer Nurs 1994; 17: 113.
15. Wyckoff J, Greenberg H, Sanderson R, Wallach P, Balducci L. Breast irradiation in the older women: a toxicity study. J Am Geriatr Soc 1994; 42: 150.
16. Lindeman RD, Tobin JD, Shock NW. Longitudinal studies on the rate of decline in renal function with age. J Am Geriatr Soc 1985; 33: 278–285.
17. Cockcroft DW, Gault MH. Prediction of creatinine clearance from serum creatinine. Nephron 1986; 16: 31–41.
18. Russell RM. Changes in gastrointestinal function attributed to ageing. Am J Clin Nutr 1992; 55: 1203–1207.
19. Durnas C, Loi C, Cusack BJ. Hepatic drug metabolism and ageing. Clin Pharmacokinetic 1990; 17: 236–263.
20. Hussain M. Neurotoxicity of antineoplastic agents. Crit Rev Oncol Hematol 1993; 14: 61–75.
21. Preece PE, Wood RAB, Mackie CR, Cushiere A. Tamoxifen as initial sole treatment of localised breast cancer in elderly patients. BMJ 1982; 284: 869–70.
22. Helleberg A, Lumdgren B, Norin T, Sander S. Treatment of early breast cancer in elderly patients by tamoxifen. Br J Radiol 1982; 15: 511–5.
23. Bradbeer J, Kyngdon J. Primary treatment of breast cancer in elderly women with tamoxifen. Clin Oncol 1983; 9: 31–4.
24. Allan SG, Rodger A, Smyth JF, Leonard RCF, Chetty U, Forrest APM. Tamoxifen as primary treatment of breast cancer in elderly or frail patients: a practical management. BMJ 1985; 290: 358.
25. Horobin JM, Preece PE, Dewar JA, Wood RAB, Cuschieri A. Long-term follow up of elderly patients with loco-regional breast cancer treated with tamoxifen only. Br J Surg 1991; 78: 213–7.
26. Kantorowitz DA, Poulter CA, Sischy B et al. Treatment of breast cancer among elderly women with segmental mastectomy or segmental mastectomy plus postoperative radiotherapy. Int J Radiat Oncol Biol Phys 1988; 15: 263.
27. Clark RM, McCulloch PB, Levine MN et al. Randomized clinical trial to assess the effectiveness of breast irradiation following lumpectomy and axillary dissection for node-negative breast cancer. J Natl Cancer Inst 1992; 84: 683.
28. Reed MW, Morrison JM. Wide local excision as the sole primary treatment in elderly patients with carcinoma of the breast. Br J Surg 1989; 76: 898.
29. Veronesi U, Luini A, Del Vecchio M et al. Radiotherapy after breast preserving surgery in women with localised cancer of the breast. N Engl J Med 1993; 328: 1587.
30. Bates T, Riley DL, Houghton J, Fallowfield L, Baum M. Breast cancer in elderly women: a Cancer Research Campaign trial comparing treatment with tamoxifen and optimal surgery with tamoxifen alone. The Elderly Breast Cancer Working Party. Br J Surg 1991; 78: 591.
31. Mustacchi G, Milani S, Plunchinotta A, De Matteis A, Rubagotti A, Perrota A. Tamoxifen or surgery plus tamoxifen as primary treatment for elderly patients with operable breast cancer: the G.R.E.T.A. trial group for Research on Endocrine Therapy in the Elderly. Anticancer Res 1994; 14: 2197.
32. Keen JC, Dixon JM, Miller EP, Cameron DA, Chetty U, Hanby A, Bellamy C, Miller WR. The expression of Ki-S1 and BCL-2 and the response to primary tamoxifen therapy in elderly patients with breast cancer. Breast Cancer Res Treat 1997; 44 (2): 123–133.
33. Dixon JM, Love CDB, Tucker S, Bellamy C, Cameron DA, Miller WR, Leonard RCF. Letrozole as primary medical therapy for locally advanced and large operable breast cancer. Breast Cancer Res Treat 1997; 46 (suppl): 54.
34. Anonymous. Tamoxifen for early breast cancer: an overview of the randomised trials. Early Breast Cancer Trialists' Collaborative Group. Lancet 1998; 351: 1451.

35. Anonymous. Polychemotherapy for early breast cancer: an overview of the randomised trials. Early Breast Cancer Trialists' Collaborative Group. Lancet 1998; 352: 930.

36. Goldhirsch A, Glick JH, Gelber RD, Senn H-J. Meeting highlights: International Consensus Panel on the treatment of primary breast cancer. J Natl Cancer Inst 1998; 90: 1601.

Breast Cancer: Diagnosis and Management
J.M. Dixon (Ed.)

CHAPTER 47

Treatment of Paget's disease

Mario Rietjens, Omar Youssef and Jean Yves Petit

1. Introduction

Paget's disease of the breast was first described by Sir James Paget in 1874 and it is an unusual presentation of breast cancer starting with characteristic changes in the nipple. The main clinical aspect of Paget's disease is nipple eczema, and is frequently associated with an underlying breast carcinoma, which is either in situ or infiltrating. The choice of surgical treatment depends on the extension of the underlying carcinoma and the breast dimension. A conservative treatment can be proposed in cases of small or large tumors in large breasts. On the other hand, a mastectomy with immediate reconstruction is a good option in cases of small tumors in small breasts. The goal of the surgical treatment is to obtain histologically negative margins and good cosmetic results.

2. Surgical techniques of conservative treatment

Different types of surgical techniques can be proposed depending on the shape of the breast. A central quadrantectomy is necessary with excision of the nipple and areola complex and a cylindrical glandular excision until the pectoralis major muscle.

A *periareolar technique* can be used in cases of small and non ptotic breasts. A central quadrantectomy can be performed by a periareolar incision and breast reshaping is obtained by 2 or 3 glandular "purse string" sutures to close the defect and increase the central projection of the breast. The skin can be also closed with a subcuticular "purse string" sutures and the final scar will disappear when the nipple and areola complex will be reconstructed over the scar. Usually, this technique doesn't require a contralateral mammaplasty to achieve symmetry [1].

Reduction mammaplasty techniques can be used in cases of large and ptotic breast. There are two main techniques that can be indicated depending on type of breast ptosis. In cases with vertical breast ptosis, the central quadrantectomy defect can be repaired by an inferior posterior dermo-glandular flap, with the preservation of a round piece of skin in the top to replace the areola. This pedicle has a good blood supply, and this technique is derived from the traditional inferior pedicle reduction mammoplasty [2,3]. In cases of lateral breast ptosis, the defect can be repaired by an inferior lateral dermo-glandular flap, also with preservation of a round piece of skin on the top and rotate it to the central quadrant of the breast [4]. Both techniques require a contralateral mammoplasty to achieve symmetry [5].

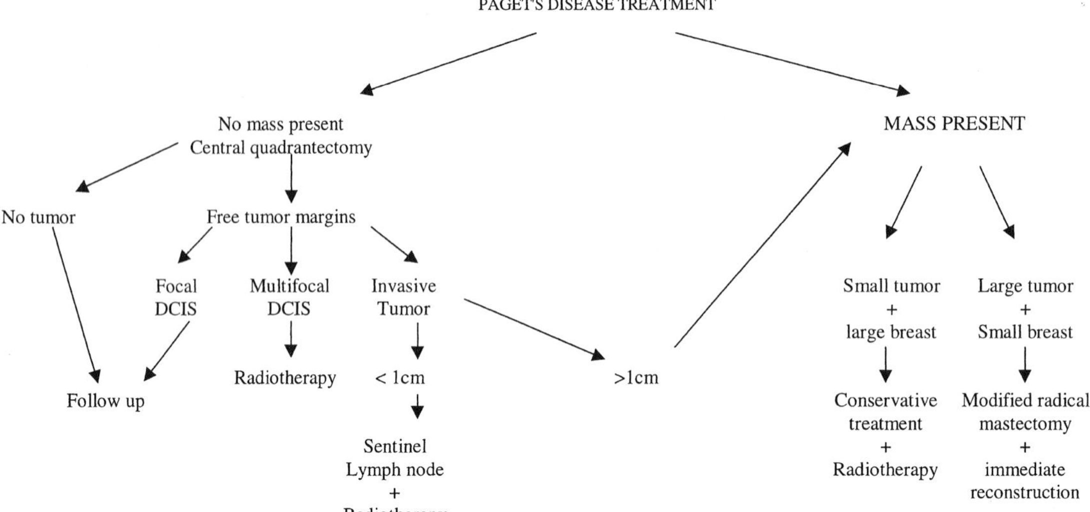

Fig. 1. Scheme for the management of Paget's disease of the breast.

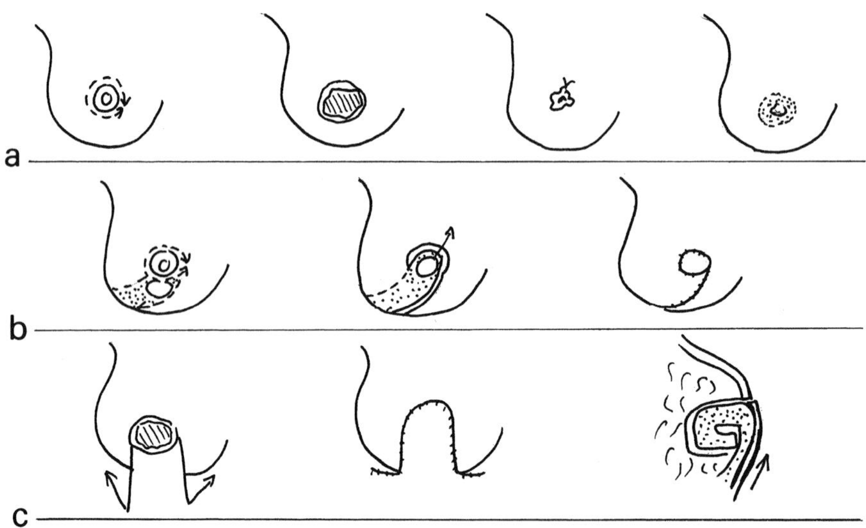

Fig. 2. Methods of partial reconstruction after central quadrantectomy: (a) With "purse string" sutures. (b) With a rotation of the infero lateral dermo-glandular flap. (c) With an infero posterior dermo-glandular flap.

3. Surgical techniques of mastectomy

The mastectomy is indicated in cases of large palpable masses or diffuse microcalcifications, and the skin-sparing mastectomy with complete conservation of the breast skin is very diffused now, because it allows a better cosmetic results in cases of immediate breast reconstruction. The axillary dissection is indicated in cases of infiltrating carcinoma. An immediate breast reconstruction can be proposed with the traditional techniques: Tissue expanders, definitive implants or myocutaneous flaps [6].

References

1. Garusi C, Petit JY, Rietjens M, Lanfrey E. La place de la chirurgie plastique dans le traitement conservateur du cancer du sein. Ann Chir Plast Esthet 1997; 42: 168–176.
2. Robbins TH. A reduction mammoplasty with the areola-nipple based on an inferior dermal pedicle. Plast Reconstr Surg 1977; 59: 64.
3. Ribeiro L. A new technique for reduction mammoplasty. Plast Reconstr Surg 1975; 12: 110.
4. Galimberti V, Zurrida S, et al. Central small size breast cancer: how to overcome the problem of nipple and areola involvement. Eur J Cancer 1993; 29: 1093.
5. Rietjens M, Petit JY, Contesso G, Bertin F, Gilles R. The role of reduction mammaplasty in oncology. Eur J Plast Surg 1997; 20: 246–250.
6. Petit JY, Veronesi U, Nahai F, Rietjens M. Chirurgie du cancer du sein. Diagnostique, curative et reconstructive. Paris: Arnette, 1997.

Breast Cancer: Diagnosis and Management
J.M. Dixon (Ed.)

CHAPTER 48

Male breast cancer

Paolo Veronesi and Roberto Gennari

1. Introduction

Although breast cancer is seen infrequently in men, it can cause significant morbidity and mortality. Its frequency is very low and accounts for less than 0.5% of all breast cancer. In the United States in 1998, an estimated 1600 new cases of male breast cancer occurred among a total breast cancer incidence of 180,300; there were 400 deaths from male breast cancer in 1998 [1]. It accounts for less than 1% of male malignancies [1].

From the epidemiological point of view there are many differences between male and female breast cancer. The incidence of male breast cancer has remained relatively stable in most countries [2,3] while female breast cancer has risen in incidence throughout the world [4,5].

The risk of male breast cancer increases with age as in females but lacks the early premenopausal peak. For this reason, the average age at diagnosis in men is 60 years, approximately 10 years later than in females. The annual incidence increases steadily from 35 years of age, with 0.1 cases per 100,000 men to 11.1 cases at age 85 years or greater.

The incidence varies with geographic location, being higher in countries such as USA and Great Britain, where in the female sex incidence is high, and it is lower in countries such as Japan, where incidence is also low in women [6]. In parts of Africa, the incidence of male breast cancer is relatively high. Zambia and Egypt, for example, have an incidence rate 15 and 12 times, respectively, that of the USA [7,8]. A plausible explanation for such elevated rates is the increased incidence of liver disease in these countries, with its associated high oestrogen levels.

Male breast cancer accounts for approximate rates of 1 in 200 or less of all breast cancers.

2. Aetiology

Although the aetiology of male breast cancer is still poorly understood, an alteration in the oestrogen/testosterone ratio is probably involved. The factors related to male breast cancer cause an imbalance in the hormonal status in men with relative androgen deficiency and includes Klinefelter's syndrome, undescended testes, orchiectomy, orchitis, late puberty, infertility, obesity, hypercholesterolaemia, oestrogen use or exposure and liver cirrhosis [9–14].

In recent years, family history has been appreciated as an important factor [15]. The BRCA2 gene is associated with an increased risk of breast cancer in men and it is a marker for identifying certain males at increased risk [16].

Alterations in the oestrogen/testosterone ratio and a family history of breast cancer in females and males predisposes to male breast cancer.

3. Diagnosis

The mean age at presentation of male breast cancer is approximately 60 years, and it is exceptional under 30 years. A painless lump, occasionally associated with nipple discharge, retraction, erosion or ulceration, is the chief symptom being present in 80–90% of patients [17,18]. Its location is most frequently in the central subareolar region [19]. Examination usually shows a hard, ill-defined, non-tender mass beneath the nipple or areola. Gynaecomastia not uncommonly precedes or accompanies breast cancer in men. Nipple discharge is an uncommon presentation for breast cancer in man, as it is in women [18]. However, nipple discharge in men is an ominous finding associated with carcinoma in nearly 75% of cases. The presence of palpable enlarged abnormal feeling axillary nodes, present in about half of the cases, gives a clue to the correct diagnosis.

Bilateral mammography should be performed as part of the preoperative evaluation, even if the diagnosis is clear, to assess the contralateral breast and exclude the presence of non-palpable masses or microcalcifications. Also ultrasonography using a high frequency probe can help to establish the diagnosis. The use of fine needle aspiration biopsy usually confirms the presence of carcinoma, therefore avoiding the need for excisional biopsy [20]. From the cytological point of view there are no differences between male and female breast cancer [21]. Core biopsy is an alternative to cytology.

Breast cancer staging is the same in men as in women, while the effectiveness of tumour markers such as CEA and CA15.3 has not been yet evaluated. Gynaecomastia and metastatic cancer from another site (e.g. prostate or lung) must be considered in the differential diagnosis of a breast lesion in a male.

4. Pathology and prognostic factors

Infiltrating ductal carcinoma is the most frequent histological subtype, as it is in women, and accounts for about 70% of all male breast cancers [17–19]. All other subtypes can occur in men, but the frequency of infiltrating lobular carcinoma is lower than in women at less than 1%. About 15% of reported cases are classified ductal carcinoma in situ (DCIS). DCIS in men occurs at an older age than women and displays a different distribution of morphologic subtypes compared with the same lesion in females. Histologically the most frequent type is low grade papillary carcinoma and with cribriform, solid or micropapillary types occurring occasionally. High grade comedo DCIS is rare and is usually associated with an invasive component [22].

Oestrogen receptors are usually present in cancers in men [19,23] and this is why they are responsive to hormonal treatment. The same prognostic factors used in female breast cancer, such as epidermal growth factor receptor, flow cytometry, DNA ploidy, S-phase fraction, thymidine labelling index, nuclear grade, HER-2 oncogene and p53 expression have not been investigated yet in males [24].

Staging according to TNM system is the most important prognostic factor. In non-disseminated disease the size of the tumour and the nodal status are the most important factors in predicting survival. The expression of c-erbB-2 is lower in male breast cancer than in females, but it seems to be associated with a poorer prognosis [25].

5. Treatment

Modified radical mastectomy, with preservation of both pectoral muscles and complete axillary dissection, is the surgical treatment of choice for invasive cancer, whereas simple mastectomy is considered standard treatment for DCIS. Less invasive procedures, such as subcutaneous mastectomy, are not appropriate because of the high risk of local recurrence. Radical mastectomy is indicated only in locally advanced cases with invasion of the muscle and where primary medical treatment is not being considered. The efficacy of sentinel node biopsy to avoid axillary dissection in patients with clinically negative nodes has not yet been tested. Postoperative radiotherapy to the chest wall has been shown to reduce local recurrences in selected series, although no benefit in overall survival has been demonstrated [17]. The same principles of the use of radiotherapy in women are followed and radiotherapy is given in locally advanced cancer or when there are multiple lymph node metastases with perilymphatic invasion.

Adjuvant treatment in patients with operable disease is usually hormonal therapy with tamoxifen. Although randomised studies are not available, the large majority of male breast cancers express hormonal receptors, and patients do appear to benefit from such a treatment [26]. Standard CMF (Cyclophosphamide, Methotrexate, 5-Fluorouracil) chemotherapy has efficacy when used as adjuvant treatment of stage II or stage III disease [27] as does the FAC (5-Fluorouracil, Adriamycin, Cyclophosphamide) regimen [28]. Nevertheless lack of randomised studies does not allow definite conclusions to be drawn on their use. Locally advanced cases or inflammatory cancers may benefit of preoperative chemotherapy, with the indications being the same as those in women.

Metastatic spread in men is similar to that of women, with involvement of bone, liver, lung, brain and other sites. Hormonal treatment in receptor-positive tumours is the treatment of choice and consists of tamoxifen as first line therapy, which has a response rate of 80% [29]. Patients who relapse on tamoxifen can be treated with another hormonal agent, such as ketoconazole, oestrogen, cyproterone acetate, androgens, progestins, aromatase inhibitors and buserelin. Patients with metastatic receptor-negative breast cancer are treated as their female counterparts, with combination chemotherapy.

References

1. Landis SH, Murray T, Bolden S et al. Cancer statistics in 1998. CA Cancer J Clin 1998; 48: 6–29.
2. Ewertz M, Holmberg L, Karajalainen S et al. Incidence of male breast cancer in Scandinavia, 1943–1982. Int J Cancer 1989; 43: 27–31.
3. La Vecchia C, Levi F, Lucchini F. Descriptive epidemiology of male breast cancer in Europe. Int J Cancer 1992; 51: 62–66.
4. Ewertz M. Epidemiology of breast cancer: the Nordic contribution. Eur J Surg 1996; 162: 97–99.
5. Devesa SS, Blot WJ, Stone BJ et al. Recent cancer trends in the United States. J Natl Cancer Inst 1995; 87: 175–182.
6. Schotterfield D, Lilienfeld AM. Some epidemiologic features of breast cancer among males. Am J Public Health 1963; 53: 890–897.
7. El-Gazayerli MM, Adbel-Aziz AS. On bilharziasis and male breast cancer in Egypt. Br J Cancer 1963; 17: 556–571.
8. Bhagwandin SS. Carcinoma of the male breast in Zambia. East Afr Med J 1972; 49: 176–179.
9. Sasco AJ, Lowenfels AB, Pasker-De Jone P. Epidemiology of male breast cancer. A meta-analysis of published case-control studies and discussion of selected etiologic factors. Int J Cancer 1993; 53: 538–549.
10. Lenfant-Pejovic MH, Mlika-Cabanne N, Bouchardy C et al. Risk factors for male breast cancer: a Franco–Swiss case-control study. Int J Cancer 1990; 45: 661–665.
11. Mabuchi K, Bross DS, Kessler I. Risk factors in male breast cancer. J Natl Cancer Inst 1985; 74: 371–375.
12. Thomas DB, Jiminez LM, McTiernan A. Breast cancer in men: risk factors with hormonal implications. Am J Epidemiol 1992; 135: 734.
13. Casagrande JT, Hanische R, Pike M, A case control study of male breast cancer. Cancer Res 1988; 48: 1326–1330.
14. Eldar S, Nash E, Abrahamson J. Radiation carcinogenesis in the male breast. Eur J Surg Oncol 1989; 15: 274–278.
15. Anderson DE, Badzioch MD. Breast cancer risks in relatives of male breast cancer patients. J Natl Cancer Inst 1992; 84: 1114–1117.
16. Thorlacius S, Tryggvadottir L, Olafsdottir GH et al. Linkage to BRCA2 region in hereditary male breast cancer. Lancet 1995; 346: 544–545.
17. Erlichman C, Murphy KC, Elhakim T. Male breast cancer: a 13-year review of 89 patients. J Clin Oncol 1984; 2: 903–909.
18. Borgen PI, Wong GY, Vlamis V et al. Current management of male breast cancer: a review of 104 cases. Ann Surg 1992; 215: 451–459.
19. Goss PE, Reid C, Pintilie M et al. Male breast carcinoma. A review of 229 patients who presented to

the Princess Margaret Hospital during 40 years: 1955–1996. Cancer 1999; 85: 629–639.
20. Salvadori B, Saccozzi R, Manzari A et al. Prognosis of breast cancer in males: an analysis of 170 cases. Eur J Cancer 1994; 30A: 930–935.
21. Sneige N, Holder PD, Katz RL et al. Fine needle aspiration cytology of the male breast in a cancer center. Diagn Cytopathol 1993; 9: 691–697.
22. Hittmair AP, Lininger RA, Tavassoli FA. Ductal carcinoma in situ (DCIS) in the male breast. Cancer 1998; 83: 2139–2149.
23. Cutuli B, Lacroze M, Dilhuydy JM et al. Male breast cancer: results of the treatments and prognostic factors in 397 cases. Eur J Cancer 1995; 31A: 1960–1964.
24. Ravandi-Kashani F, Hayes TG. Male breast cancer: a review of the literature. Eur J Cancer 1998; 34: 1341–1347.
25. Joshi MG, Lee AKC, Loda M et al. Male breast carcinoma: an evaluation of prognostic factors contributing to a poorer outcome. Cancer 1996; 77: 490–498.
26. Ribeiro G, Swindell R. Adjuvant tamoxifen for male breast cancer. Br J Cancer 1992; 65: 252–254.
27. Bagley CS, Wesley MN, Young RC et al. Adjuvant chemotherapy in males with cancer of the breast. Am J Clin Oncol 1987; 10: 55–60.
28. Patel HZ, Buzdar AU, Hortobagyi GN. Role of adjuvant chemotherapy in male breast cancer. Cancer 1989; 64: 1583–1585.
29. Jaiyesimi IA, Buzdar AU, Sahin AA et al. Carcinoma of the male breast. Ann Intern Med 1992; 117: 771–777.

Breast Cancer: Diagnosis and Management
J.M. Dixon (Ed.)

CHAPTER 49

Treatment of breast cancer during pregnancy

Antonella Surbone, Jeanne A. Petrek and Violante E. Currie

1. Introduction

Pregnancy-associated breast cancer is defined as the diagnosis of breast cancer developing during or within one year of pregnancy. The estimated incidence is between 0.2 and 3.8%, as reported in an overview of 32 series [1] and it occurs in between 1 : 3,000 and 1 : 10,000 pregnancies [2,3]. Its incidence is similar to that of uterine cancer during pregnancy [4]. Pregnancy-associated breast cancer is an issue of growing importance as more women are delaying childbearing for personal or professional reasons to their 30s or 40s [5] when there is already a higher age-related incidence of breast cancer. Pregnancy-associated breast cancer is an extremely difficult issue for a woman who has to choose between her own health and the possible risks to the foetus. Moreover, it is also associated with difficult psychological and ethical implications for her relatives and for the medical team, as the coming of a new life appears almost incompatible with the diagnosis of a possibly lethal disease. Yet, breast cancer during pregnancy can be treated and does not inevitably carry an ominous prognosis. Both diagnosis and treatment are, however, more complex in the pregnant woman. The anatomical changes in the breast of a pregnant woman, as well as other changes in her body and fluid distribution, affect treatment options. Furthermore, for the foetus, the risks of teratogenicity and/or abnormal foetal development need to be considered.

Pregnancy-associated breast cancer has traditionally been defined as the diagnosis of breast cancer made during or within one year of pregnancy.
Pregnancy-associated breast cancer carries difficult psychological and ethical implications for the patient, her relatives and the medical team.

2. Pathogenesis

The pathogenesis of breast cancer during pregnancy is unknown, and so is the precise role of gestational hormones. It is very likely that breast cancer during pregnancy represents the clinical appearance of an occult malignancy, which has been present already for some time before pregnancy. According to predictions from laboratory [6] and mathematical models [7] there is a prolonged period of subclinical growth of breast cancer before it reaches the critical number of 10^9 cells needed to give rise to a detectable tumour.

Epidemiological data support a protective effect of pregnancy on breast cancer [8] and laboratory studies have explored the possible protective effect of oestriol, the oestrogen that rises disproportionately during pregnancy. Oestriol is a relatively weak oestrogen and appears to antagonize both oestrone and oestradiol [9].

On the contrary, the effect of gestational hormones in the presence of established breast cancer appears to be a stimulatory one. In the production of hormone-sensitive rat mammary tumours following dimethylbenzanthracene (DMBA), intercurrent pregnancy enhances both the induction and the growth of such tumours [10]. These data would support the concern for promotion of an already established breast cancer in pregnant women.

Pregnancy has a protective effect against breast cancer.
Gestational hormones may, however, negatively affect an already established breast cancer.

3. Prognosis

Almost all reports note a worse prognosis for pregnancy-associated breast cancer. However, when compared with non-pregnant young controls at the same stage of disease and with the same number of involved nodes, the pregnancy-associated group has an equivalent survival rate. It is therefore still unclear whether pregnancy itself negatively impacts on the aggressivity of breast cancer secondary to its biological effects, or whether the worse prognosis in pregnant women is only a consequence of delayed diagnosis and treatment which approximates to one year in most cases of pregnancy-associated breast cancer.

A 1994 study of young breast cancer patients at nine American and European cancer centres demonstrated that a recent previous pregnancy (up to four years before diagnosis) was associated with a worse prognosis, and for each additional year of interval between pregnancy and a breast cancer diagnosis, the risk of dying decreased by 15% [11]. This study supports the promotional influence of gestational hormones on existent but subclinical cancer, and these data could also indirectly account for some of the worse prognosis observed in younger women affected by breast cancer. Two additional studies have found a significantly decreased survival in patients with a shorter interval between breast cancer diagnosis and previous pregnancy [12,13] and two other studies have failed to find a similar effect when accounting for completed pregnancies, abortions and other factors [14,15].

The earliest reports from more than a century ago noted a dismal prognosis, with 5-year survival ranging from 0% [16] to 8.6% [17] to 17% [18]. A study conducted at the Mayo clinic in 1937 [19] found a 61% 5-year survival rate among pregnancy-associated breast cancer with negative lymph nodes.

As noted in recent reviews patients diagnosed with breast cancer during pregnancy have more advanced stages of disease compared to similar women who are not pregnant [20,21]. Considering nodal status as an indication of advanced disease status, the literature shows great differences between pregnant and non-pregnant women at diagnosis. The reported rate of node-negative breast cancer in pregnant women in different series has ranged from 26% to 39% over the past three decades [21–27] (the converse is true for non-pregnant young women where node-negativity predominates). Not only is node-positivity a much more common event in pregnancy-associated breast cancer, the frequency of nodal involvement has not changed during the past three decades. The high incidence of node-positivity in pregnancy-associated breast cancer while not necessarily reflecting a more aggressive behaviour of pregnancy-associated breast cancer per se, strongly points to a delay in diagnosis in pregnant women [28–31].

Tumour size also varies in pregnant versus non-pregnant patients. In the Memorial Sloan–Kettering Cancer Center series from 1960 to 1980, only 31% of 56 pregnant patients were found to have a T1 breast cancer at diagnosis, while the T1 category was found in 50% of 166 matched non-pregnant women [21]. The Memorial series compared AJC stages I/II/III pregnant patients with non-pregnant patients from a consecutive mastectomy series of the same age, undergoing similar diagnostic and treatment procedures by the same group of physicians. A more recent publication from Memorial confirmed these findings [27]. Unquestionably diagnostic and therapeutic delays secondary to pregnancy have a potential negative affect on the course of the disease.

In the Memorial series 10-year survival was 77% for node-negative pregnant patients, and 75% for non-pregnant patients [21]. The 10-year survival for node-positive pregnant women was 25%, while it was 41% for the non-pregnant women. King reported a 10-year survival of 71% in node-negative pregnant patients [26], similar to that in the non-pregnant node-negative women and Ribeiro and Palmer also found similar survival rates [24]. There are, however, two recent case-control studies indicating that pregnancy is an independent negative risk factor for survival [32,33].

> *Pregnancy-associated breast cancer bears a worse prognosis, since it is regularly associated with more advanced disease at presentation.*
> *Worse prognosis is related to:*
> *(1) delayed diagnosis secondary to the breast changes of pregnancy,*
> *(2) a more aggressive growth pattern secondary to the biological effects of pregnancy, or*
> *(3) a combination of the two.*

4. Diagnosis

The clinical presentation of breast cancer during pregnancy does not differ from other symptomatic women. Generally, the patient first notices a palpable mass. This is often accompanied by a certain degree of nipple discharge, which may however be physiologic unless it is clearly bloody and persistent. Mammography is contraindicated during pregnancy, and it is also of little help since the breast density is increased during pregnancy, making detection or identification of abnormalities difficult. Ultrasound and MRI are more helpful in pregnancy-associated breast cancer.

While some oncologists feel comfortable with fine-needle aspiration and consider its results reliable enough, most believe that any suspicious palpable abnormality in a pregnant woman should be evaluated histologically either by a core or an open biopsy performed under local anaesthesia. These procedures are safe at all times during pregnancy and should not be delayed.

Staging procedures should be minimised, as radiologic investigations are contraindicated during pregnancy. Haematology and chemistry profiles are not always helpful, due to physiologic changes during pregnancy. There are scanty data on the reliability of markers, such as CEA and CA 15-3 in pregnancy-associated breast cancer.

There is no absolute contraindication to a chest X-ray, which is sometimes performed with abdominal and pelvic shielding. Late in pregnancy, with the gravid uterus directly under the diaphragm, foetal shielding will obscure the lower lung parenchyma. Therefore, exposing the third-trimester foetus to a chest X-ray is a decision to be made by the medical–obstetrical team on an individual basis.

As regards evaluation for bone metastases, serum alkaline phosphatase is elevated due to pregnancy itself. Conventional radiography, excluding the pelvis and abdomen, can be performed (e.g. skull, long bones) if absolutely needed, but there is no adequate substitute for a bone scan in pregnancy-associated breast cancer. A recent article suggests possible modification of the bone scanning technique for pregnant patients [34]. If the results of the bone scan will not change the immediate treatment, then it should be omitted or delayed until after delivery.

Magnetic resonance imaging is accurate and appears safe for the foetus, although the Safety Committee of the Society for the Magnetic Resonance Imaging states "the safety of MR imaging during pregnancy has not been proven" [35] Recent reports on its usage for foetal imaging in prenatal diagnosis contain limited follow-up of the infants with no untoward effects reported [36,37]. It may be particularly useful for the diagnosis or confirmation of bone metastases, liver metastases, or even brain metastases. Furthermore, there is increasing experience of the use of breast MRI instead of mammography.

5. Local treatment: surgery

One of the major achievements of oncology is the ability to offer women with breast cancer a choice between lumpectomy (or quadrantectomy) followed by radiation therapy or mastectomy. While in most cases the choice rests with the patient (where the outcomes are expected to be comparable in terms of survival), the preferred local management of breast cancer during pregnancy has been modified radical mastectomy, since radiation therapy is contraindicated in pregnancy for the developing foetus. Immediate reconstruction of the breast should not be performed in the pregnant woman, since the procedure requires substantial increase in the operative time (hence in the exposure to anaesthesia). Moreover, it is not recommended from a cosmetic point of view, and should therefore be postponed. There are large numbers of various surgical procedures performed annually on pregnant women, leading to much experience regarding pregnancy and general anaesthesia. The issue of general anaesthesia in pregnancy has been evaluated in a population-based study from Sweden, where 5,405 non-obstetric operations during pregnancy were compared to 720,000 pregnancies that had not had general anaesthesia. Adverse effects reported included low birth weight, prematurity, intrauterine growth retardation and early neonatal death, but most of these were thought to correlate with the underlying condition leading to the surgical procedure rather than to the anaesthesia itself. The incidence of congenital anomalies was not increased in women who had general anaesthesia even during the first trimester [38]. A recent review gives indications for the most appropriate anaesthesiology procedures in pregnant women [39].

In order to consider breast conservation in the pregnant woman, lumpectomy followed by radiation therapy after delivery has been suggested. To advocate this approach one must extrapolate from data obtained in the non-pregnant woman; however, the pregnant woman's breast is very different. The increase in size of the ducts, as well as the increased blood supply during pregnancy may predispose to lengthy intraductal spread. Therefore, it is not certain that local control will be the same as that in the non-pregnant woman. There has been a recent limited experience of nine women with pregnancy-associated breast cancer who were treated conservatively [40]. The median follow-up was only 24 months and, although there were no local recurrences in this series, the anatomical differences between non-pregnant and pregnant women are even greater than the differences in the breasts of pre and postmenopausal women [41]. Moreover, delay in starting radiation therapy may negatively affect outcome although there is no proven evidence that delaying radiation therapy for a few weeks has a negative impact on the prognosis of breast cancer. The choice of limited surgery followed by delivery and then by radiation therapy can thus be considered in the third trimester.

The preferred local management of pregnancy-associated breast cancer is modified radical mastectomy.
Possible adverse effects of general anaesthesia include low birth weight, prematurity, intrauterine growth retardation, and early neonatal death.
Limited series have been reported on breast conservation followed by radiation therapy after delivery, and therefore, at present it is unknown whether it is as successful as in the non-pregnant woman.

6. Local treatment: radiation therapy

Radiation therapy is absolutely contraindicated during pregnancy because of the risk of teratogenicity and of subsequent anomalies in the foetal development. Although the risk of congenital abnormalities is the most common concern, intrauterine growth retardation, premature birth, as well as subsequent neoplasia in the newborn pose a significant risk. The risk to the foetus depends on the period of gestation during the exposure. The standard breast radiotherapy course of 5000 cGy to 6000 cGy will expose the foetus to between 10 cGy, early in pregnancy, and 200 or more cGy late in pregnancy. The developing foetus receives from several tenths of a percent to several percent of the total breast dose. The radiation leakage from the radiotherapy unit should not exceed 0.1% of the direct beam exposure rate, as measured at a distance of 1 m from the radiation source [42]. During the pre-implantation period (from conception to day 10–14), the predominant effect is embryo death. The period of organogenesis (second through the eighth week) is the most sensitive period and poses the greatest risk for congenital malformations. Radiation exposure beyond 8 weeks is less likely to produce abnormalities; however, some delayed neurological problems have been reported and there is a subsequent increased risk of childhood cancers [43].

Unfortunately, the atomic bomb experience at Hiroshima and Nagasaki led to the conclusion that 5 cGy is the dose level during early pregnancy at which radiation-induced anomalies increase in frequency. Standard breast radiotherapy will expose the foetus to between 10 cGy, early in pregnancy, and 200 cGy or more late in pregnancy, and cannot therefore be considered a treatment option. Chest wall irradiation after mastectomy poses the same hazard to the foetus and should also be delayed until after childbirth [44].

Standard breast radiotherapy produces an unacceptable rate of foetal anomalies and childhood cancers so both breast and chest wall irradiation should be delayed until after childbirth.
A larger amount of radiation reaches the foetus from internal scatter through the mother's tissues. The quantity of such radiation depends on (1) the distance from the field centre to the foetus, (2) the field size, and (3) the energy source of the radiation.

7. Chemotherapy

The decision to recommend chemotherapy to a pregnant woman is difficult. Chemotherapeutic drugs exert their effect by inhibiting cell division. The physiologic changes of pregnancy on blood volume, glomerular filtration rate and other parameters may affect maternal chemotherapy and drug metabolism, and there are few pharmacokinetic studies of chemotherapy in pregnant patients. Detailed studies of transplacental passage of chemotherapeutic agents to human foetuses are also not available, and almost all drugs cross the placental barrier. The potential adverse effects of antineoplastic agents on the foetus and neonate involve immediate effects, such as spontaneous abortion, teratogenesis or organ damage and delayed effects, such as growth retardation or gonadal dysfunction. Organogenesis and limb formation primarily occur within the first ten weeks of pregnancy. The delivery of chemotherapy in the first trimester is associated with an increased incidence in the rate of stillbirths and congenital malformations [45]. In one series of 13 women exposed to chemotherapy during the first trimester, there were 4 spontaneous abortions, 4 therapeutic abortions and two major foetal malformations among the five term infants [46]. Because central nervous system development continues during the second trimester, there is some theoretical concern that chemotherapy may interfere with this process and result in cognitive problems in later life. During the third trimester chemotherapy is feasible when truly needed. In all instances, long-term follow-up of children exposed to in utero chemotherapy during maternal treatment for breast cancer is mandatory for both clinical and research purposes.

The chemotherapy agents most commonly used in a woman with breast cancer (such as cyclophosphamide, doxorubicin and 5-fluorouracil) are relatively safe to administer during the second and third trimesters. Drugs that have been given after the first trimester without a reported increased risk of birth defects include cyclophosphamide, [47] doxorubicin, [48] and 5-FU [49]. Because folic acid antagonists such as methotrexate are known to cause foetal abnormalities in the first trimester, and because there is a concern about the metabolism of methotrexate in the third space provided by the amniotic fluid, most oncologists prefer to avoid prescribing methotrexate during pregnancy. Taxanes and growth factors (e.g. G-CSF) have not been studied. Since laboratory studies have suggested that tamoxifen is teratogenic, it is contraindicated during pregnancy.

A recent prospective study of 24 women with breast cancer treated with a uniform chemotherapy regimen during the second and third trimesters of pregnancy is particularly informative. Twenty-two women were treated for primary breast cancer, primarily Stages II or III, including two women with inflammatory breast cancer. Two women had metastatic disease.

Cyclophosphamide, doxorubicin and 5-fluorouracil were given every 21 to 28 days for a maximum of 4 treatments with no evidence of foetal compromise, complications of delivery or adverse effects on newborn development. The disease-free survival of the mothers was similar to that of non-pregnant patients and was dependent on the stage of the breast cancer at diagnosis [49].

In planning chemotherapy for a pregnant woman, it is preferable to allow at least two weeks between the last dose and delivery. This minimizes the risk of delivering a neutropenic infant from a neutropenic mother. In addition, foetal drug metabolism switches from the placenta to the kidney and liver at delivery. If the foetus is delivered soon after chemotherapy, the drugs may persist for a prolonged period in the newborn [50]. Women who have recently received chemotherapy should be advised against breast-feeding. Wherever possible in women with good prognostic factors, such as negative nodes or a few involved nodes, adjuvant chemotherapy should be postponed until after delivery. All antineoplastic agents are classified as category D in terms of foetal risk. Category D is defined as follows: "there is positive evidence of human foetal risk, but the benefits from use in pregnant women may be acceptable despite the risk (e.g. if the drug is needed in a life-threatening situation or for a serious disease for which safer drugs cannot be used or are ineffective)" [51]. Most obstetricians and neonatologists would feel comfortable in administering steroids to induce foetal lung maturity [52] and delivering at 34–36 weeks of gestation when the potential complications for the newborn are substantially decreased [52]. A decision to bring forward delivery, however, is never an easy one, either for the mother or her obstetric team.

Chemotherapy in the 1st trimester is associated with an increased risk of stillbirths and congenital malformations.
Certain drugs such as doxorubicin and cyclophosphamide can be administered in the second and third trimesters.
The timing of childbirth must be planned carefully to avoid delivering a neutropenic infant.
In low risk patients, adjuvant chemotherapy can be delayed until after delivery.
Chemotherapy for the pregnant woman should be delivered by an experienced multidisciplinary team of specialists.

8. Conclusion

Pregnancy is an important and a very special event for a woman and her family, and reproductive choices are extremely delicate and personal. The first duty of the health care team is therefore to present the different, albeit limited, options to the patient and her relatives in a very honest way. The discussion should be open and the information accurate but hope should never be removed, and the informed decision of each patient should be respected [53,54]. To make the final choice of local and systemic treatment the management of the pregnant woman with breast cancer requires a close collaboration between all the members of the medical team involved in her care including obstetricians, surgical, radiation and medical oncologists, neonatologists, psychologists and social workers. A discussion of risks to the foetus compared with possible maternal benefits is crucial.

In the past, therapeutic abortion was almost always recommended, in conjunction with oophorectomy [17]. Today authors who advocated this previously have revised their recommendations [55], as most recent data fail to show any benefit for therapeutic abortion [44,49]. Therapeutic abortion often combined with bilateral oophorectomy, is still recommended if the breast cancer is very advanced because of the potential foetal damage from the proposed chemotherapy or radiation treatments, although there is no clear evidence that abortion improves the mother's survival [49]. Treatment is obviously simplified with therapeutic abortion early in pregnancy, but it is the mother who must take such a decision.

Another example of the need for team effort is the difficult interpretation of oestrogen receptors in the pregnant woman, as the accuracy and the value of steroid hormone receptor status during pregnancy are not clear. Routine ligand binding assays (without exchange techniques) depend upon the availability of unbound receptors and in pregnancy all binding sites may already be occupied by endogenous hormones. In the non-pregnant state, on the contrary, only up to 35% of cytosol receptors are occupied by endogenous steroid, so that most is available for assay [56]. Immunohistochemical assays should be accurate in the pregnant woman since both the occupied and unoccupied receptor are stained. One recent report compared the receptor status by immunohistochemistry to ligand binding assay of pregnant to non-pregnant women and suggested that some ER-negative tumours in pregnancy-associated breast cancer may have oestrogen mediated protein products [57].

Management of breast cancer during pregnancy requires a collaborative effort of all members of the medical team working for the patient's good [58].

The therapy of pregnancy-associated breast cancer requires a multi-disciplinary approach and a collaboration among all members of the health care team.
The reproductive choices of any woman should always be respected.
Doctors must work with the patient and her family to make the most appropriate decisions for the patient's good.

Acknowledgements

We are deeply indebted to Mrs. Kristine Salerno for her most valuable assistance in the preparation of the manuscript.

References

1. Wallack MK, Wolf JA Jr, Bedwinek J et al. Gestational carcinoma of the female breast. Curr Probl Cancer 1983; 7: 1–58.
2. Saunders CM, Baum M. Breast cancer and pregnancy: a review. J R Soc Med 1993; 86: 162–5.
3. Anderson JM. Mammary cancers and pregnancy. BMJ 1979; 1: 1124–7.
4. Allen HH, Nisker JA. Cancer in pregnancy: therapeutic guidelines. In: Allen HH, Nisker JA (Eds), Cancer in Pregnancy: An Overview. New York: Futura, 1988: 3.
5. Ventura SJ. First births to older mothers 1970–1986. Am J Public Health 1989; 79: 1675–84.
6. Moolgavkar SH, Day NE, Stevens RG. Two-stage model for carcinogenesis: epidemiology of breast cancer in females. J Natl Cancer Inst 1980; 65: 559–69.
7. Surbone A, Gilewski T, Norton L. Cytokinetics of

tumors. In: Holland JF, Frei III E, Bast R Jr., Kufe D, Morton D, Weichselbaum R (Eds), Cancer Medicine 4th ed. Philadelphia, PA: Lea Fabinger, 1996, pp. 769–798.

8. Kelsey JL, Berkowitz GS. Breast cancer epidemiology. Cancer Res 1988; 48: 5615–23.
9. Lemon HM. Antimammary carcinogenic activity of 17-alpha-ethinyl estriol. Cancer 1987; 60: 2873–81.
10. McCormick GM, Moon RC. Effect of pregnancy and lactation on growth of mammary tumors induced by 7, 12-dimethylibenz-(A)-anthracene (DMBA). Br J Cancer 1965; 19: 160–8.
11. Guinee VF, Olsson H, Moller T et al. Effects of pregnancy on prognosis for young women with breast cancer. Lancet 1994; 343: 1587–9.
12. Kroman N, Wolfahrt J, Andersen KW, Mouridsen HT, Westergaard T, Melbye, M. Time since childbirth and prognosis in primary breast cancer: population based study. BMJ 1997; 315: 851–5.
13. Olson SH, Zauber AG, Tang J, Harlap S. Relation of time since last child birth and parity to survival of young women with breast cancer. Epidemiology 1998; 9: 669–71.
14. Von Schoultz E, Johansson H, Wilking N, Rutqvist L. Influence of prior and subsequent pregnancy on breast cancer prognosis. J Clin Oncol 1995; 13(2): 430–4.
15. Ewertz M, Gillanders S, Meyer L, Zedeler K. Survival of breast cancer patients in relation to factors which affect the risk of developing breast cancer. Int J Cancer 1991; 49: 526–30.
16. Kilgore AR, Bloodgood JC. Tumors and tumor-like lesions of the breast in association with pregnancy. Arch Surg 1929; 18: 2079.
17. Haagensen CD, Stout AP. Carcinoma of the breast: criteria of operability. Ann Surg 1943; 118: 859.
18. White TT. Carcinoma of the breast and pregnancy. Ann Surg 1954; 139: 9.
19. Harrington SW. Carcinoma of the breast: Results of surgical treatment when the carcinoma occurred in course of pregnancy or lactation and when pregnancy occurred subsequent to operation, 1910–1933. Ann Surg 1937; 106: 690.
20. Gallenberg MM, Loprinzi CL. Breast cancer and pregnancy. Semin Oncol 1989; 16: 369–376.
21. Petrek JA, Dukoff R, Rogatko A. Prognosis of pregnancy-associated breast cancer. Cancer 1991; 67: 869.
22. Nugent P, O'Connell TX. Breast cancer and pregnancy. Arch Surg 1985; 120: 1221–4.
23. Holleb AI, Farrow JH. The relation of carcinoma of the breast and pregnancy in 283 patients. Surg Gynecol Obstet 1962; 115: 65.
24. Ribeiro G, Jones DA, Jones M. Carcinoma of the breast associated with pregnancy. Br J Surg 1986; 73: 607–9.
25. Deemarsky LJ, Neishtadt EL. Breast cancer and pregnancy. Breast 1980; 7: 17.
26. King RM, Welch JS, Martin JL et al. Carcinoma of the breast associated with pregnancy. Surg Gynecol Obstet 1985; 160: 228–32.
27. Anderson BO, Petrek JA, Byrd DR, Senie RT, Borgen PI. Pregnancy influences breast cancer stage at diagnosis in women 30 years of age and younger. Ann Surg Oncol 1996; 3: 204.
28. Zemlickis D, Lishner M, Degendorfer P et al. Maternal and fetal outcome after breast cancer in pregnancy. Am J Obstet Gynecol 1992; 166: 781.
29. Ishida T, Yokoe T, Kasumi F et al. Clinicopathologic characteristics and prognosis of breast cancer patients associated with pregnancy and lactation: analysis of case-control study in Japan. Jpn J Cancer Res 1992; 83: 1143.
30. Lethaby AE, O'Neill MA, Mason BH, Holdaway IM, Harvey VJ. Overall survival from breast cancer in women pregnant or lactating at or after diagnosis. Auckland Breast Cancer Study Group. Int J Cancer 1996; 67: 751.
31. Ezzat A, Raja MA, Berry J et al. Impact of pregnancy on non-metastatic breast cancer: a case control study. Clin Oncol 1996; 8: 367.
32. Tretli S, Kvalheim G, Thoresen S, Host H. Survival of breast cancer patients diagnosed during pregnancy or lactation. Br J Cancer 1988; 58: 382.
33. Bonnier P, Romain S, Dilhuydy JM et al. Influence of pregnancy on the outcome of breast cancer: a case-control study. Société Française de Sénologie et de Pathologie Mammaire Study Group. Int J Cancer 1997; 72: 720.
34. Baker J, Ali A, Groch MW et al. Bone scanning in pregnant patients with breast carcinoma. Clin Nucl Med 1987; 12: 519.
35. Kanal E. Pregnancy and the safety of magnetic resonance imaging. Magn Reson Imaging Clin N Am 1994; 2: 309.
36. Adzick NS, Harrison MR. The unborn surgical patient. Curr Probl Surg 1994; 31: 1.
37. Mattison DR, Angtuaco T. Magnetic resonance imaging in prenatal diagnosis. Clin Obstet Gynecol 1988; 31: 353.
38. Mazze RI, Kallen B. Reproductive outcome after anesthesia and operation during pregnancy: a registry study of 5405 cases. Am J Obstet Gynecol 1989; 161: 1178.
39. Pederson H, Finster M. Anesthetic risks in the pregnant surgical patient. Anesthesiology 1979; 51: 439.
40. Kuerer HM, Cunningham JD, Bleiweiss IJ et al. Conservative surgery for breast carcinoma associated with pregnancy. Breast J 1998; 4: 171.
41. Veronesi U, Luini A, Del Vecchio M et al. Radiotherapy after breast-preserving surgery in women with localized cancer of the breast. N Engl J Med 1993; 328: 1587–91.
42. National Council on Radiation Protection and Mea-

surements. Report #39: basic radiation protection criteria. Washington, DC, NCRP, 1971.

43. Woo SY, Fuller LM, Cundiff JH et al. Radiotherapy during pregnancy for clinical stages IA–IIA Hodgkin's disease. Int J Radiat Oncol Biol Phys 1992; 23: 407–12.
44. Petrek JA. Breast cancer and pregnancy. In: Harris JR, Lippman ME, Morrow M (Eds), Diseases of the Breast. Philadelphia, PA: JB Lippincott, 1996, 1st ed, pp. 896–901.
45. Doll DC, Ringenberg S, Yarbro JW. Antineoplastic agents and pregnancy. Semin Oncol 1989; 16: 337–46.
46. Zemlickis D, Lishner M, Degendorfer P et al. Fetal outcome after in utero exposure to cancer chemotherapy. Arch Intern Med 1992; 152: 573–6.
47. Glantz JC. Reproductive toxicology of alkylating agents. Obstet Gynecol Surv 1994; 49: 709–15.
48. Turchi JJ, Villasis C. Anthracyclines in the treatment of malignancy in pregnancy. Cancer 1998; 61: 435–40.
49. Berry DL, Theriault RL, Holmes FA. Management of breast cancer during pregnancy using as a standardized protocol. J Clin Oncol 1999; 17: 855–61.
50. Buekers TE, Lallas TA. Chemotherapy in pregnancy. Obstet Gynecol Clin N Am 1998; 25: 323–9.
51. Briggs, GG, Freeman, RK, Yaffe SJ. Drugs in Pregnancy and Lactation: a Reference Guide to Fetal and Neonatal Risk. Baltimore: Williams and Wilkens, 1998, 5th ed, xxii.
52. Danforth's Obstetrics and Gynecology. Scott JR et al. (Eds), Philadelphia, PA: JB Lippincott, 7th ed, 1994.
53. Surbone A, Petrek JA. Childbearing issues in breast carcinoma survivors. Cancer 1997; 79: 1271–8.
54. Surbone A, Petrek J. Pregnancy after breast cancer. The relationship of pregnancy to breast cancer development and progression. Crit Rev Oncol Hematol 1998; 27: 169–178.
55. Haagensen CD. The treatment and results in cancer of the breast at the Presbyterian Hospital, New York. Am J Roentgenol 1949; 62: 328.
56. Sakai F, Saez S. Existence of receptors bound to endogenous estradiol in breast cancers in premenopausal and postmenopausal women. Steroids 1976; 27: 99–110.
57. Elledge RM, Ciocca DR, Langone G, McGuire WL. Estrogen receptor, progesteron receptor and Her-2/neu protein in breast cancers from pregnant patients. Cancer 1993; 71: 2499–506.
58. Pellegrino ED, Thomasma DC. For the Patient's Good: The Restoration of Beneficence in Health Care. New York: Oxford University Press, 1988.

Breast Cancer: Diagnosis and Management
J.M. Dixon (Ed.)

CHAPTER 50

Locally advanced breast cancer

J.M. Dixon

1. Introduction

Locally advanced breast cancer is characterised by clinical features which suggest infiltration or involvement of the skin of the breast or the chest wall [1,2]. It also includes patients with ipsilateral fixed axillary lymph nodes [2] (Table 1). Large operable breast cancers and tumours involving fascia or chest wall muscles underlying the breast such as the pectoralis major should not be considered locally advanced.

Locally advanced breast cancer may arise because of position in the breast, for example, in peripheral parts of the breast where the depth of the parenchyma is less, so skin involvement may occur early in the growth of such a tumour [2]. It can occur because of neglect (some patients do not present to hospital for months or even years after they notice a mass) or it can develop because the tumour is biological aggressive. The most aggressive of all locally advanced breast cancers are those that present with diffuse breast swelling (peau d'orange) and overlying erythema (inflammatory cancers) [3]. These are fast growing tumours and have the worst prognosis of all locally advanced breast cancers.

Locally advanced breast cancer is characterised by features suggesting infiltration or involvement of breast skin or the chest wall.

Table 1. Clinical features of locally advanced breast cancer

Skin
- Ulceration
- Dermal infiltration
- Erythema over tumour
- Satellite nodules
- Peau d'orange

Chest wall
Tumour fixation to
- Ribs
- Serratus anterior
- Intercostal muscles

Axillary Nodes
- Nodes fixed to one another or to other structures

2. Frequency

Between 5 and 30% of patients presenting to breast clinics have tumours which are locally advanced [4–7]. The reason for this wide variation include the availability of breast screening, differences in definition between different centres, the local availability of health care and delays in presentation which vary from country to country.

The frequency varies between 5 and 30% depending on definition and there are wide variations in frequency between countries.

Table 2. Results from radical mastectomy in patients subdivided according to features present at the time of initial diagnosis

	5 yr local recurrence %	5 yr disease free survival %
Extensive peau d'orange	61	0
Satellite nodules	57	0
Inflammatory cancer	60	0
Ulceration	14	36
Skin involvement	17	45
Chest wall fixation	40	5
Patients without these factors	16	45

3. Previous treatments

Historically all patients with locally advanced breast cancer were treated by radical mastectomy whenever possible. Haagensen identified the features of skin involvement and fixation of the tumour to the chest wall as features which correlated with a high incidence of treatment failure (Table 2). It was from this observation that the features of inoperability outlined in Table 1 were defined. Subsequently patients with inoperable locally advanced breast cancer were treated by radiation therapy alone or in combination with surgical resection and radiotherapy [8–10]. However large doses of radiotherapy were necessary to maintain local control and at these doses radiation therapy produced severe side effects and long term problems including skin and chest wall necrosis, brachial plexopathy and lymphoedema of the arm [11–13]. With more modern techniques and smaller but radical doses of radiotherapy high rates of local remission are possible in the breast and axilla but with radiotherapy alone only 30% of patients remain free from locoregional disease at death. Furthermore, large numbers of patients succumb to metastatic disease.

Historically these patients were treated by mastectomy but this produces poor local control rates and large numbers of patients die from metastatic disease.

4. Systemic therapy

In the early 1970s a number of centres started to use systemic therapy in the management of locally advanced breast cancer [14]. From the outset, combination chemotherapy was used to treat what was perceived as aggressive and large bulk disease. These initial studies demonstrated response rates for combination chemotherapy similar to those seen in metastatic breast cancer. Responses were documented in between 50 and 90% of patients in early reports [15–17] and occurred rapidly, with detectable reduction in tumour volume often apparent after a single cycle. Although clinical response rates were high in these early studies, the number of complete clinical remissions remained low at approximately 20% [18–21] with only half to two thirds of these patients achieving a complete pathological response in the primary tumour and regional nodes [22]. There were also occasional patients who were thought clinically to have residual disease who on pathological assessment had no viable tumour [23]. The use of imaging studies, particularly ultrasound has improved assessment of response and it is recommended that patients now have both clinical and imaging assessments during primary systemic therapy [24].

Introduction of endocrine therapy to the management of locally advanced breast cancer started in elderly patients. This was based on the view that elderly patients would tolerate this treatment better than chemotherapy and that elderly patients were more likely to have hormone responsive disease [25,26]. Many of these early studies were performed in the absence of hormone receptor data. Overall, about a third of unselected patients treated with endocrine therapy achieved an objective remission and another third achieved a substantial period of stability. The response rates increased if only patients with oestrogen receptor positive tumours were treated [27].

In adjuvant therapy it is now quite common to combine chemotherapy and hormone therapy and data from studies of early breast cancer suggest

Table 3. Factors affecting choice of systemic treatment for locally advanced breast cancer

Chemotherapy
- Inflammatory cancer
- ER-negative cancer
- Rapidly progressive cancer

Hormonal treatment
- Slow growing or indolent disease
- ER-positive cancer
- Elderly or unfit patients

that combinations are more effective than either treatment alone [28]. Few studies have looked at this in the locally advanced disease setting.

5. Choice of systemic therapy

Systemic therapy should be administered as part of a planned programme of combined systemic and local therapy. Factors affecting the choice of systemic therapy for locally advanced breast cancer are outlined in Table 3.

Treatment should be administered as part of a planned programme.

5.1. Chemotherapy

The most commonly used regimens for the management of locally advanced breast cancer contain an anthracyline (either doxorubicin or epirubicin) and an alkylating agent usually cyclophosphamide. Response rates to chemotherapy with these regimens are high (Table 4) [29]. Many of the trials have used a three drug combination of 5-fluorouracil (FU), doxorubicin and cyclophosphamide (FAC), a regime with established efficacy in metastatic breast cancer. More recently epirubicin has been substituted for doxorubicin to reduce the cardiac toxicity of this regimen. A minority of trials have used the cyclophosphamide, methotrexate and 5-FU – the CMF regimen which is in widespread use in adjuvant therapy. The relative efficacy of different regimens in locally advanced breast cancer has not been established. There are some data which suggest that greater response rates in regimens which contain 5-fluorouracil can be obtained by giving the 5-FU as a continuous infusion [17]. This is used in either the FAC regimen or combined with epirubicin and cisplatin as ECF.

Overall response rates to chemotherapy are high.
Initial treatment should usually consist of combination chemotherapy or hormonal therapy depending on disease state, patient age and hormone receptor status.
Pre-operative (neoadjuvant) chemotherapy produces high response rates and in between 50 and 100% of patients.
The relative efficacy of different chemotherapy regimens in locally advanced breast cancer has not been established.

Several new agents have been introduced into the management of locally advanced breast cancer. These include the taxanes, paclitaxel (Taxol) and docetaxel (Taxetere) [30] and the vinca alkyloid vinorelbene (Navelbine) [31]. Individually

Table 4. Summary of studies and response rate using different chemotherapeutic regimens used in locally advanced breast cancer

Chemotherapy regimen	No of studies	No of courses	No of patients	% Response rate	% complete responses
FAC	7	2–4	576	31–87	8–30
Other adriamycin regimen	13	2–11	1506	50–91	2–52
CMF	2	3–4	139	47–70	8
Mitomycin regimens	2	4	114	51–94	7–44

these agents produce objective responses in 50 to 70% of patients with metastatic breast cancer not previously exposed to chemotherapy. These drugs have usually been given in combination with other drugs or added sequentially following other drugs. Few data on their effect in locally advanced breast cancer have been published. Work is currently underway to assess whether intensifying drug dosage (increasing the dose of drug given during each treatment period) is worthwhile in women with locally advanced breast cancer and whether intensification produces an improvement in operability rates, local control and survival.

Several new agents have been introduced into the management of breast cancer including the taxanes and vinorelbine. Few data of their efficacy in locally advanced breast cancer have been published.
Work is currently underway to establish whether intensifying drug dosage is worthwhile in locally advanced breast cancer.

5.2. Hormonal therapy

Primary hormonal therapy can be given to patients with locally advanced breast cancer providing that their cancers are oestrogen receptor positive and appear to be relatively slow growing or indolent [27]. The options for hormonal treatment are outlined in Table 5. Tamoxifen is the most widely used agent in locally advanced breast cancer. Results of the use of hormonal therapy in locally advanced breast cancer are presented in Chapter 51. Newer agents including the aromatase inhibitors and new anti-oestrogens are currently being assessed in locally advanced breast cancer [32,33]. Whether combinations of agents are more effective than single hormonal interventions is not entirely clear. At present, tamoxifen (20 mg per day) given alone or in combination with polychemotherapy remains the most widely used hormonal treatment in locally advanced breast cancer. However new studies suggest that response rates may be higher with the new aromatase inhibitors. It is not clear whether hormonal and cytotoxic treatments should be administered simultaneously or sequentially.

If hormonal therapy is given, tamoxifen given in a dose of 20mg/day is currently the most widely used.
Responses are seen with hormonal therapy in approximately 75% of patients whose tumours are oestrogen receptor rich (>20 fmol/mg cytosol protein, histoscore >80).

6. Timing of systemic therapy

What is not clear is whether the timing of the administration of systemic therapy in relation to local treatment modifies long term outcome. Studies comparing systemic therapy prior to or following surgery or radiotherapy have only been performed in patients with stage II/III operable breast cancer. To date the majority of these have shown equivalent results in terms of progression free and overall survival although two trials have shown a survival advantage for patients treated with primary chemotherapy compared with adjuvant chemotherapy [34,35]. The largest reported trial to date, NSABP B-18, has not yet shown

Table 5. Options for hormonal treatment in locally advanced breast cancer

Premenopausal	LHRH agonist if patient has not have a previous oophorectomy. If a response is obtained then this can be followed by surgical oophorectomy or radiation to the ovaries Tamoxifen alone or in combination with LHRH agonists is an alternative
Postmenopausal	Tamoxifen Anastrozole, letrozole, exemestane and the new pure antioestrogen are being tested in this situation

any difference in progression free or overall survival when comparing primary versus adjuvant chemotherapy [36].

Preoperative chemotherapy produces marked reduction in tumour volume which can result in substantial downstaging and provide the opportunity for breast conserving surgery in some patients with locally advanced breast cancer who initially were ineligible for any surgical procedure [36–38]. The response to primary chemotherapy is also a useful indicator of long term survival [23,39].

7. Duration of pre-operative chemotherapy

Table 6 shows how local and systemic therapies can be combined in the management of patients with inflammatory breast cancer. The optimal duration of systemic therapy remains a point of debate. Many published series have used three or four cycles of chemotherapy followed by surgery or radiotherapy with an additional four to six cycles of chemotherapy being given following local therapy. Only one randomised trial has investigated the need and usefulness of 'adjuvant' chemotherapy following primary systemic chemotherapy. In this trial following three cycles of primary (neoadjuvant) chemotherapy a further six cycles of chemotherapy was given after surgery or radiotherapy [42]. The administration of these extra six cycles prolonged both progression free and overall survival. The current trend in clinical trials is to introduce a second chemotherapy regimen in the 'adjuvant' setting following primary chemotherapy. The second regimen is selected so as not to be cross resistant and is given in an attempt to eradicate resistant tumour cells which remain following neoadjuvant chemotherapy.

> *The optimal duration of pre-operative chemotherapy is unknown.*
> *There seems to be some advantage to continuing chemotherapy after local treatment such as surgery or radiotherapy.*

8. Local control and results of treatment

The addition of systemic therapy to local treatments has improved progression free and overall survival of patients with locally advanced breast cancer compared to similar patients treated without systemic therapy. Local control remains a significant problem for patients with locally advanced breast cancer. After primary systemic therapy, the majority of patients become operable and are rendered free of clinically detectable disease. There is ongoing controversy regarding the utilisation of surgery and/or radiotherapy [40]. Published information suggests that the use of both surgery and radiotherapy after chemotherapy leads to a higher local control rate than when chemotherapy is combined with surgery and/or radiotherapy alone (Table 6). However, this issue is complex. Risk of recurrence varies considerably between different subgroups of patients with locally advanced breast cancer [23,41]. Local control rates are highest in patients who achieve a complete remission with induction chemotherapy and are lowest for patients who progress through induction chemotherapy, even if the same approach to loco-regional therapy is used thereafter.

> *Pre-operative chemotherapy followed by both surgery and radiotherapy appears to give the highest rate of local control.*

9. Radiotherapy

Radiotherapy is generally well tolerated even by elderly frail patients. It can be given concurrently with systemic hormonal treatment or it can be given after a course of primary chemotherapy. The breast skin should be given full dose and this will result in temporary erythema and possible desquamation. Palpable tumour masses should receive tumour boosts (Table 7).

Table 6. Response and survival rate of patients given primary or post-operative or post-radiotherapy chemotherapy

Author	Treatment timing	No. of pts	Response rate	Median follow up (months)	% disease-free	% alive
Pierga	Primary	200	64	36	68	93
	Post-operative	*190*	*NA*		*66*	*86*
Ragaz	Primary	69	NS	48	57	69
	Post-operative	*30*	*NA*		*47*	*60*
Scholl	Primary	196	82	54	59	86*
	Post-operative	*194*	*NA*		*55*	*78*
De Oliveira	Primary	81	NS	60	68	*82*
	Post-operative	*90*	*NA*		*66*	71
Rubens	Primary	12	50	40	50	50
	Post-radiotherapy	*12*	*NA*		*42*	*50*
Semiglazov	Primary	137	69	53	86*	86
	Post-radiotherapy	*134*	*61*		*72*	*79*
Mauriac	Primary	133	63	34	80	95
	Post-operative	*134*	*NA*		*79*	*88*
Olsen	Primary	119	77		NS	19
		119		96		
	Post-radiotherapy		*76*		*NS*	19
Fisher	Primary	747	80	60	67	80
	Post-operative	*759*	*NA*		*67*	*80*
Schaake-Koning	Primary	39	NS	66	20	41
	Post-radiotherapy	*34*	*NA*		*20*	*40*

Data taken from Ref. [45].

Radiotherapy is generally well tolerated. The breast skin should be given full dose and palpable tumour masses should receive tumour boosts.

Table 7. Radiotherapy for locally advanced breast cancer

Treatment areas
- Breast
- Axilla and supraclavicular fossa

Treatment
- Megavoltage X-rays
- Technique for enhancing skin dose
- 40–50 Gy in 15–25 fractions over 3–5 weeks
- Boost to tumour mass if possible by external beam or radioactive implant of 10–20 Gy

Toxicity
- Lethargy
- Skin erythema and small areas of moist desquamation
- Temporary mild dysphagia
- <3% risk of pneumonitis

10. Role of surgery

Some patients who have cancers with direct skin involvement either because of the position in the breast or due to neglect, are suitable for primary surgical treatment and the outcome both in terms of local control and survival is little different from the majority of patients with operable breast cancer (Table 2) (1). Surgery is now commonly employed after primary systemic (neoadjuvant) chemotherapy and it is sometimes possible to perform wide local excision although mastectomy is the most common operation performed [38]. Both wide excision and mastectomy should be combined with axillary node dissection to ascertain axillary node status following primary systemic therapy because the number of involved nodes is the single most important predictor of subsequent survival (Fig. 1) [43,44]. Mastectomy or wide excision is usually followed by radiotherapy either to the remaining breast or to the chest wall. Toilet

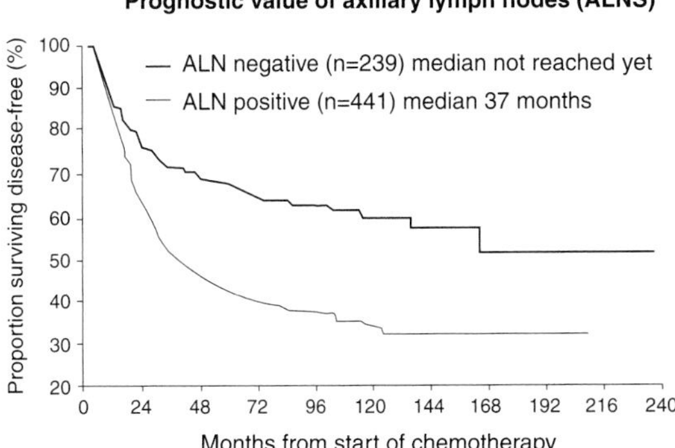

Fig. 1. Prognostic value of number of involved axillary lymph nodes after primary chemotherapy for locally advanced breast cancer. Data from Rahman et al. [44].

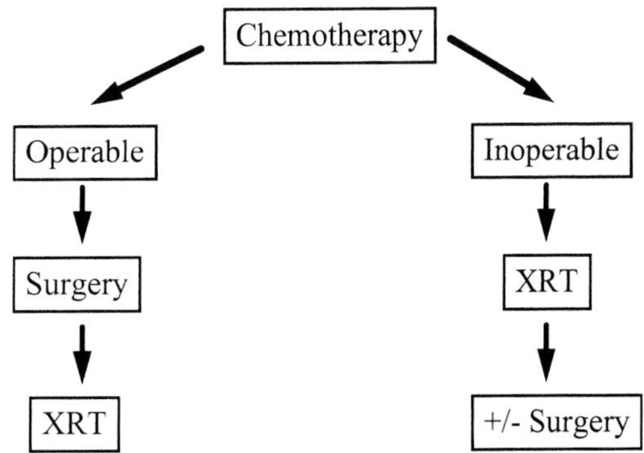

Fig. 2. Outline of the management of inflammatory breast cancer.

surgery used in an effort to control a fungating tumour, a local recurrence on the chest wall or progression of local disease is often ineffective. It can however palliate fungating and malodorous cancers.

> *Surgery is commonly employed after neoadjuvant chemotherapy; it is sometimes possible to conserve the breast although mastectomy is the commonest operation performed.*
> *The most important prognostic factor in locally advanced breast cancer is axillary lymph node status obtained at surgery following primary systemic (neoadjuvant) therapy.*
> *Toilet mastectomy used in an effort to control fungating cancer or recurrence is usually ineffective but can be used to palliate malodorous cancers.*

11. Combining treatments

A suggested outline for the treatment of inflammatory breast cancer is shown in Fig. 2. Selection of surgery or radiotherapy following neo-adjuvant chemotherapy depends on initial response to chemotherapy. Patients who become operable are treated by surgery followed by radiotherapy whereas those who still have signs of local advancement are treated by radiotherapy with surgery reserved for any residual disease.

Residual disease in the breast following chemotherapy and radiotherapy can be excised by salvage mastectomy, ideally followed by a myocutaneous flap (latissimus dorsi or transverse rectus abdominus) (Fig. 3) [2].

> *Salvage mastectomy is appropriate for patients who have residual disease followed systemic therapy and radiotherapy.*

12. Prognostic factors

While initial tumour size, tumour grade and the presence or absence of lymph node involvement remain important in the prognosis of locally advanced breast cancer, the response to chemotherapy and the extent of residual disease after chemotherapy are more important predictors of long term outcome [43,44]. The status of the axillary lymph nodes following chemotherapy appears a particularly potent prognostic factor. Hormone receptor status is a predictor of response to therapy rather than a major prognostic factor.

> *Response to neoadjuvant chemotherapy predicts for survival.*

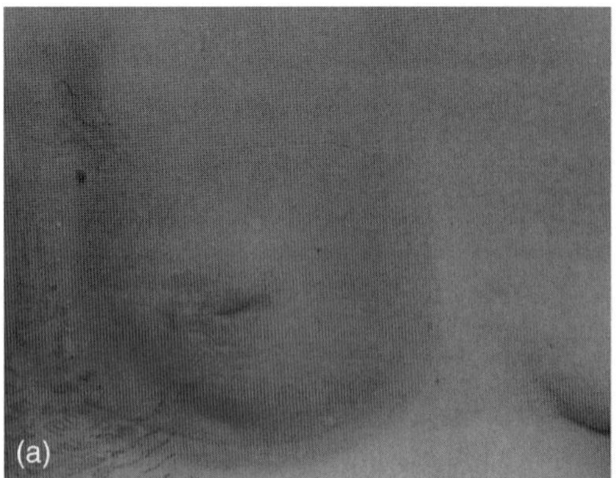

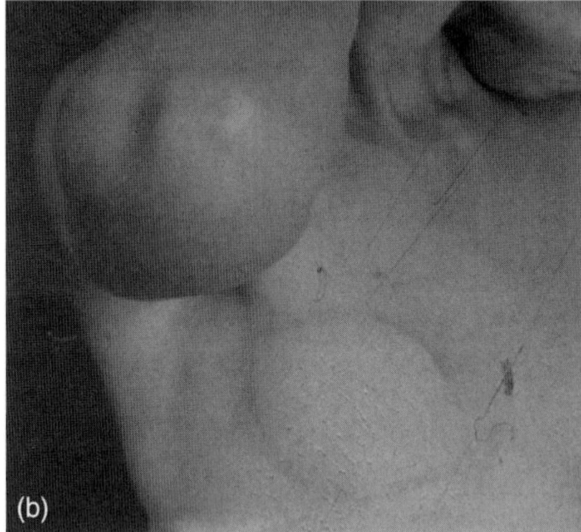

Fig. 3. Patient with an inflammatory breast cancer (a) treated initially with chemotherapy and radiotherapy and then a salvage mastectomy with a latissimus dorsi flap reconstruction (b).

References

1. Haagensen CD, Stout AP. Carcinoma of the breast: criteria for inoperability. Am Surg 1943; 118: 859–866.
2. Rodger A, Leonard RCF, Dixon JM. ABC of breast diseases: Locally advanced breast cancer. Br Med J 1994; 309: 1431–1433.
3. Jaiyesimi IA, Buzdar AU, Hortobagyi G. Inflammatory breast cancer: a review. J Clin Oncol 1992; 10: 1014–1024.
4. Hortobagyi GN, Buzdar AU. Locally advanced breast cancer: a review including the MD Anderson experience. In: Ragaz J, Ariel IM (Eds.) High-Risk Breast Cancer. Berlin, Springer-Verlag, 1991, pp 382.
5. Seidman H, Gelb SK, Silverberg E et al. Survival experience in the Breast Cancer Detection Demonstration Project. CA Center J Clin 1987; 37: 258.
6. Zeichner GI, Mohar BA, Ramirez UMT. Epidemiologia del cancer de Mama en el Instituto Nacional de Cancerologia (1989–1990). Cancerologia 1993; 39: 1825.
7. Moisa FC, Lopez J, Raymundo C. Epidemiologia del carcinoma del seno mamario en Latino America. Cancerologia 1989; 35: 810.
8. Hortobagyi GN, Buzdar AU. Locally advanced breast cancer: a review including the MD Anderson experience. In: Ragaz J, Ariel IM (Eds.) High-Risk Breast Cancer. Berlin, Springer-Verlag, 1991, pp 382.
9. Zucali R, Uslenghi C, Kenda R et al. Natural history and survival of inoperable breast cancer treated with radiotherapy and radiotherapy followed by radical mastectomy. Cancer 1976; 37: 1422.
10. Harris JR, Sawicka J, Gelman R et al. Management of locally advanced carcinoma of the breast by primary radiation therapy. Int J Radiat Oncol Biol Phys 1983; 9: 345.
11. Baclese F. Roentgen therapy as the sole method of treatment of cancer of the breast. Am J Roentgenol 1949; 62: 311.
12. Fletcher GH, Montague ED. Radical irradiation of advanced breast cancer. Am J Roentgenology 1965; 93: 573.
13. Spanos WJ, Montague ED, Fletcher FH. Late complications of radiation only for advanced breast cancer. Int J Radiat Oncol Biol Phys 1980; 61: 1473.
14. Kennedy BJ, Kelley RM, White G et al. Surgery as an adjunct to hormone therapy of breast cancer. Cancer 1957; 10: 1055.
15. Hortobagyi GN, Buzdar AU. Locally advanced breast cancer: a review including the MD Anderson experience. In: Ragaz J, Ariel IM (Eds.) High-Risk Breast Cancer. Berlin, Springer-Verlag, 1991, pp 382.
16. Hortobagyi GN, Singletary SE, McNeese MD. Treatment of locally advanced and inflammatory breast cancer. In: Harris JR, Lippman ME, Morrow M, Hellman S (Eds.) Diseases of the Breast. Philadelphia, Lippincott-Raven, 1996, pp 585–599.
17. Smith IE, Walsh G, Jones A et al. High complete remission rates with primary neoadjuvant infusional chemotherapy for large early breast cancer. J Clin Oncol 1995; 13: 424–429.
18. Hobar PC, Jones RC, Schouten J et al. Multimodality treatment of locally advanced breast carcinoma. Arch Surg 1988; 123: 951.
19. Cocconi G, di Blasio B, Bisagni G et al. Neoadjuvant chemotherapy or chemotherapy and endocrine therapy in locally advanced breast carcinoma. Am J Clin Oncol 1990; 13: 226.
20. Lippman Me, Sorace RA, Bagley CS et al. Treatment of locally advanced breast cancer using primary induction chemotherapy with hormonal synchronisation

followed by radiation therapy with or without debulking surgery. Natl Cancer Inst Monogr 1986; 1: 153.
21. Schwartz GF, Cantor RI, Biermann WA. Neoadjuvant chemotherapy before definitive treatment for stage III carcinoma of the breast. Arch Surg 1987; 122: 1430.
22. Hortobagyi GN, Singletary SE, McNeese MS. Treatment of locally advanced and inflammatory breast cancer. In: Diseases of the Breast. Harris JR, Lippman ME, Morrow M, Hellman S (Eds.) Philadelphia, Lippincott-Raven, 1996, pp 585–599.
23. Hortobagyi GN, Ames FC, Buzdar AU, Kau SW, McNeese MD, Paulus D et al. Management of stage III primary breast cancer with primary chemotherapy, surgery and radiation therapy. Cancer 1988; 62: 2507–2516.
24. Forouhi P, Walsh JS, Anderson TJ, Chetty U. Ultrasonography as a method of measuring breast tumour size and monitoring response to primary systemic treatment. Br J Surg 1994; 81: 223–5.
25. Pearlman NW, Guerra O, Fracchia AA. Primary inoperable cancer of the breast. Surg Gynecol & Obstet 1976; 143: 909–913.
26. Rubens RD, Bartelink H, Engelsman E, Hayward JL, Rotmensz N, Sylvester R et al. Locally advanced breast cancer: the contribution of cytotoxic and endocrine treatment to radiotherapy. Eur J Cancer 1989; 25: 667–678.
27. Keen JC, Dixon JM, Miller EP, Cameron DA, Chetty U, Hamby A, Bellamy C, Miller WR. Expression of Ki-S1 and BCL-2 and the response to primary tamoxifen therapy in elderly patients with breast cancer Breast Cancer Research and Treatment 1997; 44: 123–133.
28. Early Breast Cancer Trialists' Collaborative Group. Systemic treatment of early breast cancer by hormonal, cytotoxic or immune therapy: 113 randomised trials involving 31,000 recurrences and 24,000 deaths amongst 75,000 women. Lancet 1992; 339: 1–15 and 71–85.
29. Hortobagyi GN. Treatment of locally advanced breast cancer. In: JM Dixon (Ed.) Surgery: Breast and Endocrine. Mosby, London, 1998, in press.
30. Verweij J, Clavel M, Chevallier B. Paclitaxel (Taxol) and Docetaxel (Taxotere): Not simply two of a kind. Ann Oncol 1994; 5: 495–505.
31. Johnson SA, Harper P, Hortobagyi GN, Pouillart P, Vinorelbine: an overview. Cancer Treat Rev 1996; 22: 127–142.
32. Dixon JM. Letrozole as primary medical therapy for locally advanced and large operable breast cancer. Breast Cancer Research and Treatment 1997; 46 (suppl): 54.
33. DeFriend DJ et al. Investigation of a new pure antioestrogen (ICI 182780) in women with primary breast cancer. Cancer Research 1994; 54: 408–414.
34. Scholl SM, Asselain B, Beuzeboc P, Dorval T, Garcia-Giralt E, Jouve M et al. Improved survival rates following first line chemotherapy in operable breast cancer, 4 year results of a randomised trial. Proc 4th International Congress on Anti-Cancer Chemotherapy 1993; 64.
35. Semiglazov VF, Topuzov EE, Bavli JL, Moiseyenjo VM, Ivanova OA, Seleznev IK et al. Primary (neoadjuvant) chemotherapy and radiotherapy compared with primary radiotherapy alone in stage IIb–IIIa breast cancer. Ann Oncol 1994; 5: 591–595.
36. Fisher B, Broan A, Mamounas E, Wieand S, Robidoux A, Margolese RG et al. Effect of preoperative chemotherapy on local–regional disease in women with operable breast cancer: findings from National Surgical Adjuvant Breast and Bowel Project B-18. J Clin Oncol 1997; 15: 2483–2493.
37. Jacquillat C, Weil M, Baillet F, Borel C, Auclerc G, de Maublanc MA et al. Results of neoadjuvant chemotherapy and radiation therapy in the breast-conserving treatment of 250 patients with all stages of infiltrative breast cancer. Cancer 1990; 66: 119–129.
38. Singletary SE, McNeese MD, Hortobagyi GN. Feasibility of breast-conservation surgery after induction chemotherapy for locally advanced breast carcinoma. Cancer 1992; 69: 2849–2852.
39. Scholl SM, Pierga JY, Asselain B, Beuzeboc P, Dorval T, Garcia-Giralt E et al. Breast tumour response to primary chemotherapy predicts local and distant control as well as survival. Eur J Cancer 1995; 31a: 1969–1975.
40. Pierce LJ, Lippman M, Ben-Baruch N, Swain S, O'Shaughnessy J, Bader JL et al. The effect of systemic therapy on local–regional control in locally advanced breast cancer. Int J Radiation Oncol Biol Phys 1992; 23: 949–960.
41. Thoms WW, McNeese MD, Fletcher GH, Buzdar AU, Singletary SE, Oswald MJ. Multimodal treatment for inflammatory breast cancer. Int J Radiation Oncol Biol Phys 1989; 17: 739–745.
42. DeLena M. Zucali R, Viganotti G, Valagussa P, Bonadonna G. Combined chemotherapy–radiotherapy approach in locally advanced (T3b-T4) breast cancer. Cancer Chemother Pharmacol 1978; 1: 53–59.
43. McCready DR, Hortobagyi GN, Kau SW, Smith TL, Buzdar AU, Balch CM. The prognostic significance of lymph node metastases after preoperative chemotherapy for locally advanced breast cancer. Arch Surg 1989; 124: 21–25.
44. Rahman Z, Buzdar AU, Singletary E, Hortobagyi GN. Selection of systemic therapy: is axillary lymph node status important? Seminars in Breast Disease 1998; in press.
45. Hortobagyi GN. Treatment of locally advanced breast cancer. In: Surgery. Mosby International, London, 1998, in press.

Breast Cancer: Diagnosis and Management
J.M. Dixon (Ed.)

CHAPTER 51

The role of hormonal treatment for locally advanced breast cancer

B.R. Pieters and H. Bartelink

1. Introduction

1.1. Hormonal therapy

In the presence of Haagensen's clinical criteria of inoperability breast cancer has traditionally been considered as locally advanced disease (Table 1). In contrast to the numerous trials investigating the role of chemotherapy in locally advanced breast cancer, few trials have been performed to explore the value of hormonal treatment. Hormonal treatment has been more extensively studied in early stage breast cancer where results demonstrate a relative reduction in death hazard rates of about 20% [1].

At the end of the 19th century, Beatson noticed that oestrogenic hormonal manipulation had an effect on breast cancer growth. He observed that when performing a bilateral oophorectomy in women with recurrent or locally advanced breast cancer, the disease regressed [2]. Nowadays ovarian ablation is still frequently used as adjuvant or as the sole hormonal treatment for premenopausal patients with early stage or (locally) advanced breast cancer. Similar results to oophorectomy have been reported with bilateral adrenalectomy [3]. However, due to side effects and advances in hormonal treatments this type of treatment has been abandoned.

The most extensively studied medical hormonal treatment in locally advanced breast cancer is tamoxifen. Tamoxifen is an anti-oestrogen, which acts by competitively inhibiting the binding of oestrogen to oestrogen receptors [4]. Other antitumour activity of tamoxifen may be by inhibition of angiogenesis [5,6] and induction of apoptosis [7]. Tamoxifen is usually reserved for postmenopausal women, who have a low level of endogenous oestrogens. Premenopausal women in contrast have a high level of circulating oestrogens. Instead of prolonged treatment with hormonal medication, ovarian ablation is an alternative. For treatment of stage II breast cancer ovarian ablation is superior to adjuvant chemotherapy for patients with an oestrogen receptor positive cancer [8].

At the Princess Margaret Hospital, Toronto, Canada and the Imperial Cancer Research Fund, London, UK the effect of ovarian irradiation with or without prednisolone on recurrence and survival was investigated for stages I–III breast cancer [9]. Premenopausal women had the greater benefit when ovarian irradiation was combined with prednisolone treatment. The mechanism by which prednisolone acts on breast carcinoma cells is not clear, and other clinical trials have failed to show any beneficial effect of corticosteroids on breast cancer [8,10–12].

In inflammatory breast cancer oestrogen and progesterone receptors are expressed in about 40% and 30% of cases, respectively [13,14]. Hor-

Table 1. Haagensen's clinical criteria of inoperability

- Extensive skin edema
- Skin nodules
- Inflammatory carcinoma
- Parasternal lymph node metastasis
- Supraclavicular lymph node metastasis
- Edema of the arm
- Distant metastasis
- Presence of two or more of the following grave signs:
  - skin ulceration
  - skin edema limited to 1/3 of the breast
  - chest wall fixation
  - axillary lymph nodes of 2.5 cm or more
  - fixed axillary lymph nodes

monal therapy is of little value in the treatment of these cancers, except for infrequent cases where hormonal receptors are expressed.

2. Phase-II trials

One of the first studies reporting the efficacy of tamoxifen for locally advanced breast cancer was conducted by Veronesi et al. In a pilot study of 46 postmenopausal women with inoperable breast cancer, including cases with inflammatory signs, were treated with tamoxifen for 6 weeks. The objective response rate was 30%. The median survival was 10 months and was much better for responders than for non-responders [15]. At the same time, Williams et al. reported a series of 43 patients treated primarily with tamoxifen. Seventy-six percent had a positive oestrogen receptor. A response rate of 44% was observed and in 30% the disease remained stable for 6 months [16]. Compared to the results achieved with chemotherapy, lower response rates were observed. Survival was however not negatively influenced, being 73% at 36 months.

Tamoxifen alone produces response rates in locally advanced breast cancer of 30–44% of unselected patients.

3. Chemotherapy vs hormonal intervention (Table 2)

The first reported trial comparing chemotherapy and hormonal therapy as primary treatment for locally advanced breast cancer was conducted by Alagaratnam et al. from Hong Kong. In this small randomised study, 71 postmenopausal women were included with stage III breast cancer. All patients underwent a simple mastectomy and loco-regional irradiation. No information was available on hormonal receptor status. Patients were further randomly allocated to systemic therapy either tamoxifen until recurrence of disease or 10 courses of CAF (cyclophosphamide, adriamycin, 5-fluorouracil) chemotherapy. Disease-free survival in both arms were identical. The conclusion was that tamoxifen had the same effect on tumour recurrence as polychemotherapy but with less toxicity [17].

A comparable study was reported by Gazet et al. [18], the only difference being that premenopausal women were included and systemic therapy was given before and after loco-regional therapy. Patients were randomised to receive 4 cycles of chemotherapy (mitoxantrone, methotrexate, mitomycin-C) or hormonal therapy. Postmenopausal women received 4-hydroxyandrostenedione (aromatase-inhibitor) as hormonal treatment and premenopausal women had goserelin (luteinizing hormone releasing hormone analogue) prescribed. After 12 weeks of treatment, patients were restaged. All 60 patients also received loco-regional therapy which consisted of wide local excision or radical mastectomy if operable, or radiotherapy if inoperable. In cases of partial remission or stable disease, systemic treatment was continued following loco-regional treatment. Chemotherapy was continued for a further 4 cycles and hormonal therapy for a further 65 weeks. For only 13 patients was hormonal status assessed. The majority were oestrogen receptor positive. With chemotherapy a greater response was observed. However, no significant difference in metastasis rate or survival were detected. Willsher et al. performed a randomised trial in 108 women of multimodal therapy compared with initial hormonal therapy [19]. Multimodal therapy consisted of mitoxantrone, methotrexate, mitomycin-C chemotherapy followed by mastectomy and radiotherapy to the chest wall. Tamoxifen was given as hormonal therapy supplied with goserelin if the patient was premenopausal. The more aggressive multimodal therapy did not appear to be superior to hormonal treatment alone in terms of metastasis free rate of survival. Loco-regional control was worse for the hormone group compared to the multimodal therapy group (22% vs 60%) but salvage treatment was successful in the majority of cases. Oestrogen receptor positive tumours were more likely to respond to hormonal therapy.

Hormonal therapy appears equivalent to chemotherapy in locally advanced breast cancer in terms of metastases free survival in studies published to date.

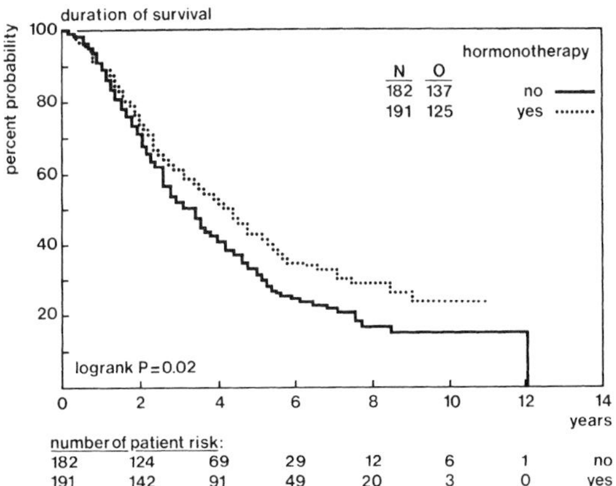

Fig. 1. Kaplan–Meier survival curves whether or not receiving hormonal treatment. From Bartelink H et al., Hormonal therapy prolongs survival in irradiated locally advanced breast cancer: A European Organisation for research and Treatment of Cancer randomised phase III trial, J Clin Oncol 1997; 15 (1): 207–215.

4. Combination chemotherapy with hormonal therapy (Table 2)

Schaake-Koning et al. studied a combination of chemotherapy and hormonal therapy in a randomised phase III Trial of 118 patients with a locally advanced breast carcinoma [20]. Patients entered included those with a positive apical axillary node; patients with inflammatory breast cancer were also entered. Radiotherapy to the breast and regional node areas was compared with radiotherapy combined with CMF chemotherapy and tamoxifen or CMF alternating with AV(adriamycin and vincristine) before and after radiotherapy and tamoxifen. In both arms tamoxifen was restricted to the treatment period. Data on hormonal receptors was incomplete and therefore not analysed. Multimodality therapy did not show any improvement when compared to radiotherapy alone regarding survival and relapse free survival. The largest and most complete study on the role of hormonal treatment in locally advanced breast cancer was conducted by the EORTC (European Organisation for Research and Treatment of Cancer). This study assessed the role of adjuvant hormonal treatment (HT) and the role of adjuvant chemotherapy (CT) [12]. This study comprised 410 patients accrued over 6 years. All patients received radiotherapy (RT) to the breast and regional lymph nodes. Patients were randomised to chemotherapy (12 course of CMF and prednisolone for 5 years) or to hormonal therapy depending on their menopausal status; premenopausal patients were treated with ovarian irradiation and postmenopausal patients were prescribed tamoxifen for 5 years. Randomisation was by a 2 × 2 factorial design; i.e. RT vs RT + CT vs RT + HT vs RT + CT + HT. Shortly after closure of the trial a highly significant difference in survival was noticed in favour of patients receiving chemotherapy. However, with a longer follow-up the benefit of chemotherapy disappeared. Eight years after closure of the trial it became apparent that patients benefited most from hormonal therapy. For patients receiving hormonal therapy the median duration of survival was prolonged

Table 2. Randomised studies of hormonal treatment for locally advanced breast cancer

Ref.	Stage	Treatment scheme	Patients	FU	Recurrences	Survival	Loco-regional control
20	II (positive axillary apex) + III	RT vs RT + CMF + Tamoxifen vs RT + CMF/AV + Tamoxifen	118	median 5.5 years	Relapse-free survival at 2 years: 38% vs 54% vs 44% $p =$ ns		
17	III	CAF vs Tamoxifen	71	median 33 months	Recurrent disease: 40% vs 50% $p =$ ns		
18	III	MMM vs Hormonal treatment Premenopausal: 4-Hydroxyandrostenedion Postmenopausal: Goserelin	60	minimal 65 weeks or until death	Disease free at 65 weeks: 67% vs 57% $p =$ ns		
19	III	MMM vs HT Premenopausal HT: Tamoxifen + Goserelin Postmenopausal HT: Tamoxifen	108	median 30 months	Metastasis rate: 45% vs 43% $p =$ ns	Median survival: >60 months vs 43 months $p =$ ns	Local control rate: 60% vs 22% $p < 0.001$
12	II (positive axillary apex) + III	RT vs RT + CMF vs RT + HT vs RT + CMF + HT Premenopausal HT: ovarian ablation + prednisolone Postmenopausal HT: Tamoxifen	410	median 8 years		Median duration survival HT vs non-HT: 4.3 years vs 3.3 years $p = 0.02$ CT vs non-CT: 3.8 years vs 3.6 years $p = 0.17$	Loco-regional recurrence rate HT vs non-HT: 47% vs 61% CT vs non-CT: 48% vs 59%

RT = Loco-regional radiotherapy; HT = hormonal treatment; CT = chemotherapy; CMF = cyclophosphamide, methotrexate, 5-fluorouracil; AV = adriamycin, vincristine; CAF = cyclophosphamide, adriamycine, 5-fluorouracil; MMM = mitoxantrone, methotrexate, mitomycin-C.

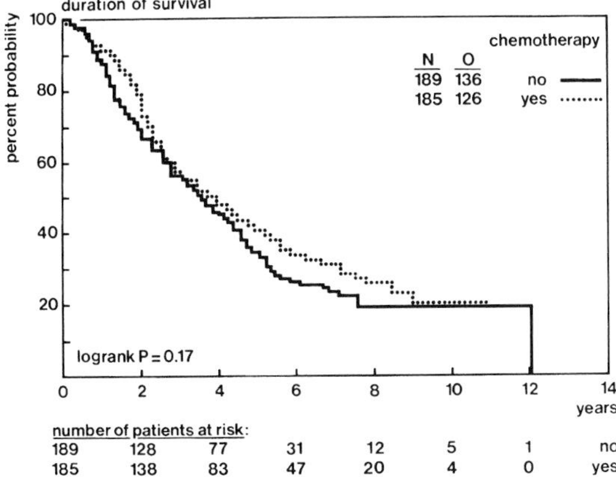

Fig. 2. Kaplan–Meier survival curves whether or not receiving chemotherapy. From Bartelink H et al., Hormonal therapy prolongs survival in irradiated locally advanced breast cancer: A European Organisation for research and Treatment of Cancer randomized phase III trial, J Clin Oncol 1997; 15 (1): 207–215.

by 1 year (3.3 vs 4.3 years) (Fig. 1). In contrast patients receiving chemotherapy had only an improvement of 2.4 months (3.6 vs 3.8 years) (Fig. 2). The reduction in death hazard associated with hormonal therapy was 25% and was constant following trial closure for 8 years thereafter. The largest therapeutic effect was seen for patients receiving chemotherapy and hormonal therapy. Loco-regional control was greatly improved when systemic therapy was combined with local irradiation. The improvements seen with chemotherapy and hormonal therapy in loco-regional control was of the same magnitude. With chemotherapy the loco-regional recurrence rate was reduced from 59% to 48% at 6 years, and from 61% to 47% in patients who received hormonal therapy, both highly significant. Of all patients who developed a loco-regional recurrence after adjuvant systemic treatment, salvage mastectomy and/or axillary dissection was only needed in 5% of cases.

> *Combining hormonal and chemotherapy with radiotherapy with or without surgery in locally advanced breast cancer improves local control and prolongs survival compared with local treatment alone or one systemic therapy alone.*

References

1. Early Breast Cancer Trialists' Collaborative Group. Systemic treatment of early breast cancer by hormonal, cytotoxic or immune therapy. Lancet 1992; 339: 1–15.
2. Beatson GT. On the treatment of inoperable cases of carcinoma of the mamma: suggestions for a new method of treatments, with illustrative cases. Lancet 1896; 2: 104–107; 162–165.
3. Dao TL, Huggins C. Metastatic cancer of the breast treated by adrenalectomy. Evaluation and the five-year results. JAMA 1957; 165: 1793–1797.
4. Osborne CK, Elledge RM, Fuqua SAW. Estrogen receptors in breast cancer therapy. Sci Med 1996; 3: 32–41.
5. Gagliardi A, Collins CD. Inhibition of angiogenesis by antiestrogens. Cancer Res 1993; 53: 533–535.
6. Haran EF, Maratzek AF, Goldberg I, Horowitz A, Begani H. Tamoxifen enhances cell death in implanted MCF7 breast cancer by inhibiting endothelium growth. Cancer Res 1994; 54: 5511–5514.
7. Ellis PA, Saccani-Jotti G, Clarke R et al. Induction of apoptosis by tamoxifen and ICI 182780 in primary breast cancer. Int J Cancer 1997; 72: 608–613.
8. Scottish Cancer Trials Breast Group and ICRF Breast Unit. Adjuvant ovarian ablation versus CMF chemotherapy in premenopausal women with pathological stage II breast carcinoma: the Scottish trial. Lancet 1993; 341: 1293–1298.
9. Meakin JW, Hayward JL, Panzarella T, et al. Ovarian irradiation and prednisone following surgery and radiotherapy for carcinoma of the breast. Breast Cancer Res. Treat. 1996; 37: 11–19.
10. Fentiman IS, Howell A, Hamed H et al. A controlled trial of adjuvant tamoxifen, with or without prednisolone, in post-menopausal women with operable breast cancer. Br J Cancer 1994; 70: 729–731.
11. Rodger A, Jack WJL, Hardman PDJ, Kerr GR, Chetty U, Leonard RCF. Locally advanced breast cancer: report of phase II study and subsequent phase III trial. Br J Cancer 1992; 65: 761–765.
12. Bartelink H, Rubens RD, van der Scheuren E, Sylvester R. Hormonal therapy prolongs survival in irradiated locally advanced breast cancer: a European Organisation for Research and Treatment of Cancer randomised phase III trial. J Clin Oncol 1997; 15: 207–215.
13. Paradiso A, Tommasi S, Brandi M et al. Cell kinetics and hormonal receptor status in inflammatory breast carcinoma. Comparison with locally advanced disease. Cancer 1989; 64: 1922–1927.
14. Charpin C, Bonnier P, Khowzami A et al. Inflammatory breast carcinoma: an immunohistochemical study using monoclonal anti-pHER-2/neu, pS2, cathepsin, ER and PR. Anticancer Res 1982; 12: 591–598.

15. Veronesi A, Frustaci S, Tirelli U et al. Tamoxifen therapy in postmenopausal advanced breast cancer: efficacy at the primary tumour site in 46 evaluable patients. Tumori 1981; 67: 235–238.
16. Williams MR, Gibson D, Marsh L et al. The early results from a randomised study of radiotherapy versus Nolvadex (tamoxifen) as initial treatment for stage III breast cancer. Eur J Surg Oncol 1988; 14: 235–240.
17. Alagaratnam TT, Wong J. Tamoxifen versus chemotherapy as adjuvant treatment in stage III breast cancer. Aust N Z J Surg 1986; 56: 39–41.
18. Gazet JC, Ford HT, Coombes RC. Randomised trial of chemotherapy versus endocrine therapy in patients presenting with locally advanced breast cancer (a pilot study). Br J Cancer 1991; 63: 279–282.
19. Willsher PC, Robertson JFR, Chan SY, Jackson L, Blamey RW. Locally advanced breast cancer: early results of a randomised trial of multimodal therapy versus initial hormone therapy. Eur J Cancer 1997; 33: 45–49.
20. Schaake-Koning C, Hamersma van der Linden E, Hart G, Engelsman E. Adjuvant chemo- and hormonal therapy in locally advanced breast cancer: a randomised clinical study. Int J Radiat Oncol Biol Phys 1985; 11: 1759–1763.

Breast Cancer: Diagnosis and Management
J.M. Dixon (Ed.)

CHAPTER 52

Endocrine therapy of breast cancer

R.E. Coleman

1. Introduction and historical overview

The use of hormonal therapy for breast cancer began a hundred years ago when Beatson reported tumour regression after oophorectomy in pre-menopausal women with advanced disease [1]. In post-menopausal women oestrogens were introduced in the 1930s, and prior to the introduction of tamoxifen ablative procedures such as adrenalectomy and hypophysectomy were frequently performed. In the 1970s major advances were made in our understanding of the endocrine basis of treatment in breast cancer, with recognition of how hormone receptors mediate oestrogen dependence and predict those likely to benefit from treatment, along with the development of new classes of hormonal agents and the results of the first trials testing endocrine therapy in the adjuvant setting.

Today, hormonal therapy is appropriate treatment for all stages of oestrogen or progesterone receptor-positive breast cancers requiring systemic treatment. In metastatic disease, endocrine treatments achieve tumour shrinkage in around one third of all patients, while in the adjuvant setting tamoxifen and oophorectomy have been shown to significantly reduce disease recurrence and mortality [2,3].

2. Oestrogen and the oestrogen receptor

The oestrogen receptor (ER) was identified in 1967. ER is a member of a family of receptor proteins found in the nucleus which bind to steroid hormones to act as DNA transcription factors. Most biological effects of oestrogen in the breast are mediated by ER and high concentrations of ER are found in approximately half of all human breast cancers. The classic oestrogen receptor (ERα) is composed of 595 amino acids and has two transcriptional domains. Oestrogen binds to the carboxy-terminal end of the molecule (AF2) causing the receptor to undergo confirmational change. This complex binds to DNA at promoter regions of oestrogen responsive elements (EREs) which are then transcribed. The ultimate effect of oestrogen action is to promote cell division through the activation of cyclin-dependent kinases. Additionally, tamoxifen may inhibit apoptosis by increasing levels of the anti-apoptotic bcl-2 protein [4].

3. Prediction of response

Until the discovery of ER and its subsequent measurement, the possible benefits of hormonal therapy were based on clinical judgements. Patients with a long disease free interval, soft tissue rather than visceral metastases, increasing age and response to previous hormonal treatments are likely to show endocrine responsiveness. Measurement of ER, however, clearly improves the prediction of response. Numerous studies have shown that patients with metastatic breast tumours containing ER have a 50–70% chance of responding to hormonal therapy. Additionally the absence of ER is a very strong predictor for lack of response with response frequencies of less than 5% in ER-negative tumours. Additionally the higher the ER level, the more likely a response will be achieved [5]. The presence of progesterone receptors (PR) in breast cancers indicates a functional oestrogen receptor and therefore also predicts for response with ER+/PR+ tumours being the most likely to benefit from endocrine treatment.

The mechanisms underlying a lack of response in 30–50% of ER-positive tumours remains unclear and other factors are being evaluated including cerb-B2 — the epidermal growth factor receptor, PS2 protein and P53.

ER is the best predictor of response to endocrine therapy but only 50–70% of ER +ve cancers will respond.

4. Adjuvant endocrine treatments

The value of systemic adjuvant therapy in women with operable breast cancer is well established with the choice of treatment depending on the risk of recurrence, the age of the patient and the presence of ER. In pre-menopausal women endocrine treatment options include ovarian ablation/suppression, tamoxifen or a combination of the two, while for post-menopausal women tamoxifen is the only endocrine agent currently of proven benefit.

The Early Breast Cancer Trialists Collaborative Group (EBCTCG) has confirmed that in women under 50 years of age, overall survival and recurrence free survival are significantly improved following ovarian ablation [3]. Indeed some of the considerable benefit seen following adjuvant chemotherapy for pre-menopausal women is probably mediated through cytotoxic induced ovarian suppression. For women with ER-positive tumours the development of amenorrhoea after chemotherapy predicts for improved survival [6] and several recent studies have shown the magnitude of benefit from ovarian suppression is similar to that achieved with chemotherapy [7,8] while a number of trials are in progress to investigate whether ovarian suppression adds to the benefits of chemotherapy ± tamoxifen.

Table 1. Benefits of adjuvant tamoxifen in ER+ tumours

Duration of tamoxifen		Odds of recurrence at 10 years	Odds of death at 10 years
1 year		−21%	−12%
2 years		−29%	−17%
5 years	all patients	−47%	−26%
	node positive	−43%	−28%
	node negative	−49%	−25%

The 1995 EBCTCG overview analysis has confirmed the benefits of adjuvant tamoxifen in women with ER-positive tumours (Table 1) [2]. Tamoxifen benefits both pre- and post-menopausal women, is of added benefit even in the presence of combination chemotherapy, and has a sustained effect lasting at least 15 years. The duration of tamoxifen administration is important with 5 years adjuvant tamoxifen being superior to 1–2 years. The value of continuing tamoxifen beyond 5 years is not established with some suggestion from relatively small trials that prolonging tamoxifen beyond 5 years does not have additional benefits, perhaps due to the partial oestrogen agonist activity of tamoxifen on dormant breast cancer cells [9].

Hormonal therapies have been shown in randomised adjuvant trials to reduce both the risk of disease recurrence and death.

5. Endocrine treatment of advanced disease

Advanced breast cancer is incurable and the aims of treatment are palliation with prolongation of survival and maintenance of quality of life. For these reasons endocrine treatment is preferred as the initial systemic treatment for metastatic disease except in patients known to have ER-negative tumours or with life-threatening visceral disease such as liver metastases with abnormal liver function or lymphangitis carcinomatosa. In these situations a rapid response is required to salvage the situation and chemotherapy is usually preferred.

No single class of hormonal agents has been shown to be consistently superior in the treatment of metastatic disease so the choice of treatment is dictated by toxicity and effects on quality of life. In post-menopausal women tamoxifen is currently the treatment of choice unless metastatic disease has developed during, or shortly after, exposure to adjuvant tamoxifen therapy. In pre-menopausal women both ovarian suppression and ablation or tamoxifen are effective. However recent data suggest that combined ovarian suppression and tamoxifen (total oestrogen blockade) may be more effective than either treatment alone [10].

Patients experiencing a response or more than 6 months of stable disease have approximately a 30% chance of responding to a second line endocrine treatment. Here the choice of potential treatments is much wider (Table 2). Responses to third, and even subsequent, endocrine treatments may be seen in some patients, sometimes delaying the need for palliative chemotherapy for many years.

The median duration of response to first line endocrine treatment is 12–18 months with response durations to second and third line treatment on average becoming progressively shorter.

Table 2. Endocrine treatments in breast cancer

Pre-menopausal women	
Ovarian ablation:	
Oophorectomy	++++
Ovarian irradiation	++++
LHRH analogues	++++
Anti-oestrogens:	
Tamoxifen	++++
Post-menopausal women	
Anti-oestrogens:	
Tamoxifen	+++++
Toremiphene	+++
Newer SERMS (e.g. raloxifene)	?
Pure anti-oestrogens (e.g. Faslodex)	?
Aromatase inhibitors:	
Aminoglutethimide	+
Testolactone	+
Anastrozole	++++
Letrozole	++++
Formestane	++
Exemestane	+++
Progestins:	
Megestrol acetate	++
Medroxyprogesterone acetate	++
Norethisterone acetate	+
Oestrogens	(+)
Androgens	(+)
Glucocorticoids	+

+++++ First line treatment of choice.
++++ Highly effective/2nd line treatment of choice.
+++ Proven efficacy.
++ Useful in certain circumstances/3rd line alternatives.
+ Occasional use.
(+) Active but outdated.
? Under development.

6. Anti-oestrogens

6.1. Tamoxifen

Tamoxifen is a derivative of tri-phenyl-ethylene which is rapidly absorbed with a half life of 4–7 days allowing once daily dosage. Steady state serum concentrations are achieved after about 4 weeks therapy while the tissues concentrations of tamoxifen metabolites may be up to a hundred fold higher than those in serum and persist for many weeks after the drug is stopped. Tamoxifen has many biological effects acting as an anti-oestrogen on the tumour but it has oestrogen agonist effects on bone and the endometrium. Tamoxifen's activity is mediated through the ER but also a variety of effects on growth factor expression, oestrogen metabolism, as well as effects on apoptosis and angiogenesis. In advanced breast cancer most breast tumours that initially respond to tamoxifen develop resistance to the drug. The mechanisms of tamoxifen resistance are an area of considerable research but it is most likely that within hormone-dependent ER-positive breast cancers cells exist that contain mutated ER receptors which are resistant, or indeed even stimulated, by continued exposure to tamoxifen [11].

Tamoxifen has now been established in the treatment of breast cancer for more than 20 years and none of the alternative agents have yet been shown to be more effective. Additionally tamoxifen is generally very well tolerated. Hot flushes, amenorrhoea, vaginal bleeding and discharge are the most common side effects along with weight gain and occasional fluid retention and mild nausea. Long term toxicities are rare but include ocular toxicity with reversible retinal lesions and macular oedema and cataracts. More importantly prolonged exposure to tamoxifen (usually in the adjuvant setting) doubles the risk of the development of uterine cancer (2 per 1000 per year for tamoxifen versus 1 per 1000 per year for controls) [2]. The majority of tamoxifen-induced uterine cancers present at an early stage but this is an important, albeit long term complication of tamoxifen. Concern over the possibility of excess numbers of colon cancers or liver tumours has proven unfounded. The oestrogenic effects of tamoxifen do have beneficial side-effects including a reduction in serum chloresterol and low density lipoproteins, and a reduction in bone mineral loss in post-menopausal women although bone loss does occur with tamoxifen in the pre-menopausal age range [12]. Tamoxifen also reduces the frequency of new breast tumours and overall the risk benefit ratio for tamoxifen is heavily in favour of its use in all stages of the disease.

Tamoxifen acts mainly through the ER. It doubles the risk of endometrial cancers but the number of contralateral breast cancers it prevents outweighs the problem with endometrial cancer.

6.2. Toremifene

Toremifene is a tamoxifen analogue with a somewhat lower oestrogen agonist activity, particularly with regard to the uterus. However its anti-tumour activity and subjective toxicities are very similar to tamoxifen [13] and at present it is not widely prescribed.

6.3. Selective oestrogen receptor modulators (SERMs)

There has been intense research by the pharmaceutical industry to develop more selective ER modulators with differences in their relative agonist and antagonist properties on normal and malignant tissues. The best established is raloxifene which, like tamoxifen, has oestrogenic effects on bone and lipids but differs in not having any significant oestrogenic effects on the endometrium. Raloxifene is available for the prevention of osteoporosis but its activity in the treatment of breast cancer is not yet defined. In the large osteoporosis trials raloxifene decreased the frequency of breast cancer in comparison to placebo [14] and is currently being evaluated as a chemopreventive agent in normal women at high risk of breast cancer.

6.4. Pure anti-oestrogens

A number of pure anti-oestrogens are in development which have shown clinical activity against tamoxifen-resistant breast cancer [15] and offer the potential for more prolonged anti-tumour effects through the downregulation of ER. These agents will have both good and bad effects on the normal tissues, and comparative trials with tamoxifen will be required to determine the risk/benefit ratio.

6.5. *Aromatase inhibitors*

Aromatase is an enzyme belonging to the cytochrome P450 family which catalyses conversion of androgens into oestrogens. In pre-menopausal women the ovary is the site of most oestrogen synthesis, but in the post-menopausal age range small amounts of oestrogen are produced, particularly in fat tissues, through the aromatisation of androgens produced by the adrenal glands. Breast cancers themselves may also show aromatase activity. Inhibition of aromatase is therefore a reliable way of reducing post-menopausal oestradiol levels and both non-competitive "suicide" steroidal androgen analogues and competitive non-steroidal inhibitors of aromatase have been developed and are now established as second line treatment for post-menopausal breast cancer or as first-line therapy when recurrence has developed during or shortly after adjuvant tamoxifen [16].

Table 3. Summary of results of phase III trials of third generation aromatase inhibitors

Comparisons with megestrol acetate — 4 studies, $n = 2459$:
Anastrozole 1 mg and 10 mg
Letrozole 0.5 mg and 2.5 mg
Vorozole [a] 2.5 mg
Exemestane 25 mg
Comparisons with aminoglutethimide — 2 studies, $n = 1113$:
Letrozole 0.5 mg and 2.5 mg
Vorozole 2.5 mg
Aromatase inhibitors better tolerated:
less weight gain
fewer thrombo-embolic problems
Aromatase inhibitors more effective:
more frequent or more durable responses
survival advantage of several months
Clinical consequences:
Megestrol displaced as second-line choice
Aminoglutethimide use now outdated
Clinically relevant differences between third generation compounds not yet established
Role in adjuvant setting under evaluation

[a] Vorozole no longer in development.

6.6. *Non-steroidal inhibitors*

Aminoglutethimide was the first aromatase inhibitor to be developed. In general the non-steroidal competitive aromatase inhibitors act by binding to aromatase but aminoglutethimide has a number of other actions including inhibition of adrenal desmolase. The drug was originally introduced as a medical inhibitor of adrenal function and at high dose (1000 mg/day) requires glucocorticoid replacement. Thereafter it was appreciated that the drug was effective against breast cancer at much lower doses through its effect on peripheral aromatase and that it does not require adrenal hormone replacement for anti-tumour activity. In numerous studies aminoglutethimide has been shown to have similar activity to tamoxifen but its use was limited by significant side-effects including lethargy, confusion, skin rashes, dizziness and nausea.

More recently the highly selective aromatase inhibitors anastrazole and letrozole have been developed which reduce circulating oestradiol to almost undetectable levels. Because of their highly specific actions the drugs are well tolerated and in randomised clinical trials have been shown to be superior in activity to both aminoglutethimide [17] and the progestin [18,19], megestrol acetate, as well as having more favourable toxicity profiles (Table 3).

In these large, carefully performed, randomised phase III trials anastrazole 1 mg was shown to have equivalent response rates and time to treatment failure but was associated with a statistically significant survival advantage over megestrol acetate [19] while letrozole 2.5 mg had a higher response rate than megestrol acetate and a superior time to treatment failure [18]. Both agents were associated with a lower incidence of cardiovascular side-effects, weight gain and dyspnoea, although nausea and headache were more common. Letrozole and another non-steroidal aromatase inhibitor, vorozole, have been compared to the parent compound aminoglutethimide [17,20] and have been shown to be superior both in terms of anti-tumour activity as well as tolerability.

Both letrozole and anastrozole are currently being compared with tamoxifen as first line treatment in metastatic disease and in the adjuvant setting as a potential alternative or addition to tamoxifen.

6.7. Steroidal suicide aromatase inhibitors

These steroidal analogues of androgen bind irreversibly to the aromatase enzyme leading to its inactivation. Testolactin was the first suicide inhibitor developed but it has relatively low activity against advanced breast cancer. Subsequently 4-hydroxy-androstenedione (formestane) was developed and this has similar activity to both tamoxifen [21] and megestrol acetate [22]. Formestane is given by intramuscular injection every two weeks, causing some discomfort at the injection site and has largely been superceded by the more recently introduced oral agents. These include exemestane which has recently also been shown to be superior to megestrol acetate in a randomised trial [23].

> *The aromatase inhibitors anastrozole and letrozole are the most commonly used second line hormonal agents and have advantages with less toxicity and greater efficacy when compared to the progestins. The use of these agents as first line treatment is being evaluated.*

6.8. Progestins

Progesterone analogues have been used in the treatment of advanced breast cancer for more than 30 years. Despite this their mechanism of anti-tumour action remains uncertain. Progestins probably have direct effects on ER, they may downregulate ER and may interact with androgen receptors. Additionally they reduce oestrogen levels through their glucocorticocoid-like effects on the pituitary adrenal axis causing suppression of plasma levels of gonadotrophins and adrenal androgen precursors of oestrogen.

The two most widely used progestins are megestrol acetate and medoxyprogesterone acetate with the latter available as a depot intramuscular injection as well as by mouth. Progestins have clear activity in advanced breast cancer and in some studies were suggested to be more active than tamoxifen but their use was limited to second and third line treatment because of their toxicity profile which includes weight gain, dyspnoea and fluid retention.

> *Progestins are now used mainly as third line treatment. They can be valuable in patients with poor appetite and weight loss.*

6.9. Ovarian ablation and gonadotrophin-releasing hormone analogs (GnRH)

In pre-menopausal women pituitary secretion of gonadotrophins stimulates ovarian production of oestrogens. Suppression of pre-menopausal oestrogen levels can therefore be obtained by either removal of the ovaries (oophorectomy), irradiation of the ovaries or administration of gonadotrophin-releasing hormone analogues (GnRH).

Surgical oophorectomy obviously has immediate effects on oestrogen levels but involves both an anaesthetic and an operation although laparoscopic oophorectomy has reduced the recovery period from this operation considerably. The ovaries are relatively sensitive to the effects of ionising radiation and ovarian ablation can be achieved following a short course of external beam radiotherapy usually with 1200–1500 cGy administered over 4–5 days. Following ovarian irradiation, oestradiol levels fall steadily over 4–6 weeks to castrate levels but occasionally, and particularly in very young women, partial recovery of ovarian function may occur. The GnRH analogues act on the hypothalamic pituitary axis by a process known as receptor downregulation [24]. Normally pituitary secretion of the gonadotrophins FSH and LH results from the pulsatile secretion of LHRH by the hypothalamus. GnRH analogues bind in the pituitary, initially causing a surge of LH production and a transient rise in oestradiol levels, but subsequently the receptors cease to function, LH levels fall and production of oestrogen is suppressed over 2–4 weeks to post-menopausal levels essentially causing a medical castration.

Depot formulations of GnRH analogues with durations of action from 1 to 3 months have been developed and achieve a 30–45% rate of anti-tumour response lasting for a median of 9 months, results which are comparable to surgical castration. There may also be GnRH receptors in breast cancer cells and this may explain the occasional response to GnRH analogues of ER-negative and post-menopausal breast cancers. Their clinical use should be restricted to women with ER-positive pre-menopausal breast cancers.

The Gnrh analogues have extended the use of ovarian ablation.

7. Other treatments

Androgens, oestrogens and glucocorticoids have been widely used in the past to treat advanced breast cancer but are now, perhaps with the exception of glucocorticoids, rarely prescribed. This decline in popularity has nothing to do with their activity which is significant, but reflects their toxicity profiles and the availability of much more specific well tolerated compounds.

8. Combined endocrine treatments

In general most studies comparing combination endocrine treatments with sequential use have found no advantage to the combination therapies. However an overview analysis of 4 trials comparing ovarian suppression with or without tamoxifen has suggested a significant survival benefit from combination therapy [10] and studies of this strategy in the adjuvant setting are in progress. Similarly in post-menopausal women total oestrogen blockade with a combination of tamoxifen and an aromatase inhibitor is being evaluated in large randomised trials.

Combinations of endocrine treatments with chemotherapy have been shown to improve survival in ER-positive patients in the adjuvant setting [25] but in advanced breast cancer, although response rates may be increased by combining both modalities, time to progression and overall survival are not influenced.

Trials suggest that combinations of Gnrh analogues and tamoxifen in advanced breast cancer may be better than either agent alone.

9. Endocrine prevention of breast cancer

The demonstration in adjuvant clinical trials that tamoxifen administration reduces the frequency of contralateral breast cancer has led to the hypothesis that tamoxifen may play a role in breast cancer prevention. As a result several studies were set up, both in the United States and Europe, to assess the value of tamoxifen in high risk women. The results have been inconsistent but in the largest trial, conducted by NSABP, tamoxifen reduced the risk of invasive breast cancer by 49% (Table 4) [26]. However whether this strategy reduces breast cancer deaths, is cost-effective, and worth the uncommon but definite long-term side-effects of tamoxifen remains a matter of debate, at least in Europe where placebo-controlled prevention trials continue to recruit women [27,28]. In the United States, tamoxifen is an accepted strategy for breast cancer prevention and now the long-term health benefits (both on cancer and other clinical endpoints) of raloxifene and tamoxifen are being compared.

Table 4. Summary of results from the NSABP P1 Tamoxifen prevention trial

	Tamoxifen	Placebo	
No. of women studied	6681	6707	
Person years of follow-up	26154	26247	
Invasive breast cancers	89	175	$p < 0.00001$
Non-invasive breast cancers	35	69	$p < 0.002$
Cancer deaths	23	42	
Breast cancer deaths	3	6	
Non-cancer deaths	34	29	
Endometrial cancers	36	15	
Fractures	111	137	
Ischaemic heart disease	71	62	
Stroke/TIA	57	49	
Pulmonary embolus/DVT	53	28	

The results of the NSABP tamoxifen prevention study are consistent with the reduction in the rate of contralateral breast cancer seen in the tamoxifen overviews.

Raloxifene has less agonist activity on the endometrium and is being compared in randomised prevention trials with tamoxifen.

References

1. Beatson GT. On the treatment of inoperable cases of carcinoma of the mamma. Suggestions for a new method of treatment with illustrative cases. Lancet 2: 104–107, 1896.
2. Early Breast Cancer Trialists' Collaborative Group. Tamoxifen for early breast cancer: an overview of the randomised trials. Lancet 351: 1451–1467, 1998.
3. Early Breast Cancer Trialists' Collaborative Group. Ovarian ablation in early breast cancer: overview of the randomised trials. Lancet 348: 1189–1196, 1996.
4. Jensen EV. Hormone dependency of breast cancer. Cancer 47: 2319–2326, 1981.
5. Osborne CK, Yochmowitz MG, Knight WA III, McGuire WL. The value of oestrogen and progesterone receptors in the treatment of breast cancer. Cancer 46: 2884–2888, 1980.
6. Powles T. Prognostic impact of amenorhoea after adjuvant chemotherapy. Eur J Cancer 34: 603–605, 1998.
7. Scottish Cancer Trials Breast Group and ICRF Breast Unit. Adjuvant ovarian ablation versus CMF chemotherapy in premenopausal women with pathological stage II breast carcinoma: the Scottish trial. Lancet 341: 1293–1298, 1993.
8. Ejlertson B, Dombernowsky P, Henning T et al. Comparable effects of ovarian ablation and CMF chemotherapy in premenopausal hormone-receptor positive breast cancer patients ASCO Proceedings 18: 66a, abstr 248; 1999.
9. Fisher B, Dignam J, Bryant J et al. Five versus more than 5 years of tamoxifen therapy for breast cancer with negative lymph nodes and oestrogen receptor positive tumours. J.N.C.I. 88: 1529–1542, 1996.
10. Klijn JGM, Seynaeve C, Beex L et al. Combined treatment with buserelin (LHRH-A) and tamoxifen vs single treatment with each drug alone in premenopausal metastatic breast cancer: preliminary results of EORTC study 10881. ASCO Proceedings 15: 117, 1996.
11. Locker GY. Hormonal therapy of breast cancer. Cancer Treat Rev 24: 21–240, 1998.
12. Powles TJ, Hickish T, Kanis JA et al. Effect of tamoxifen on bone mineral density measured by dual energy X-ray absorptiometry in healthy premenopausal and postmenopausal women. J Clin Oncol 14: 78–84, 1996.
13. Hayes DF, van Zyl JA, Hacking A et al. Randomised comparison of tamoxifen and two separate doses of toremifene in post-menopausal patients with metastatic breast cancer. J Clin Oncol 13: 2556–2566, 1995.
14. Cummings SR, Norton L, Eckert S et al. Raloxifene reduces the risk of breast cancer and may decrease the risk of endometrial cancer in post-menopausal women. Two year findings from the Multiple Outcomes of Raloxifene Evaluation (MORE) trial. ASCO Proceedings 17: 2a, 1998.
15. Howell A, DeFreind D, Robertson J et al. Response to a specific anti-oestrogen ICI 182780 in tamoxifen-resistant breast cancer. Lancet: 345: 29–30, 1995.
16. Dowsett M. Aromatase inhibitors come of age. Ann Oncol 8: 631–632, 1997.
17. Marty M, Gershanovich M, Campos B et al. Letrozole, a new potent, selective aromatase inhibitor superior to aminoglutethimide (AG) in postmenopausal women with advanced breast cancer previously treated with antioestrogens [abstract]. ASCO Proceedings 16: 156, 1997.
18. Dombernowsky P, Smith I, Falkson G et al. Letrozole, a new oral aromatase inhibitor for advanced breast cancer: double-blind randomised trial showing a dose effect and improved efficacy and tolerability compared with megestrol acetate. J Clin Oncol 16: 453–461, 1998.

19. Buzdar A, Jonat W, Howell A. Anastrozole, a potent and selective aromatases inhibitor, versus megestrol acetate in post-menopausal women with advanced breast cancer: results of overview analysis of two phase III trials. J Clin Oncol 14: 2000–2011, 1996.
20. Bergh J, Boneterre J, Houston SJ et al. Vorozole (Rivizor) versus aminoglutethimide (AG) in the treatment of postmenopausal breast cancer relapsing after tamoxifen [abstract]. ASCO Proceedings 16: 156, 1997.
21. Perez–Carrion R, Alberola Candel V, Calabresi F et al. Comparison of the selective aromatase inhibitor fromestane with tamoxifen as first-line hormonal therapy in post-menopausal women with advanced breast cancer. Ann Oncol 5: (Suppl 7): S19–S24, 1994.
22. Dowsett M, Coombes RC. Second generation aromatase inhibitors — 4-hydroxy-androstenedione. Breast Cancer Res Treat 30: 81–87, 1994.
23. Bajetta E, Dirix LY, Fein LE et al. Survival advantage of examestane (Aromasin) over megestrol acetate in postmenopausal women with advanced breast cancer refractory to tamoxifen: results of a phase III randomised double-blind study. Eur J Cancer 35: suppl 4; S85, Abstr 271, 1999.
24. Jonat W. Luteinizing hormone-releasing analogues — the rationale for adjuvant use in premenopausal women with early breast cancer. Br J Cancer 78 (suppl 4): 5–8, 1998.
25. Early Breast Cancer Trialists' Collaborative Group. Polychemotherapy for early breast cancer: an overview of the randomised trials. Lancet 352: 930–942; 1998.
26. Fisher B, Constantino JP, Wickerham DL et al. Tamoxifen for the prevention of breast cancer: Report of the NSABP P-1 study. J.N.C.I. 90: 1371–1388, 1998.
27. Powles T, Eeles R, Ashley S, Easton D, Chang J, Dowsett M et al. Interim analysis of the incidence of breast cancer in the Royal Marsden Hospital tamoxifen randomised chemoprevention trial. Lancet 352: 98–101, 1998.
28. Veronesi U, Maosonneuve P, Costa A et al. Prevention of breast cancer with tamoxifen: preliminary findings from the Italian randomised trial among hysterectomised women. Italian Tamoxifen Prevention Study. Lancet 352: 93–93, 1998.

Breast Cancer: Diagnosis and Management
J.M. Dixon (Ed.)

CHAPTER 53

The role of chemotherapy in metastatic disease

Mark J. Allen and Ian E. Smith

1. Introduction

Survival of patients with metastatic breast cancer is very variable ranging from a few months to many years but cure is rarely if ever achieved, even in patients who attain a complete remission following treatment [1]. It follows that the two main aims of chemotherapy for metastatic disease are first to provide symptom relief and improve quality of life and second to prolong survival, if possible (Inset 1).

Inset 1

- Effective palliation
- Survival benefit (probably)

Randomised trials have shown that chemotherapy improves quality of life in patients with metastatic breast cancer [2] and there is evidence to suggest that tumour response to chemotherapy, although not a critical clinical endpoint in itself, is usually a reliable surrogate marker for symptom palliation [2–4].

Improved survival with chemotherapy is more difficult to demonstrate. Trials of chemotherapy versus best supportive care have not been carried out, and would nowadays be considered unethical on the basis of established symptom relief. Circumstantial evidence for benefit comes from an overview of trials comparing "effective" (reasonable response rates) with "ineffective" chemotherapy (very low response rates) which show a significant survival benefit for the effective treatment [5]. In addition it is well established clinically that some patients with life threatening visceral metastases can obtain remissions lasting many months with chemotherapy and it seems self-evident that such patients have achieved survival prolongation.

The aim of treatment of metastatic breast cancer is primarily to provide symptom relief and improve quality of life and secondly if possible to improve survival.

2. Standard chemotherapy schedules

2.1. Anthracycline combinations

Anthracyclines, and in particular doxorubicin and epirubicin, are the most active standard chemotherapeutic agents against breast cancer with response rates in the range of 40–60% [6]. Randomised trials have shown that response rates are superior when used in combination rather than as single agents [7–9] with an associated trend towards survival improvement. These findings were confirmed by a recent meta-analysis of chemotherapy and endocrine therapies for breast cancer [10]. This analysis also failed to demonstrate convincingly that single agent chemotherapy had fewer side effects (apart from increased neurotoxicity with vincristine-containing regimens).

Typical anthracycline-containing regimens include FAC (5-FU, adriamycin [doxorubicin], cyclophosphamide), FEC (adriamycin replaced by epirubicin which has less cardiotoxicity) and AC (adriamycin and cyclophosphamide) (Inset 2). 50–80% of patients achieve an objective response to FAC [11] and in ECOG trials FAC has provided a reproducible high response rate of around 60% with a median survival of around 20 months [12]. Studies have shown that anthracycline combinations are more effective than CMF (see below). An anthracycline may not of course be suitable for all patients: some may have relapsed rapidly after receiving anthracyclines as part of adjuvant treatment and others may be near to the safe cumulative dose and be at significant risk of cardiomyopathy if given more anthracyclines. For a few patients the higher risk of alopecia with anthracyclines may be unacceptable, although scalp cooling may be useful to present this. For such patients both older and newer chemotherapy options may be available.

Inset 2

Typical anthracycline combinations	
• FAC	5-FU 600 mg/m^2 iv Adriamycin 60 mg/m^2 iv Cyclophosphamide 600 mg/m^2 iv q. 3 weekly
• FEC	5-FU 600 mg/m^2 Epirubicin 60–75 mg/m^2 Cyclophosphamide 600 mg/m^2 q. 3 weekly
• AC	Adriamycin 60 mg/m^2 Cyclophosphamide 600 mg/m^2 q. 3 weekly

Anthracyclines are the most widely used and most efficacious of the chemotherapy drugs used to treat advanced breast cancer.

2.2. CMF schedules

CMF (Cyclophosphamide, methotrexate and 5-fluorouracil) (Inset 3) was for many years the most widely used chemotherapy combination in the treatment of breast cancer. Response rates for this regimen are in the range of 40–60%. In general, CMF is less active than anthracycline regimens. A National Cancer Institute randomised trial compared FAC with CMF and found that the overall response rate for CMF was 60% and 82% for FAC [13]. Another study showed median survival of 16 months for CMF compared with 26 months for FAC [14], and an overview analysis has demonstrated a small benefit in terms of response and survival for anthracycline-containing combinations over CMF [15].

Inset 3

CMF	
Cyclophosphamide*	100 mg/m^2 orally days 1–14
Methotrexate	35–40 mg/m^2 iv days 1 and 8
5-FU	600 mg/m^2 iv days 1 and 8
q. 4 weekly	

* or 600 mg/m^2 iv days 1 and 8

Anthracycline regimens appear superior to CMF in advanced breast cancer.

2.3. Other older drugs

Several other cytotoxic drugs also have useful clinical activity against breast cancer.

2.3.1. Mitozantrone

This drug is structurally related to doxorubicin. In a series of previously untreated patients a response rate of 35% was achieved [16]. Subsequent randomised trials have shown that mitozantrone has a lower response rate than doxorubicin [17,18] but this has to be set against less toxicity including less alopecia and cardiotoxicity [18]. Moreover no survival difference has emerged between the two agents. Mitozantrone has therefore been incorporated into a number of chemotherapy schedules, particularly in Europe, and is a useful drug to consider if a patient is keen to avoid alopecia. It has been used in regimens such as MMM (mitozantrone, methotrexate, mitomycin C) (Inset 4) which has similar efficacy to anthracycline regimens [19] and CMF [20], although it may be associated with greater myelosuppression.

Inset 4

MMM	
• Mitozantrone	8 mg/m^2 iv
• Methotrexate	35 mg/m^2 iv
• Mitomycin C	6 mg/m^2 iv courses 1, 2, 4, 6
q. 3 weekly	

MM	
• Mitozantrone	11 mg/m^2 iv
• Methotrexate	35 mg/m^2 iv
q. 3 weekly	

2.3.2. Cisplatin

This drug has significant activity when used as first-line treatment against breast cancer, but is rarely effective as second-line therapy [21]. The combination of epirubicin with cisplatin (used at a dose of 60 mg/m^2) and continuous infusional 5-FU has been shown to have high response rates in advanced breast cancer with only a moderate increase in toxicity compared with conventional schedules [22] (Inset 5). Experience at the Royal Marsden Hospital has shown that another combination, MVP (mitomycin C, vinblastine, cisplatin), commonly used in non-small cell lung cancer, has response rates approaching 50% in a phase II study and is generally well-tolerated [23]. Such a combination may be considered in those patients for whom other drugs are felt to be unsuitable.

Inset 5

EcisF	
Epirubicin	60 mg/m^2 iv bolus
Cisplatin	60 mg/m^2 iv bolus
5-FU	200 mg/m^2/24 hours iv continuously

2.3.3. Etoposide

This is a very active agent in the treatment of small cell lung cancer, germ cell tumours, and lymphomas, and has useful bioavailability when taken orally. A series of small studies have generally shown low activity in previously treated patients with metastatic breast cancer although one series of 43 patients reported a response rate of 35% [24].

2.3.4. Mitomycin C

This anti-tumour antibiotic was shown many years ago to have significant activity in previously treated patients with metastatic breast cancer [25] and it has been used particularly in the United Kingdom in the MMM combination along with methotrexate and mitozantrone. In the short term the drug is well tolerated, but it can cause cumulative myelosuppression, thrombocytopenia and pulmonary toxicity. With the development of newer agents (see below) it is likely that mitomycin C will cease to have a major role in the treatment of this disease.

2.3.5. Infusional 5-FU

Continuous infusional 5-FU delivered by ambulatory pump and Hickman line is an active although not widely used approach that has activity in around 30% of patients relapsing after prior chemotherapy [26] and provides symptom palliation in over 40% of such patients.

2.4. Newer drugs

In the last few years several active new drugs have become available for treatment of breast cancer including in particular the taxanes — paclitaxel

(Taxol) and docetaxel (Taxotere), and the vinca alkaloid vinorelbine (Navelbine). These are already established as useful second-line chemotherapy in metastatic disease and are currently being assessed as first-line therapy and in adjuvant treatments.

2.4.1. Paclitaxel (Taxol)

In phase II trials, paclitaxel (Inset 6) has shown response rates of 30–40% as first-line chemotherapy for metastatic disease and around 20% in relapsed (including anthracyline-resistant) disease [27]. Phase I/II trials of the combination of doxorubicin and paclitaxel have demonstrated high response rates (83%) [28], but at the expense of greater toxicity, including cardiotoxicity [29]. A phase III trial demonstrated that the combination of doxorubicin and paclitaxel was more effective than either single agent with respect to response rate and median time to progression but a survival advantage was not seen [30].

The optimal schedule of administration remains to be established. Side effects of treatment include alopecia, myalgia, peripheral neuropathy and myelosuppression.

Inset 6

New agents

- Paclitaxel (Taxol)
  175–225 mg/m^2 iv in 3 hr infusion q. 3 wkly
- Docetaxel (Taxotere)
  75–100 mg/m^2 iv q. 3 wkly
- Vinorelbine (Navelbine)
  25–30 mg/m^2 iv days 1 and 8, q. 3 wkly

2.4.2. Docetaxel (Taxotere)

Currently data suggest that Taxotere (Inset 6) is probably more active than Taxol in the treatment of metastatic breast cancer. As a trade-off, however, it is associated with greater myelosuppression and it is our own impression that Taxotere is also associated with a greater degree of fatigue. Phase II trials have reported response rates of around 50%, even in patients with anthracycline-resistant disease [31,32]. A phase III trial in patients who relapsed following anthracycline treatment for metastatic disease showed an advantage for docetaxel over the combination of mitomycin C and vinblastine (response rates 30 vs. 11.6%; median survival 11.4 vs. 8.7 months) [33]. Another phase III trial has reported improved response rates and survival for the combination of doxorubicin and docetaxel compared with doxorubicin and cyclophosphamide [34].

> *Ongoing studies are evaluating whether taxanes should be used as first line agents alone or in combination with anthracyclines in advanced breast cancer.*

2.5. Vinorelbine (Navelbine)

This is a so called third generation vinca alkaloid which, unlike its parent compounds, has considerable activity in metastatic breast cancer with response rates of 40–60%, given in a dose of 25 mg/m^2 iv days 1 and 8, three-weekly [35,36] (Inset 6). An attractive feature of vinorelbine as palliative therapy for metastatic disease is its low side effects profile: its principal toxicities are neutropenia and local discomfort at the site of intravenous injection. In contrast alopecia, fatigue and significant nausea and vomiting are rare.

In phase III randomised trials vinorelbine combined with doxorubicin has shown similar response rates to a standard FAC schedule [37] but with 15% grade IV neutropenia, and vinorelbine with mitozantrone has similar response rates to FAC or FEC with significantly higher response rates in patients previously pre-treated with adjuvant therapy [38].

2.5.1. Oral 5-FU derivatives

Results with continuous infusional chemotherapy have stimulated interest in a series of oral 5-FU derivatives or prodrugs which have high and predictable oral bioavailability and which aim to mimic the pharmacokinetics of continuous infusional 5-FU. These include Eniluracil (Glaxo), in combination with 5-FU (UFT; Bristol Myers Squibb), and capecitabine (Roche), which is currently the most advanced of the agents in clinical development. Potentially, the development of these simple, low toxicity, oral cytotoxic agents would offer obvious advantages in palliative therapy.

3. Dose–response effects

A continuing debate in the chemotherapy of metastatic breast cancer (and indeed elsewhere in cancer medicine) is whether higher doses are more effective. Randomised trials have emphasised the need not to "under-dose": a Canadian trial comparing conventional with low dose CMF demonstrated that standard dose therapy achieved higher response rates, longer survival and better symptom control [39]. This does not necessarily imply continuing benefit with further dose escalation. Several retrospective analyses have shown a correlation between dose intensity and tumour response [40–43], but the increased toxicity involved with dose escalation does not usually translate into survival benefit (Inset 7).

Inset 7

Dose escalation

- Higher response rates
- Greater toxicity
- Survival benefit doubtful

4. Conclusions

Chemotherapy can provide effective palliation in patients with metastatic breast cancer, but not cure. Anthracycline combinations are currently the most effective, but a series of new agents offer useful second-line therapy, and may prove more effective as first-line treatment.

References

1. Greenberg PA, Hortobagyi GN, Smith TL, Ziegler LD, Frye DK, Buzdar AV. Long-term follow-up of patients with complete remission following combination chemotherapy for metastatic breast cancer. J Clin Oncol 1996; 14: 2197–205.
2. Coates A, Gebski V, Bishop JF et al. Improving the quality of life during chemotherapy for advanced breast cancer. A comparison of intermittent and continuous treatment strategies. N Engl J Med 1987; 317: 1490–5.
3. Coates A, Gebski V, Signorini D et al. Prognostic value of quality-of-life scores during chemotherapy for advanced breast cancer. J Clin Oncol 1992; 10: 1833–38.
4. Hayes DF, Henderson IC, Shapiro CL. Treatment of metastatic breast cancer: Present and future prospects. Semin Oncol 1995; 22: 5–21 (suppl 5).
5. A'Hern RP, Ebbs SR, Baum MB. Does chemotherapy improve survival in advanced breast cancer? A statistical overview. Br J Cancer 1988; 57: 615–8.
6. Honig SF. Treatment of metastatic disease. In: Harris JR, Lippman ME, Morrow M, Hellman S (Eds), Diseases of the Breast. Philadelphia, PA: Lippincott–Raven, 1996, pp. 669–734.
7. Anderson M, Daugaard S, von der Maase H et al. Doxorubicn versus mitomycin versus doxorubicin plus mitomycin in advanced breast cancer: A randomised study. Cancer Treat Rep 1986; 70: 1181–6.
8. Ingle JN, Maillard JA, Schaid DJ et al. Randomized trial of doxorubicin alone or combined with vincristine and mitomycin C in women with metastatic breast cancer. Am J Clin Oncol 1989; 12: 474–80.
9. French Epirubicin Study Group. A prospective randomized trial comparing epirubicin monochemotherapy to two fluorouracil, cyclophosphamide, and epirubicin regimens differing in epirubicin dose in advanced breast cancer. J Clin Oncol 1991; 9: 305–12.
10. Fossati R, Confalonieri V, Torri E et al. Cytotoxic and hormonal treatment for metastatic breast cancer: a systematic review of published randomized trials involving 31,510 women. J Clin Oncol 1998; 16: 3439–60.
11. Henderson IC. Chemotherapy for metastatic disease. In: Harris JR, Helman S, Henderson IC, Kinne DW (Eds), Breast Diseases. Philadelphia, PA: J.B. Lippincott, 1991, 2nd ed, pp. 604–65.
12. Falkson G, Gelman RS, Tormey DC et al. The Eastern Cooperative Oncology Group experience with cyclophosphamide, adriamycin and 5-fluorouracil (CAF) in patients with metastatic breast cancer. Cancer 1985; 56: 219–24.
13. Bull JM, Tormey DC, Shou-Hua L et al. A randomised comparative trial of doxorubicin versus methotrexate

in combination drug therapy. Cancer 1978; 41: 1649–57.
14. Aisner J, Weinberg V, Perloff M et al. Chemotherapy versus chemo-immunotherapy (CAF v CAFVP v CMF each ± MER)for metastatic carcinoma of the breast: a CALGB study. J Clin Oncol 1987; 5: 1523–33.
15. A'Hern RP, Smith IE, Ebbs SR. Chemotherapy and survival in advanced breast cancer: the inclusion of doxorubicin in Cooper type regimens. Br J Cancer 1993; 67: 801–5.
16. Cornbleet MA, Stuart–Harris RC, Smith IE et al. Mitoxantrone for the treatment of advanced breast cancer: single agent therapy in previously untreated patients. Eur J Cancer Clin Oncol; 20: 1141–6.
17. Neidhart JA, Gochnour S, Roach RW et al. Mitoxantrone versus doxorubicin in advanced breast cancer: a randomised cross-over trial. Cancer Treat Rev 1983; 10: 41–6.
18. Henderson IC, Alegra JC, Woodcock T et al. Randomised clinical trial comparing mitoxantrone with doxorubicin in previously treated patients with metastatic breast cancer. J Clin Oncol 1989; 7: 560–71.
19. Powles TJ, Jones AL, Judson IR et al. A randomised trial comparing combination chemotherapy using mitomycin C, mitoxantrone and methotrexate (3M) with vincristine, anthracycline and cyclophosphamide (VAC) in advanced breast cancer. Br J Cancer 1991; 64: 406–10.
20. Jodrell DI, Smith IE, Mansi JL et al. A randomised comparative trial of mitoxantrone/methotrexate/mitomycin C (MMM) and cyclophosphamide/methotrexate/5-fluorouracil (CMF)in the treatment of advanced breast cancer. Br J Cancer 1991; 63: 794–8.
21. Smith IE, Talbot DC. Cisplatin and its analogues in the treatment of advanced breast cancer: a review. Br J Cancer 1992; 65: 787–93.
22. Jones AL, Smith IE, O'Brien MER et al. Phase II study of continuous infusion fluorouracil in combination with epirubicin and cisplatin in patients with metastatic and locally advanced breast cancer: an active new regimen. J Clin Oncol 1994; 12: 1259–65.
23. Mendes R, Verrill M, Webb A, Eisen T, Johnston S, Smith IE. MVP (mitomycin C, vinblastine, cisplatin) salvage chemotherapy (CT) in anthracycline-pre-treated advanced breast cancer in a phase II study. Breast Cancer Res Treat 1998; 50: 266.
24. Martin M, Lluch A, Casado A et al. Clinical activity of chronic oral etoposide in previously treated metastatic breast cancer. J Clin Oncol 1994; 12: 986.
25. Van Oosterom AT, Powles TJ, Hamersma E et al. A phase II study of mitomycin C in refractory advanced breast cancer. A multi-centre pilot study. In: Mouridsen HT, Palshof T (Eds), Breast Cancer in Experimental and Clinical Aspects. Proc 2nd EORTC Breast Cancer Conference, Copenhagen, Pergamon Press, 1979.
26. Cameron DA, Gabra H, Leonard RCF. Continuous 5-fluorouracil in the treatment of breast cancer. Br J Cancer 1994; 70: 120–4.
27. Seidman AD, Tiersten A, Hudis C et al. Phase II trial of paclitaxel by 3-hour infusion as initial and salvage chemotherapy for metastatic breast cancer. J Clin Oncol 1995; 13: 2575–81.
28. Gehl J, Boesgaard M, Paaske T et al. Combined doxorubicin and paclitaxel in advanced breast cancer: effective and cardiotoxic. Ann Oncol 1996; 7: 687–93.
29. Dombernowsky P, Boesgaard M, Andersen E, Jensen BV. Doxorubicin plus paclitaxel in advanced breast cancer. Semin Oncol 1997; 24: suppl 17.
30. Sledge GW Jr, Neuberg D, Ingle J, et al. Phase III trial of doxorubicin versus paclitaxel versus doxorubicin plus paclitaxel as first-line therapy for metastatic breast cancer: An intergroup trial. Proc Am Soc Clin Oncol 1997; A2.
31. Ravdin PM, Burris HA III, Cook G et al. Phase II trial of docetaxel in advanced anthracycline-resistant or anthracenedione-resistant breast cancer. J Clin Oncol 1995; 13: 2879–85.
32. Valero V, Holmes FA, Walters RS et al. Phase II trial of docetaxel: a new, highly effective antineoplastic agent in the management of patients with anthracycline-resistant metastatic breast cancer. J Clin Oncol 1995; 13: 2886–94.
33. Nabholtz JM, Senn HJ, Bezwoda D et al. Prospective randomized trial of docetaxel versus mitomycin plus vinblastine in patients with metastatic breast cancer progressing despite previous anthracycline-containing chemotherapy. J Clin Oncol 1999; 17: 1413–24.
34. Nabholtz JM, Falkson G, Campos D et al. A phase III trial comparing doxorubicin (A) and docetaxel (T) (AT) to doxorubicin and cyclophosphamide (AC) as first line chemotherapy for metastatic breast cancer. Proc Am Soc Clin Oncol 1999; A485.
35. Weber BL, Vogel CL, Jones S et al. Intravenous vinorelbine as first-line and second-line therapy in advanced breast cancer. J Clin Oncol 1995; 13: 2722–30.
36. Canobbio L, Boccardo F, Pastorino G et al. Phase II study of navelbine in advanced breast cancer. Semin Oncol 1989; 16: 33–36.
37. Blajman C, Balbiani L, Coppola F et al. Phase III study: navelbine (N) plus adriamycin (A) versus fluorouracil (F) plus cyclophosphamide (C) in advanced breast cancer (ABC). Ann Oncol 1996; 7 (suppl 5): 112P.
38. Namer M, Soler-Michel P, Mefti F et al. Is the combination FAC/FEC always the best regimen in advanced breast cancer (ABC)? Utility of mitoxantrone (M) and vinorelbine (V) association as an alternative

in some situations. Results from a phase III prospective randomized trial. Breast Cancer Res Treat 1997; 46: A406.

39. Tannock IF, Boyd NF, DeBoer G et al. A randomised trial of two dose levels of cyclophosphamide, methotrexate and fluorouracil chemotherapy for patients with metastatic breast cancer. J Clin Oncol 1988; 6: 1377–87.
40. Frei E. Dose response for adjuvant chemotherapy of breast cancer: experimental and clinical considerations. Recent Results Cancer Res 1989; 115: 25–7.
41. Fountizilas G, Skarlos D, Pavlidis N et al. High dose epirubicin as a single agent in the treatment of patients with advanced breast cancer. A Hellenic Cooperative Oncology Group Study. Tumour 1991; 77: 232–6.
42. Bezwoda WR, Dansey R, Seymour L. High dose 4'epi-adriamycin for the treatment of breast cancer refractory to standard dose anthracycline chemotherapy: achievement of second responses. Oncology 1990; 47: 4–8.
43. Clemons M, Gharif R, Howell A. The value of dose intensification of standard chemotherapy for advanced breast cancer using colony-stimulating factors alone. Cancer Treat Rev 1998; 24: 173–84.

Breast Cancer: Diagnosis and Management
J.M. Dixon (Ed.)

CHAPTER 54

Bone metastases and impending pathological fractures

Robert E. Coleman

1. Introduction

The skeleton is the most common organ to be affected by metastatic breast cancer, and the site of disease which produces the greatest morbidity. Additionally, metastatic disease may remain confined to the skeleton with the decline in quality of life and eventual death due entirely to skeletal complications. With in excess of 250,000 deaths worldwide each year from breast cancer, strategies to reduce the incidence of bone metastases or palliate established skeletal disease are clearly of tremendous clinical importance. Rapid developments are occurring in skeletal imaging, reconstructive orthopaedic surgery, radiotherapy — particularly through the development of bone-seeking radiopharmaceuticals, new endocrine and cytotoxic treatments, and increasing use of bisphosphonates to prevent and treat skeletal complications.

The skeleton is the most common organ affected by metastasis in breast cancer.

2. Bone metabolism in cancer

There is now a much greater understanding of the mechanisms underlying the development of bone metastases and the interdependence between cancer cells and bone [1]. Tumour cells within the bone marrow cavity secrete a variety of paracrine factors which stimulate bone cell function. This stimulation of osteoclast function is of particular importance, resulting in osteolysis and is typically associated with disruption of the normal coupling between osteoblast and osteoclast function. These effects on bone cell function may in turn influence serum and urinary levels of biochemical markers of bone metabolism.

In addition to the well recognised release of bone cell activating factors from the tumour, it is now appreciated that release of bone derived growth factors and cytokines from resorbing bone can both attract cancer cells to the bone surface and facilitate their growth and proliferation. Inhibition of bone resorption could therefore have an effect on the development and progression of metastatic bone disease. Bone metastases are typically referred to as "lytic", "sclerotic" or "mixed", according to the radiographic appearances of the lesions. Where bone resorption predominates, with little new bone formation, focal bone destruction occurs and the metastases have a lytic appearance. Conversely, in bone metastases characterized by increased osteoblastic activity, the lesions appear sclerotic. However, this classification is simplistic and typically both processes are accelerated in the affected bone. This may be evident on the radiograph as illustrated by the

Table 1. Clinical, radiological and biochemical features of bone metastases

Clinical features	Radiological	Biochemical
Pain common	Bone scan very rarely completely normal	Alkaline phosphatase usually elevated
Usually multiple sites	Discrete lytic or sclerotic lesions on radiographs	Increased urinary markers of bone resorption
Axial skeletal involvement typical	Fracture/vertebral pedicle destruction common	Hypercalcaemia common
	Soft tissue extension on CT/MRI	Tumour markers often elevated

appropriately termed mixed lesion, histologically with evidence of increased osteoclast activity and resorption cavities even within sclerotic lesions, and more recently on biochemical evaluation of bone resorption rates in patients with bone metastases [2].

> *Breast cancer metastases to bone influence the balance of bone formation by osteoblasts and bone destruction by osteoclasts by a variety of mechanisms.*

3. Diagnosis of bone metastases

70% of patients with bone metastases will experience pain and this should prompt investigation. A radionuclide bone scan is the most sensitive imaging technique for the detection of bone metastases. Focal increase in tracer uptake will occur at sites of increased blood flow or osteoblast activity. However, bone scan appearances are non-specific and radiological confirmation is usually required. Considerable destruction of the normal bony architecture is necessary for a lesion to be identified on a plain radiograph; consequently computerised tomography (CT) or magnetic resonance imaging (MRI) are occasionally required to confirm the diagnosis. Tumour marker determinations may also aid in the diagnosis of metastatic bone disease (Table 1).

4. Prognosis and clinical course

In marked contrast to a median survival of less than six months in women with first recurrence of breast cancer in the liver, the median survival after first recurrence of breast cancer in bone is approximately two years [3]. The probability of survival with bone metastases in advanced breast cancer is influenced by the subsequent development of metastases at extra-osseus sites; those patients with additional organ involvement have a median survival of 1.6 years compared to 2.1 years for those with disease remaining clinically confined to the skeleton ($p =< 0.001$) [4]. Patients with bone only disease are more likely at diagnosis to be older, post-menopausal and have invasive lobular carcinoma, presenting initially with little or no involvement of axillary lymph nodes; they are less likely to have poorly differentiated grade III ductal tumours.

> *The median survival for patients with breast cancers involving bone is two years.*

5. Skeletal complications

Bone metastases cause considerable morbidity (Table 2). This includes pain, hypercalcaemia, pathological fracture, and spinal cord or nerve

Table 2. Complications of metastatic bone disease

Pain often requiring opiates and/or radiotherapy
Reduced mobility
Pathological fracture of long bone
Vertebral collapse
Hypercalcaemia of malignancy
Spinal cord compression
Bone marrow infiltration

root compression. From randomised trials in advanced breast cancer [5,6] it can be seen that one of these major skeletal events occurs on average every 3–4 months. In one study of 498 patients with first relapse in bone from breast cancer, 145 (29%) developed one or more major complications of metastatic bone destruction, with hypercalcaemia in 86 (17%), pathological long bone fracture in 78 (16%) and spinal cord compression in 13 (3%) [4].

> *Patients with bone metastases from breast cancer develop a major skeletal event approximately every 3–4 months.*

6. Treatment of bone metastases

6.1. Systemic anticancer treatment

In selecting systemic anti-tumour treatment for metastatic bone disease, the biological characteristics of the tumour are most important. Tumours expressing hormone receptors are generally treated with endocrine treatment, with chemotherapy being reserved for endocrine refractory disease. However, chemotherapy may be more hazardous in patients with skeletal disease due to bone marrow infiltration by tumour and damage from previous radiotherapy.

There have been numerous recent developments in endocrine and cytotoxic treatments which are of relevance to the patient with metastatic bone disease. In premenopausal women, total oestrogen blockade with ovarian suppression and tamoxifen is probably superior to either treatment alone [7], while in posmenopausal women, the new highly specific aromatase inhibitors letrozole and anastrozole are both superior in efficacy and better tolerated than the older agents, megestrol acetate and aminoglutethimide [8]. In the context of palliative chemotherapy, early reports suggest that more durable palliation is possible with taxane based chemotherapy [9].

6.2. Bisphosphonates

It is now clear that the bisphosphonates provide an additional treatment strategy to the known benefits of both external beam radiotherapy and systemic endocrine and cytotoxic treatments, which reduces both the symptoms and complications of bone involvement. Ongoing research is aimed at trying to define the optimum route, dose, schedule and type of bisphosphonate.

All bisphosphonates are characterized by a P–C–P containing central structure, which promotes their binding to the mineralized bone matrix, and a variable R' chain. Following administration, bisphosphonates bind avidly to exposed bone mineral around resorbing osteoclasts leading to very high local concentrations of bisphosphonate in the resorption lacunae (up to 1000 μM). On release from the bone surface, bisphosphonates are internalised by the osteoclast, where they cause disruption of the biochemical processes involved in bone resorption [10].

Other actions of the bisphosphonates include effects on the generation of new osteoclasts by inhibition of the fusion of precursor cells and their subsequent maturation, disturbance of production by osteoblasts of both osteoclast-inhibitory and stimulatory coupling factors, and inhibition of bone-resorbing cytokine release from macrophages adjacent to the bone surface [11]. Bisphosphonates also cause osteoclast apoptosis, with the appearance of distinctive changes in cell and nuclear morphology [12]. Although the molecular targets responsible for promoting this apoptosis are unknown, the bisphosphonates have recently been shown to inhibit enzymes of the mevalonate pathway [13] which are ultimately responsible for events that lead to the post-translational modification of GTP-binding proteins such as Ras. These observations raise the intriguing possibility that bisphosphonates may modulate the behaviour of cells other than osteoclasts. Sasaki et al. [14] have shown that the potent third generation bisphosphonate risedronate may reduce tumour burden and prevent further metastasis in a murine model of metastatic bone disease, while other amino-bisphosphonates can inhibit the adhesion of breast cancer cells to bone matrices in vitro [15] Recently, a preliminary report has indicated that the bisphosphonate ibandronate promotes apoptosis in bone metastases derived from an intra-ventricular inoculation of nude mice with the MDA-231 human breast cancer cell line [16].

Bisphosphonates act by disrupting bone resorption by osteoclasts.

6.3. Bisphosphonates as adjunctive therapy in metastatic bone disease

In 1983, a small study from Elomaa and colleagues reported that oral clodronate could inhibit osteoclastic activity and result in symptomatic improvement in patients with metastatic breast cancer [17]. This study stimulated other investigators, particularly in Europe, to evaluate either regular intravenous infusions of pamidronate, enteric coated oral pamidronate, or either oral or parenteral clodronate in advanced breast cancer. In addition to the effects on bone pain, sclerosis of lytic lesions was seen following intravenous pamidronate and a reduction in skeletal morbidity reported in oral bisphosphonate studies [12].

Subsequently other randomised trials have been performed (Table 3), including in advanced breast cancer a study comparing chemotherapy plus intravenous pamidronate 45 mg every three weeks with chemotherapy alone. This study reported a 48% improvement in time to progression in bone (249 vs 168 days) in favour of combination therapy [10], and was followed by the large placebo-controlled studies performed in the USA, Canada and Australasia of endocrine therapy with and without pamidronate [5] and chemotherapy with and without pamidronate [6]. These trials have shown that bisphosphonates significantly reduce skeletal morbidity in advanced breast cancer. Differences began to show after 3 months treatment and were maintained for two years. No significant effects on survival have yet been seen.

Bisphosphonates significantly reduce skeletal morbidity in patients with bone metastases from breast cancer.

In advanced breast cancer, the recently published BASO guidelines suggest the use of bisphosphonate is prioritised, with patients with endocrine resistant, symptomatic, predominantly bone only disease with relatively indolent disease being of the highest priority, while those with rapidly progressing visceral disease, even in the presence of bone metastases, are of a lower priority [20]. Once started, bisphosphonates should generally be continued indefinitely as their effects on bone metabolism wane within a couple of months. However, a patient achieving a good response to systemic treatment could very reasonably have a break from treatment and restart again on symptomatic progression.

Table 3. Effects of bisphosphonate treatment on skeletal morbidity; summary results of randomised trials

Breast cancer	n	Agent	Route	Results
Van Holten et al., 1987 [a]	161	Pamidronate	po	Reduced skeletal morbidity rate — 94 vs 52 ($p =< 0.01$)
Paterson et al., 1993	173	Clodronate	po	Reduced vertebral fractures and hypercalcaemia
Conte et al., 1996 [a,b]	295	Pamidronate	iv	Increased time to bone progression — 249 vs 168 days ($p = 0.02$)
Hortobagyi et al., 1996	382	Pamidronate	iv	Proportion experiencing SRE — 46% vs 65% ($p =< 0.001$)
Hultborn et al., 1996	401	Pamidronate	iv	Median time to skeletal progression — 9 vs 14 months ($p =< 0.01$)
Theriault et al., 1997	374	Pamidronate	iv	Proportion experiencing SRE —56% vs 67% ($p = 0.027$)

[a] Not placebo-controlled study.
[b] Evaluation blinded.

6.4. New bisphosphonates

At present clodronate, usually given orally, and infusions of pamidronate are the two most widely used bisphosphonates in oncology. As impressive as the clinical trial data are, both compounds have significant drawbacks to their more general use. Only a small percentage (<5%) of an oral dose of clodronate is absorbed, and for some patients the size and number of capsules required limits compliance, while infusions of pamidronate are time consuming and place additional demands on already overworked intravenous therapy units. The development of more potent bisphosphonates could be expected to simplify treatment and possibly improve the therapeutic effectiveness of bisphosphonate therapy.

6.5. Bisphosphonates for maintenance of skeletal health

6.5.1. The normal skeleton

Many patients with cancer are at increased risk of osteoporosis because of the endocrine changes induced by cancer treatments. This is a particularly important long term problem in women with breast cancer for whom there are concerns about the safety of hormone replacement therapy. Osteoporosis can be both prevented and treated effectively with bisphosphonates [21] and their use should be seriously considered in women experiencing a premature menopause.

> *Bisphosphonates prevent and treat osteoporosis associated with breast cancer treatments.*

6.5.2. Prevention of bone metastases

There are numerous animal studies indicating that bisphosphonates can prevent the development of metastatic bone disease, but we do not yet know with any certainty whether prophylactic bisphosphonates will be useful in the human situation. A number of clinical studies with the bisphosphonate clodronate suggest that the promising results in animals do translate into the human situation [22,23], although conflicting results have recently been reported [24]. Powles et al. have reported a reduction in the development of bone metastases in a study of 1079 women with primary operable breast cancer. After a median follow-up of around 4 years, only 28 (5.2%) patients on clodronate had developed definite bone metastases compared with 44 (8.1%) on placebo ($p = 0.054$) [22].

Subsequently, Diel et al. reported a study in 302 patients without overt evidence of metastatic disease, but selected on the basis of breast cancer cells in the bone marrow identified by immunocytochemistry, who were randomised to receive oral clodronate or allocated to a control group. After a median follow-up of 36 months, those randomised to clodronate had a reduced incidence of bone metastases (11 vs 25, $p =< 0.002$) and, most surprisingly, a reduction in extra-skeletal metastases (19 vs 42, $p =< 0.001$) as well [23]. The effects on extraskeletal metastases are difficult to explain but suggest that, in these patients with "in transit" micrometastases, the growth factors and cytokines normally released from bone are necessary for tumour cell survival and/or their biological capability to establish a metastatic focus. However, a very similar size study of 299 women receiving adjuvant systemic treatment with or without oral clodronate has produced conflicting results and should temper enthusiasm for use outside the clinical trial setting. In this Finnish study [24], a higher incidence of both bone and extraskeletal metastases occurred and both disease-free (52% vs 69%) and overall (68% vs 81%) five year survival figures were significantly worse in clodronate treated patients.

Although there may be differences in the molecular targets of bisphosphonates, particularly between clodronate and the amino-bisphosphonates [13], animal data suggest that the inhibition of bone metastases is a class-effect. Perhaps even more impressive results could be obtained with more potent bisphosphonates. Certainly patient compliance could be improved by the development of a simple, occasional, parenteral administration or a more potent oral formulation.

Studies of use of bisphosphonates in the adjuvant setting have produced conflicting results.

7. Complications of bone metastases

7.1. Pain

Bone pain is often poorly localised and has a deep boring quality which aches or burns accompanied by episodes of stabbing discomfort. It frequently interferes with activity and sleep and is improved by bed rest. Non-steroidal anti-inflammatory drugs (NSAIDs) are used as first line treatment. Combination with an opioid may be necessary but the NSAIDs should be continued. Radiotherapy is the treatment of choice for localised bone pain. The efficacy of irradiation in relieving pain from bone metastases is well established. Single doses of 4–8 Gy are effective with more patients experiencing pain relief following the higher dose. About 50% of patients achieve pain relief within the first two weeks, rising to around 80% at 4 weeks. The duration of response is usually several months.

For widespread bone pain, hemibody irradiation (HBI) may be useful. Response rates following 6 to 8 Gy are around 80%, with some patients responding within 24 hours of receiving treatment. Again no relation to pathological type is seen. HBI is associated with more toxicity than localised fields, with temporary gastrointestinal toxicity and bone marrow suppression in most patients. Because of the increased toxicity from HBI, systemic radioisotopes have been developed to deliver radiation to multiple sites of bone disease. Strontium^{89m} and Samarium^{153m} have been shown in placebo controlled trials to provide useful palliation, with osteosclerotic metastases responding best [25].

Radiotherapy is the treatment of choice for localised bone pain related to bony metastatic disease.

8. Bisphosphonates for bone pain

High doses of intravenous bisphosphonates, may provide useful symptomatic relief for patients with either diffuse bone pain or localised pain no longer amenable to radiotherapy. Reduced pain and analgesic consumption coupled with improved mobility and quality of life is seen in approximately one half of patients [18]. The magnitude and duration of effect appears to be related to the dose and potency of the bisphosphonate administered. The majority of studies have been with pamidronate, but clodronate will also relieve pain although, because of the relatively short duration of action in comparison to pamidronate [26], infusions of clodronate every 10–14 days are probably necessary to provide durable symptom control whereas pamidronate is given every 4–8 weeks [27]. To obtain optimal effects, the intravenous route is necessary, at least until more potent and well tolerated oral bisphosphonates have been developed, as it has not been demonstrated that any of the currently available oral bisphosphonates, in the absence of systemic anticancer treatment, can significantly reduce metastatic bone pain.

The effect of bisphosphonates on pain seems to be independent of the nature of the underlying tumour or radiographic appearance of the metastases, with sclerotic lesions responding similarly to lytic metastases. Additionally, there appear to be an important link between metastatic bone pain and the rate of bone resorption, with subjective response correlating with biochemical response [28]. The aim of bisphosphonate treatment should be to restore the rate of bone resorption to normal. With the currently available bisphosphonates patients with bone metastases and a very high rate of bone resorption respond poorly [27]. Ongoing studies are in progress to evaluate both more potent bisphosphonates and more dose-intensive schedules of pamidronate.

More potent bisphosphonates may not be clinically superior but simply enable more convenient intravenous bolus administration. It needs to be kept in mind that to obtain more complete inhibition of skeletal morbidity may require more than even the 'perfect' bisphosphonate can provide. There are data from animal studies to indicate that the metalloproteinase inhibitors increase the inhibitory effects of bisphosphonates on the development of metastases. Additionally a specific regulator of osteoclast development and differentiation, osteoprotegerin, has recently been identified [29] and is entering clinical evaluation. It is quite possible that in the future a combined attack on bone cell function will be recommended.

Bisphosphonates are effective for diffuse bone pain and bone pain no longer amenable to radiotherapy.

9. Hypercalcaemia of malignancy

Hypercalcaemia is the most common metabolic complication of malignancy producing many unpleasant gastrointestinal and neurological symptoms. Focal osteolysis by tumour cells, generalised osteolysis by humoral factors secreted by the tumour, increased renal tubular reabsorption of calcium and impaired renal glomerular function may all contribute to the pathophysiology. Intravenous bisphosphonates, in conjunction with rehydration, are now established as the treatment of choice for hypercalcaemia. 70–90% of patients will achieve normocalcaemia resulting in relief of symptoms and improved quality of life [30].

Intravenous bisphosphonates and rehydration with saline is the treatment of choice for hypercalcaemia.

10. Pathological fracture and spinal cord compression

Pathological fracture, particularly of weight bearing bones, is best managed with internal surgical fixation followed by post-operative irradiation [20]. Radiotherapy is indicated also for bones which are not amenable to surgical fixation such as the ribs, limb girdle bones and vertebrae. The role of radiotherapy in the prevention of pathological fracture is controversial. Spinal cord or cauda equina compression is the most devastating complication of bone metastases. The prognosis depends on the degree of neurological dysfunction rather than the type of treatment employed. Immediate high dose steroids followed by urgent radiotherapy is the treatment of choice in most cases, with surgery recommended in otherwise reasonably fit patients with very sudden deterioration in neurological function. Such patients typically have an ischaemic component and/or major structural damage to the spine which radiotherapy will not influence. Both decompression and stabilisation of the spine are required.

Surgery with bone fixation or joint replacement should be considered for patients with bony metastases who are at risk of or who have developed a pathological fracture.

11. Conclusions

During the next five years, skeletal morbidity from metastatic bone disease can be expected to decline as the use of bisphosphonates increases. Randomised trials indicate that bisphosphonates have an important influence on the course of metastatic bone disease. Further cost-benefit data would be helpful, but it can probably already be stated that bisphosphonate treatment should now be part of the standard therapy for most patients with bone metastases from breast cancer.

To confirm the potential use of bisphosphonates for prevention of bone metastases adequately will require very large randomised trials. However, confirmation, coupled with the known positive effects of bisphosphonates on bone mass, would make routine prescription of adjuvant bisphosphonate treatment a very high priority for further studies.

References

1. Coleman RE, Rubens RD. Bone metastases. In: Clinical Oncology, 2nd edition, Abeloff MD, Armitage JO, Lichter AS, Niederhuber JE, editors, Churchill Livingstone: New York, 1999, in press.
2. Coleman RE. Monitoring of bone metastases. Eur J Cancer, 34/2: 252–259, 1998.
3. Coleman RE, Rubens RD. The clinical course of bone metastases from breast cancer. Br J Cancer, 55: 61–66, 1987.
4. Coleman RE, Smith P, Rubens RD. Clinical course and prognostic factors following recurrence from breast cancer. Br J Cancer, 17: 336–340, 1998.
5. Hortobagyi GN, Theriault RL, Porter L, Blayney D, Lipton A, Sinoff C et al. Efficacy of pamidronate in reducing skeletal complications in patients with breast cancer and lytic bone metastases. N.E.J.M., 335: 1785–1791, 1996.
6. Theriault RL, Lipton A, Hortobagyi GN, Leff R, Gluck S, Stewaet JF et al. Pamidronate reduces skeletal morbidity in women with advance breast cancer and lytic bone lesions: A randomised, placebo-controlled trial. J Clin Oncol, 17: 846–854, 1999.
7. Boccardo F, Blamey RW, Kljn JMG, Tominaga T, Duchateau L, Sylveter R. LHRH-agonist + tamoxifen versus LHRH Agonist alone in premenopausal women with advanced breast cancer. Results of a meta-analysis of four trials. ASCO Proceedings, 18: 110a, 1999.
8. Dowsett M. Aromatase inhibitors come of age. Ann Oncol, 8: 631–632, 1997.
9. Nabholtz J-M, Falkson G, Campos D, Szanto J, Martin M, Chan S et al. A phase III trial comparing doxorubicin (A) and docetaxel (T) (AT) to doxorubicin and cyclophosphamide (AC) as first line chemotherapy for metasatic breast cancer. ASCO Proceedings, 18: 127a, 1999.
10. Rogers MJ, Xiong X, Ji X, Monkkonen J et al. Inhibition of growth of Dictyostelium discoideum amoeboe by bisphosphonates is dependent on cellular uptake. Pharmacol Res, 14: 625–630, 1997.
11. Rogers MJ, Watts DJ, Russell RGG. Overview of bisphosphonates. Cancer, 80/8 (suppl): 1652–1660, 1997.
12. Hughes DE, Wright KR, Uy HL et al. Bisphosphonates promote apoptosis in murine osteoclasts in vitro and in vivo. J Bone Miner Res, 10: 1478–1487, 1995.
13. Luckman SP, Coxon FP, Russell RGG, Rogers MJ. Nitrogen-containing bisphosphonates inhibit the mevalonate pathway and prevent post-translational prenylation of GTP-binding proteins, including Ras. J Bone Miner Res, 13: 581–589, 1998.
14. Sasaki A, Boyce BF, Story B et al. Bisphosphonate risedronate reduces metastatic human breast cancer burden in bone in nude mice. Cancer Res, 55: 3551, 1995.
15. Van der Pluijm G, Vloedgraven H, van Beek E et al. Bisphosphonates inhibit the adhesion of breast cancer cells to bone matrices in vitro. J Clin Invest, 98: 698, 1996.
16. Hiraga T, Williams PJ, Kawakatsu H et al. The bisphosphonate ibandronate increases apoptosis of metastatic breast cancer cells as well as osteoclasts. Proc. Am Soc Bone Miner Res, S192: A1183, 1998.
17. Elomaa I, Blomqvist C, Grohn P, Porkka L, Kairento AL, Selander K et al. Long-term controlled trial of bisphosphonate in patients with osteolytic bone metastases. Lancet, 1: 146–149, 1983.
18. Van Holten–Verzantvoort AT, Bijvoet OLM, Cleton FJ, et al. Reduced morbidity from skeletal metastases in breast cancer patients during long term bisphosphonate (APD) treatment. Lancet, ii: 983–985, 1987.
19. Conte PF, Mauriac L, Calabresi F, Santos R et al. Delay in progression of bone metastases treated with intravenous pamidronate: Results from a multicentre randomised controlled trial. J Clin Oncol, 14; 2552–2559, 1996.
20. The Breast Specialty Group of the British Association of Surgical Oncology. The management of metastatic bone disease. Eur J Surg Oncol, 25: 3–23, 1999.
21. Saarto S, Blomqvist C, Valimaki M, Makela P, Sarna S, Elomaa I. Chemical castration induced by adjuvant cyclophosphamide, methotrexate, and fluorouracil chemotherapy causes rapid bone loss which is reduced by clodronate: A randomised study in premenopausal patients. J Clin Oncol, 15: 1341–1347, 1997.
22. Powles TJ, Paterson AHG, Nevantaus A, Legault S, Pajunen M, Tidy VA et al. Adjuvant clodronate reduces the incidence of bone metastases in patients with primary operable breast cancer. ASCO Proceedings, 17: 468a, 1998.
23. Diel I, Solomayer E-F, Costa SJ et al. Reduction in new metastases in breast cancer with adjuvant clodronate treatment. N Engl J Med, 339: 357–363, 1998.
24. Saarto T, Blomqvist C, Virkkunen P, Elomaa. No reduction of bone metastases with adjuvant clodronate treatment in node-positive breast cancer patients ASCO Proceedings, 18: 128a, 1999.
25. Serafini AN, Houston Sj, Resche I, Quick DP, Grund FM, Ell P et al. Palliation of pain associated with metastatic bone cancer using Samarium-153 Lexidronam: a double-blind placebo-controlled trial. J Clin Oncol, 16: 1574–1581, 1998.
26. Vinholes JJ, Purohit OP, Abbey ME, Eastell R, Coleman RE. Evaluation of new bone resorption markers in a randomized comparison of pamidronate or clodronate for hypercalcaemia of malignancy. J Clin Oncol, 15: 131–138, 1997.
27. Vinholes JJ, Purohit OP, Abbey ME, Eastell R, Coleman RE. Relationships between biochemical and symptomatic response in a double-blind trial of

pamidronate for metastatic bone disease. Ann Oncol, 8: 1243–1250, 1997.
28. Vinholes JJ, Guo C-Y, Purohit OP, Eastell R, Coleman RE. Metabolic effects of pamidronate in patients with metastatic bone disease. Br J Cancer, 73: 1089–1095, 1996.
29. Kong Y-Y, Yoshida H, Sarosi O, Tan H-L, Timms E et al. OPGL is a key regulator of osteoclastogenesis, lymphocyte development and lymph-node organogenesis. Nature, 397: 315–323, 1999.
30. Coleman RE. Pamidronate Disodium in the treatment and management of hypercalcaemia. Rev Contemp Pharmacother, 9: 147–164, 1998.

Breast Cancer: Diagnosis and Management
J.M. Dixon (Ed.)

CHAPTER 55

Management of metastases at other sites — pleural effusions

Fiona E. Nussey and David A. Cameron

1. Introduction

Pleural effusions are a common problem associated with breast carcinoma, and may affect up to 50% of patients at some stage during their illness [1,22]. Once a patient with a pre-existing malignant disease develops a pleural effusion median survival time in most cancers is only of the order of a few months [6] but patients with breast carcinoma may survive for a number of years [2].

> *Pleural effusions affect up to 50% of patients with breast cancer.*

2. Aetiology

Pleural effusions related to cancer can be classified into three broad categories. The first occurring because of a co-morbid condition such as cardiac failure. The second known as the paramalignant effusions, i.e. those which are related to tumour, but are not related to direct pleural involvement by the malignancy. Examples include mediastinal lymph node involvement causing lymphatic obstruction, or hypoalbuminaemia from cachexia or liver metastases. The third group is malignant effusions caused by direct involvement of the pleura by tumour [3,4]. Any pleural effusive process can be exacerbated by conditions which are more likely to occur in a patient with cancer such as pulmonary embolism, pneumonia and prior mediastinal or thoracic radiotherapy [5].

Several mechanisms are thought to be responsible for the production of pleural effusions in malignancy. Lymphatic and capillary obstruction leads to reduced absorption of fluid and protein, chemical mediators cause increased capillary permeability and direct erosion of blood vessels and hypoproteinaemia also occur [10].

> *The most common presentation of a pleural effusion is with breathlessness.*

3. Presentation

The commonest symptom is breathlessness, but patients can present with cough and chest discomfort. Only a small proportion are found incidentally. Examination usually reveals reduced chest expansion on the affected side along with reduced tactile vocal fremitus, dullness to percussion and reduced air entry. If the effusion is large then there may be evidence of tracheal deviation away from the affected side.

4. Diagnosis

A chest X-ray shows blunting of the costophrenic angle when as little as 175 ml of fluid have accumulated, and a decubitus view is able to detect volumes of as little as 100 ml [6]. An X-ray which does not show the classical appearances of blunting of the costophrenic angle does not however exclude the possibility of a subpulmonary effusion and ultrasound can delineate this fluid more clearly. Pleural aspiration and examination of the fluid by cytology is the method most commonly used to evaluate a pleural effusion. It however only results in a definitive diagnosis in 50 to 70% of cases [28]. Pleural effusions are divided into two groups based on certain characteristics; protein, glucose and lactate dehydrogenase levels, with exudates being more common in a malignant effusion [27]. Closed pleural biopsy can confirm the diagnosis of a malignant effusion but sampling the correct areas is a problem and the procedure is not without risk and morbidity. Thoracoscopy and biopsy under direct vision increases the diagnostic yield up to as high as 96% [6].

Diagnosis by pleural aspiration and cytology of fluid shows malignant cells in between 50 and 70% of patients with malignant pleural effusion [28].

Other assays have been used to increase the chances of a positive diagnosis of malignant pleural effusion including lactate dehydrogenase isoenzymes [7,8], pleural fluid haptoglobin levels [9], the relationship between serum and pleural fluid complement [9], pleural fluid tumour markers [5,10] and cytogenetic analysis [5]. Telomerase, an enzyme involved in the stabilisation of telomere length, can be measured in pleural fluid and this may have a clinical application in selecting patients in whom a malignant cause for their effusion is likely [11].

5. Management

For most patients with a malignant pleural effusion the priority is good palliation of symptoms with minimal morbidity or inconvenience (Fig. 1). The presence of fluid on the chest X-ray in a patient with no, or minimal symptoms, is not necessarily an indication for intervention [2]. Where life expectancy is less than a few weeks it may be most appropriate merely to perform a thoracocentesis and administer oxygen and morphine for symptom relief.

Thoracocentesis. This relieves symptoms and provides the opportunity to confirm the diagnosis of a malignant effusion. Unfortunately fluid can begin re-accumulating in as little as 4 days and there is an approximately 98% chance of recurrence at 30 days [5]. Some advocate performing this on a repeated basis but it is associated with risk of adhesions and loculation which makes further management more difficult [6]. There is also a risk of pneumothorax or empyema, and loss of albumin can be a problem [3].

Simple aspiration is associated with an approximately 98% chance of recurrence within 30 days.

Chest Drain. The insertion of an intercostal drain is an effective method of removing the fluid and allows instillation of various therapeutic agents. Guidelines have been issued for a method of insertion of intercostal drains, which is associated with a smaller risk of serious complications [29]. Recently there has been a move towards the use of smaller bore drains (of between 10 and 14 French gauge) for patients with malignant pleural effusions. Several studies have found these to be as good as larger drains, better tolerated and with a lower rate of complications [13–15]. They also mean that out patient treatment may be possible.

Ambulatory Sclerotherapy. In a group of 19 patients having ambulatory sclerotherapy there was a 79% complete or partial response rate (in terms of re-accumulation of fluid) following bleomycin insertion. There were no readmissions in the study period, and pain associated with the procedure responded to simple analgesia [16]. This approach has a great deal to offer to patients with advanced cancer as it minimises time spent in hospital, and merits direct formal comparison with the more traditional treatments. Other drains are being de-

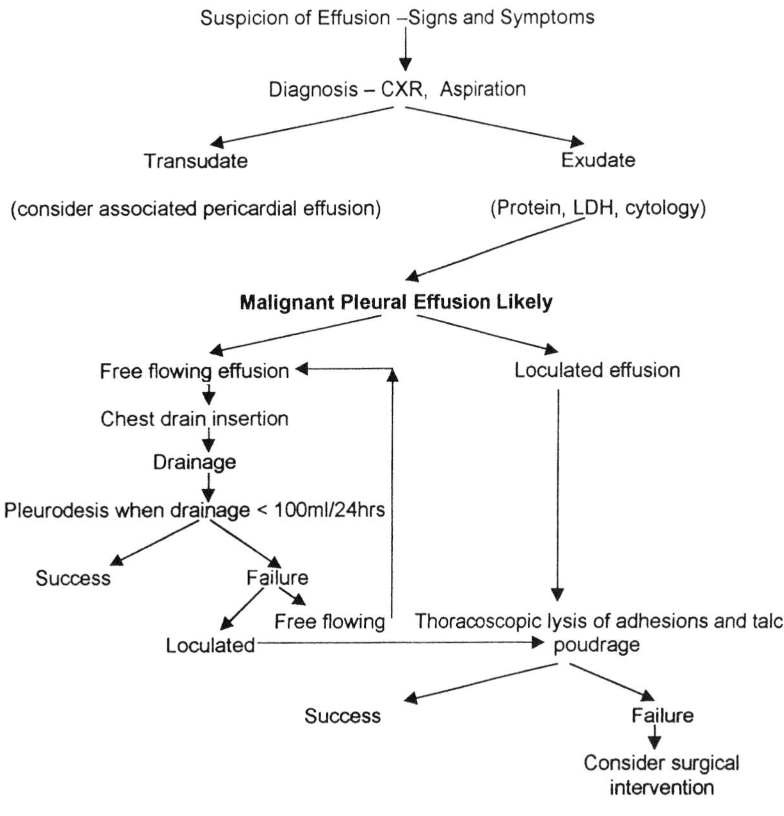

Fig. 1.

veloped in an attempt to optimise fluid drainage prior to pleurodesis [17].

Chemical Pleurodesis. This is thought to work by causing an intense inflammatory reaction, which results in reduced fibrinolytic activity, mesothelial cell injury and a fibroblast proliferation [19]. This causes the parietal and visceral pleurae to fuse together [18] obliterating any potential space for fluid to re-accumulate.

A number of prognostic factors have been identified as being helpful in defining determining indications for pleurodesis. Negative factors include a pleural fluid pH of less than 7.2, a glucose of less than 60 mg/dl, LDH of greater than 600 u/l, Karnofsy performance status of less than 70%, massive effusion and the presence of additional CXR abnormalities. These factors which were significantly associated with a high probability of failure with pleurodesis using tetracycline of bleomycin are likely to reflect an abnormal pleural surface not apparently affected by sclerosing agents and may reflect a large area of pleural involvement by tumour [12].

Many different agents have been investigated since talc was first used in 1935 [18]. There remains controversy as to which agent produces the best results, but what has become clear is that the rate of drainage should be less than 100 ml in 24 hours before pleurodesis is attempted.

Tetracycline has the added advantage of having additional prophylactic antimicrobial activity. The parenteral form is no longer being manufactured and it is becoming increasingly difficult to obtain. It is thought to work by fibroblast growth factor like activity from both direct and indirect mesothelial cell activation [20].

Treatment of malignant effusion is drainage of fluid with a chest drain followed by pleurodesis.

Talc is in common use and is believed to be the best available sclerosant, and it is relatively cheap. It is reported to have up to a 98% success rate. It is however associated with pain and fever post instillation and there have been reports of ARDS, pneumothorax and pneumonitis in association with its use. It can be made into a slurry with sterile saline or given by poudrage at thoracoscopy. This latter procedure usually requires a general anaesthetic, which may not be possible or desirable in patients with advanced malignancy. A recent report described the use of bedside thoracoscopy and this gets round the problems of needing a general anaesthetic [21]. An ongoing randomised controlled trial in the USA is designed to establish whether talc poudrage is better than talc slurry [5].

Bleomycin is one of the most commonly used agents and is cytotoxic. It is given in a dose of 1 mg/kg (maximum dose of 40 mg/m^2) into the drain and left in situ for some hours before being drained out. Toxicity has been reported (alopecia, mucositis and alveolar injury) but mainly in patients with impaired renal function who have reduced excretion of what is a predominantly renally excreted drug [19]. Other side effects include fever following instillation. It has a 31 to 85% response rate and can be used in combination with other chemotherapeutic agents, as it does not cause marrow suppression [6].

A variety of agents have been used to achieve pleurodesis including tetracycline, talc and bleomycin.

Various biological agents have been shown to be effective and include bacterial extracts (*Corynebacterium parvum*) interferon, tumour necrosis factor and interleukin-2 [6,20,23–25].

Despite the wide variety of agents available, successful control of effusion is possible in only 80% of patients [20]. Each agent has its own advantages and disadvantages, and the choice of agent should be based on cost, how easily the agent is to obtain locally and available clinical expertise [20,26].

Surgical Options. For those who are fit enough for surgery, or whose effusions are not controlled by pleurodesis, certain surgical procedures can be useful. Pleurectomy is effective and with the advent of video assisted techniques has become safer [6], although there is still a 10% mortality [2]. The place of pleuroperitoneal shunting has not as yet been defined, but there are suggestions that it may be useful if there is a thickened restrictive cortex encasing the lung which prevents apposition of visceral and parietal pleural surfaces [2]. It does however require a well motivated patient as the reservoir requires to be pumped 400 times per day [6]. An intrapleural Tenckhoff catheter is undergoing testing which allows the patient to periodically drain their own effusions [4].

About 20% of effusions are not controlled by drainage and installation of sclerosants and in these resistant cases pleurectomy is an option.

References

1. D. Greenwald, C. Philips, J. Bennet. Management of Malignant Pleural Effusions. J Surg Oncol 1978; 10: 361–368.
2. M. Tattersall. Management of malignant pleural effusion. Aust NZ J Med 1998; 28: 394–396.
3. I. Smith, S. Heys, O. Eremin. Surgical management of patients with advanced cancer. J Surg Oncol 1997; 23(2): 178–82.
4. M. Fiocco, M. Krasna. The management of malignant pleural and pericardial effusions. Haematol Oncol Clin N Am 1997; 11(2): 253–264.
5. M. DeCamp, S. Mentzer, D. Sugarbaker. Malignant effusive diseases of the pleura and pericardium. Chest 1997; 112(4)s: 291–295s.

6. C. Belani, T. Pajeau, C. Bennett. Treating malignant pleural effusions cost consciously. Chest 1998; 113(1)s: 79–83s.
7. N. Cobben, A. van Belle, H. Pennings, P. Mulder, M. van Deijer-Viser, E. Wouters, M. Drent. Diagnostic value of lactate dehydrogenase isoenzyme pattern in pleural effusions. Eur J Clin Chem Biochem 1997; 359(7): 523–528.
8. I. Lassos, R. Breuer, O. Intrator, M. Somerblick. Differential diagnosis of pleural effusion by lactate dehydrogenase isoenzyme analysis. Chest 1997; 111(3): 649–651.
9. M. Alexandrakis, S. Colulcheri, D. Kyriakou et al. Diagnostic Value of ferritin, haptoglobin, alpha 1 antitrypsin, lactate dehydrogenase and complement C3 and C4 in pleural effusion differentiation. Resp Med 1997; 91: 517–523.
10. M. San Jose, D. Alvarez, L. Valden, A. Sarandesen, J. Valle, P. Perela. Utility of tumour markers in the diagnosis of neoplastic pleural effusion. Clin Chim Acta 1997; 265: 193–205.
11. C. Yang, M. Lee, R. Lan, J. Chen. Telomerase activity in pleural effusions; diagnostic significance. J Clin Oncol 1998; 16(2): 567–573.
12. E. Martinez-Moragon, J. Aparicio, J. Sanchis, R. Menedez, M.C. Rogado, F. Sanchis. Prognostic factors for survival and response to chemical pleurodesis in a series of 120 cases. Respiration 1998; 65: 567–573.
13. E. Patz, H.P. McAdam, J. Erasmas et al. Sclerotherapy for malignant pleural effusions. A prospective randomised trial of bleomycin versus doxycycline with small bore catheter drainage. Chest 1998; 113(5): 1305–1310.
14. E. Marmon, E. Patz, J. Erasmus, H. McAdams, P. Goodman, J. Herndon. Treatment with small bore catheter thoracostomy and talc pleurodesis. Radiology 1999; 210: 277–281.
15. P. Clementsen, T. Evald, G. Grode, M. Hansen, G. Kragy Jacobsen, P. Faurschou. Treatment of malignant pleural effusion; pleurodesis using a small percutaneous catheter. A prospective randomised study. Resp Med 1998; 92: 593–596.
16. E. Patz. Malignant pleural effusions. Recent advances and ambulatory sclerotherapy. Chest 1998; 113(1s): 745–775.
17. H. Ishikawa, H. Satoh, Y. Hamashota et al. Curved chest tube for drainage of malignant pleural effusion. Resp Med 1998; 92: 633–637.
18. F. Rodriguez-Paradero, V. Anthony. Pleurodesis; state of the art. Eur Resp J 1997; 10: 1648–1654.
19. P. Zimmer, M. Hill, K. Casey, E. Harvey, D. Low. Prospective randomised trial of talc slurry versus bleomycin in pleurodesis for symptomatic malignant pleural effusions. Chest 1997; 112(2): 430–434.
20. Y. Aelony. Cost effective pleurodesis. Chest 1998; 113(6): 1731–1732.
21. Y. Aelony, R. King, C. Boutin. Thoracoscopic talc poudrage in malignant pleural effusions. Effective pleurodesis despite low pleural pH. Chest 1998; 113(4): 1007–1012.
22. A. Van Belle, G. ten Velde, E. Wouters. Chemical pleurodesis in the management of malignant effusions. Eur J Cancer 1997; 34(1): 205–206.
23. H. Wilkins, M. Connoly, P. Grays, G. Manquez, D. Nelson. Recombinant interferon alpha 2b in the management of malignant pleural effusions. Chest 1997; 111(6): 1597–1599.
24. G. Stathopoulos, C. Baxevaris, N. Papadopoulos et al. Local immunotherapy with interferon alpha in metastatic pleural and pericardial effusions; correlation with immunologic parameters. Anticancer Res 1996; 16: 3855–3860.
25. G. Rauthe, J. Sistermanns. Recombinant tumour necrosis factor in the local therapy of malignant pleural effusion. Eur J Cancer 1996; 33(2): 226–231.
26. E. Martinez-Maragan, J. Aparicio, M. Rogado, J. Sanchis, F. Sanchis, V. Gil-Suay. Pleurodesis in malignant pleural effusions; a randomised study of tetracycline versus bleomycin. Eur Respir J 1997; 10: 2380–2383.
27. R. Light, W. Ball. Lactate dehydrogenase isoenzymes in pleural effusions. Am Rev Resp Dis 1973; 108: 660–664.
28. W. Salyer, J. Eggleston, Y. Erozan. Efficacy of pleural needle biopsy and pleural fluid cytopathology in the diagnosis of malignant neoplasm involving the pleura. Chest 1975; 67: 536–539.
29. M. Tomlinson, T. Treasure. Insertion of a chest drain: how to do it. Br J Hosp Med 1997; 58(6): 248–252.

Breast Cancer: Diagnosis and Management
J.M. Dixon (Ed.)

CHAPTER 56

Management of metastases at other sites: brain metastases

A. Rodger

1. Introduction

1.1. Incidence and risk factors

While it is difficult to ascertain from the published literature the overall incidence of brain metastases in breast cancer patients, with the incidence varying from as low as 5.9% to 39% [1], several series agree that these metastases are commoner in pre- or perimenopausal women [2,3], in tumours which are oestrogen receptor negative [4], if adjuvant systemic therapy has not been given [2,4,5] and in patients who present initially with more advanced disease [2,3,5]. Brain metastases are also more likely to be associated with a short initial disease free interval and a more advanced phase of metastatic relapse.

> *Brain metastases are more common in pre- or perimenopausal patients; in patients who present with more advanced disease; and in oestrogen receptor negative tumours.*

2. Presenting clinical features

The signs and symptoms which suggest the presence of brain metastases from breast cancer are the same as those for primary intracranial neoplasms or secondary deposits from any other solid tumour. A brain metastasis can produce signs and symptoms from direct destruction of neurological tissue or it can raise intracranial pressure (ICP). The latter may result from tumour associated cerebral oedema or tumour volume increase. Raised ICP can result in a shift of cerebral structures leading to herniation.

Table 1.

Major presenting features for brain metastases [3,6]	
Motor deficits	70%
Headache	45%–52%
Nausea	35%
Seizures	20%
Behaviourial/mental changes	33%

NB: patients may present with more than one feature.

Specific signs and symptoms will depend on the anatomical site of metastases, local direct effects and more distant indirect effects (such as herniation). Metastases from breast cancer are rarely haemorrhagic so sudden onset of catastrophic signs are rare. Symptoms tend to develop slowly and insidiously. The predominant early signs and symptoms are listed in Table 1. Clinical signs may be minimal and papilloedema may only be present in 15% of patients [6].

> *Clinical suspicion of brain metastases is raised when there are signs and/or symptoms of raised intracranial pressure; focal neurological signs; sudden onset of seizure; and/or behaviourial or mental changes.*

3. Confirming the diagnosis

When signs and/or symptoms suggest the presence of brain metastases, confirmation is best made by careful clinical examination paying particular attention to a full neurological examination — which may detect evidence of extracranial CNS involvement — and fundoscopy. The most useful initial radiological investigation is CT with contrast enhancement. Radio-isotope scanning is of no value and cerebral angiography is rarely of any value. Metastases usually appear on pre-contrast CT scans as rounded areas of increased density and after administration of intravenous contrast, lesions generally enhance due to surrounding oedema. Metastases are usually multiple although solitary lesions may be seen.

If no metastatic lesions are identified or if only a solitary lesion is seen on CT, a MRI scan, preferably utilising gadolinium enhancement, should be performed. MRI may detect smaller lesions than can be seen on CT and can, therefore, detect lesions which are not visible on CT or where CT reveals only a solitary lesion. MRI is superior for imaging the posterior fossa [7] and in differentiating metastases from meningiomas [8].

Biopsy — either by incisional/excisional biopsy or core biopsy — is rarely required unless the patient has either been disease free for a considerable time, has had a previous non breast primary cancer, e.g. melanoma, or the CT and MRI images give rise to diagnostic doubts, e.g. where a primary brain tumour cannot be excluded.

> *A contrast enhanced CT is required when brain metastases are suggested; an MRI with gadolinium enhancement should be performed if the CT is negative or shows only a solitary lesion; biopsy is rarely required to confirm the diagnosis.*

4. Treatment

The treatment of cerebral metastases depends on a number of factors: whether the intracranial disease is a solitary lesion or there are multiple metastases; the extent of any extracranial breast cancer; the previous history of the disease and in particular the likely response of the total disease profile to further treatment; the performance status of the patient including the extent of any neurological deficit; and whether or not this is the first manifestation of cerebral disease.

When the diagnosis has been made and if cerebral oedema is present, treatment should be initiated with dexamethasone 16 mg per day in divided doses. Oral administration is generally appropriate although treatment may be initiated intravenously.

The toxicity of such steroid therapy can be minimised with judicious use of such medications as ranitidine and prompt application of antifungals when oral candidiasis is noted. Patients must be warned about such possible side effects and the likelihood of proximal myopathy and the Cushingoid effects of steroids. Such steroid therapy will generally produce prompt and impressive reduction in symptoms due to raised ICP.

> *When raised ICP is diagnosed, dexamethasone 16 mg/day in divided doses should be prescribed with full attention to and warning about its toxicity.*

Anticonvulsants are required if seizures have occurred. Intravenous Mannitol may be required if herniation has occurred or is impending.

While the mainstay of local therapy for brain metastases has been and remains radiotherapy, surgery may play a role to confirm a diagnosis by biopsy (see above) or in the management of an accessible solitary lesion. The evidence is conflicting even in randomised trials of the value of surgical resection of a solitary lesion in addition to the whole brain radiotherapy (WBRT). Mintz et al. in a Canadian study found no benefit for resection plus WBRT versus WBRT alone [9] Others have reported a better survival for the combination [10,11] while Patchell [10] showed that surgery plus WBRT improved quality of life and led to fewer in brain recurrences. In these latter studies radiotherapy doses were higher than those in the Canadian study. In these trials patients with breast cancer were a minority but there is no evidence that in principle patients with breast cancer behave any differently. All studies emphasise that results are likely to be better and such invasive treatments warranted when extracranial disease is absent, controlled or amenable to further treatment. Otherwise WBRT alone is indicated.

> *Surgical resection should be attempted if:*
> *a solitary accessible lesion is identified and confirmed on MRI*
> *extracranial primary and metastatic disease is absent, controlled or amenable to further treatment*
> *WBRT is given postoperatively to a dose of over 30 Gy.*

An alternative to surgical resection is stereotactic radiosurgery (SRS) which is a single fraction of high dose stereotactically focused small beam radiotherapy or stereotactic radiotherapy (SRT) which is delivered in a number of fractions.

There are, as yet, no results of randomised comparisons of surgery and SRS/SRT and accrual to such trails has been slow. However, The Joint Centre for Radiation Therapy in Boston claims results similar in terms of both survival and CNS local control for SRS alone [12]. Factors associated with poor survival are age over 60 years and, again, active extracranial disease.

While SRS can be considered in place of surgery for a solitary lesion, it may play a role when that lesion is inaccessible to the surgeon. Generally WBRT has been prescribed before or after SRS if surgery is not performed. However, retrospective nonrandomised data have questioned the need for WBRT in these patients [13]. Sneed's data suggest that SRS alone with at least 15 Gy to each lesion (maximum 4 lesions) is as good as SRS plus a variety of WBRT doses in terms of survival and freedom from intracranial progression. SRS alone also allowed salvage therapy to be given after progression. SRS is demanding financially and of other resources. Its role in managing patients with brain metastases needs further study in randomised trials.

> *Stereotactic radiosurgery (SRS) is playing an increasing role in the treatment of solitary brain metastases and when only a few lesions (up to 4) are identified.*
> *The value of SRS as a less invasive alternative to surgery needs to be explored in trials.*

The majority of patients presenting with brain metastases from breast cancer have evidence of multiple metastases and generally have widespread extracranial metastases and, less often, uncontrolled locoregional disease. Local treatment of the brain metastases is palliative and by WBRT.

Steroids should be continued during the WBRT but can be gradually reduced, symptoms allowing, to about 4 mg/day. After completion of WBRT attempts should be made to reduce steroids to zero gradually, but this is not always possible.

Megavoltage radiotherapy (to reduce skin reactions) is preferred using two opposed fields, each treated daily. The fields for WBRT should encompass the whole brain. Simple immobilisation systems should be employed to ensure accuracy of set up. Treatment head rotation is used to irradiate the temporal fossae but without irradiating the upper cervical spine (a common site of bone metastases requiring irradiation) and the eyes and eyebrows. Simple blocking with custom made blocks or multileaf collimation may be useful.

> *Whole brain radiotherapy (WBRT) should avoid the eyes and the upper cervical spine but cover all brain tissue utilising simple immobilisation and blocking techniques.*

The patient should be advised that hair loss will occur and warned about skin reactions which are dose dependent but include erythema and dry desquamation of part of the scalp.

There is controversy over appropriate doses and fractionation even though a number of randomised trials have been reported. A series of RTOG trials addressed this issue and failed to show any benefit for protracted high dose treatment (50 Gy over 4 weeks) when compared with 20 Gy in 1 week (5 fractions) [14–16]. Even shorter courses of 10 Gy in 1 day [17] or 12 Gy in 2 fractions [18]. appear to give similar benefits in terms of initial responses but duration of response may be less than with higher doses over longer periods.

Commonly used and acceptable doses are 20 Gy in 5 fractions over 1 week or 30 Gy in 10 fractions over 2 weeks prescribed at the midplane. After surgical resection a dose of at least 30 Gy is recommended but higher doses, utilising boosts may be useful.

> *Radiation doses (WBRT)*
> *NO SURGERY — FIT — OPTIONS*
> • *20 Gy in 5 fractions over 1 week*
> • *30 Gy in 10 fractions over 2 weeks*
> *NO SURGERY — POOR PERFORMANCE STATUS OR POOR PROGNOSIS — OPTIONS*
> • *10 Gy in single fraction (1 day)*
> • *12 Gy in 2 fractions (2 days)*
> *POSTOPERATIVE — OPTIONS*
> • *30 Gy in 10 fractions over 2 weeks followed by boost of 6 Gy in 3 fractions in 3 days to excision area*
> • *40 Gy in 20 fractions over 4 weeks*
> *POSTSTEREOTACTIC RADIOSURGERY (15–18 Gy)*
> • *40 Gy in 20 fractions over 4 weeks*

Relief of symptoms is obtained in 70–93% of patients but in about 20% symptoms will recur in 6 months, and 35% in 12 months [19]. The median survival after x-ray therapy is 3–6 months but 15% survive 1 year and 5–10% live for more than 2 years [19]. Breast cancer patients have a longer survival than those with lung cancer [14].

For those whose disease recurs or progresses within the brain, steroids are usually increased or reintroduced. Further radiotherapy may be considered depending on time since previous treatment and dose/fractionation. SRS may also be considered for solitary or a limited number of lesions.

> *Recurrent or progressive CNS disease may be considered for further radiotherapy with caution.*
> *SRS may be appropriate.*

Patients of exceedingly poor prognosis or performance status should receive best supportive care with steroids and analgesics. As with all patients with metastatic breast cancer which is likely to respond to hormonal manipulation (receptor positive) appropriate changes to hormonal therapy should be made in conjunction with local therapy.

> *If a response to hormone therapy is likely, appropriate hormone therapy changes should be made.*

Systemic chemotherapy has generally had little role to play in managing intracranial disease. Meningeal involvement can be treated by intrathecal methotrexate which must not be given in conjunction with cranial irradiation. (In rare circumstances protracted craniospinal radiotherapy alone can be considered). Systemic chemotherapy for extracranial disease may be required for symptom control.

> *Systemic chemotherapy has little role to play in managing intracranial disease.*
> *Intrathecal methotrexate for meningeal disease must not be given concurrently with cranial irradiation.*

Other forms of CNS disease may also be amenable to urgent local radiotherapy, e.g. spinal cord compression, choroidal metastases and cranial nerve compressive syndromes due to bone metastases. Doses of 20 Gy in 5 fractions are usually sufficient (Fig. 1).

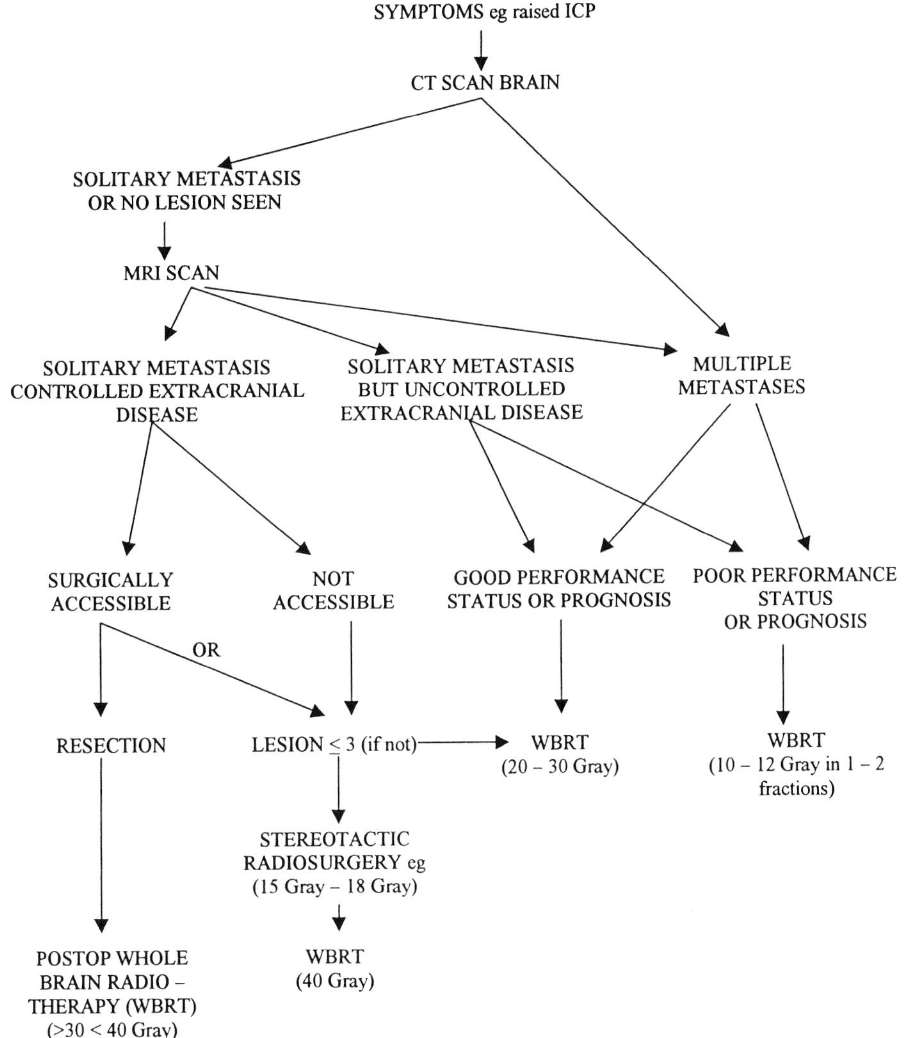

Fig. 1.

> *Choroidal metastases, spinal cord compression and compressive cranial nerve metastases are amenable to urgent palliative radiotherapy.*

5. Case scenario

A 45 year old woman develops headaches, nausea and visual blurring four years after treatment for node positive, receptor positive breast cancer treated by wide local excision and radiotherapy and systemic adjuvant chemotherapy (CMF) and tamoxifen. Papilloedema is noted on fundoscopy. Full clinical examination is negative. A CT brain is requested and shows a solitary enhancing lesion with oedema in the right cerebral hemisphere.

She should have an MRI to exclude other lesions. An MRI with gadolinium contrast enhancement reveals four other scattered small lesions.

Her general condition is excellent with a normal performance status. She should receive dexamethasone 4 mg four times daily orally and a full explanation of all possible side effects including dyspepsia, peripheral myopathy, weight gain, fat redistribution and sleep disturbances. She is not suitable for surgery or stereotactic radiosurgery. She should have radiotherapy planned and her disease fully staged by CT chest and abdominal scanning (CT or ultrasound), bone scan, FBE, LFTs, calcium.

These are negative. Radiotherapy is prescribed as 2 parallel opposed megavoltage fields to a midplane dose of either 20 Gy in 5 daily fractions or 30 Gy in 10 fractions over 2 weeks delivered with immobilisation using a lightweight moulded cast. She will be told to expect epilation.

Her tamoxifen should be stopped. She menopaused with CMF. An aromatase inhibitor should be prescribed.

Acknowledgements

I gratefully acknowledge the advice and assistance of Drs Michael Dally and Andrew Hui in the William Buckland Radiotherapy Centre.

References

1. Glass JP, Foley KM. Brain metastases in patients with breast cancer. In: Harris JR, Hellman S, Henderson IC, Kinne DW (Eds) Breast Disease. 2nd ed. Philadelphia: JB Lippincott Company 1991; 679–688.
2. Sparrow GEA, Rubens RD. Brain metastases from breast cancer: clinical course, prognosis and influence of treatment. Clin Oncol 1981; 7: 291–301.
3. Snee MP, Rodger A, Kerr GR. Brain metastases from carcinoma of breast: a review of 90 cases. Clin Radiol 1985; 36: 365–367.
4. Stewart JF, King RJB, Sexton S et al. Oestrogen receptors, sites of metastatic disease and survival in recurrent breast cancer. Eur J Cancer Clin Oncol 1981; 17: 449 *et seq.*
5. DiStefano A, Yap HY, Hortobaggi GN et al. The natural history of breast cancer patients with brain metastases. Cancer 1979; 44: 1913–1918.
6. Gamache FW, Galicich JH, Posner JB. Treatment of brain metastases by surgical extirpation. In: Weiss L, Gilbert HA. Posner JB (Eds) Brain Metastases. Boston: GK Hall 1980; 390–414.
7. Kent DL, Larson FB. Magnetic resonance imaging of the brain and spine. Ann Intl Med 1988; 108: 402–424.
8. Sze G, Shin J, Karl G et al. Intraparenchymal brain metastases: MR imaging versus contrast — enhanced CT. Radiology 1988; 168: 187–194.
9. Mintz AH, Kestle J, Rathbone MP, Gaspar L et al. A randomised trial to assess the efficacy of surgery in addition to radiotherapy in patients with single cerebral metastases. Cancer 1996; 78: 1470–1476.
10. Patchell RA, Tibbs PA, Walsh JW, Dempsey RJ et al. A randomised trial of surgery in the treatment of single metastases to the brain. New Engl J Med 1990; 322: 494–499.
11. Noordijk EM, Vecht CJ, Haaxma-Reiche H, Padberg GW et al. The choice of treatment of single brain metastases should be based on extracranial tumour activity and age. Int J Radiat Oncol, Biol Phys 1994; 29: 711–717.
12. Loeffler JS, Shrieve DC. What is appropriate therapy for a patient with a single brain metastasis? Int J Radiat Oncol, Biol Phys 1994; 915–917.
13. Sneed PK, Lamborn KR, Forstner JM, McDermott MW et al. Radiosurgery for brain metastases: is whole brain radiotherapy necessary? Int J Radiat Oncol, Biol Phys 1999; 43: 549–558.
14. Borgelt B, Gelber R, Kramer S, Brady L et al. The palliation of brain metastases: final results of the first two studies by the Radiation Therapy Oncology Group. Int J Radiat Oncol, Biol Phys 1980; 6: 1–19.
15. Borgelt B, Gelber R, Larson M, Hendrickson F et al. Ultrarapid high dose irradiation schedules for the palliation of brain metastases: final results of the first two studies of the RTOG. Int J Radiat Oncol, Biol Phys 1981; 7: 1633–1638.
16. Kurtz J, Gelber R, Brady L, Carella R et al. The palliation of brain metastases in favourable patient population: a randomised clinical trial by the RTOG. Int J Radiat Oncol, Biol Phys 1981; 7: 891–895.
17. Aaronson NK. Quality of life research in cancer clinical trials: a need for common rules and language. Oncology 1990; 4(5): 59–66.
18. Priestman TJ, Dunn J, Brada M, Rampling R et al. Final results of the Royal College of Radiologists' trial comparing two different radiotherapy schedules in the treatment of cerebral metastases. Clin Oncol 1996; 8: 308–315.
19. Coia LR, Aaronson N, Linggood R, Loeffler J et al. A report of the consensus workshop panel on the treatment of brain metastases. Int J Radiat Oncol, Biol Phys 1992: 23: 223–227.

Breast Cancer: Diagnosis and Management
J.M. Dixon (Ed.)

CHAPTER 57

Breast cancer: delivering the diagnosis

Peter Maguire

1. Introduction

Most cancer patients want to know if they have breast cancer, their likely treatments, side effects and prognosis [1]. However, a minority of women do not wish to know if they have cancer, especially those who are elderly, have advanced disease and come from socio-economically deprived areas.

2. General principles

The extent to which patients with breast cancer perceive that the information they are given at the time of diagnosis is adequate to their needs affects their later psychological adjustment [2]. Patients who feel they are given information appropriate to their needs adjust well psychologically while those who feel they are given too much or too little information have a much higher risk of developing a major depressive illness or generalised anxiety disorder within the first follow-up year. So, the challenge for surgeons having to deliver the diagnosis of cancer is how to tailor what they say to what the patient is ready to hear.

Most women who attend with breast symptoms will have considered that they may have cancer but hope otherwise. They may also have worried that if they have cancer they may need more aggressive treatments like mastectomy and chemotherapy. So, when the bad news is broken their concerns may be confirmed and new ones provoked. There is a strong link between the number of concerns of moderate severity or severe degree patients are left with after bad news consultations and the later risk of developing a depressive illness and/or generalised anxiety disorder [3]. So, a key task of the doctor breaking bad news is to ensure that patient's concerns are elicited, and where possible, resolved.

> *Psychological adjustment is maximised when*
> *Patients needs for information are elicited,*
> *The information given is tailored to their needs and*
> *Their concerns prior to and following hearing the diagnosis are elicited and resolved*

3. Specific guidelines

Girghis and Sanson-Fisher [4] drew up guidelines on the basis of a literature review and the recommendations of a consensus panel of doctors and cancer patients about how bad news should be broken (Table 1).

A systematic review of the literature by Miller and Maguire [5] came to similar conclusions about the guidelines but disagreed about the use of euphemisms. They considered these had a place in the minority of patients who had no awareness that they had cancer. The use of euphemisms allows

Table 1. Guidelines for breaking bad news

- Ensure privacy and adequate time
- Assess patient's understanding of the nature of their disease and prognosis
- Provide information about diagnosis and prognosis simply and honestly
- Avoid using euphemisms like growth or tumour
- Encourage patients to express their feelings about the news
- Be empathic
- Give a broad but realistic time frame concerning prognosis

clinicians to test whether patients are ready to hear the full diagnosis or merely wish to hear what might be done for them. Given these general principles and specific guidelines about breaking bad news a key question is what happens in practice.

Breaking bad news requires privacy and adequate time.

4. Behaviours in practice

In a study of experienced cancer specialists, including breast cancer surgeons, breaking bad news consultations have been recorded and analysed to see whether these principles are followed [6]. In most consultations patient's thoughts and feelings about the likely diagnosis and treatment were not first elicited. The news about the cancer diagnosis was given in a routinised way. It was assumed that patients wished to know the diagnosis, the evidence for it, the need for further tests, the likely treatments to be given and probable outcomes. There was no attempt to check which issues patients wanted to consider first. For example, it was common for surgeons working in screening clinics to start the process of delivering bad news by showing patients mammograms to illustrate where their cancers were. Many patients did not want to look at their x-rays and when they saw them found it hard to distinguish the cancer from other similar white areas in their breasts. This led them to fear that cancer had affected the whole breast.

The work showing a link between the concerns provoked by bad news and later distress, anxiety and depression argues strongly the need for doctors to actively elicit patient's concerns once they have given the bad news. However, this objective scrutiny of consultations showed that patients were given little opportunity to disclose their concerns. As soon as they delivered the bad news the clinicians genuinely believed that their main aim was to reassure patients by moving into information and advice mode. Patients were not actively invited to say how they were feeling on hearing the bad news or what their concerns were. Consequently, most concerns remained undisclosed and patients remained preoccupied with them. Because of this preoccupation they did not assimilate much of the information offered even when it was presented carefully and categorised by diagnosis, treatment and prognosis. When patients were left with undisclosed concerns they were more likely to develop an unduly negative appraisal of their predicament which increased the risk of later psychiatric disorder.

It has been argued that what patients want to know varies by culture. This has been used as an argument, at least in Europe, for avoiding telling patients the truth [7]. However, recent work suggests that such views are untrue with most patients preferring to hear the diagnosis [8].

A major question is why doctors who are dedicated to their patients offer immediate reassurance instead of acknowledging their patient's distress and eliciting their concerns before determining and responding to individual patient's information needs.

Doctors should actively elicit patient's concerns after giving bad news.

5. Fear of asking questions

They worry that if they ask patients how they are feeling after breaking bad news it will be perceived as a stupid question ("Of course I am distressed, what do you expect"). In reality, overt acknowledgement of patient's distress ("I am sorry to have to tell you you have cancer and I can see it has made you very upset") makes it legitimate for patients to disclose how worried they are. It also allows the surgeon a chance to explore the reasons for the patient's upset and elicit the underlying concerns. Yet, most surgeons fear that if they ask patients directly about their concerns ("What exactly is making you upset at the moment?") they will unleash strong emotions like despair or anger. They fear that they will not be able to contain these, that it will harm the patient psychologically and take up too much time. Moreover, it might encourage patients to ask difficult questions like "Why wasn't it diagnosed sooner or How long have I got?" They also fear that such enquiry may get them too close emotionally to their patients, hamper their ability to make objective decisions and threaten their own emotional survival. Offering immediate and positive reassurance after breaking bad news is, therefore, perceived as an optimal strategy.

Offering reassurance after breaking bad news is not an optimal strategy.

5.1. Reasons for fears

They say their fears derive from a lack of training in key communication skills during their undergraduate and postgraduate training. They claim they were never trained to explore patient's concerns or feelings and had little help in learning how to manage common difficult communication tasks like breaking bad news, handling uncertainty and dealing with difficult questions [9].

6. Picking up the pieces

Many doctors console themselves that if they break bad news in this routine way it will not matter because the patient will be assessed by other people, notably specialist cancer nurses or general practitioners Any misunderstandings will then be resolved. This ignores the strong programming effect their behaviour has on patients during the bad news consultation. When they do not actively elicit patient's concerns and feelings patients assume that other health professionals who see them subsequently will be no more interested in these issues than the doctor.

The reasons for fear of eliciting patient's concerns are shown in Table 2.

It is important to realise that patients also actively withhold their concerns. The reason they do so are summarised in Table 3.

Table 2. Fears of eliciting patient's concerns

- It will unleash strong emotions
- They will not be able to contain these
- The patient will be harmed psychologically
- They will be faced with difficult questions
- It will take too much time
- They will get too close to the patient
- It will threaten their survival

Table 3.

- They believe their concerns are inevitable
- Nothing can be done to resolve them
- If they reveal them they will be viewed as pathetic and inadequate
- Patients do not wish to burden doctors they respect and like with their concerns
- They feel it is not legitimate to mention their worries because they are not asked direct questions about them
- Their cues about problems are not picked up

7. How to break bad news

7.1. Checking awareness

First establish patient's perceptions of their situation by asking, after taking a history of their presenting symptoms, "What are your views about what might be wrong?" and then "How do you feel about it?" Showing such direct interest in patient's perceptions and feelings educates them that you are interested in them as persons. They are much more likely to disclose their concerns both before hearing the bad news and afterwards. Most patients with breast symptoms will then indicate they are worried it could be cancer. When you come to break bad news it will be a matter of confirming what they fear rather than breaking it from new.

Surgeon: When you found your lump did you have any thought as to what it might be?

Patient: I immediately thought it could be cancer.

Surgeon: Any other reason for that?

Patient: Well, my mother had breast cancer and died of it.

Surgeon: So, it is not surprising then you are worried it could be cancer. I am afraid I have to tell you on the basis of our tests that it is.

In 10% of patients your questions about their perceptions will indicate they have little awareness of what it wrong. It is important to check whether they are ready to know the truth by giving them a warning shot.

Surgeon: When you found the lump what did you think it was?

Patient: I thought it was a cyst.

Surgeon: Why did you think that?

Patient: I've had several lumps before and they have all been cysts. I did not think there was any need to worry.

Surgeon: I am afraid it looks more serious than that.

Patient: What do you mean.

Surgeon: When we did the biopsy it showed some abnormal cells.

Patient: What do you mean abnormal cells?

The surgeon: then proceeds to explain she has cancer.

The patient might have responded by saying "I don't want to know the details. Just tell me whether you can treat me." In this situation the patient's wishes should be respected as her response indicate she is not ready to hear the truth.

Check whether the patient is aware of the likely cause of her lump.

7.2. Acknowledging patient's distress and eliciting their concerns

There is no way that bad news can be softened. Once you voice it most patients will assimilate it and show signs of verbal or non verbal distress. It is important that you acknowledge this distress and invite the patient to say exactly why she is distressed. You should avoid offering reassurance, information and advice until you have elicited all the patient's main concerns.

Surgeon: I am sorry to have had to confirm that you have cancer as you thought. I can see it has distressed you. Would you mind telling me just what exactly is distressing you just now.

Patient: I have always equated cancer with death. I have got two young children and I want to live long enough to see them grow up.

Surgeon: Before I deal with those worries, are there any other concerns.

Patient: I am only 34, the last thing I want is to have to lose a breast.

Surgeon: Any other concerns?

Patient: No.

Surgeon: Which of these concerns would you like me to deal with first?

Patient: Whether you can do anything to treat the cancer.

The surgeon then explained that on the basis of the investigations he had done so far she could be treated with a wide local incision and radiotherapy since the lymph nodes were negative.

When he later asked how she was feeling she said she was reassured because she thought her cancer was terminal when she entered the consultation. He then dealt with her remaining concerns before asking "Is there any other information you would like?"

While patients need to feel that the nature and extent of their main concerns about their predicament will be elicited and understood it needs to be emphasised that they are not looking for immediate resolution of all of them. Less important concerns can be left to subsequent consultations.

> *Elicit all the patient's concerns and deal with their main concerns.*

8. Factors affecting the breaking of bad news

Ideally, bad news should be broken in private and negotiation should take place with patients about whether they wish to speak to the doctor alone or with a relative present. If a relative is present it may stop patients disclosing key concerns because they wish to protect their relatives from undue distress. It is better to talk to patients on their own first and elicit their concerns before checking if they wish to have relatives present to talk through their concerns and treatment options. When bad news is broken effectively it may provoke patients to ask questions which highlight the uncertainty of their predicament so it is important to know how this uncertainty can be managed.

9. Managing uncertainty

It is important to acknowledge the reality of their uncertainty by saying "I am sorry, at this stage we just don't know. Until we have done the tests I have discussed I simply can't tell you what the likely outcome is." It is important then to emphasise "I appreciate that not knowing more at this point must be very frustrating for you. However, I will give you the information as soon as possible."

10. Involving patients in treatment decisions

Recent studies have shown that patients differ in the extent to which they wish to be involved in treatment decisions [10]. Some prefer to take the lead, some want to leave it to the clinician to decide while others prefer to share in decision making. In general only half of patients with cancer achieve their preferred level of decision making [10]. It is obviously difficult to identify and respond to patient's needs within busy consultations. So, additional aids to communication like audio-tape recordings and letters have been advocated to allow patients to review what was said, consider the implications and share the information with family and key friends. However, in one study comparing the effects of providing an audiotape consultation of a general information tape or no tape [11] no difference in psychological adjustment was found in patients at follow-up according to the condition they were assigned to. Those given a general information tape fared worse.

Moreover, there has been no evidence of any substantial reduction in anxiety and depression from using tapes or summaries. In one study patients with a poor prognosis were more distressed after listening to the consultation tape [12]. So, it may be that the quality of the original bad news consultation is the key to helping patients adjust.

11. Monitoring subsequent reactions

Patients are more likely to disclose their concerns when followed up after the bad news consultation if the doctor asks open directive questions (how have you been getting on since I saw you last?), asks about the patient's perceptions (how do you see things working out?), feelings (how are you feeling about all this?), clarifies the responses (you say things are not going to work out, what do you mean?), you said you were devastated, can you say more about that?). When doctors summarise what they have heard (can I just recap, you say you are optimistic your cancer can be cured but worried about the side effects of chemotherapy) it educates patients they have been listening and promotes disclosure of their concerns. The use of empathy (I can see it was the last thing you were expecting) and educated guesses (as we have talked I have got the feeling that you have been very upset by this) makes patients feel the doctor is concerned about them as a person

Table 4. Behaviours facilitating disclosure

- Open directive questions
- Questions about patient's perceptions
- Questions about patient's feelings
- Clarifying cues about perceptions and feelings
- Summarising
- Being empathic
- Negotiating
- Making educated guesses

Table 5. Behaviours inhibiting disclosure

- Closed questions
- Use of multiple questions
- Use of leading questions
- Offering premature advice and reassurance
- Ignoring cues about feelings and perceptions

even if the guesses are wrong. It is not easy to tell if patients will find talking about their feelings too painful. So, they should be asked (negotiation) (can you bear to tell me how you felt about having a colostomy?). These behaviours are summarised in Table 4 [13].

Behaviours that inhibit disclosure are shown in Table 5 [13]. Closed questions which seek a yes or no answer, asking several questions at once, inviting a particular answer (you've had no problems since your surgery?), giving information and advice before key concerns have been identified inhibit disclosure [13].

Closed questions which seek a yes or no answer inhibits disclosure of concerns.

12. Improving the breaking of bad news

Constructive feedback of actual performance when interviewing patients is known to lead to the acquisition of key skills and relinquishing of inhibitory behaviours [14].

References

1. Meredith C, Symonds P, Webster L, Lamont D, Ryper L, Gillis CR, Fallowfield L. Informational needs of cancer patients in West Scotland: cross sectional survey of patient's views. BMJ 1996: 313; 724–726.
2. Fallowfield LJ, Hall A, Maguire GP, Baum M. Psychological outcomes of different treatment policies in women with early breast cancer outside a clinical trial. BMJ 1990: 301; 575–580.
3. Parle M, Jones B, Maguire P. Maladaptive coping and affective disorders in cancer patients. Psychol Med 1996: 26; 735–744.
4. Girghis A, Sanson-Fisher RW. Breaking bad news: consensus guidelines for medical practitioners. J Clin Oncol 1995: 13; 2449–2456.
5. Miller S, Maguire P, Thomson J. Breaking bad news to adult cancer patients: A review of the evidence.
6. Maguire GP. Study of senior doctors breaking bad news.
7. Arraras KI, Illaramendi JJ, Valerdi JJ, Wright SJ. Truth-telling to the patient in advanced cancer: family information filtering and prospect for change. Psycho-Oncology 1995: 4; 191–196.
8. Fielding R, Hung J. Preferences for information and involvement in decisions during cancer care among a Hong Kong Chinese population. Psycho–Oncology 1996: 5; 321–329.
9. Maguire P, Faulkner A. How to improve the counselling skills of doctors and nurses in cancer care. BMJ 1988: 297; 847–849.
10. Degner LF, Kristjanson LJ, Bowman et al. Information needs and decisional preferences in women with breast cancer. JAMA 1997: 1485–1491.
11. Dunn SM, Butow PN, Tattersall MHN. General information tapes inhibit recall of the cancer consultation. J Clin Oncol 1993: 11; 2279–2285.
12. McHugh P, Lewis S, Ford S. et al. The efficacy of audio tapes in promoting psychological well-being in cancer patients: A randomised controlled trial. Br J Cancer 1995: 71; 388–393.
13. Maguire P, Faulkner A, Booth K. et al. Helping cancer patients disclose their concerns. Eur J Cancer 1996: 32A; 78–81.
14. Maguire P, Booth K, Elliott C, Jones B. Helping health professionals involved in cancer care acquire key interviewing skills in the impact of workshops. Eur J Cancer 1996: 32A; No. 9, 1486–1489.

Breast Cancer: Diagnosis and Management
J.M. Dixon (Ed.)

CHAPTER 58

Palliative care for patients with breast cancer

Jeremy Keen

1. Introduction

"Pray for me, O my friends; a visitant
Is knocking his dire summons at my door,
The like of whom, to scare me and to daunt,
Has never, never come to me before . . . "

Cardinal Newman *The Dream of Gerontius*

For the vast majority the receipt of a diagnosis of cancer amounts to the "signing of a death warrant". Improvements in the management of breast cancer mean that this is not as true as it once was, but the diagnosis of metastatic disease certainly brings to the mind of the patient a "visitant" with "dire summons". The modern hospice movement and the development of the specialty of palliative care has at its core an aim of alleviating some of the fear associated with living with progressive incurable illness. Such fear may be associated with or exacerbated by physical symptoms, social concerns or psychological and spiritual problems. In an attempt to acknowledge such a multifactorial dependency of the experience of patients with advanced disease, palliative care has been defined in various ways. Many definitions have been unfortunately pretentious and frankly offensive to other specialties looking after dying patients. However it is hoped hospices provide rather more than "designer deaths" — a definition supplied by a general surgeon at a recent meeting. The World Health Organisation has defined palliative care as "the active total care of patients whose disease is not responsive to curative treatment" [1]. Many have adopted this as a definition of specialist palliative care but to do so is misleading as this simply defines the aim of most specialists. The editors of The Oxford Textbook of Palliative Medicine define specialist palliative care as "The study and management of patients with active, progressive, far-advanced disease for whom the prognosis is limited and the focus of care is on the quality of life" [2]. Immediately one seeks further definition of "active, progressive, far-advanced disease" and this is likely to differ between individual patients, different cancers and different non-malignant conditions. A fundamental point of specialist palliative care is potential access to specialist palliative care clinicians immediately it is accepted that the patient is no longer curable. The vast majority of patients with proven metastatic breast cancer will continue to receive cytotoxic chemotherapy, hormonal manipulation or radiotherapy and these agents extend and improve quality of life and thus provide palliative care. However, what can multidisciplinary specialist palliative care services offer for individual patients?

Palliative care is the study and management of patients with active, progressive, far-advanced disease for whom the prognosis is limited and the focus of care is on the quality of life.

2. The provision of specialist palliative care

2.1. Specialist palliative care in-patient units

There are, at present, 236 Palliative Care Units and Hospices providing inpatient services throughout the UK and an ever increasing number of facilities worldwide [3]. Most units will discharge between 30% and 45% of their patients with an average duration of admission being between two and three weeks. Patients who are discharged have usually been admitted either for symptom control or for respite for their immediate carers. The mechanism of referral for in-patient care varies from unit to unit but is usually arranged by the General Practitioner (primary care physician) or Hospital Consultant.

2.2. Home care services

Pioneered and funded in the main by Macmillan Cancer Relief the whole of the UK is serviced by a network of Community Palliative Care Nurses. Their role is seen as complimentary to that of the community nursing service. The usual volume of their caseloads means that they cannot commit to regular "hands-on" nursing care of individual patients. Their role is therefore more to provide specialist advice on symptom control issues, to be a counsellor and advocate for the patient and most often to spend time with patients and their families. Additionally, they give time to listen to the fears and frustrations of patients and take time to explain the significance of what is happening to them. Home Care nurses are often closely linked to in-patient palliative care units and can access expertise for advice or consideration of admission.

There is potential for overlap between these community services and similar provision within the acute hospital. This is true for patients with breast cancer with many specialist units having their own counsellors or Breast Care Nurse Specialists. Patients will often visit the unit regularly for many years, undergoing multiple courses of chemotherapy and radiotherapy and close relationships are often built with counsellors and breast care nurses. It is often therefore inappropriate to involve additional services until a much later stage of the illness.

A very few specialist palliative care units are beginning to experiment with a more comprehensive home care nursing service involving 24 hour multidisciplinary palliative care within a patient's own home. Such a service carries obvious resource implications, but would enable many patients to stay at home longer and to die at home if that is their wish.

Home care nursing services for patients are available in many countries in Europe.

2.3. Day care services

Many specialist palliative care units (SPCUs) operate day centres to provide rehabilitative/adaptive activities for patients along with access to nursing, medical and paramedical services. The respite provided for carers also helps to maintain patients in the community for longer periods.

2.4. Hospital support teams

Palliative care teams operating within acute hospitals have been the latest evolution of the palliative care/hospice movement. After the birth of the modern hospice movement in the late 1960's the need for specialist palliative expertise in acute hospitals was quickly recognised. The first such team was founded in 1976 [4] and there are, at present, 209 palliative care teams in hospitals throughout the UK [3]. The teams usually comprise nurse specialists, physicians, social workers and occasionally psychologists and chaplains. The major remit of such teams is to advise individual patients and their families, on pain and symptom control and to offer emotional and psychospiritual support. Help with end-of-life decision making has been identified as a major reason for referral [5]. The provision of formal and informal education programmes by palliative care teams to all carers within hospitals helps to ensure that some of the perceived lack of knowledge and skills, reported by carers themselves, is being addressed.

> *A range of palliative care is available including home support, day care services, hospital support teams and in-patient facilities.*

3. Common problems in the palliative care of patients with breast cancer

Major symptoms in patients in the terminal stages of breast cancer include pain, weakness, anorexia, nausea, dyspnoea, weight loss, constipation and cough.

Table 1 lists the most frequent problems encountered in patients with breast cancer referred to one unit. The management of these common problems is considered but more details can be obtained from one of the comprehensive texts now available [2,6–8]. Whilst pain is the most frequent symptom in a palliative care population dyspnoea is the most persistent and least-well controlled symptom [9,10].

Table 1. Symptoms reported by 200 consecutive patients with breast cancer admitted to St. Columba's Hospice, UK

Main problem on admission	Percentage of 200 admissions
Pain	67
Weakness	55
Anorexia	30
Nausea	27
Dyspnoea	22
Weight loss	19
Constipation	16
Vomiting	14
Cough	13
Peripheral oedema	10
Ulcerated tumour	10

Table 2. Principal pain type(s) on admission to St. Columba's Hospice (some patients had more than one pain type rate as a 'principal pain')

Pain type	No. of admissions (%)
Bone	63
Neuropathic	28
Visceral	17

4. Pain

Pain is a cortical response comprising the perception of a sensation and the emotional reaction to it. Control of pain is totally dependent on adequate assessment of the type and likely cause of the pain and the emotional context in which it is being expressed.

The study of pain management has produced several possible classification systems but here the most common types of pain reported by patients with breast cancer is used (Table 2). In any one individual several different types of pain may be reported simultaneously making adequate assessment vital for efficient management.

4.1. Bone pain

Pain from metastatic lesions within bone is the most common form of pain reported in breast cancer (Table 2). Treatment may be approached in several ways and usually a combination of all modalities are required during the course of the illness. Bone pain is treated by a combination of anti-tumour therapy, bisphosphonates, non-opioid and opioid analgesics. Local anaesthetic procedures and surgery also play role in the care of some patients.

Treatment of metastatic bone pain
• *Anti-tumour therapy — Systemic chemotherapy or hormonal manipulation*
Radiotherapy to individual sites or, under investigation, the use of radioisotopes
• *Bisphosphonates — Mechanism uncertain*
• *Non-opioid analgesics — Principally non-steroidal anti-inflammatory drugs (NSAIDs) and corticosteroids*
• *Opioid analgesics*
• *Anaesthetic techniques — Peripheral nerve blocks, epidural or intrathecal infusions*
• *Surgery — Stabilisation of long bones and relief of vertebral compression*

4.2. *Anti-tumour therapy*

The use of chemotherapy hormonal manipulation and radiotherapy must always be considered for patients with breast cancer. The decision not to treat further with systemic agents can often be very difficult [11]. It requires a good working knowledge of the ratio of likely benefit versus likely side effects for both the antitumour agent and alternative methods of pain control. The use of radiotherapy is one of the cornerstones of treatment of painful bony metastases and should be considered in all cases [12,13]. The use of radioisotopes such as strontium-89 is well established in the treatment of bone metastases from prostatic carcinoma and preliminary results of trials in breast cancer are encouraging [14].

4.3. *Bisphosphonates*

Pamidronate and clodronate are now licensed for the treatment of bone pain in breast cancer with evidence from randomised controlled trials of efficacy [15,16]. The analgesic effect appears to be dose-dependent and they have a variable duration of activity. Studies of bisphosphonates in hypercalcaemia suggest an average duration of effect of four weeks for pamidronate. The same drug given in one study, at a dose of 120 mg intravenously produced an analgesic effect in 59% of patients for a median of twelve weeks [17]. A recent review of the evidence for the use of bisphosphonates in bone pain recommended an IV infusion of 60–90 mg of pamidronate every three to four weeks for advanced cancer patients with painful lytic metastases [18]. An alternative is the use of oral clodronate at a dose of 1600 mg per day. There is evidence to suggest that not only can such agents relieve the pain from bone metastases but also delay development of new areas of bone involvement and even the incidence of pathological fractures [19,20]. The mechanism of action of bisphosphonates as analgesics is largely unknown. Vinholes et al. noted a correlation between reductions in pain scores and markers of bone resorption in patients treated with pamidronate [21]. Additionally, inhibition of cytokine secretion from peripheral monocytes has been noted in vitro after exposure to Ibandronate, a new bisphosphonate [22]. If similar effects on tumour associated macrophages occur in vivo this may, in part, explain the relatively rapid analgesic effects that have been reported in some studies. Indeed, relief of pain has been noted, in one study, as early as two to three days after an infusion of clodronate but can take up to two weeks to become evident [23]. Bisphosphonates are becoming an established part of therapy for breast cancer patients with bone metastases. New, more potent bisphosphonates such as Ibandronate and Zoledronate have been given, in trials, at lower oral doses and by IV bolus with fewer side effects and easier patient management [18]. There is a considerable potential financial burden associated with the regular prescription of these agents to a large patient population. If there is a reduction in skeletal morbidity with bisphosphonates with a resulting reduced requirement for in-patient care then such costs may well be largely recuperated. This has been confirmed, by a cost-benefit analysis for the use of bisphosphonates in myeloma [24].

Table 3. 'Strong' opioids, and the preparations available, for the treatment of cancer pain

- Morphine — mu opioid receptor agonist and the strong opioid of choice. Available in a variety of oral preparations and for parenteral use.
- Diamorphine — Activity at the mu opioid receptor and possibly a distinct, as yet unidentified, receptor site. Greater solubility means this is opioid of choice for the parenteral route where it is available (UK only).
- Hydromorphone — mu agonist and analogue of morphine with similar pharmacokinetic properties.
- Oxycodone — mu agonist with similar properties to morphine, introduced in the UK in 2000.
- Fentanyl — Transdermal route allows continuous delivery of this short acting mu receptor agonist. Investigation of oral formulations ongoing.
- Methadone — Agonist activity at both mu and delta opioid receptors and antagonist at NMDA receptors. Potentially useful in neuropathic pain and opioid tolerance. Long and unpredictable half life.

4.4. Non-opioid analgesics

The role of Non Steroidal Anti-inflammatory Drugs (NSAIDs) in the management of bone pain has been the subject of a certain degree of controversy. Their efficacy in metastatic bone pain is not fully supported by good quality evidence [25]. However, NSAIDs, when used in combination with opioids, have been shown to improve pain control and additionally allow reduction of the dose of opioid whilst maintaining pain control [26,27]. This effect is particularly useful in the treatment of incident (movement-related) bone pain when therapy with opioids is often limited by side effects. There have been interesting reports confirming the tolerability and effectiveness of ketorolac, administered by continuous subcutaneous infusion, in pain that has proved difficult to control with opioids and oral NSAIDs [28,29]. The introduction of new COX-2 selective NSAIDs should reduce the incidence of gastric and renal complications which sometimes limits the use of this class of agents [30]. The role of NSAIDs in cancer pain in general has been recently and usefully reviewed [31].

Corticosteroids, alternative anti-inflammatory agents, are often quoted as useful co-analgesics in bone pain [32]. Whilst anecdotally this appears to be the case there is no satisfactory evidence, as yet, to confirm their value.

4.5. Opioid analgesics

Metastatic bone pain is relieved by appropriate use of opioids in the vast majority of cases. It is fortunate that there is now a range of opioids available for use as strong analgesics, several of which are available in both short and long acting preparations and in formulations suitable for alternative routes of administration (Table 3). Evidence suggests that in cases where good pain control cannot be achieved with one opioid because of side effects, a change to an alternative may allow acceptable control to be obtained [33]. These findings have fostered a closer examination of the use of opioids and particularly the incidence and manifestations of opioid side effects and toxicity (Table 4). The recognition that even mild opioid toxicity is potentially avoidable by using alternative opioids and other measures

Table 4. Opioid side effects

Sedation
Constipation
Dry mouth
Nausea
Gastroparesis
Hypotension
Itch
Delirium
Hallucinations
Agitation
Myoclonus
Hyperalgesia

should keep us vigilant for the development of such toxicities in our patient population.

The high incidence of "terminal restlessness" observed in patients with end stage cancer is often a manifestation of hyperactive delirium associated with myoclonus and cutaneous hyperalgesia from opioid toxicity. Unfortunately this is often unrecognised and is often treated with increased doses of opioids which exacerbates the problem. Opioid toxicity develops because of a reduction in renal clearance of metabolites associated with reduced fluid intake in dying patients. The appropriate management is either reduction of the opioid dose or maintenance of hydration. Hydration in the palliative care setting is often provided by nightly subcutaneous infusion of fluid. This avoids the potential complications of maintaining intravenous access and allows the patient and their family the freedom from hydration lines during the daytime. Additionally, and particularly important for some families, such treatment protocols can be managed successfully in the home setting.

Some bone pain does not completely respond to opioids alone. Two areas are worthy of mention. Firstly when the localised bone pain is associated with a neuropathic pain. This combination is often the presenting symptom of vertebral metastases. The treatment of neuropathic pain is a controversial issue particularly with respect to the definition of such pain and the role of opioid analgesics in its management [34]. The management of neuropathic pain is discussed further below. Incident or "movement-related" pain is probably the most difficult bone pain to manage and is often difficult to control with opioids alone. A regular opioid dose high enough to provide pain relief on movement often results in undue side effects at rest when there is no longer a painful stimulus. Such pain always requires a management plan that maximises the use of additional co-analgesic drugs and procedures. Radiotherapy should always be considered and in the short term, while waiting for the benefits of radiotherapy, a local anaesthetic procedure may be required. One option to enable some incident pains to be controlled by opioids alone is to use psychostimulants to relieve sedation if this is the only side effect of the opioid [35]. Methylphenidate at doses of between 2.5 mg and 10 mg given early morning and at midday may allow the dose of opioid to be increased to a sufficiently high enough to provide pain control on movement.

4.6. Local anaesthetic procedures

Some sites of painful metastases are amenable to peripheral neural blockade. Intercostal or paravertebral blocks can afford good pain control for rib metastases or direct invasion. Intraosseus injection of local anaesthetic, steroid and in some instances phenol can bring immediate relief to small single painful metastatic sites [36]. An epidural infusion of local anaesthetic alone, or in combination with an opioid, may afford good pain relief in the short-term management of incident pain related to the vertebral column whilst other modalities are introduced and titrated. Long-term epidural or intrathecal infusions or even a neurosurgical procedure such as a cordotomy may be the only way of affording relief in severe incident pain in some patients.

4.7. Surgery

In incidences where painful bone metastases are seen to involve the cortex of long bones the insertion of a pin or nail may produce analgesic benefit and avoid an unstable pathological fracture. Reconstruction of major joints may be indicated where the presence of metastatic deposits is resulting in pain and the risk of joint failure. Mixed bone and neuropathic pain from vertebral metastases and consequent spinal instability can be alleviated by surgical spinal stabilisation in certain instances. Such surgery not only alleviates pain but can enable patients to maintain a degree of independence which is vital for those patients who survive for many months and years.

5. Neuropathic pain

The management of neuropathic pain has been the subject of several reviews and multiple adjuvant analgesic trials over the past two decades. Trials, almost without exception, have been carried out in patients with non-malignant pain. Anecdotal evidence however, would suggest similar analgesic effects of these drugs in patients with malignant disease. Common presentations of neuropathic pain in patients with breast cancer relate either to vertebral metastases and a radiculopathy or to a brachial plexopathy. The latter often occurs as a direct result of tumour invasion or secondary to damage from surgery or radiotherapy.

It is generally agreed that neuropathic pain is less responsive to opioids than bone pain with higher doses of opioid required to obtain an analgesic effect. Such high doses are often not achieved before the onset of intolerable side effects, although in any individual switching opioids may improve the therapeutic index. There is increasing evidence that *N*-methyl-D-aspartate (NMDA) receptor antagonists, of which ketamine is a well known example, appear to be effective analgesics in neuropathic pain [37,38]. Methadone, a potent opioid receptor agonist also has NMDA receptor antagonist activity [39] and therefore theoretically would be the ideal opioid in mixed bone and neuropathic pain. Evidence for the efficacy of methadone in neuropathic pain is, as yet, limited to individual case-reports [40]. Initiation of methadone can be complicated by a great individual variability in half-life and is probably best done with assistance from a palliative care or chronic pain service. There are likely to be new combined preparations of NMDA antagonists and opioids on the market in the near future which, although possessing all the limitations of fixed dose combinations, may be easier to use than methadone.

Despite opioids, optimal control of neuropathic pain often requires the addition of an adjuvant analgesic. The list of adjuvant analgesics which may provide additional benefit is lengthy but the mainstays of treatment are the antidepressants and anticonvulsants. Systematic reviews of trials involving both these classes of agents have demonstrated little difference in their analgesic benefit or the incidence of related adverse effects [41,42]. In practice, treatment is usually commenced with a tricyclic antidepressant and an anticonvulsant added if there is failure to achieve satisfactory pain relief. Increasing experience with NMDA antagonists has resulted in the earlier introduction of these agents in pain management protocols.

Treatment of neuropathic pain often requires adjuvant analgesics; tricyclic antidepressants and/or anticonvulsants being the drugs of choice.

6. Visceral pain

The most frequent form of visceral pain experienced by patients with metastatic breast cancer is liver capsular pain. Effective pain relief can usually be achieved by opioids used alone or in combination with corticosteroids and/or NSAIDs. If such an approach does produce adequate analgesia or is limited by side effects then recent evidence suggests that NMDA antagonists may have a role in visceral pain [43]. Alternatively coeliac or hypogastric nerve plexus block can be considered where the facilities exist for such procedures to be performed.

7. Dyspnoea

Dyspnoea during the final stages of breast cancer is often the most distressing symptom not only for the patient to experience, but also for the family and professional carer to observe. Dyspnoea, like pain is a cortical perception of an increase in the work of breathing. It is therefore particularly influenced by emotional and psychological factors. Patients with a life threatening condition such as advanced breast cancer often perceive the development of dyspnoea as the final stage in their illness. There is evidence to suggest that development of dyspnoea does indeed indicate a poor prognosis [44] nonetheless, reassurance and relaxation techniques are fundamental to clinical management. Formal training programmes to teach new breathing and relaxation techniques to patients with primary lung tumours have proved successful in the management of dyspnoea [45]. Elements of such programmes may also be helpful for patients with pulmonary metastases from other primary tumours.

The approach to control of dyspnoea should involve identification of the causal factors. In one study of breast cancer patients presenting to a casualty department with dyspnoea, pleural effusions were the most common cause (31%) followed by left ventricular failure (11%) and "pneumonitis" (11%) [46]. Pleural or pericardial effusions should be drained, heart failure, anaemia, embolic phenomena and infections treated appropriately and adequate analgesia provided for chest wall pain. In breast cancer a frequent cause of extremely distressing end stage dyspnoea is related to the development of lymphangitis carcinomatosa. This is difficult to treat although corticosteroids may give prompt but usually only short-lived relief. Evidence suggests a steroid induced myopathy of the respiratory musculature, with resultant potential exacerbation of symptoms, can be detected as early as 15 days after commencement of treatment [47]. Steroids should therefore be used with care and reviewed frequently. Symptomatic treatment of dyspnoea usually involves oxygen, opioids and either benzodiazepines or phenothiazines.

Control of dyspnoea in end-stage illness often requires the use of opioids and/or anxiolytics with a trial of oxygen given if there is evidence of hypoxia.

7.1. Oxygen

The role of oxygen therapy in reducing dyspnoea in advanced cancer remains controversial. The positive effect of breathing either air or oxygen through a face mask seems clear but the results of published studies are divided on the evidence of a significant effect of oxygen [48,49]. The wider availability of pulse oximetry may allow better selection of patients who benefit from oxygen and help to avoid psychological dependence. Evidence from one study suggests that in cancer patients improvement in dyspnoea on oxygen could not be predicted from the level of hypoxia prior to treatment [49]. Oxygen should be humidified to decrease exacerbating the underrated symptom of a dry mouth that often complicates opioid therapy.

7.2. Opioids

Evidence from several studies demonstrates a clear beneficial effect of systemic opioids in the relief of dyspnoea [50,44]. Although several possible mechanisms of action on central and peripheral sites have been postulated, the exact mode of action of opioids remains unclear. In one uncontrolled study, morphine produced a subjective relief of dyspnoea without significantly decreasing the respiratory rate or increasing end tidal carbon dioxide concentration [51]. Additionally, the improvement in dyspnoea appeared to be of shorter duration than analgesic effects (approximately 2 hours rather than 4 hours). Such evidence would suggest that long acting preparations or short dosing intervals of immediate release opioid preparations are most appropriate.

There has been a vogue for the use of nebulised morphine in the treatment of dyspnoea. The evidence for a beneficial effect of the nebulised route of administration of opioids is largely anecdotal or based on results of small-scale trials. A recent review concluded that such evidence does not support the use of nebulised morphine in dyspnoea from cancer [52]. In practice many patients are receiving opioids for pain and an increase in dose of 30 to 50% will usually provide relief of dyspnoea.

7.3. Psychotropic drugs

Short acting benzodiazepines such as lorazepam can be useful in relieving symptoms of dyspnoea exacerbated by acute episodes of anxiety. Beneficial effects on dyspnoea have been observed with the use of phenothiazines alone and in combination with opioids for patients with non-malignant respiratory disease. Buspirone, a relatively new anxiolytic has been reported to be useful in dyspnoea associated with malignant disease [43]. Further trials with this group of agents are warranted.

8. Conclusions

Palliative care has been said to start from the moment a diagnosis of a potentially life threatening illness is made. Very often this may be in terms of emotional and psychological support for an individual who may be facing the realisation of their mortality for the first time. Fortunately over recent years nurse counsellors from specialist cancer units have increasingly provided such support for patients with breast cancer.

The timing of referral to specialist palliative care services remains a major difficulty not only for clinicians but also for patients themselves. Such a difficulty often represents a lack of knowledge of the services that are available. Additionally, there is often close involvement of the oncology unit with patients with advanced breast cancer having received multiple courses of chemotherapy. Such a special relationship is sometimes best maintained until death without involvement of new personnel. A particular danger of this is the potential of missing opportunities to allow individuals to begin to acknowledge and prepare for impending death. Whilst still rooted in the philosophy of the hospice specialist, palliative care is evolving as a medical and nursing subspecialty and is developing ever closer links with established cancer services. The introduction of palliative care teams into the hospital setting has helped in education of clinicians, patients and their relatives and has begun to smooth the transition to specialist palliative care for those for whom it is appropriate.

Physical symptom control will always constitute a major part of palliative care. Problematic pain control is still the most frequent reason for referral to palliative care services and patients with breast cancer can present particular difficulties. Bone is a common site of metastases and patients may survive several years with progressive disease and pain. The increasing availability of different opioid, non-opioid and adjuvant analgesics and an improved awareness of opioid side-effects, in particular, has led to a refinement in prescribing policies. The development of new research methodologies to study management of symptoms, such as pain and dyspnoea, in a patient population with advanced disease is a challenge. Specialist palliative care does not seek to de-skill cancer physicians and surgeons and must complement existing services. Such an integrated service must ensure that every patient with breast cancer has access to the particular services that enable her/him to live with the maximum quality for the longest period. The provision of security of care and opportunities to allay some of the fears of incurable illness can only enhance the likelihood of achieving such aims.

References

1. World Health Organisation. Cancer pain relief and Palliative Care. Technical Report Series 804. Geneva, Switzerland 1990; p. 11.
2. Doyle D, Hanks GWC, MacDonald N: Introduction. In Doyle D, Hanks GWC, MacDonald N, eds. Oxford Textbook of Palliative Medicine. Oxford, England. Oxford University Press 1993, p. 3.
3. 1999 Directory of Hospice and Palliative Care Services. The Hospice Information Service at St. Christopher's. London, UK.
4. Bates TD, Hoy AM, Clarke DG, Laird PP. The St Thomas Hospital Terminal Care Support Team — a new concept of hospice care. Lancet 1981; I: 1201–

1203.
5. Weissman D, Griffie J. The Palliative Care Consultation Service of the Medical College of Wisconsin. J Pain Symptom Manage 1994; 9: 474–479.
6. Saunders C, Sykes N, eds. The Management of Terminal Malignant Disease. 1993 Edward Arnold, Great Britain.
7. Twycross R. Pain Relief in Advanced Cancer. 1994 Churchill Livingstone, Edinburgh, UK.
8. Twycross R. Symptom Management in Advanced Cancer. 1997 Radcliffe Medical Press Ltd, Oxford, UK.
9. Higginson I, McCarthy M. Measuring symptoms in terminal cancer: are pain and dyspnoea controlled? J R Soc Med 1989; 82: 264–267.
10. Reuben DB, Mor V. Dyspnea in terminally ill cancer patients. Chest 1986; 89: 234–236.
11. Stockler M, Wilcken N, Coates A. Chemotherapy for metastatic breast cancer — when is enough enough? Eur J Cancer 1997; 33: 2147–2148.
12. Rasmusson B, Vejborg I, Jenson AB, et al. Irradiation of bone metastases in breast cancer patients: a randomised study with 1-year follow-up. Radiother Oncol 1995; 34: 179–184.
13. McQuay HJ, Carroll D, Moore RA. Radiotherapy for painful bone metastases: a systematic review. Clin Oncol 1997; 9: 150–154.
14. Robinson RG, Preston DF, Schiefelbain BHS, Baxter K. Strontium-89 therapy for the palliation of pain due to osseous metastases. JAMA 1995; 274: 420–424.
15. Van Holten-Verzantvoort ATM, Kroon HM, Bijvoet OLM, et al. Palliative pamidronate treatment in patients with bone metastases from breast cancer. J Clin Oncol 1993; 11: 491–498.
16. Paterson AHG, Powles TJ, Kanis J, et al. Double-blind controlled trial of oral clodronate in patients with bone metastases from breast cancer. J Clin Oncol 1993; 11: 59–65.
17. Purohit OP, Anthony C, Radstone CR, et al. High dose IV pamidronate for metastatic bone pain. Br J Cancer 1994; 70(3): 554–558.
18. Fulfaro F, Casuccio A, Ticozzi C, Ripamonti C. The role of bisphosphonates in the treatment of painful metastatic bone disease: a review of phase III trials. Pain 1998; 78: 157–169.
19. Conte PF, Latreille J, Mauriac F, et al. Delay in progression of bone metastases in breast cancer patients treated with intravenous pamidronate: results from a multi-national randomised control trial. J Clin Oncol 1996; 14: 2552–2559.
20. Hortobagyi GN, Theriault RL, Porter L, et al. Efficacy of Pamidronate in reducing skeletal complications in patients with breast cancer and lytic bone metastases. N Engl J Med 1996; 335: 1785–1791.
21. Vinholes JJ, Guo C-Y, Purohit OP, et al. Metabolic effects of Pamidronate in patients with metastatic bone disease. Br J Cancer 1996; 7: 1089–1095.
22. Crouch S, Lyons A, Wilcock A. Investigating the analgesic action of intravenous biphosphonates: in vitro effect of BM 21.0955 (Ibandronate) on macrophage production of inflammatory cytokines. Palliat Med 1997; 11: 64.
23. Ernst DS, MacDonald N, Paterson AHG, et al. Double-blind crossover trial of IV clodronate in metastatic bone pain. J Pain Symptom Manage 1992; 7: 4–11.
24. Laasko M, Lahtinen R, Virkkunen P, Elomaa I. Subgroup and cost-benefit analysis of the Finnish multicentre trial of Clodronate in multiple myeloma. Br J Haematol 1994; 87: 725–729.
25. Eisenberg E, Berkey CS, Carr DB, et al. Efficacy and safety of non-steroidal anti-inflammatory drugs for cancer pain: a meta-analysis. J Clin Oncol 1994; 12: 2756–2765.
26. Joishy SK, Walsh D. The opioid-sparing effects of intravenous ketorolac as an adjuvant analgesic in cancer pain: Application in bone metastases and the opioid bowel syndrome. J Pain Symptom Manage 1998; 16: 334–339.
27. Bjorkman R, Ullman A, Hedner J. Morphine-sparing effect of diclofenac in cancer pain. Eur J Clin Pharmacol 1993; 44: 1–5.
28. Blackwell N, Bangham L, Hughes N, et al. Subcutaneous ketorolac. A new development in pain control. Palliat Med 1993; 7: 63–65.
29. DeConno F, Zeeca E, Martini C, et al. Tolerability of ketorolac via continuous subcutaneous infusion for cancer pain. A preliminary report. J Pain Symptom Manage 1994; 9: 119–121.
30. Hawkey CJ. COX-2 inhibitors. Lancet 1999; 353: 307–314.
31. Jenkins CA, Bruera E. Nonsteroidal ant-inflammatory drugs as adjuvant analgesics in cancer patients. Palliat Med 1999; 13: 183–196.
32. Watanabe S, Bruera E. Corticosteroids as adjuvant analgesics. J Pain Symptom Manage 1994; 9: 442–445.
33. De Stoutz ND, Bruera E, Suarez-Almazor M. Opioid rotation for toxicity reduction in terminal cancer patients. J Pain Symptom Manage 1995; 10: 378 384.
34. Dellemijn P. Are opioids effective in relieving neuropathic pain? Pain 1999; 80: 453–462.
35. Bruera E, Fainsinger R, MacEarchen, Hanson J. The use of methylphenidate in patients with incident cancer pain receiving regular opiates. A preliminary report. Pain 1992; 50: 75–77.
36. Rowell NP. Intralesional methylprednisolone for rib metastases: an alternative to radiotherapy? Palliat Med 1988; 2: 153–155.
37. Backonja M, Arndt G, Gombar KA, et al. Response of chronic neuropathic pain syndromes to ketamine: a preliminary study. Pain 1994; 56: 51–57.
38. Mercadente S. Ketamine in cancer pain: an update. Palliat Med 1996; 10: 225–230.

39. Ebert B, Andersen S, Krogsgaard-Larsen P. Ketobemidone, methadone and pethidine are non-competitive *N*-methyl-D-aspartate (NMDA) antagonists in the rat cortex and spinal cord. Neurosci Lett 1995; 187: 165–168.
40. Galer BS, Coyle N, Pasternak GW, Portenoy RK. Individual variability in the response to different opioids: report of five cases. Pain 1992; 49: 87–91.
41. McQuay HJ, Tramer M, Nye BA, et al. A systematic review of antidepressants in neuropathic pain. Pain 1996; 68: 217–227.
42. McQuay HJ, Carroll D, Jadad AR, et al. Anticonvulsant drugs for management of pain: a systematic review. Br Med J 1995; 311: 1047–1052.
43. Olivar T, Laird JM. Differential effects on *N*-methyl-D-aspartate receptor blockade on nociceptive somatic and visceral reflexes. Pain 1999; 79: 67–73.
44. Ripamonti C, Fulfaro F, Bruera E. Dyspnoea in patients with advanced cancer: incidence, causes and treatments. Cancer Treat Rev 1998; 24: 69–80.
45. Bredin M, Corner J, Krishnasamy M, et al. Multicentre randomised controlled trial of nursing intervention for breathlessness in patients with lung cancer. Br Med J 1999; 318: 901–904.
46. Escalante CP, Martin CG, Elting LS, et al. Dyspnea in cancer patients. Etiology, resource utilisation, and survival. Implications in a managed care world. Cancer 1996; 78: 1314–1319.
47. Batchelor TT, Taylor LP, Thaler HT, et al. Steroid myopathy in cancer patients. Neurology 1997; 48: 1234–123.
48. Bruera E, de Stoutz N, Velasco–Leiva A, et al. The effects of oxygen on the intensity of dyspnea in hypoxemic terminal cancer patients. Lancet 1993; 342: 13–14.
49. Booth S, Kelly MJ, Cox NP, et al. Does oxygen help dyspnea in patients with cancer? Am J Respir Crit Care Med 1996; 153: 1515–1518.
50. Bruera E, MacEachern T, Ripamonti C, Hanson J. Subcutaneous morphine for dyspnoea in cancer patients. Ann Int Med 1993; 119: 906–907.
51. Bruera E, Macmillan K, Pither J and MacDonald N. Effects of morphine on the dyspnea of terminal cancer patients. J Pain Symptom Manage 1990; 5: 341–344.
52. Davis CL. Breathlessness, cough, and other respiratory problems. Br Med J 1997; 315: 931–934.

Subject Index